Veterinary Periodontology

Veterinary Periodontology

Brook A. Niemiec, DVM
Diplomate, American Veterinary Dental College
Fellow, Academy of Veterinary Dentistry
Southern California Veterinary Dental Specialties
San Diego, CA, 92123, USA

WILEY-BLACKWELL
A John Wiley & Sons, Inc., Publication

Wiley-Blackwell is an imprint of John Wiley & Sons, formed by the merger of Wiley's global Scientific, Technical and Medical business with Blackwell Publishing.

Editorial Offices
2121 State Avenue, Ames, Iowa 50014-8300, USA
The Atrium, Southern Gate, Chichester, West Sussex, PO19 8SQ, UK
9600 Garsington Road, Oxford, OX4 2DQ, UK

For details of our global editorial offices, for customer services and for information about how to apply for permission to reuse the copyright material in this book please see our website at www.wiley.com/wiley-blackwell.

Library of Congress Cataloging-in-Publication Data

Niemiec, Brook A.
Veterinary periodontology / Brook A. Niemiec.
p. ; cm.
Includes bibliographical references and index.
ISBN 978-0-8138-1652-4 (hardback : alk. paper)
1. Veterinary dentistry. 2. Periodontics. 3. Periodontal disease. I. Title.
[DNLM: 1. Periodontal Diseases–veterinary. SF 867]
SF867.N54 2012
636.089′7–dc23
2012015385

A catalogue record for this book is available from the British Library.

Wiley also publishes its books in a variety of electronic formats. Some content that appears in print may not be available in electronic books.

Cover design by Nicole Tuet

Set in 10.5/13pt Minion by SPi Publisher Services, Pondicherry, India

Contents

Contributors

Brett Beckman, **DVM, FAVD, DAVDC, DAAPM**
Florida Veterinary Dentistry, Punta Gorda, FL
Atlanta Veterinary Dentistry, Sandy Springs, GA
Affiliated Veterinary Specialists, Orlando, FL

Robert Furman, **BVMS, MRCVS**
Chief Resident
Southern California Veterinary Dental Specialties
Irvine, CA

Jerzy Gawor, **DVM, PhD, FAVD**
Klinika Weterynaryjna Arka, Kraków, Poland

Colin E. Harvey, **BVSc, FRCVS, DACVS, DAVDC**
Professor of Surgery and Dentistry
Department of Clinical Studies, School of Veterinary Medicine
University of Pennsylvania
Philadelphia, PA

James E. Hinrichs, **DDS, MS**
Diplomate, American Board of Periodontology
Professor and Director of Advanced Education in Periodontology
University of Minnesota
Minneapolis, MN

R. Michael Peak, **DVM, DAVDC**
Chief of Dentistry
Tampa Bay Veterinary Specialists
The Pet Dentist of Tampa Bay, Inc.
www.thepetdentist.com

Kevin Stepaniuk, **BSc, DVM, FAVD, DAVDC**
Veterinary Clinical Sciences
College of Veterinary Medicine
University of Minnesota
St. Paul, MN

Paul Theuns, **DVM**
Goudenregenstraat 29
3353 VA Papendrecht
Netherlands

Reviewers

Ruth E. Bartel, DAVDC
Daniel T. Carmichael, DAVDC
Johnathon R. Dodd, DAVDC
Jerzy Gawor, FAVD
Barron P. Hall, DAVDC
Christopher J. Snyder, DAVDC
Jason W. Soukup, DAVDC
Tammy L. White, DAVDC

Preface

Veterinary dentistry has been practiced for centuries, but only really developed into proper performance on small animal patients since the 1980s. Thanks to veterinary dental pioneers such as Emily, Mulligan, Williams, Grove, and Ross, this field has since become a recognized specialty with a growing reputation. Although we are still called "doggy dentists" and often work in obscurity, we are indeed coming into our own.

More and more clients are seeking options for the "best care" for their "four-legged children." This includes proper dental treatment, especially as trends are turning toward smaller breeds, which are typically even more prone to periodontal disease. Furthermore, with trends of increasing life spans for our small animal patients, dental disease is becoming more severe and problematic. Moreover, the significant local and particularly systemic disease is a growing concern as a consequence of unchecked periodontal disease. These trends have resulted in a collectively marked increase in the number of clients interested in proper periodontal therapy and all options available for maintaining teeth and health (dental and overall).

Throughout the growth in our field, we have leaned heavily on the human side of dentistry for our information and treatment modalities. While this has certainly been invaluable, we have learned that dogs and cats are not small humans. Although the basic tenets of periodontal disease and treatment are the same between our patients and their human counterparts, there are significant differences in the anatomy and physiology as well as common disease states. I have made every attempt to point out these differences within this text. On occasion, this is based on unpublished "experience" of mine and that of my colleagues, which is noted for the reader when necessary. I believe these comments and sections are an important advantage to the reader and are therefore some of the most important aspects of this book.

This text is of value to anyone who has interest in veterinary dentistry, overall veterinary practice, and even human dentistry. Clients and front office staff will benefit from the chapters on local and systemic disease, so they can understand the disease process. In addition, the chapters on basic periodontal care (prophylaxis, nonsurgical treatment, and homecare) will help them to understand what happens in the dental operatory of general practices. Technicians, students, and inexperienced veterinarians will enjoy these sections as well as those on pathogenesis and progression of disease, radiology, antimicrobial therapy, pain management, and equipment. Experienced practitioners will also benefit from all those chapters, but they may use the surgical section to start exploring more advanced procedures as well. I expect this text to be especially valuable for those practitioners pursuing dentistry certificates, as it provides all the current research and techniques in one book with easy-to-follow, high-quality step-by-step graphics. Finally, seasoned specialists can utilize this book to review the research and potentially glean information from some of the newer techniques from either the author's experience or from my foray deep into the literature.

It is critical to note that although many of the procedures in this text seem straightforward, hands-on training is essential to proper therapy. This includes techniques that are seemingly basic such as dental radiology, periodontal probing, and scaling (both hand and ultrasonic techniques). (Please see appendix 4, "Resources," for a list of courses.)

Above all, however, my main goal in writing this book is to improve periodontal care in general veterinary practices. In my time of almost 20 years in practice, the quality of veterinary dentistry within our specialty and within high-end general practices has improved exponentially. However, the quality of dental care within the average veterinary practice is still very poor. In my estimation, the number of general practices that perform complete subgingival scaling, ever use a periodontal probe, provide dental radiographs, or have a DVM perform an oral examination is less than 10%. As such, the vast majority of veterinary dental care is significantly substandard.

It is my hope that this text will inspire veterinarians to continue advancing their knowledge and skills regarding periodontal disease and therapy, thereby resulting in superior care for all veterinary patients. As a final note, I have also learned a great deal during the writing of this text, which has improved my patient care and greatly benefited my practice.

Best regards,
Brook A. Niemiec, DVM
Diplomate, American Veterinary Dental College
Fellow, Academy of Veterinary Dentistry

SECTION 1

Understanding the disease process

1

The structure and function of the periodontium

Kevin Stepaniuk and James E. Hinrichs

Periodontium

The supporting apparatus of the tooth is known as the periodontium. The gingiva, periodontal ligament (PDL), cementum, and alveolar bone are the tissues of the periodontium (Figure 1.1). This unique collection of tissues has a functional role in the oral cavity beyond anchoring the tooth in the bone. Understanding the structural, functional, biochemical, immunological, and molecular aspects of the periodontium is necessary to understand the pathophysiology of periodontal disease, periodontal treatments, periodontal regeneration, and periodontal repair. The hard tissues (cementum and bone) and the soft tissues (PDL and gingiva) of the periodontium play active rolls in the local inflammatory and immune response by synthesizing and releasing cytokines, growth factors, and enzymes. This fascinating interrelation of tissues, along with the normal apoptosis of the cells of the periodontium, provides the backdrop for the continued battle between periodontal health and disease.

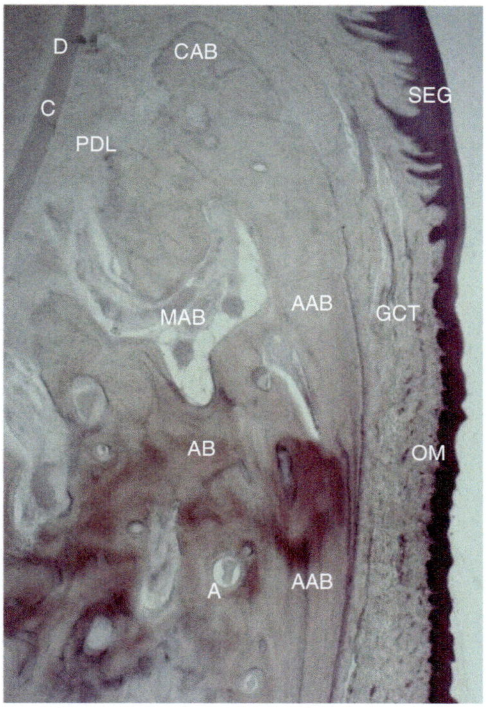

Figure 1.1 Histological image of the periodontium depicting dentin (D), cementum (C), periodontal ligament (PDL), alveolar bone (AB), apposition of buccal alveolar bone (AAB) associated with insertion of dental alveolar fiber, coronal crest of alveolar bone (CAB), medullary alveolar bone (MAB), arteriole (A), gingival connective tissue (GCT), stratified epithelium of gingiva (SEG), and oral mucosa (OM).

Odontogenesis and the periodontium

Odontogenesis is the embryological events in tooth development. Complete tooth development is described elsewhere.[1] However, the development of the tooth is not isolated from development of the periodontal tissues. During enamel development an outer enamel epithelium (OEE), inner enamel epithelium (IEE), and stellate reticulum are present. Adjacent to the enamel epithelium are the ectomesenchymal cells that form the dental follicle and papilla. The dental follicle gives rise to the cementum, PDL, and some alveolar bone.[2] This ectomesenchymal embryonic tissue forming the dental papilla and follicle is derived from neuroectoderm.[2]

The tooth root forms after the crown has developed, but before it is completely mineralized. The OEE and IEE, without the stellate reticulum, develop into *Hertwig's epithelial root sheath* (HERS). HERS proliferates into the underlying connective tissue to form the root. The dental papilla is stimulated to form odontoblasts, which

Veterinary Periodontology, First Edition. Brook A. Niemiec.

produce dentin. At this stage, the root sheath breaks up and cementoblasts are formed from the adjacent ectomesenchymal tissue. This inductive, interactive ectodermal-ectomesenchymal pattern of tooth and periodontium development is conserved in most higher vertebrate species.[3] HERS cells can remain trapped in the periodontal ligament and are known as the epithelial rests of Malassez (ERMS) (Figures 1.2 and 1.3). These cells, if stimulated later in life, may become cysts or possibly odontogenic tumors.[4,5] However, it is debated whether the ERMS are sources of odontogenic tumors.

The enamel epithelium proliferates into a thick reduced enamel epithelium that fuses with the oral epithelium.[6] The gingiva forms as the crown of the tooth penetrates into the oral epithelium and erupts into the oral cavity. A dentogingival junction is created and the junctional epithelium is established.

Repair and/or regeneration of the periodontium share many of the same events that occur during development of these unique tissues. A complete understanding of these chemical messengers and cell origins may provide a basis for periodontal repair and regeneration. However, the complete biochemical and molecular changes and the origins of cells, particularly cementoblasts, are not fully understood. It may be argued that periodontal tissue cannot be regenerated (restored to normal architecture), rather it is repaired.[2] For example, there is little evidence to support that acellular (primary) cementum reforms. Instead, when repair occurs, cellular cementum is deposited; this is argued to not be a true odontogenic tissue.[2] In many regeneration studies, the newly formed cementum is cellular with low numbers of fibers resulting in a new attachment may be weaker than the normal acellular extrinsic fiber cementum.[7] Similarly, repair as opposed to complete regeneration of a PDL occurs following damage.[8]

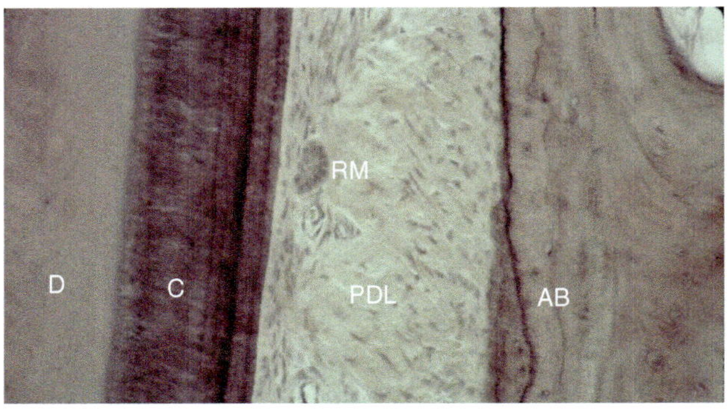

Figure 1.2 Epithelial rests of Malassez: dentin (D), cementum (C), periodontal ligament (PDL) with rests of Malassez (RM), and incremental apposition lines in alveolar bone (AB).

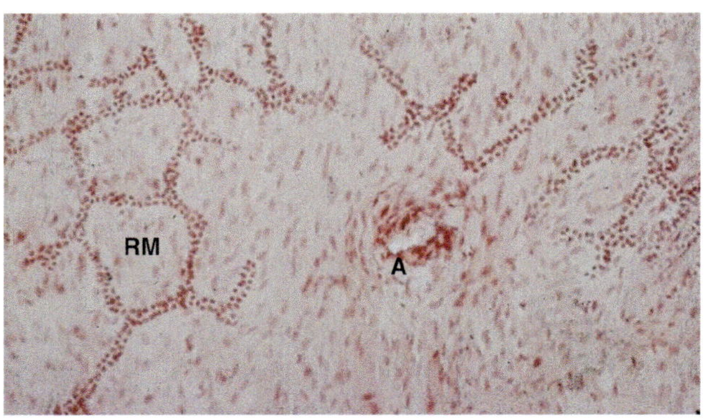

Figure 1.3 Connective tissue with an arteriole (A) with epithelial rests of Malassez (RM) displayed as a mosaic pattern.

Gingiva

The oral mucosa is classified into specialized mucosa (dorsum of tongue), the non-keratinized alveolar mucosa and the keratinized masticatory mucosa. The masticatory mucosa includes the hard palate mucosa and the gingiva. The gingiva is demarcated from the alveolar mucosa by the mucogingival junction (Figure 1.4).

General histology of the gingiva

A stratified squamous epithelium and deeper connective tissue (collagen fibers and ground substance) are the components of the gingiva. Gingival connective tissue consists of collagen fibers (type I and III collagen), fibroblasts, nerves, blood vessels, lymphatics, macrophages, eosinophils, neutrophils, T and B lymphocytes, and plasma cells.[1,9,10] This connective tissue is called *lamina propria* with a superficial papillary layer and deeper reticular layer. There are some variations in the lamina propria in relation to the type of gingiva. In the attached gingiva, the lamina propria has a papillary layer interdigitating with *rete pegs* of

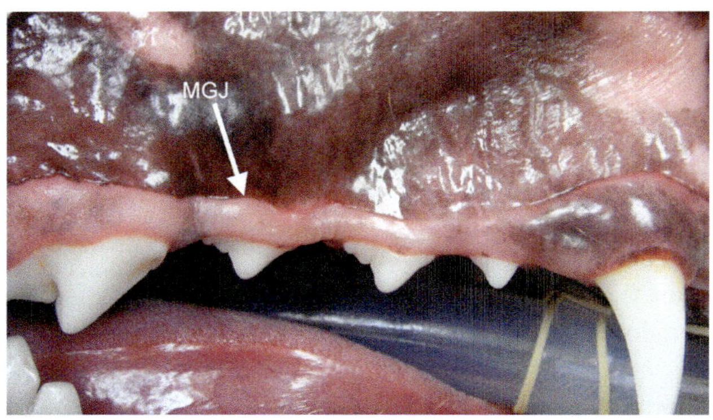

Figure 1.4 A photograph showing part of a dog's right maxillary arcade. The mucogingival junction (MGJ) demarcates between keratinized gingiva and non-keratinized alveolar mucosa.

the epithelium and a reticular layer adjacent to the periosteum of the alveolar bone.

The *keratinocyte* is the main cell type of the gingival epithelium.[11] The keratinocytes proliferate via mitosis in the basal layer of the epithelium. As cells migrate to the surface epithelium, they differentiate. The keratinization process includes flattening of the cuboidal cells, production of keratohyaline granules, and disappearance of the nucleus. The majority of gingival epithelium is parakeratinized and consists of the stratum basale, stratum spinosum (prickle cell layer), and stratum corneum. Pyknotic nuclei are present in the stratum corneum of *parakeratinized* epithelium. *Non-keratinized* epithelium lacks a stratum corneum and stratum granulosum with superficial keratinocytes containing nuclei. *Orthokeratinized* (complete keratinization with a *stratum granulosum*) gingiva was not observed in canine gingival samples.[12] The epithelial cells of the gingiva have cell-to-cell attachments consisting of desomosomes, adherens junctions, tight junctions, and gap junctions.[13]

Other cells found in the epithelium include *Langerhans cells*, *Merkel cells*, and *melanocytes*.[1,9–11] Melanocytes function to produce melanin granules, thereby providing a barrier to ultraviolet light damage. The melanin granules are phagocytosed and stored by melanophages in the epithelium and connective tissue.[10] Melanocytes also function as dendritic cells (antigen-presenting cells). The Langerhans cells are dendritic cells located in the suprabasal layers of the gingival epithelium. They originate from the bone marrow and function as antigen-presenting cells to the lymphocytes. Merkel cells are found in the deep layers of the gingival epithelium and are involved in tactile sensation.

The epithelium is attached to the lamina propria through the basement membrane consisting of the basal lamina (*lamina lucida* and *lamina densa*) and reticular lamina. Proteoglycans and laminin are present. Type IV and VII are the major collagens of the basement membrane.[14] Hemidesmosomes of the basal epithelial cells attach to the lamina lucida. Clinically, the distinction of the region is important. Mucous membrane pemphigoid cleavage occurs at the basement membrane, resulting in the entire epithelium, including the basal layer, cleaving off the lamina propria, whereas pemphigus vulgaris causes intraepithelial cleavage, leaving basal cells attached to the lamina propria.

Gingival fiber groups

The gingival fiber group is sometimes considered to be part of the periodontal ligament fiber group, which will be discussed later. The collagen fiber bundles of the gingiva are organized into groups (Figure 1.5):[6]

1. *Dentogingival group*: Fibers attach cervical cementum to free and attached gingiva. These are the most numerous fibers of the gingiva.
2. *Alveologingival group*: Fibers attach the alveolar bone to free or attached gingiva.
3. *Dentoperiosteal group*: Fibers attach the cervical cementum to the alveolar bone after traversing over the alveolar margin and toward the apex.
4. *Circular gingival group*: Fibers are interlaced with the other fiber groups within the marginal gingiva and encircle the tooth.

Vascular supply, nerves, and lymphatics of the gingiva

The blood supply to the gingival tissues arises from branches of the maxillary arteries and mandibular inferior alveolar arteries, terminating as supraperiosteal arterioles along the lingual and buccal surfaces of the alveolar bone, as well as from the periodontal ligament vasculature and arterioles from the marginal bone.[10] The gingival vascular system is a region of microcirculation.[15] The microvascular circulation of the human gingiva can be divided into the gingival region (where the capillaries run perpendicular to the surface) and the interdental papillae regions (where the capillaries run parallel to the surface).[16] The density of human gingival capillary loops increases with age and tends to be greater in females.[17] The vascular network in the dog gingiva was found to have a "glomerulus-like" form in the sulcular epithelium and a squamous mesh form in the junctional epithelium.[18] This network exudates fluid and allows leukocytes to pass into the gingival crevicular fluid.

These vascular networks are the primary defense against periodontal insults. The vascular beds are important in autoimmune and periodontal pathologies. The increased vascular densities in gingiva may be related to some of the first non-specific defenses against periodontitis. Capillaries of the marginal gingiva are the first vessels involved with inflammation.[15]

Innervation of the gingiva arises from the periodontal ligament and the regional trigeminal (cranial nerve V) branches. The mucosa of the oral cavity is richly innervated and primarily sensory.[1] The rich supply of neuronal axons is found in the lamina propria following the course of the vasculature in addition to nerve fibers in the vicinity of the epithelium.[19] Specialized sensory nerve endings are present (Meissner's or Ruffini's corpuscles, Krause's bulbs, and mucocutaneous endorgans) that detect heat, cold, touch, and pain.[1]

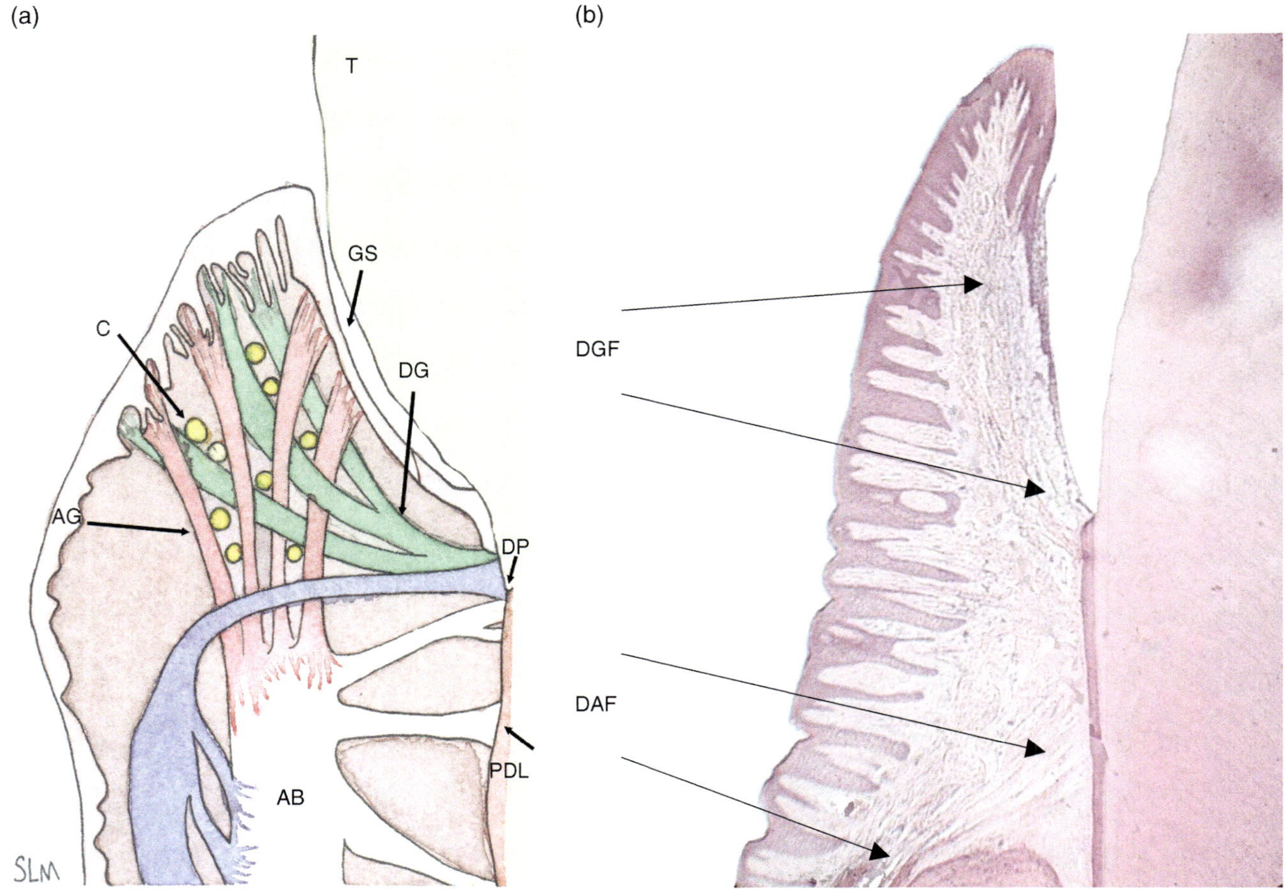

Figure 1.5 (a) Schematic drawing of the gingiva and gingival fiber groups. Dentogingival group (DG), alveologingival group (AG), dentoperiosteal group (DP), circular gingival group (C), alveolar bone (AB), periodontal ligament (PDL), gingival sulcus (GS). (Illustrated by Ms. Sarah L. Mann.) (b) Gingival fibers groups: Dentinal-gingival fibers (DGF) radiate from cementum into papilla, marginal gingival, and attached gingiva, while dentinal-alveolar fibers (DAF) radiate from cementum to insert into surface of alveolar bone.

Microscopic anatomy of periodontal lymphatics is challenging and difficult to study.[20,21] Within the oral mucosa the lymphatics play a primary role in the diffusion, control, and resolution of inflammatory processes. Lymphatics remove extracellular fluid, cellular debris, bacteria, and cells. The endothelial wall of gingival lymphatics is complex, with more intercellular junctions and intercellular channels with few open endothelial junctions.[22] The lymph of the gingival lymphatics drains into the PDL lymphatic system and follows the vasculature to a collective network, external to the periosteum of the alveolar bone, as it moves toward regional lymph nodes.[10,21]

Classification of gingiva and types of gingival epithelium

The gingiva is divided into the *free gingiva* (synonyms include marginal and unattached gingiva), *attached gingiva*, and *interdental gingiva*. The gingiva protects the underlying alveolar bone and tooth roots from mechanical trauma, and provides an epithelial barrier to help prevent bacteria from reaching the underlying tissues. The gingiva plays an active role in cellular communication, responds to infection, and integrates the innate and acquired immune responses when challenged by bacteria.[10] Epithelial cells excrete interleukin-8 and other cytokines and produce antimicrobial peptides as part of an innate defense mechanism.[13]

Free gingiva and the sulcular epithelium

The surface of the free gingiva adjacent to the tooth forms the wall of the gingival sulcus. The gingiva on the opposite side of this layer is exposed directly to the oral cavity (Figure 1.6). The epithelial layer exposed directly to the oral cavity is a parakeratinized stratified squamous epithelium. The free gingiva of young dogs is delicate

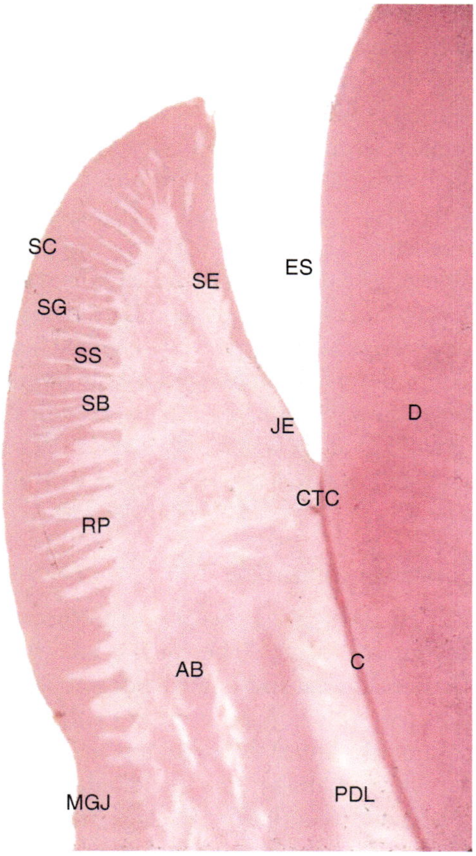

Figure 1.6 Healthy periodontium depicted with stratified squamous oral epithelium exhibiting Rete pegs (RP), stratum corneum (SC—keratinzed), stratum granulosum (SG—granular), stratum spinosum (SS—prickle cell), and stratum basalar (SB—germinativum). The sulcular epithelium (SE) consists of SB and SS with a limited amount of granulosum in coronal aspect, while junctional epithelium (JE) contains SB and SS and no granulosum. The mucogingival junction is identified as MGJ. ES represents the enamel space. CTC is the connective tissue attachment to cementum, AB the crest of the alveolar bone, PDL the periodontal ligament, C the cementum, and D the dentin, respectively.

and flat with a knife-edge marginal termination, whereas older dogs have a more curved appearance.[23] The free gingival height was measured at 1.80–1.92 mm and the width (most apically) at 1.31–1.34 mm.[23]

The gingival sulcus is lined with a non-keratinized stratified squamous epithelium that is referred to as *sulcular epithelium*. The gingival sulcus is bound by the junctional epithelium apically, the tooth, and the sulcular epithelium. Sulcular epithelium lacks rete pegs.[10] It is suggested that the non-keratinized nature of the sulcular epithelium is the result of the local irritation and inflammation within the gingival sulcus.[10]

The normal gingival sulcus depths are < *3 mm* in dogs and < *0.5 mm* in cats.[24] In plaque-free dogs and/or when plaque is well controlled, the gingival sulcus is essentially

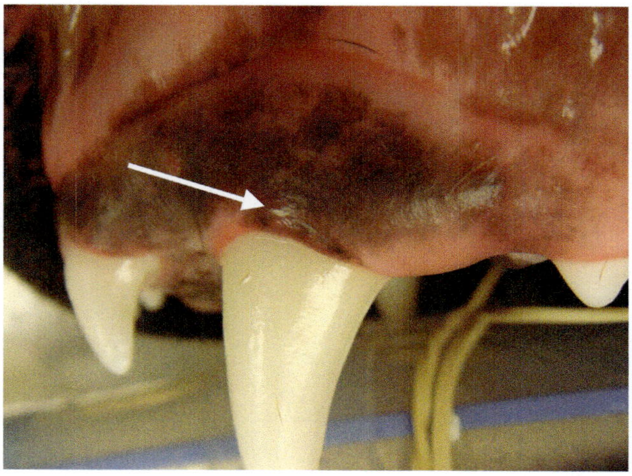

Figure 1.7 Photograph of a left maxillary canine tooth of a dog, gingiva, and alveolar mucosa. The free gingival groove within the keratinized gingiva is identified with an arrow.

absent with a probing depth close to 0 mm.[25] Clearly, there are breed variations in dogs, with giant breed dogs having deeper "normal" sulcular measurements as compared to toy breed dogs, which have shallower "normal" sulcular measurements. Likewise, in dogs without periodontal inflammation, the gingival sulcus is often minimal and there is minimal gingival crevicular fluid and leukocytes.[25] The *cementoenamel junction* (CEJ) is normally positioned just apical to the free gingival margin. In young dogs, the junctional epithelium extends from the CEJ to the oral epithelium with minimal gingival sulcus observed.[23,25]

Attached gingiva

The free gingiva is continuous to the attached gingiva and may be demarcated by a *free gingival groove* (Figure 1.7).[23] The thickness of attached gingiva in large breed dogs (as determined by transgingival probing) was measured as 1.10–2.20 mm, with the thinnest areas in the region of the incisors and the thickest regions around the canine, maxillary fourth premolar, and mandibular first molar teeth.[26] These measurements may not correlate with small and toy breed dogs. Individual variation of masticatory mucosa thickness has been observed in humans.[27] Likewise, the gingival width (as measured from the free gingival margin to the mucogingival junction) varies in the canine oral cavity with less gingival width in the region of the maxillary premolars compared to the canine tooth.[28] It has been suggested that 2 mm of attached gingiva (apical-coronal height) must be maintained for periodontal health.[29] The clinical significance of gingival width and thickness in various regions in the oral cavity is not known. It could be speculated that these thinner regions are more likely

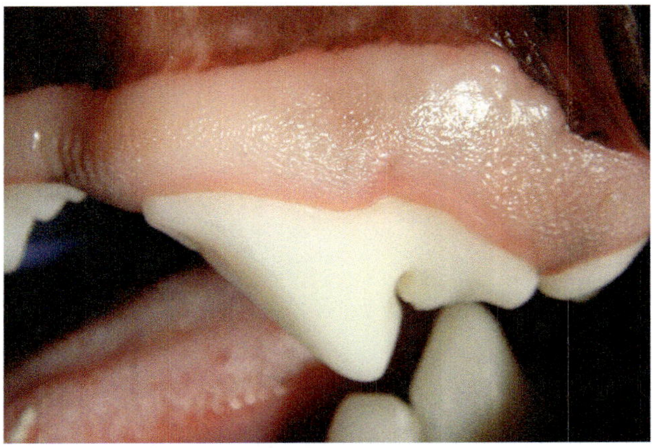

Figure 1.8 Photograph of the attached gingiva of a left maxillary fourth premolar in a young dog. Stippling illustrated within keratinized gingival tissue.

predisposed to periodontal disease, and the thicker and wider regions would be more ideal sites to use for periodontal surgical procedures (periodontal flap procedures and harvesting free gingival grafts).

The attached gingiva is a parakeratinized stratified squamous epithelium and has strong connections to the underlying periosteum of the alveolar bone. The attached gingiva is demarcated from the alveolar mucosa by the *mucogingival junction* (MGJ), which remains stationary throughout life.[10] Significant clinical loss of gingiva toward the MGJ (gingival recession) and/or probing depths of the gingival sulcus beyond the MGJ require periodontal surgery to help re-establish periodontium that can be maintained for periodontal health.

The attached gingival connective tissue and epithelium interdigitate. The connective tissue and gingival epithelial extensions are termed the *dermal papilla* and rete pegs, respectively. Well-developed rete pegs provide strong attachment to the underlying connective tissue. This well-developed interdigitation of the epithelial rete pegs and papillary layer can result in a clinical appearance of *gingival stippling* on the labial surface of attached gingiva (Figure 1.8).[12] In humans, the stippling is most prominent in the maxillary subpapillary region, whereas dogs do not have a proper interdental papillae and stippling is absent in these interdental spaces.[12] In one study, gingival stippling was found most commonly in older dogs (8–9 years of age), with younger dogs having absent stippling suggestive of less developed tissues.[23] In a more recent study, the stippling was found most commonly in middle-aged dogs and less in young and older patients.[12]

Interestingly, the most prominent signs of stippling were found at the canine teeth, upper fourth premolar, and first molar teeth with absence in the premolar teeth.[12] These are the same regions that were found to have the thickest width of attached gingiva. Therefore, the attachments will be stronger in these regions. These regions are considered to be the strategic teeth in carnivores and are challenged with the greatest mechanical forces during mastication.

In humans, stippling of the attached gingiva has been associated with the interdigitation of the rete pegs and dermal papillae.[10] This appears not to be the case in canine patients. The microscopically detectable pits in the canine gingiva do not correspond to the structures of the rete pegs and dermal papillae.[12] Loss of stippling has been suggested as a sign of gingival disease in humans.[10,12] In the dog, however, stippling can still be present in inflamed gingiva.[12] Regardless, the parakeratinized layer of the gingiva in dogs was found to be 5–10 cell layers thick whether it was in a region of stippled or unstippled gingiva.[12]

Interdental gingiva

The interdental gingiva between the teeth can form a pyramidal or col shape.[10] The col is a non-visible concavity between buccal and lingual gingival papillae. The col is covered with non-keratinized epithelium and is most commonly found between the maxillary fourth premolars and first molars, the mandibular first and second molars, and the incisors in dogs.[29] This region of non-keratinized epithelium is more susceptible to irritation and trauma, resulting in inflammation and possible early loss of periodontium.

Junctional epithelium and the gingival crevicular fluid

The gingival epithelium lining the sulcus is continuous to the *junctional epithelium* (JE) at the apical extent of the sulcus. The JE is a non-keratinized stratified squamous epithelium that attaches the gingiva to the tooth (Figure 1.9). JE contains fewer desmosomal junctions compared to other oral epithelial tissues.

JE provides a physical epithelial barrier to the apical periodontal structures. It allows passage of *gingival crevicular fluid* (GCF) and inflammatory cells (via diapedesis) into the sulcus. The JE has a rapid cell turnover rate that helps maintain a favorable host-parasite equilibrium and rapid repair of damaged tissue.[30] The JE replaces every 4–6 days, whereas the sulcular epithelium takes several more days to do so. The gingival epithelium takes 9–12 days to replace.[6,30] It has been suggested that JE cells have endocytic capacity similar to neutrophils and macrophages.[6]

Apical to the JE, the densely packed collagen bundles of the connective tissue anchor to the acellular extrinsic fiber cementum, which plays a key role in limiting the migration of the JE (Figure 1.10).[6] The apical aspect of the JE is 1–2 cell layers thick, whereas the thickness

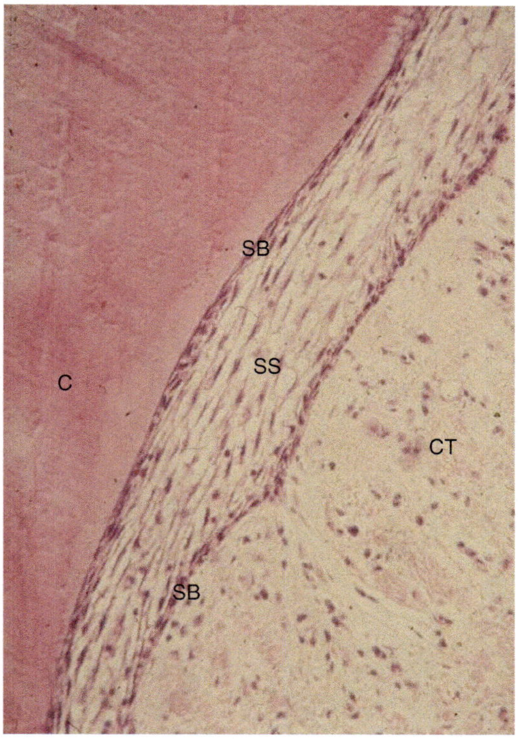

Figure 1.9 The junctional epithelium is composed of the stratum basalar (SB) and stratum spinosum (SS) and constitutes the interface between the cementum (C) and underlying connective tissue (CT).

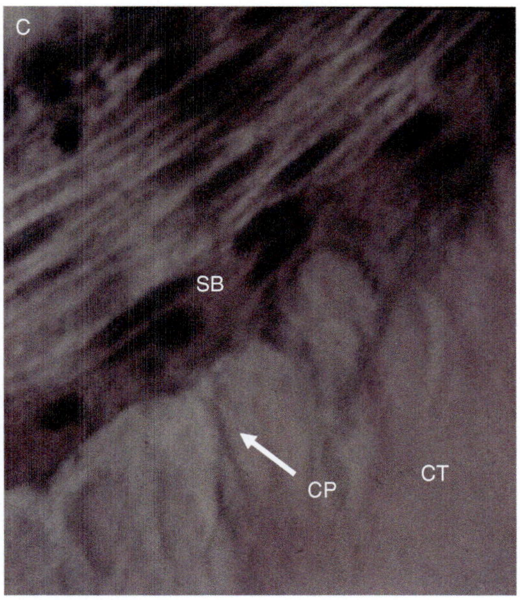

Figure 1.10 Cytoplasmic projections (CP) from the stratum basalar (SB) cells of the junctional epithelium extend into intercellular spaces of connective tissue (CT) cells and along cementum surface (C).

increases to 10–20 cells coronally.[6] It measures approximately 2 mm in apical-coronal direction. As junctional epithelial cells migrate coronally to be shed into the sulcus, a continuous attachment to the tooth surface is

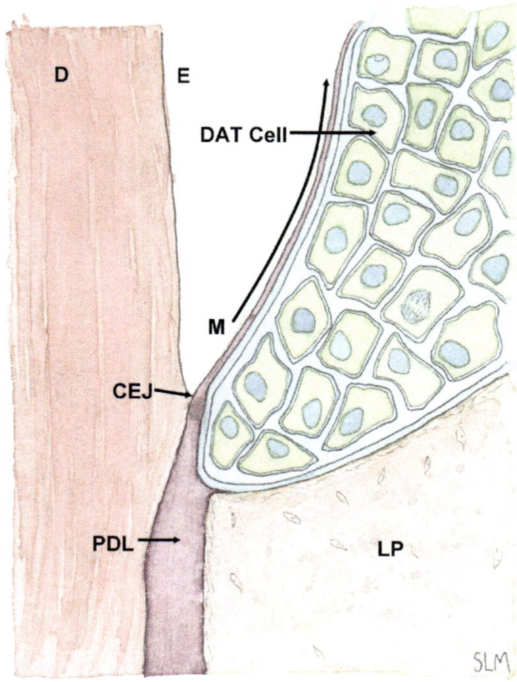

Figure 1.11 Schematic drawing of junctional epithelium. Lamina propria (LP), periodontal ligament (PDL), cementoenamel junction (CEJ), dentin (D), enamel (E), directly attached to tooth cell (DAT cell), movement of junctional epithelial cells coronally (M). (Illustrated by Ms. Sarah L. Mann.)

maintained, and these JE cells remain undifferentiated (Figure 1.11). The JE produces an internal basal lamina and anchors to this lamina via hemidesmosomes (Figure 1.12). The external basal lamina separates the JE from the gingival connective tissue.

Hemidesmosomes of the JE cells plasma membrane directly attach to the tooth (DAT cells). An internal basal lamina on the tooth surface interacts with the epithelial attachment.[30] The DAT cells synthesize the internal basal lamina, since there is no connective tissue present. The JE is a stratified epithelium with a basal layer facing connective tissue and a suprabasal layer extending to the tooth surface.[30] Interestingly, evidence suggests these DAT cells have mitotic activity, which is unique, since they are several cellular layers away from the basal layer of the epithelium.[30]

The JE vessels are fenestrated, which functions to allow exchange of substances through the openings.[18] The GCF moves through these fenestrations into the cellular spaces and then into the sulcus. The movement of GCF coronally helps clean the sulcus. Additionally, leucocytes move between the cellular gaps of the stratified squamous epithelium and into the sulcus in an organized manner.[18]

The GCF may be a transudate or exudate.[10,30] The composition of the GCF depends on the presence of a

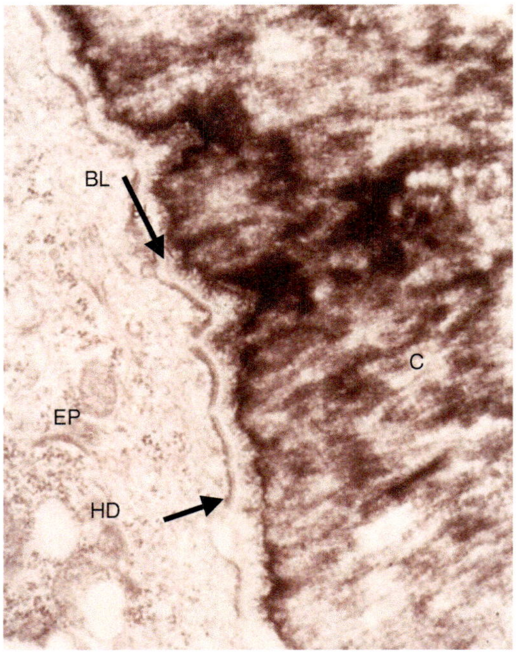

Figure 1.12 An electron microscopic image depicting hemidesmosomes on the periphery of an epithelial cell with the basal lamina (BL) consisting of the lamina densa [adjacent to cementum (C)] and lamina lucida [adjacent to periphery of epithelial cell (EP)] interspersed between the hemidesmosome and cementum (HD).

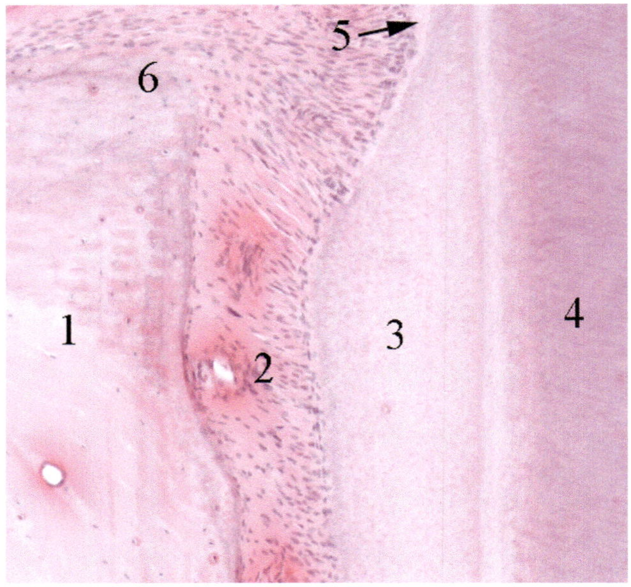

Figure 1.13 Histomicrograph of a feline periodontal ligament space. Alveolar bone (1), periodontal ligament (2), cementum (3), dentin (4), acellular afibrillar cementum (5), marginal alveolar bone (6). Reprinted with permission, Roux P, et al. Observations of the periodontal ligament and cementum in cats with dental resorptive lesions. J Vet Dent. 22(2):74–85, 2005.

plaque biofilm. Normally, there will be minimal fluid production. With inflammation, however, the fluid production increases and the GCF will contain breakdown products of connective tissue, epithelial cells, inflammatory cells, bacteria, and serum. The GCF mechanically flushes the sulcus, as well as contains antimicrobial products, immunoglobulins, and plasma proteins; the latter also assists in epithelial adhesion.[10] It is important to note that the polymorphonuclear leukocytes at the gingival margin do not remove plaque. These leukocytes provide a protective wall against bacteria.[30] The primary granules of these leukocytes contain myeloperoxidase, lysozyme, elastase, cathepsin G, urokinase, acid hydrolases, and defensins.[30] Lactoferrin, elastase, and lysozyme are found in the secondary granules.[30] (See chapter 4 for a complete discussion of GCF and its response to bacterial infection.)

Gingival tissues and age

All cells in the body and periodontium experience preprogrammed cell death (apoptosis). In particular, gingival cells and fibroblasts have a high rate of apoptosis in the normal turnover of the periodontium.[31,32] Apoptosis may play a role in different types of drug-induced gingival enlargement, particularly that caused by calcium channel blockers.[33] However, the mechanisms are multifactorial and not fully understood.[34,35] Increased collagen content of gingival connective tissue has been identified with increasing age in the dog, whereas no age-related gingival epithelial differences were found.[23] However, an earlier study found a thicker keratinized epithelial layer in the juvenile dog.[36] The most apical cells of the JE were at the CEJ in young dogs, and apical to the CEJ in older dogs with periodontal inflammation control. These findings suggest that teeth may be undergoing continued passive eruption.[23]

Periodontal ligament

The PDL is continuous with the gingival tissues, anchors the tooth in the jaw, acts as a shock absorber, and is active in periodontium maintenance (Figures 1.13 and 1.14). The PDL can be divided into a bone-related region rich in cells and vessels, a middle zone with fewer cells and thinner collagen fibrils, and a cementum-related region with dense collagen bundles.[6] Progenitor cells for fibroblasts, osteoblasts, and cementoblasts are found in the PDL.[7] The width of the buccal PDL was found to be 0.15–0.2 mm in dogs.[23] When PDL is destroyed, dentoalveolar ankylosis occurs and the adaptability of the periodontium is lost.

The principal collagenous fibers of the PDL are arranged in bundles that insert into the cementum and alveolar bone and are referred to as *Sharpey's fibers*. Type I collagen is the primary component of these principal fibers. The tensile

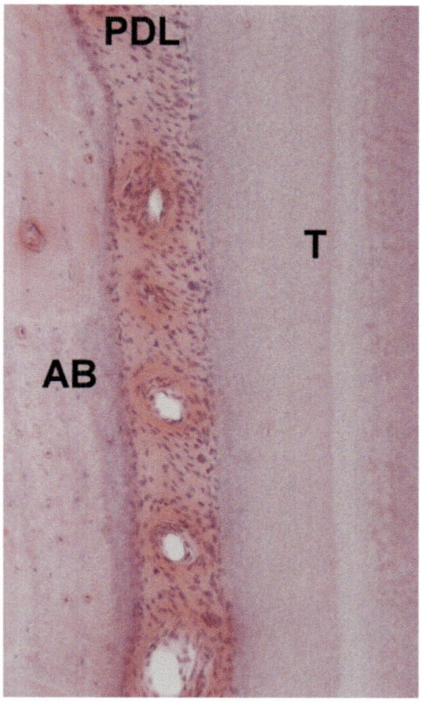

Figure 1.14 Histomicrograph of feline periodontal ligament. Alveolar bone (AB), periodontal ligament (PDL), tooth (T). Reprinted with permission, Roux P, et al. Observations of the periodontal ligament and cementum in cats with dental resorptive lesions. J Vet Dent. 22(2):74–85, 2005.

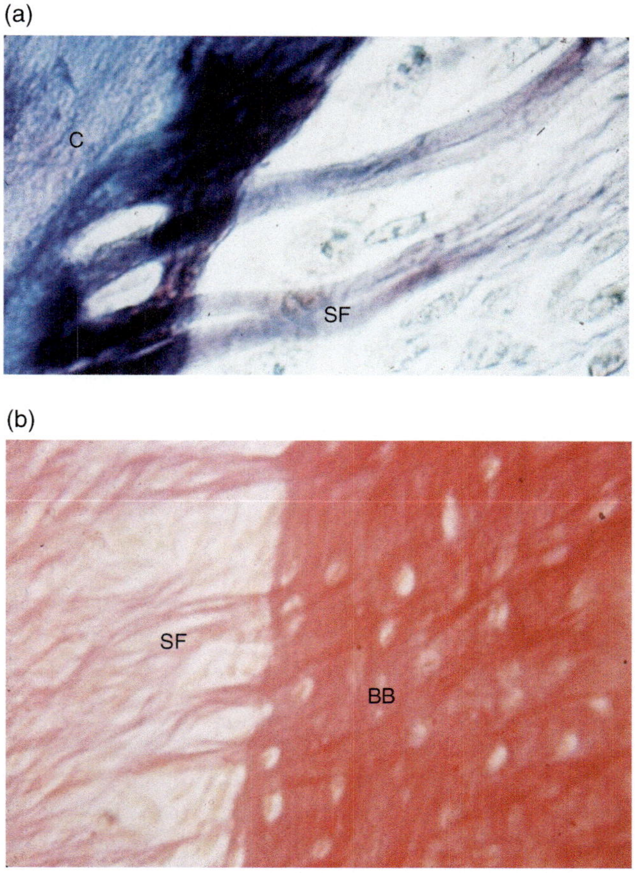

Figure 1.15 (a) Insertion of Sharpey's fibers (SF) into cementum (C). (b) Insertion of Sharpey's fibers (SF) into bundle bone (BB).

strength of these fibers has been reported to be greater than that of steel.[10] These fibers mineralize when embedded into the cementum and alveolar bone (Figure 1.15). The alveolar wall insertion of the Sharpey's fibers is the tension side of the PDL.[8] As Sharpey's fibers traverse deep into the bone, the length of penetration into the hard tissues can be much greater than the width of the PDL.[8]

The PDL acts as a shock absorber, and the viscoelastic system theory is used to explain the mechanism. As force is applied to the tooth, the fibers of the PDL tighten and blood is then forced from PDL vessels traversing the cribiform plate to the cancellous bone. The cribiform plate is most abundant in the cervical third of the tooth.[37] Additionally, mechanoreceptors, free nerve endings, pressure, and vibration sensors are found in the PDL.

Cells and connective tissue of the periodontal ligament

The cellular constituents of the PDL include epithelial rests of Malassez, immune cells, connective tissue cells, and neurovascular cells. The connective tissue cells include fibroblasts, osteoblasts, and cementoblasts. Undifferentiated cells that can differentiate into all of the above cells are also found in the PDL.[6,38] However, the exact source of the PDL is not fully understood. The fibroblasts in the PDL, similar to osteoblasts and cementoblasts, have an increased level of alkaline phosphatase activity and produce a mineralized matrix with osteopontin and bone sialoprotein.[6] It has been proposed that the maintenance of epidermal growth factor receptors on the fibroblasts of the PDL maintains these precursor cells as fibroblasts, whereas the loss of these growth factors allows differentiation into cementoblasts and osteoblasts.[6] Others have suggested HERS may give rise to cementoblasts and PDL fibroblasts.[7]

The fibroblast is the most abundant cell of the PDL and these cells are continually renewed.[8] Fibroblasts synthesize collagen and have phagocytic capacity. They remove collagen fibrils by phagocytosing the fibrils from the extracellular environment and degrading them with lysomal cysteine proteinases.[6] This lysosomal mechanism does not involve extracellular collagenase enzymes. Collagen degradation of the PDL is an intracellular phenomena following phagocytosis by periodontal fibroblasts,[8] whereas with disease, PDL breakdown is via extracellular mechanisms. The intracellular degradation allows a more specific and precise control for remodeling and replacement of the PDL under normal physiological

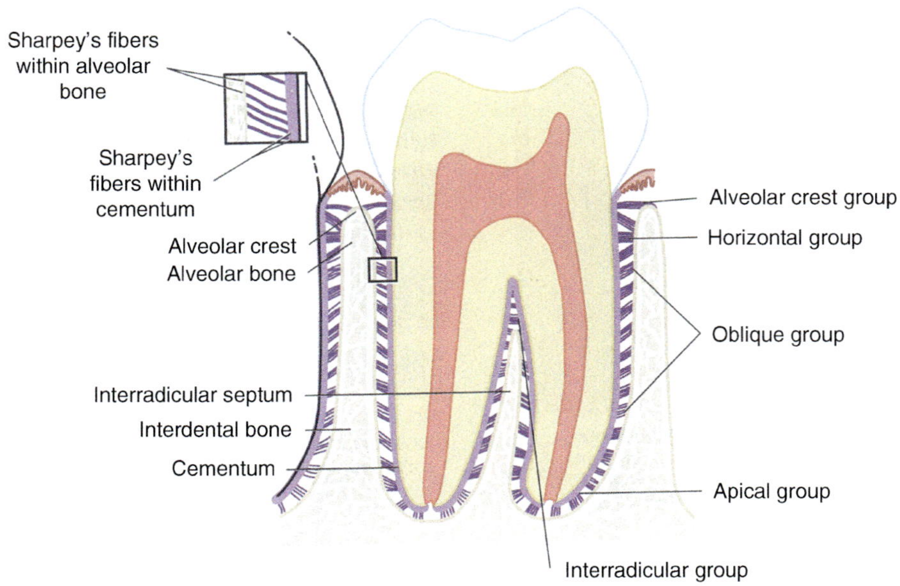

Figure 1.16 The alveolodental fiber groups of the periodontal ligament. Reprinted with permission, chapter 14, Periodontium: Cementum, alveolar bone, periodontal ligament. In: Dental Embryology, Histology, and Anatomy (Bath-Balogh M, Fehrenback MJ). 2nd ed. Copyright Elsevier Inc., 2006, p. 226.

conditions. New fibroblasts in repair of the periodontium arise from the perivascular cells in the PDL as well as from progenitor cells in the adjacent alveolar bone.[6]

Ground substance containing glycosaminoglycans (hyaluronic acid and proteoglycans), glycoproteins (fibronectin and laminin), and water fill the spaces between the cells and fibers in the PDL.[37] The extracellular components of the PDL connective tissue have a high turnover rate. Collagen has a very short half-life (several days) in the PDL, but collagenases have not been detected in the normal tissues.[8] However, the matrix metalloproteinase (MMP) enzymes are synthesized in a latent, non-active form that becomes activated by tissue and plasma proteinases, bacterial proteinases, and oxidative stress.[14] MMPs play a major role in connective tissue breakdown during disease, whereas phagocytosis degrades collagen for normal replacement, remodeling, and repair.[14]

The epithelial rests of Malassez are identified as isolated clusters of cells or interlacing strands in prepared tooth specimens.[37] The ERMS are most numerous in the apical and coronal regions and have been reported more on the mesial side of human molars compared to the distal side.[8] The exact function ERMS is not known but they do not appear to maintain the width of the PDL, prevent ankylosis, or prevent root resorption.[8]

Periodontal ligament fiber groups

Principal fiber bundles insert into bone and cementum as Sharpey's fibers. The primary collagens of the PDL are type I, III, and XII.[14] These fibers reconstruct and reinsert following periodontal damage from periodontitis, trauma, and orthodontic tooth movement. The PDL fiber groups respond to the physiological needs of the tooth.

The alveolodental fibers anchor between cementum and bone and include the following (Figure 1.16):[6]

1. *Alveolar crest fiber group* inserts in an apico-oblique direction beneath the JE and functions to resist extrusion, horizontal, rotational, and lateral tooth movement.
2. *Horizontal fiber group* inserts between cementum and bone at right angles and functions to resist horizontal and rotational tooth movement. They are located just apical to the alveolar margin.
3. *Oblique fiber group* inserts in a coronal-oblique direction (the bone insertion is positioned coronal to the cementum insertion) and functions to resist intrusive forces associated with occlusal stress and rotational tooth movement. The forces are transferred into tension of the alveolar bone. This fiber group is the largest, making up two-thirds of the fibers in the PDL.[6]
4. *Apical fiber group* inserts from the apex to the alveolar bone and functions to resist extrusion and rotational tooth movement.
5. *Interradicular fiber group* is found in multirooted teeth and connects cementum to marginal bone (Figure 1.17).
6. *Transseptal fiber group* anchors the cementum of two adjacent teeth (Figure 1.18). This group of fibers has an important role necessitating retention in orthodontics.

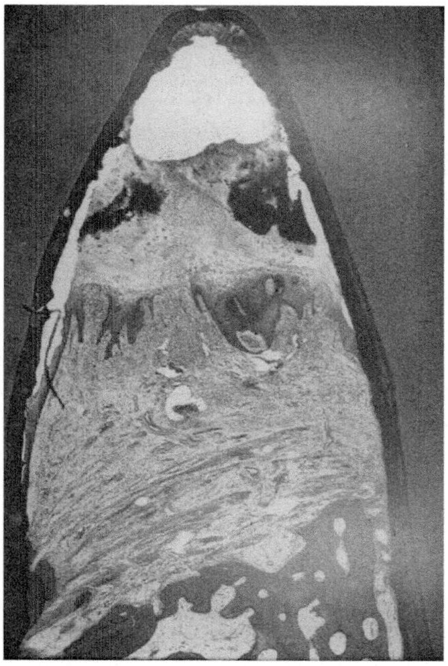

Figure 1.17 Intact interradicular periodontal fibers traverse the intraseptal bone and insert into the roots of a molar tooth despite extensive periodontitis in furcation region.

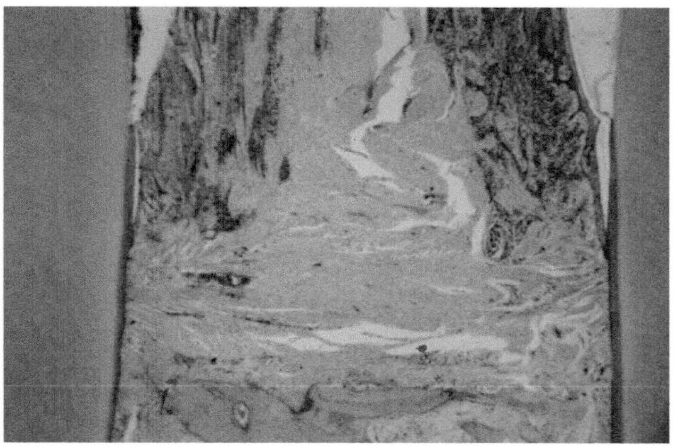

Figure 1.18 Horizontally oriented transseptal periodontal fibers lay coronal to the alveolar bone and insert into proximal surfaces of adjacent teeth.

In addition to the principal fiber groups, there is an indifferent fiber plexus of collagen inserting in all directions.[10] The PDL does not contain mature elastin but does contain two immature forms known as oxytalan and elunain.[10] *Oxytalan* fibers, similar to elastin, are found oriented in an apico-coronal direction and attach to the coronal third of the tooth.[8] It has been speculated that the function of these fibers is to provide elastic properties to the PDL, facilitate fibroblast attachment and migration, and may be involved in vascular flow.[8]

Vascular network of the periodontal ligament

The PDL has a good blood supply for a connective tissue. Branches of the maxillary and mandibular alveolar artery provide blood to the terminal branches.[39] The blood supply to the PDL arrives via (1) the alveolar bone blood supply through the Volkmann's canals (cribiform plate), (2) anastomosis with the gingival vessels, and (3) vessels arriving apically to the tooth.[18] The PDL has a polygonal mesh vascular network.[18] The movement of blood from the PDL to the alveolar bone allows the PDL to act as a shock absorber of occlusal forces. In large molars, the apical region of the vascular meshwork has a vertically longer, more elliptical shape, and adjacent capillary venules with anastomosing branches.[18] Blood vessels of the PDL provide nourishment to the cells of the PDL and osteoblasts of the adjacent alveolar bone. Lymphatics of the PDL drain into the alveolar bone in the coronal two-thirds and the apical lymphatics in the apical one-third.[20] Lymphatics were identified in the alveolar bone traversing to adjacent periodontal ligaments.[20]

The *rete venosum* in the alveolar bone may act as the reservoir for the displaced blood from the PDL vessels during occlusal force loading.[18] Additionally, there are very few valves in the venules of the PDL that traverse the Volkmann's canals.[18] Valves normally prevent backflow of blood in veins and venules. In the case of the PDL, the absence of valves can allow blood to flow back to the PDL from the alveolar bone when the occlusal forces are removed.

Cementum

Cementum, an avascular tissue with no innervations, is approximately 45–50% mineralized [hydroxyapatite, $Ca_{10}(PO_4)_6(OH)_2$], and 55–50% connective tissue. The organic matrix of cementum is mostly composed of types I (90%) and III (5%) collagen.[14,38,40] The cementum receives nourishment from the PDL.

Cementum must attach to the dentin surface of the root. In cementum, bone sialoprotein may act as an adhesion molecule to maintain cells on the root surface and initiate mineral formation.[38] It is proposed that there is a specific cementum attachment protein (a cementum-specific collagen) and a cementum-derived growth factor unique to cementum.[38]

Cementum is thinnest at the cementoenamel junction and thickest apically. Root cementum was found to be 5–10 times greater in older dogs and cementum thickness increased apically, whereas the width of the PDL remained constant.[23] In humans, approximately 60–65% of teeth have cementum overlapping enamel, 30% ending

Box 1.1 Development of the cementum

The development of the cementum is not fully understood or characterized. Although basic periodontium embryology was previously discussed, it is worthwhile to focus on the cementum more closely, as there are consequences when evaluating periodontal "repair" and "regeneration." The cementoblasts arise from the dental follicle. The disintegrating HERS does not have a secretory role in acellular cementum formation, despite some theories suggesting otherwise.[38,40] Amelogenin, an enamel matrix protein, was not found in cells of HERS.[38] Enamel matrix proteins (EMPs) have been debated as an important molecule in regeneration. However, detection of EMP expression along the root is sparse and its presence in bone and cementum is unclear.[7] Detection in some studies could be the result of dentin contamination during extraction of the EMP. Although enamel matrix protein extracts have been used for periodontal regeneration, and there is some evidence of successful "regeneration," there is no evidence they play a role during normal cementum development.[40]

EMP may promote the cementoblast activities of proliferation, migration, adhesion, and differentiation and may stimulate periodontal attachment structures during repair, but this does not necessarily result in regeneration.[38]

at the junction between enamel and cementum, and 5–10% have a space between enamel and cementum. Clinical conditions such as cemental aplasia, hypoplasia, cemental hyperplasia, and hypercementosis can occur. When cementum and the PDL are lost, the tooth can become ankylosed to the alveolar bone with resulting loss of proprioception and resistance of occlusal forces.

Types of cementum

Cementum is classified based on cells and the source of collagen fibers.[38] Unlike bone, cementum is avascular, lacks innervation, and shows little or no remodeling in the canine and feline.[38] Cementum is divided into acellular (referred to as primary) and cellular (referred to as secondary) and then further divided based on the origins of the collagen fibers from cementoblasts (intrinsic fiber cementum) and fibroblasts (extrinsic fiber cementum).[6] It is possible that acellular and cellular cementum are distinct types of cementum developing from different embryonic origins.[2]

Both acellular and cellular cementum are arranged in lamellae parallel to the long axis of the tooth representing rest periods. Acellular cementum is more mineralized than cellular, whereas cellular contains cementocytes in lacunae.[6] Cementocytes have a physiological adaptive role in tooth movement and repair of periodontal tissue.

The intrinsic fibers are arranged parallel to the root surface. Sharpey's fibers (extrinsic fibers) insert at approximately 90 degrees to the root surface, are fully mineralized in acellular cementum, and are only partially mineralized (mineralized periphery with unmineralized core) in cellular cementum. Acellular cementum forms before cellular cementum. However, cellular cementum forms at a faster rate.

1. *Acellular afibrillar cementum* (ACC): No cementocytes, extrinsic, or intrinsic fibers are present. It is a mineralized ground substance located over the enamel and dentin at the CEJ and has no role in attachment.[6,7] The precise cellular origin and function is unknown.
2. *Acellular extrinsic fiber cementum* (AEFC): Densely packed with Sharpey's fibers and lacking cementocytes. It is located on the cervical and middle third of the tooth, covering 40–70% of the root surface, and functions to anchor the PDL to the tooth root.[6] It is estimated there are 30,000 fibers/mm^2 inserting into the cementum.[7]
3. *Cellular mixed stratified cementum* (CMSC): Extrinsic and intrinsic fibers are present and it may contain cementocytes. It is found on the apical one-third of the root and in the furcation areas.[6,7] It contains layers of acellular extrinsic fiber cementum and cellular/acellular intrinsic fiber cementum.[6] The purpose is to compensate for physiological forces acting on the tooth in the alveolus.
4. *Cellular intrinsic fiber cementum* (CIFC): Cementocytes and intrinsic fibers are present with no extrinsic fibers. It is found filling resorption lacunae and root fracture sites.[7] The intrinsic fibers are not found within the PDL. CIFC has no role in tooth attachment with the fibers arranged parallel to the root surface while circling around the root.[6]
5. *Acellular intrinsic fiber cementum* (AIFC): There are no cementocytes and intrinsic fibers are only present. It is a component of the stratified layers of AIFC and CIFC that contributes to the CMSC.[7]
6. *Intermediate cementum*: This cementum is found near the cementodental junction and remnants of HERS are embedded in the calcified ground substance.

Alveolar bone

Bone is comprised of 67% inorganic material (hydroxyapatite) and 33% organic material. Collagen makes up the majority (80–90%) of the organic component of bone with greater than 95% being type I collagen and less than

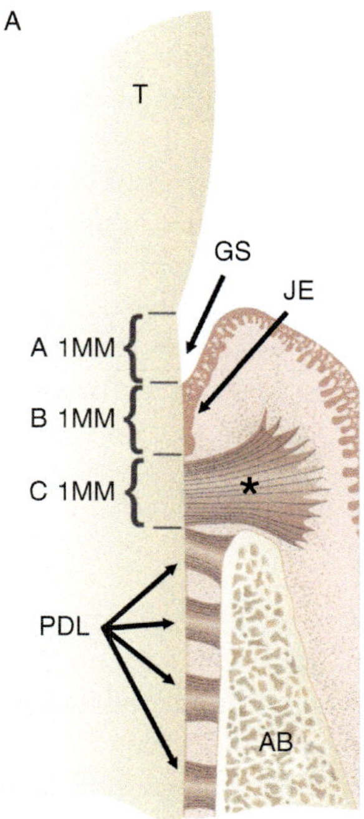

Figure 1.19 A drawing of the dentogingival interface demonstrating the biological width measured from the apical aspect of the gingival sulcus to the alveolar margin (B + C). This space is occupied by the junctional epithelium (JE) and the gingival connective tissue and gingival fibers (*). The tooth (T) is anchored in the alveolar bone (AB) by the periodontal ligament (PDL). Reprinted with permission, J Vet Dent. 25(2):86–95, 2008.

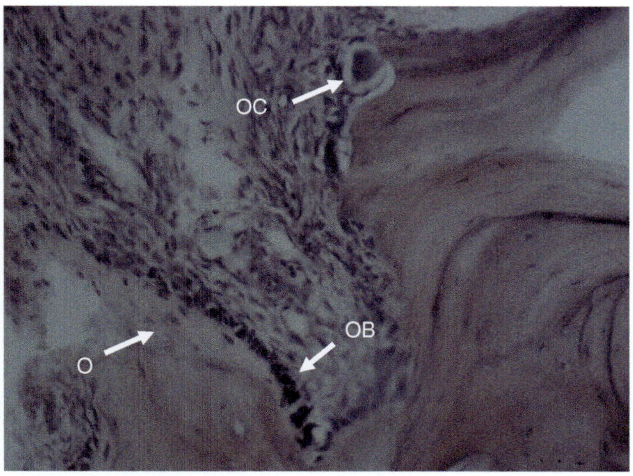

Figure 1.20 Remodeling of alveolar bone depicted by a line of osteoblasts (OB—lower center) forming new bone (O—osteoid) with entrapped osteocytes (dark nuclei). A resorption bay is noted in top center with one multinucleated osteoclast (OC).

5% type III, V, VI, XII collagen.[7,41] Osteopontin (OPN) and bone sialoprotein (BSP) are two non-collagenous proteins of bone and cementum that are present in the interfibrillar spaces.[7] The collagenous matrix called osteoid, secreted by osteoblasts, provides the scaffolding for apatite mineral deposition as well as other non-collagenous proteins.

Different types of bone are found in the maxillofacial region. Woven bone arises from a connective tissue template and a process of intramembranous ossification. The maxilla and mandible contain alveolar processes that house roots of the teeth.[6] Alveolar bone supports the tooth structure, helps distribute occlusal forces, and is continually remodeled as it responds to the forces of mastication. The alveolar bone is composed of plates of cortical (compact) bone with spongy cancellous (trabecular) bone in between. Cancellous bone is also found in the interradicular and interdental spaces between cortical bone and the alveolar wall.[42] Bone lining the alveolus, where the Sharpey's fibers insert, is referred to as *bundle bone*. Bundle bone, irregularly arranged and less dense, is produced by osteoblasts between the Sharpey's fibers.[42] The bone layers are arranged parallel to the apico-coronal direction of the tooth.[41] The inner cortical bone is radiographically dense and is radiographically referred to as the *lamina dura*. Cortical bone meets coronally at the alveolar margin and is usually 1.5–2.0 mm below the CEJ (Figure 1.19).[43]

Alveolar bone consists of lamellated and bundle bone.[6] The osteon is the structural unit of bone with a central Haversian canal and interconnecting Volkmann's canals. Histologically, a cement line can be seen between old and newly formed bone. The apical and coronal aspects of the alveolar bone (cribiform plate) have openings connecting the bone marrow to the PDL via Volkmann's canals.[6]

Alveolar bone remodeling

Bone is remodeled while under constant force. There is an interdependency of osteoblasts and osteoclasts called coupling.[37] Osteoclasts and osteoblasts interact in a paracrine and autocrine fashion. Osteoblasts and newly formed osteoid (Figure 1.20) line the region of recently resorbed bone vacated by osteoclasts. Cancellous bone trabeculae increase in number and thickness and cortical bone may be added when increased forces are placed on the jaws.[37]

Osteoclasts are responsible for resorption of bone by removing the hydroxyapatite and organic matrix. They arise from hematopoietic cells of the monocyte/macrophage lineage of the bone marrow. Osteoclasts are large multinucleated cells that produce a variety of hydrolytic enzymes that are secreted into an acidic environment. Osteoclasts are found in *Howship's lacunae* (Figure 1.21). The ruffled border of a multinucleated osteoclast creates a microenvironment for bone resorption.

Osteoblasts produce bone matrix (both collagenous and non-collagenous), which is termed osteoid. Rapidly forming bone (embryonic and juvenile growing bone, as

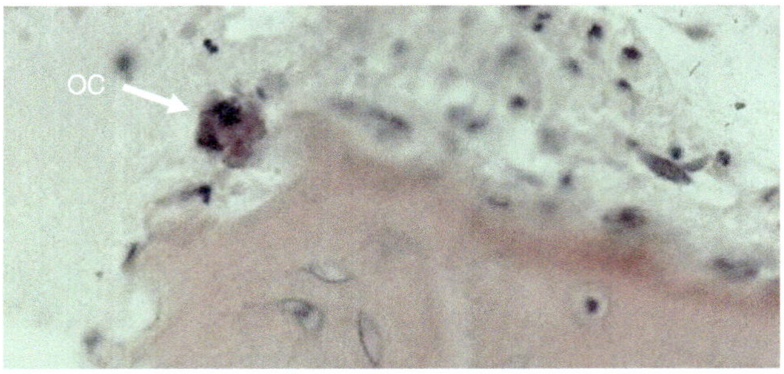

Figure 1.21 A multinucleated osteoclast (OC) in Howship's lacunae bay of resorption.

well as bone involved in repair) is called woven bone. There are large areas of interfibrillar spaces occupied by mineral crystals and large numbers of osteocytes.[7] Alkaline phosphatase, secreted by osteoblasts, starts the nucleation of hydroxyapatite crystals. More mature lamellar bone has organized collagen fiber sheets perpendicular to one another with very little interfibrillar space.[41] Osteopontin and bone sialoprotein are expressed in alveolar bone.[41] Osteopontin is located at cement lines in bones and may play a role in integrating new and old bone together.[41] Osteoblasts that do not undergo apoptosis or remain on the bone surface can be trapped in bone lacunae as osteocytes.[41]

Bone formation and resorption are closely coordinated. Osteoclasts are stimulated to resorb bone by parathyroid hormone, parathyroid-related peptide, vitamin D_3, interleukin-1, interleukin-6, tumor necrosis factor-α, transforming growth factor-α, and prostaglandin-E_2 (PGE_2).[7,41] Parathyroid hormone and vitamin D_3 influence osteoclasts indirectly by acting on osteoblasts. Osteoclasts are inhibited by calcitonin, transforming growth factor-β, estrogen, and interferon-γ.[41] Prostaglandin E_2 is a potent stimulator of osteoclasts and bone resorption.

An interesting new area of bone regulation is the RANK (receptor-activated nuclear factor $\kappa\beta$)/RANKL(receptor-activated nuclear factor $\kappa\beta$ ligand)/OPG (osteoprotegrin) system in relation to osteoclast regulation.[7] It is also necessary for macrophage-colony stimulating factor to be present along with osteoblasts and cell-to-cell contact for osteoclast regulation. RANKL/OPG balance in the bone microenvironment is crucial for osteoclast control. The stimulators of osteoclasts and subsequent bone resorption work via this system.

RANK is expressed on the plasma cell membranes of osteoclast precursor cells, whereas RANKL is expressed on the plasma cell membranes of osteoblasts. OPG produced by osteoblasts acts as a decoy receptor by binding RANKL, thereby preventing activation of RANK. The suppression of this system decreases development, formation, and activity of osteoclasts, whereas an induction of the system increases them.[7] Understanding this functional system of the alveolar bone can allow development of targeted therapies for alveolar bone loss.

It should be noted that the RANK/RANKL/OPG system is not the direct target of bisphosphonate compounds used in medicine. Bisphosphonates inhibit bone resorption by inducing osteoclast and macrophage apoptosis.[31,44] There has been bisphosphonate-related osteonecrosis of the jaws due to inhibition of osteoclasts in human patients. Yet at controlled local doses they may provide treatment of periodontitis due to control of osteoclasts.[45]

Conclusion

The periodontium is a dynamic system responding to attack from oral bacteria. Despite meticulous periodontal homecare and annual dental cleanings, periodontium is lost over time. There is increased attachment loss of the periodontium as the patient ages.[46,47]

Understanding the structure and function of the periodontium is necessary for understanding periodontal defense mechanisms, periodontal disease pathophysiology, periodontal treatments, and periodontal regeneration and repair. Regeneration implies reproduction or reconstitution of the tissues so they are completely restored (as in embryological tooth development) versus repair, which implies healing without restoration.[48]

Acknowledgment

Schematic diagrams depicted in Figures 1.5a and 1.11 were illustrated by Ms. Sarah L. Mann, University of Minnesota student.

Box 1.2 Key points

- The lining of the gingival sulcus is non-keratinized and is therefore more fragile than the outer coating of the attached gingiva. Care must be taken during subgingival cleaning.
- Dogs do not have proper interdental papillae.
- The normal gingival sulcus depths are <*3 mm* in dogs and <*0.5 mm* in cats.
- However, in plaque-free dogs and/or when plaque is well controlled, the gingival sulcus has a minimal probing depth.
- The periodontal ligament is continuous with the gingival tissues, anchors the tooth in jaw, acts as a shock absorber, and is active in maintenance of the periodontium.
- Alveolar bone supports the tooth structure, helps distribute occlusal forces, and is continually remodeled as it responds to the forces of mastication.
- The alveolar bone is composed of plates of cortical (compact) bone with spongy cancellous (trabecular) bone in between.

References

1. Nanci A. Ten Cate's Oral Histology: Development, Structure, and Function. 7th ed. Philadelphia: Mosby-Elsevier, 2008.
2. Ten Cate AR. The development of the periodontium—a largely ectomesenchymally derived unit. Periodontol 2000 13:9–19, 1997.
3. Moss ML. Phylogeny and comparative anatomy of oral ectodermal-ectomesenchymal inductive interactions. J Dent Res. 48(5):732–737, 1969.
4. Gardner DG. Epulides in the dog: A review. J Oral Pathol Med. 25(1):32–37, 1996.
5. Verstraete FJ, Ligthelm AJ, Weber A. The histological nature of epulides in dogs. J Comp Pathol. 106(2):169–182, 1992.
6. Cho MI, Garant PR. Development and general structure of the periodontium. Periodontol 2000 24:9–27, 2000.
7. Bosshardt DD. Are cementoblasts a subpopulation of osteoblasts or a unique phenotype? J Dent Res. 84(5):390–406, 2005.
8. Beertsen W, McCulloch CA, Sodek J. The periodontal ligament: A unique, multifunctional connective tissue. Periodontol 2000 13:20–40, 1997.
9. Bath-Balogh M, Fehrenbach MJ. Gingival dentogingival junctional tissues. In: Dental Embryology, Histology, and Anatomy. 2nd ed. St. Louis: Elsevier-Saunders, 2006, pp. 151–160.
10. Fiorellini, J.P., Kim, D.M., Ishikawa, S.O. The Gingiva. In: Carranza's Clinical Periodontology. St. Louis: Saunders, 2006, pp. 46–67.
11. Bath-Balogh M, Fehrenbach MJ. Oral mucosa In: Dental Embryology, Histology, and Anatomy. 2nd ed. St. Louis: Elsevier-Saunders, 2006, pp. 127–149.
12. Kyllar M, Witter K, Tichy F. Gingival stippling in dogs: Clinical and structural characteristics. Res Vet Sci. 88(2):195–202, 2010.
13. Dale BA. Periodontal epithelium: A newly recognized role in health and disease. Periodontol 2000 30:70–78, 2002.
14. Bartold PM, Narayanan AS. Molecular and cell biology of healthy and diseased periodontal tissues. Periodontol 2000 40:29–49, 2006.
15. Nuki K, Hock J. The organisation of the gingival vasculature. J Periodontal Res. 9(5):305–313, 1974.
16. Scardina GA, Fuca G, Messina P. Microvascular characteristics of the human interdental papilla. Anat Histol Embryol. 36(4): 266–268, 2007.
17. Scardina GA, Cacioppo A, Messina P. Anatomical evaluation of oral microcirculation: Capillary characteristics associated with sex or age group. Ann Anat. 191(4):371–378, 2009.
18. Matsuo M, Takahashi K. Scanning electron microscopic observation of microvasculature in periodontium. Microsc Res Tech. 56(1):3–14, 2002.
19. Lohinai Z, Szekely AD, Benedek P, et al. Nitric oxide synthase containing nerves in the cat and dog dental pulp and gingiva. Neurosci Lett. 227(2):91–94, 1997.
20. Berggreen E, Haug SR, Mkonyi LE, et al. Characterization of the dental lymphatic system and identification of cells immunopositive to specific lymphatic markers. Eur J Oral Sci. 117(1):34–42, 2009.
21. Matsumoto Y, Zhang B, Kato S. Lymphatic networks in the periodontal tissue and dental pulp as revealed by histochemical study. Microsc Res Tech. 56(1):50–59, 2002.
22. Marchetti C, Poggi P. Lymphatic vessels in the oral cavity: Different structures for the same function. Microsc Res Tech. 56(1): 42–49, 2002.
23. Berglundh T, Lindhe J, Sterrett JD. Clinical and structural characteristics of periodontal tissues in young and old dogs. J Clin Periodontol. 18(8):616–623, 1991.
24. Wiggs, R.B., Lobprise, H.B. Chapter 4, Oral Examination and Diagnosis. In: Veterinary Dentistry, Principles and Practice. Philadelphia: Lippincott-Raven, 1997, pp. 87–103.
25. Attstrom R, Graf-de Beer M, Schroeder HE. Clinical and histologic characteristics of normal gingiva in dogs. J Periodontal Res. 10(3):115–127, 1975.
26. Kyllar M, Witter K. Gingival thickness in dogs: Association with age, gender, and dental arch location. J Vet Dent. 25(2):106–109, 2008.
27. Muller HP, Schaller N, Eger T, et al. Thickness of masticatory mucosa. J Clin Periodontol. 27(6):431–436, 2000.
28. Shoukry M, Ben Ali L, Abdel Naby M, et al. Repair of experimental plaque-induced periodontal disease in dogs. J Vet Dent. 24(3):152–165, 2007.
29. Wiggs RB, Lobprise HB. Periodontology. In: Veterinary Dentistry, Principles and Practice. Philadelphia: Lippincott-Raven, 1997, pp. 186–191.
30. Pollanen MT, Salonen JI, Uitto VJ. Structure and function of the tooth-epithelial interface in health and disease. Periodontol 2000 31:12–31, 2003.
31. Satchell PG, Gutmann JL, Witherspoon DE. Apoptosis: An introduction for the endodontist. Int Endod J. 36(4):237–245, 2003.
32. Koulouri O, Lappin DF, Radvar M, et al. Cell division, synthetic capacity and apoptosis in periodontal lesions analysed by in situ hybridisation and immunohistochemistry. J Clin Periodontol. 26(8):552–559, 1999.
33. Lewis JR, Reiter AM. Management of generalized gingival enlargement in a dog—case report and literature review. J Vet Dent. 22(3):160–169, 2005.
34. Meisel P, Schwahn C, John U, et al. Calcium antagonists and deep gingival pockets in the population-based SHIP study. Br J Clin Pharmacol. 60(5):552–559, 2005.
35. Seymour RA, Ellis JS, Thomason JM. Risk factors for drug-induced gingival overgrowth. J Clin Periodontol. 27(4):217–223, 2000.
36. Matsson L, Attstrom R. Histologic characteristics of experimental gingivitis in the juvenile and adult beagle dog. J Clin Periodontol. 6(5):334–350, 1979.
37. Fiorellini JP, Kim DM, Ishikawa SO. The tooth-supporting structures. In: Carranza's Clinical Periodontology. St. Louis: Saunders, 2006, pp. 68–92.
38. Saygin NE, Giannobile WV, Somerman MJ. Molecular and cell biology of cementum. Periodontol 2000 24:73–98, 2000.
39. Evans HE. The Heart and Arteries. 3rd ed. Philadelphia: Saunders, 1993, pp. 612–620.
40. Diekwisch TG. The developmental biology of cementum. Int J Dev Biol. 45(5–6):695–706, 2001.
41. Sodek J, McKee MD. Molecular and cellular biology of alveolar bone. Periodontol 2000 24:99–126, 2000.
42. Saffar JL, Lasfargues JJ, Cherruau M. Alveolar bone and the alveolar process: The socket that is never stable. Periodontol 2000 13:76–90, 1997.
43. Bath-Balogh M, Fehrenbach MJ. Periodontium: Cementum, alveolar bone, periodontal ligamant. In: Dental Embryology, Histology, and Anatomy. 2nd ed. St. Louis: Elsevier-Saunders, 2006, pp. 207–230.
44. Mohn KL, Jacks TM, Schleim KD, et al. Alendronate binds to tooth root surfaces and inhibits progression of feline tooth resorption: A pilot proof-of-concept study. J Vet Dent. 26(2):74–81, 2009.
45. Shinoda H, Takeyama S, Suzuki K, et al. Pharmacological topics of bone metabolism: A novel bisphosphonate for the treatment of periodontitis. J Pharmacol Sci. 106(4):555–558, 2008.
46. Hoffmann T, Gaengler P. Epidemiology of periodontal disease in poodles. J Small Anim Pract. 37(7):309–316, 1996.
47. Hoffmann T, Gaengler P. Clinical and pathomorphological investigation of spontaneously occurring periodontal disease in dogs. J Small Anim Pract. 37(10):471–479, 1996.
48. Bosshardt DD, Sculean A. Does periodontal tissue regeneration really work? Periodontol 2000 51:208–219, 2009.

2

Etiology and pathogenesis of periodontal disease

Introduction

While there are many factors associated with the development of periodontal disease, the inciting etiologic agent is plaque bacteria.[1–8] Research has shown that inflammation will continue as long as the gingiva is exposed to a bacterial biofilm and will resolve after its removal.[9,10] In fact, one author emphatically states, "Forty years of experimental research, clinical trials, and demonstration projects in different geographical and social settings have confirmed that effective removal of dental plaque is essential to dental and periodontal health throughout life."[11]

Periodontal disease is described in two stages, gingivitis and periodontitis. Gingivitis is the initial, *reversible* stage of the disease process in which the inflammation is confined to the gingival tissues.[6,12] In other words, there is no inflammation involving the periodontal ligament or alveolar bone. The gingival inflammation, which is initiated by plaque bacteria, may be reversed with a thorough dental prophylaxis and consistent homecare.[12,13]

Periodontitis is the later stage of the disease process and is defined as an inflammatory disease of the deeper supporting structures of the tooth (periodontal ligament and alveolar bone) caused by microorganisms.[3,14] These conditions are discussed in detail in respective chapters. This chapter will focus on the pathogenesis of both of these diseases, which are often interrelated.

Plaque

Periodontal disease (both gingivitis and periodontitis) is initiated when oral bacteria adhere to the teeth in a substance called plaque.[1,2,6,10,15] Dental plaque is defined as a structured, resilient substance that adheres tenaciously to intraoral hard tissues.[15–17] Plaque is a biofilm which is made up almost entirely of oral bacteria, contained in a matrix composed of salivary glycoproteins and extracellular polysaccharides.[6,15,17,18] A biofilm is a unique environment in which nutrients (as well as oxygen) diffuse through the different layers, which supports changes in microbiotic composition.[15] In addition, there exists a series of fluid channels within the plaque biofilm that facilitate nutrient delivery and waste removal.[18,19] As such, these channels act as a primitive circulatory system for the biofilm. In essence, plaque is a unique organism.[18]

Adherence of plaque

The warm, moist, nutrient-rich environment of the oral cavity makes it an ideal breeding ground for bacteria. Fortunately, many of these bacteria are swallowed or "drooled" and therefore do not contribute to periodontal disease. For bacteria to initiate periodontal disease, they must remain attached to the oral tissues, and therefore adherence is an important aspect of periodontal disease. There are several niches for this to occur within the mouth, including the teeth, periodontium, buccal epithelium, tongue, and tonsils.[15] The first two are most important in the discussion of periodontal disease.

Although the periodontium is easily colonized by oral bacteria, there appears to be individual variation between animals as to the relative adherence of bacteria. In fact, it has been shown that bacterial adherence is increased in those who are predisposed to periodontal disease.[20] Fortunately, the high turnover rate of the oral soft tissues limits the level of infection.

The major niche for bacterial colonization is the teeth.[15] Teeth are particularly prone to bacterial adherence because they are hard, irregular, and non-shedding. They also create a unique and abrupt transition from the periodontal tissues. The combination of these factors

Veterinary Periodontology, First Edition. Brook A. Niemiec.

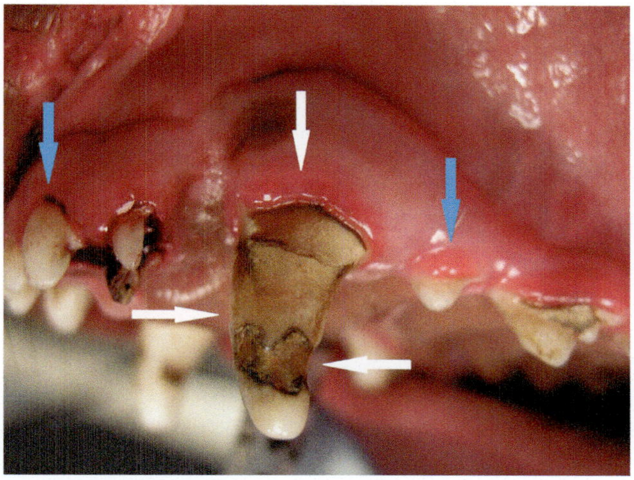

Figure 2.1 Intraoral picture of the maxillary left of a dog with widespread enamel hypocalcification. Note the significant calculus and gingival inflammation on the canine (white arrows), especially when compared with the second incisor and first premolars (blue arrows), which are unaffected.

makes the teeth very efficient bacterial colonization sites. Plaque adherence is further enhanced by many anatomic or pathologic states that may either roughen the teeth or inhibit plaque removal.[15,21] Factors associated with a roughened tooth surface include enamel hypocalcification (Figure 2.1), tooth resorption or uncomplicated crown fractures (Figure 2.2), wear (attrition or abrasion) (Figure 2.3), or presence of calculus.[3] Conditions that inhibit plaque removal (normally achieved by either natural means such as chewing or by homecare methods) include crowding (Figure 2.4), periodontal pockets (Figure 2.5), gingival foreign bodies (Figure 2.6), or gingival hyperplasia (Figure 2.7).[3] Therefore, these issues should be addressed along with standard periodontal care. Additionally, gingival inflammation has been shown to increase plaque accumulation[22] (likely due to increased crevicular fluid production and the nutrients it supplies).[15] This finding proves the critical importance of good oral hygiene.

Plaque formation

The process of plaque formation is divided into three major stages: formation of the pellicle, initial bacterial adhesion and attachment, and finally bacterial colonization and plaque maturation.[15]

The first stage is formation of the pellicle on the surface of the teeth, which starts within *nanosoeconds* of a prophylaxis.[15] The pellicle is a thin, saliva-derived layer including numerous proteins (such as glycoproteins), enzymes, and other molecules that act as attachment sites for bacteria.[6] The initial pellicle differs from saliva and therefore is thought to form by selective adsorption

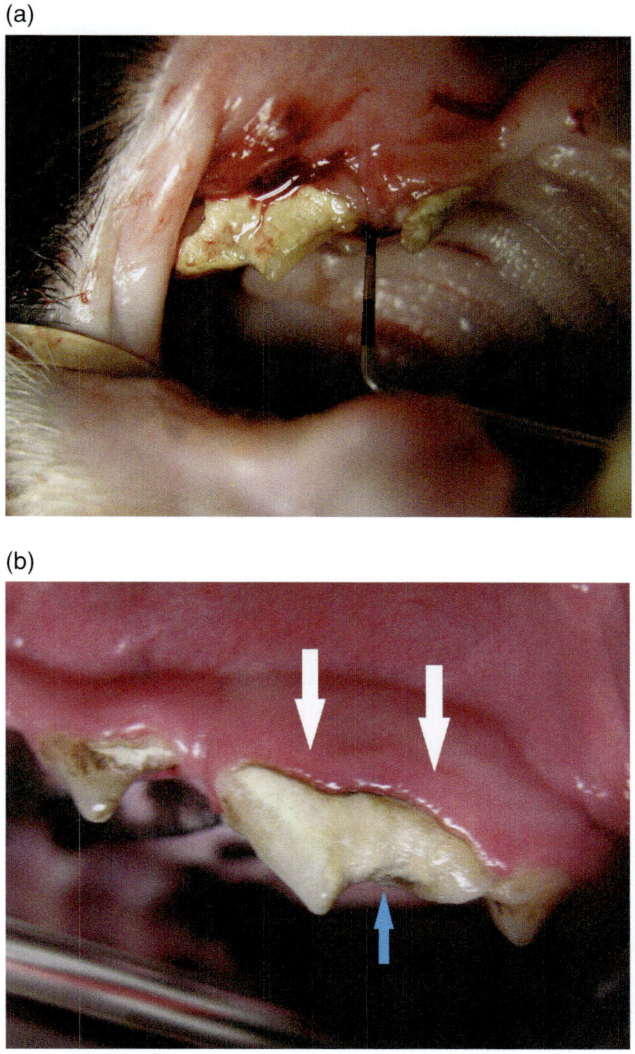

Figure 2.2 (a) Intraoral dental picture of a feline patient with tooth resorption and associated calculus. This has contributed to the periodontal loss as demonstrated by the probe. (b) Intraoral picture of the left maxillary fourth premolar (208) of a dog that has an uncomplicated crown fracture (blue arrow). Note the significant calculus present (white arrows).

of macromolecules. The physical and chemical nature of the underlying surface significantly affects the properties of the pellicle.[23,24] In addition, these characteristics can be transferred through the pellicle layer and continue to affect bacterial adhesion.[25] Therefore, the surfaces of the teeth have a significant influence on the formation of plaque.

The second stage is the initial adhesion and attachment of bacteria, which occurs within *seconds* of a prophylaxis.[26] This adhesion is not completely understood but can be thought of as occurring in three phases.[27] It should be noted that this system is similar to that in all aqueous environments from pipelines to cardiovascular devices. *Phase 1 is transportation to the surface of the*

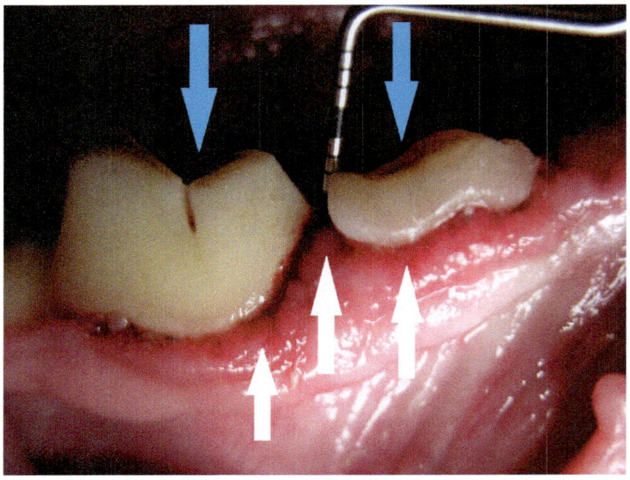

Figure 2.3 Intraoral picture of the mandibular right of a dog with widespread abrasion (blue arrows). Note the periodontal pocket as well as significant gingival inflammation (white arrows).

tooth, which occurs via random contacts, either through Brownian motion, sedimentation, liquid flow, or active bacterial movement (chemotaxis). *Phase 2 is the initial adhesion of bacteria* through an interaction between the bacteria and the tooth surface, which occurs when the distance separating them is less than 50 nm. The forces responsible for the adhesion can be broken into long- (between 2 and 50 nm) and short-range (< 1 nm) forces. Long-range forces (van der Waals and electrostatic repulsive) typically result in reversible binding. Short-range forces (hydrogen bonding, ion pair formation, steric interaction) do not often come into play (due to the need for a very close association), but when they do, they result in irreversible binding. *Phase 3 is true bacterial attachment* by specific interactions (covalent, ionic, or hydrogen bonding), which follows direct contact or bridging. This bonding occurs between specific extracellular proteinaceous components (adhesions) on the bacteria and complementary receptors on the pellicle and is species specific.

It is important to note that bacteria are separated into early and late colonizers. Early colonizers are gram-positive aerobes that bind directly to the pellicle, while secondary colonizers cannot bind to clean tooth surfaces, and thus bind only to the early colonizers.[6] Streptococci[28] and actinomyces are the typical early colonizers and each bind to specific salivary molecules.[29–33] Most of the early colonizing streptococci offer receptor molecules to the oral flora.[29]

It is critical to note that phase 3 attachment results in irreversible bonding much more readily on rough or irregular surfaces due to the fact that the bacteria are protected from shear forces (see below).

(a)

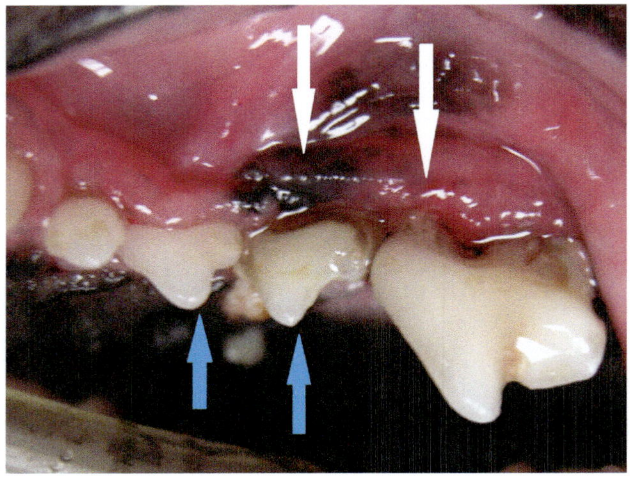

(b)

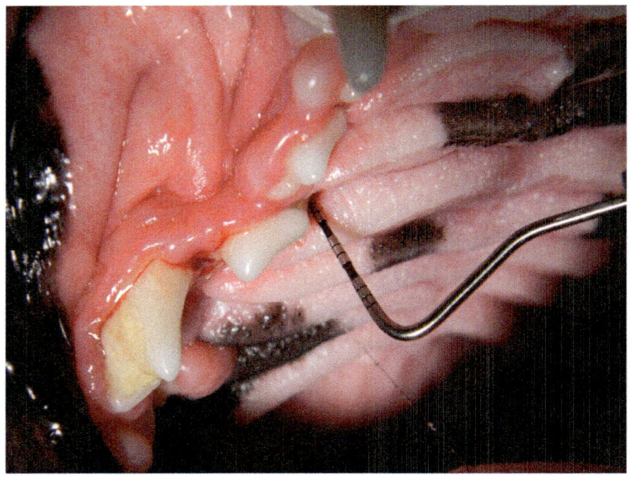

Figure 2.4 (a) Intraoral picture of the maxillary left of a dog with crowding and rotation of the second through fourth premolars (blue arrows) and secondary periodontal disease as evidenced by the gingival recession (white arrows). (b) Intraoral picture of the maxillary right of a dog with crowding and rotation of the second through fourth premolars. Note the significant periodontal loss involving the third premolar (107).

In humans at least, it appears that fusobacterium is a bridge between the early and late colonizers, as the late colonizers appear to coaggregate mostly with it as opposed to directly to early colonizers.[34]

The final step is colonization and plaque maturation, which is actually a continuation of the initial attachment above. It is initiated when the attached microorganisms multiply and create the microcolonies that make up the biofilm. These microcolonies are made up of different bacteria that typically exhibit coaggregation, defined as cell-to-cell recognition of genetically distinct partner cell types.[29,35] In fact, almost all oral bacteria possess surface

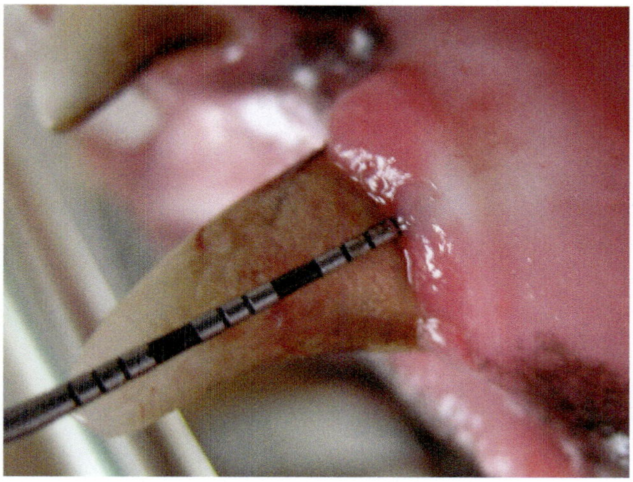

Figure 2.5 Intraoral picture of the left maxillary canine (204) of a dog with a periodontal pocket as well as significant calculus.

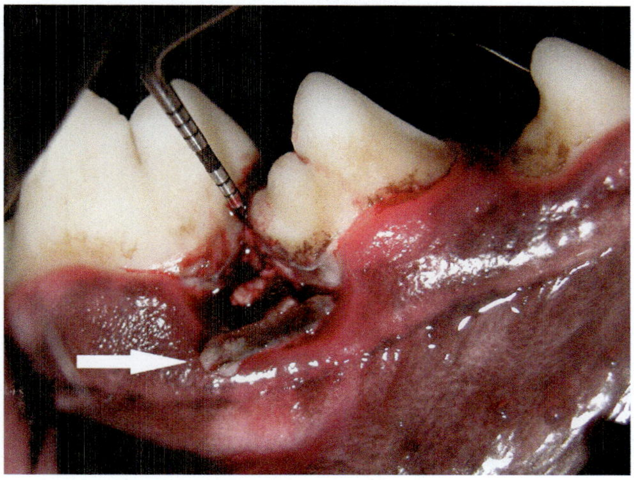

Figure 2.6 Intraoral picture of the mandibular right of a dog with an area of significant periodontal loss secondary to a gingival foreign body (wood) (white arrow).

molecules that promote cell-to-cell interaction.[28] The secondary colonizers include pathogenic strains such as prevotella and porphyromonas.

This coaggregation is strong evidence of the bacterial interdependency within a biofilm. Furthermore, the actions of the early colonizers (use of oxygen) and their byproducts (e.g., lactate, formate, and succinate) aid the periodontopathogenic secondary colonizers, such as porphyrmonas. Finally, the host inadvertently provides nutrients to the pathogenic species in the form of blood and crevicular fluid.

All of the above processes take place within 24 hours if the plaque is not disturbed. This means that pathogenic bacteria have already started colonizing the tooth *1 day* following a complete dental prophylaxis.[2,6] This first day

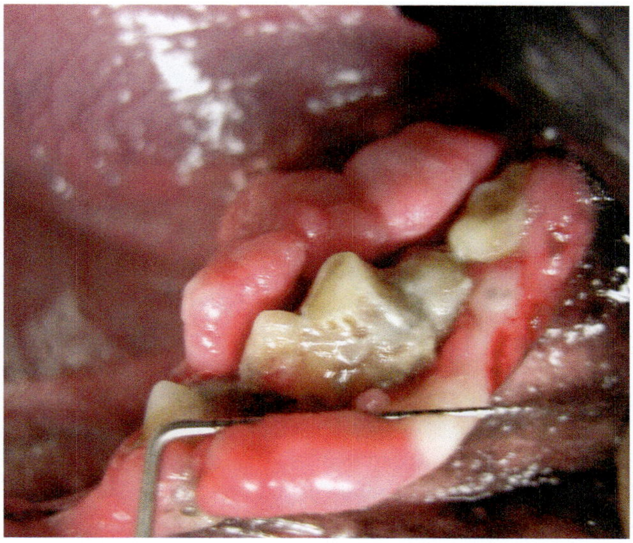

Figure 2.7 Intraoral picture of the left mandibular first molar (309) of a dog with gingival enlargement. When the gingiva is retracted, the significant underlying calculus is exposed. A gingivectomy (see chapter 15) will ameliorate this condition (at least temporarily).

results in a small amount of the tooth surface being covered, which expands greatly until day 4, when the maximum plaque coverage is attained. Mature plaque (and calculus) can contain up to 100,000,000,000 bacteria per gram.[36,37] After 4 days, plaque does not grow but the flora changes from gram positive to gram negative. It is this change in bacterial species that results in the initiation of gingivitis.[15] Importantly, plaque will return to healthy levels and flora within a few days if a plaque control regimen is established, and this in turn will result in the resolution of gingivitis.[4,9]

Bacterial behavior

It has been shown that 99% of all bacteria live within a biofilm.[38] Bacteria within a biofilm behave differently than (and in fact are phenotypically distinct from)[39] free living or "planktonic" bacteria by exerting different sigma factors, among other processes.[40] As a matter of fact, bacterial plaque is, in essence, an organism where the needs of the bacterial community are placed before the individual bacteria and the bacteria are therefore much more difficult to neutralize than individual organisms.[17,18,40] Most importantly, bacteria within a biofilm are *1,000 to 1,500 times more resistant* to antibiotics than their planktonic counterparts.[15,17,19,41] Furthermore, this protection gives plaque bacteria resistance to concentrations of antiseptics up to 500,000 times what would kill singular bacteria.[42] This resistance is due to several factors including the "slime" layer, slower growth rate,

> **Box 2.1** Key clinical point
>
> The visible plaque on the tooth surface is known as *supragingival* plaque.[6,15] Once it extends under the free gingival margin and into the area known as the gingival sulcus (between the gingiva and the teeth or alveolar bone), it becomes known as *subgingival* plaque.[15,45] Supragingival plaque is thought to affect the pathogenicity of the subgingival plaque in the early stages of periodontal disease by providing protection and reducing available oxygen.[6,15] However, once the periodontal pocket forms, the effect of the supragingival plaque and calculus is minimal.[6] Therefore, control of supragingival plaque alone is ineffective in controlling the progression of periodontal disease.[3,46,47] This is one of the major reasons that "anesthesia-free dental cleanings" are insufficient for periodontal therapy. Addressing the subgingival plaque cannot be performed adequately without anesthesia. See Box 10.2 (Non-anesthetic Dentistry).

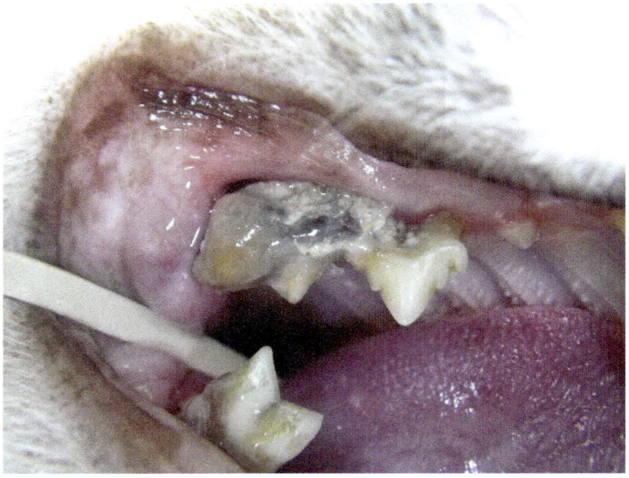

Figure 2.8 Intraoral picture of the maxillary right of a cat with significant calculus.

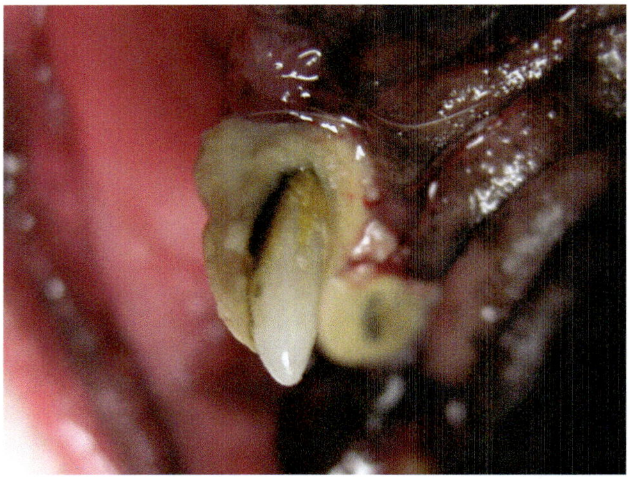

Figure 2.9 Intraoral picture of the right maxillary canine (104) of a dog with significant calculus.

concentration of antimicrobial enzymes (e.g., beta lactamase), communication between the bacteria (quorum sensing), and expressing genes for antibacterial resistance.[38,43–45] Unfortunately, the vast majority of our knowledge about bacteria (in general and in regards to a particular patient) occurs from laboratory monocultures. Therefore, it is likely not an accurate assessment of the behavior of plaque bacteria.[18] This needs to be taken into account when considering the use of antimicrobials in periodontal therapy.

Initial plaque bacteria from healthy sites consists of predominately non-motile, gram-positive, aerobic facultative rods and cocci.[6,15,48,49] Gingivitis is caused by an increase in the overall numbers of bacteria, and this increase is primarily of motile gram-negative rods (approximately 50%) and anaerobic species.[15] In established periodontal disease, gram-negative rods account for approximately 74% of the microbiotic flora.[15] In fact, anaerobic organisms compose over 90% of the bacterial species in chronic periodontal disease.[49–51] Finally, elevated numbers of spirochetes are found in periodontal pockets of dogs, as compared to healthy sites.[52] (See chapter 3 for a complete discussion of periodontal bacteriology.)

Calculus

Calculus (or tartar) is essentially bacterial plaque that has become calcified by the minerals in saliva (Figures 2.8 and 2.9).[6,53] This can occur on the first day of plaque formation (i.e., the day after a cleaning) as early as 4 hours after deposition of the plaque.[54] Calculus is 70–90% inorganic and is made up of various calcium salts, mostly in a crystalline form.[53] The most common form across all species is hydroxyapatite, and in cats is the only form encountered.[55] The minerals for calcification of the supragingival plaque are provided by the saliva, whereas the subgingival calculus minerals are provided by the gingival crevicular fluid.[53] The organic component consists of various protein-polysaccharide complexes, host cells, and microorganisms.[56]

Calculus typically attaches to the tooth surface via adhesion of a dental pellicle to the tooth enamel; however, it may also attach via mechanical interlocking and develop under surface irregularities.[53] These findings help explain why calculus levels are higher on unpolished or damaged teeth. In addition, the level of calculus formation varies quite a bit in humans, suggesting a genetic predisposition, which is certainly seen in veterinary patients as well. In addition, it appears (at least in humans) that calculus attains a maximum thickness in a

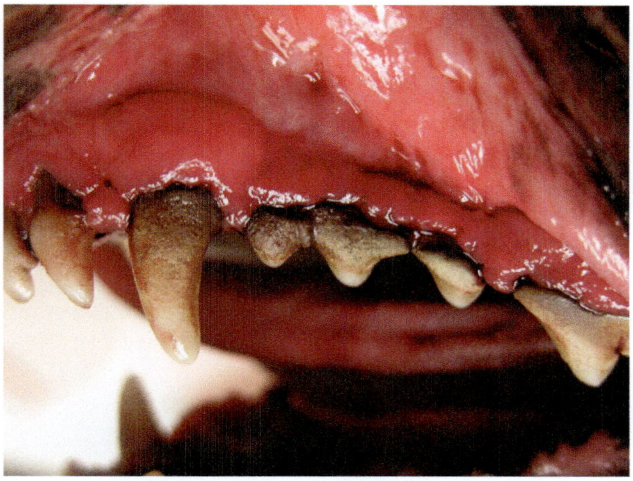

Figure 2.10 Intraoral picture of the maxillary left of a dog with significant buccal calculus.

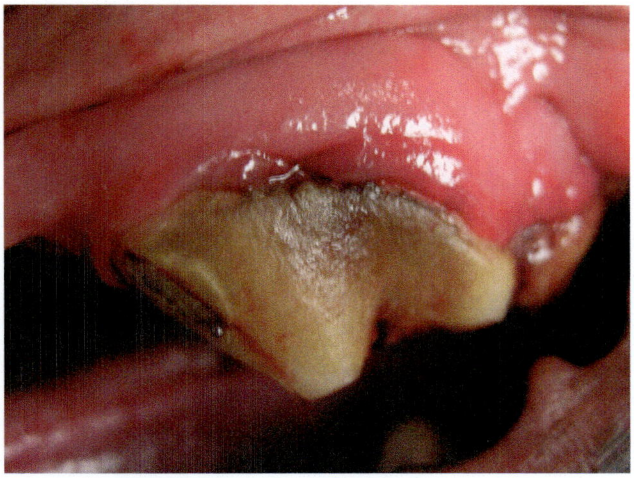

Figure 2.11 Intraoral picture of the left maxillary fourth premolar (208) of a dog with significant buccal calculus.

relatively short time (under 6 months).[57,58] This maximum thickness is likely attributed to the fact that bulky calculus may be removed by mechanical action (chewing).

In veterinary patients, calculus typically accumulates faster and in larger amounts on the buccal surface of the maxillary teeth (Figure 2.10).[59] The reason for this is unknown, but it has been postulated that the action of the tongue dislodges plaque from the lingual surface. The maxillary carnassials appear to be particularly susceptible to plaque and calculus accumulation (Figure 2.11).[49] This may be due to the fact that the parotid and zygomatic salivary ducts open over the tooth, or that the developmental groove on this tooth plays a part in plaque and calculus retention.

Calculus in and of itself is relatively non-pathogenic, providing mostly an irritant effect (See Box 2.2).[6,46] This was reported in several studies that compared wild animals with their domestic counterparts. The wild carnivores had significantly less calculus on their teeth, with a similar level of periodontal disease.[59–61] Furthermore, one human study found that clinical attachment gains were not related to the degree of residual calculus;[62] and it has also been proven that complete calculus removal is not possible, regardless of method used.[63]

Despite the fact that calculus is not inherently pathogenic, it is still critical to achieve as clean as possible tooth surfaces. Calculus is coated with a thin layer of plaque,[53] which keeps the key etiologic agent of periodontal disease in close association with the gingiva, thus allowing for continued periodontal inflammation.[6,53,64] Furthermore, the presence of calculus leads to more plaque accumulation by providing rough surfaces as well as creating protected areas for plaque retention that both increase plaque attachment and retention.

Other predisposing factors

Factors within the oral cavity

In addition to dental calculus, there are several other factors that increase plaque accumulation and therefore hasten periodontal disease. The most important of these factors is tooth roughness (especially in the subgingival area).[3,65,66] Tooth roughness can occur secondary to developmental problems (such as enamel hypocalcification) or tooth trauma (such as attrition, abrasion, or fracture; see above). In addition, iatrogenic causes (such as poor restorations [Figure 2.16],[21,67] especially overhangs,[68] or lack of/improper polishing following a dental prophylaxis) can have a significant effect on periodontal disease (Figure 2.17).[3,6] These issues can usually be rectified with a properly placed restoration and/or polishing. The importance of proper polishing should be emphasized, as the lack of this is one of the many reasons that "anesthesia-free" cleanings are ineffective. Finally, gingival recession will increase calculus deposition as the exposed cementum is rougher than normal enamel (Figure 2.18).

Oral malocclusions (especially crowding) may also disrupt natural cleaning ability and inhibit homecare, leading to increased plaque accumulation (Figure 2.19).[3,69,70] In these cases, selective extractions or odontoplasty may be indicated to improve periodontal health.

Persistent deciduous teeth have also been proven to predispose the patient to periodontal disease,[71,72] partially due to the resultant crowding, which decreases natural healing ability (as above) (Figure 2.20). In addition, the deciduous tooth shares the same gingival collar as the erupting permanent, thus not allowing for normal periodontal attachment development. The combination

Box 2.2 The role of calculus in periodontal disease is overstated

The fact that supragingival calculus is only minimally pathogenic is a very important point, as the need for professional therapy is typically determined by the calculus index, which may or may not be indicative of the level of disease present. For instance, patients commonly present with relatively clean tooth crowns but with significant subgingival disease (Figure 2.12), and vice versa with thick concentrations of calculus and yet little to no disease (Figure 2.13). In addition, one author asserts that subgingival calculus may be a *product* rather than a cause of periodontal pockets.[53] The thought is that the initial inflammation was caused by plaque, resulting in the pocket, which the calculus then invaded. Therefore, the level of gingival inflammation is likely a much better indicator of the level of periodontal disease. Even this, however, can be difficult to interpret in patients with darkly pigmented gums (Figure 2.14). Furthermore, evaluation of the lingual surfaces of the teeth and the molar teeth in a conscious (awake) patient is often insufficient, especially for small and toy breed dogs (Figure 2.15). Consequently, regular exams under general anesthesia are required for comprehensive periodontal care, regardless of the conscious exam findings.

(a) (b) (c) (d)

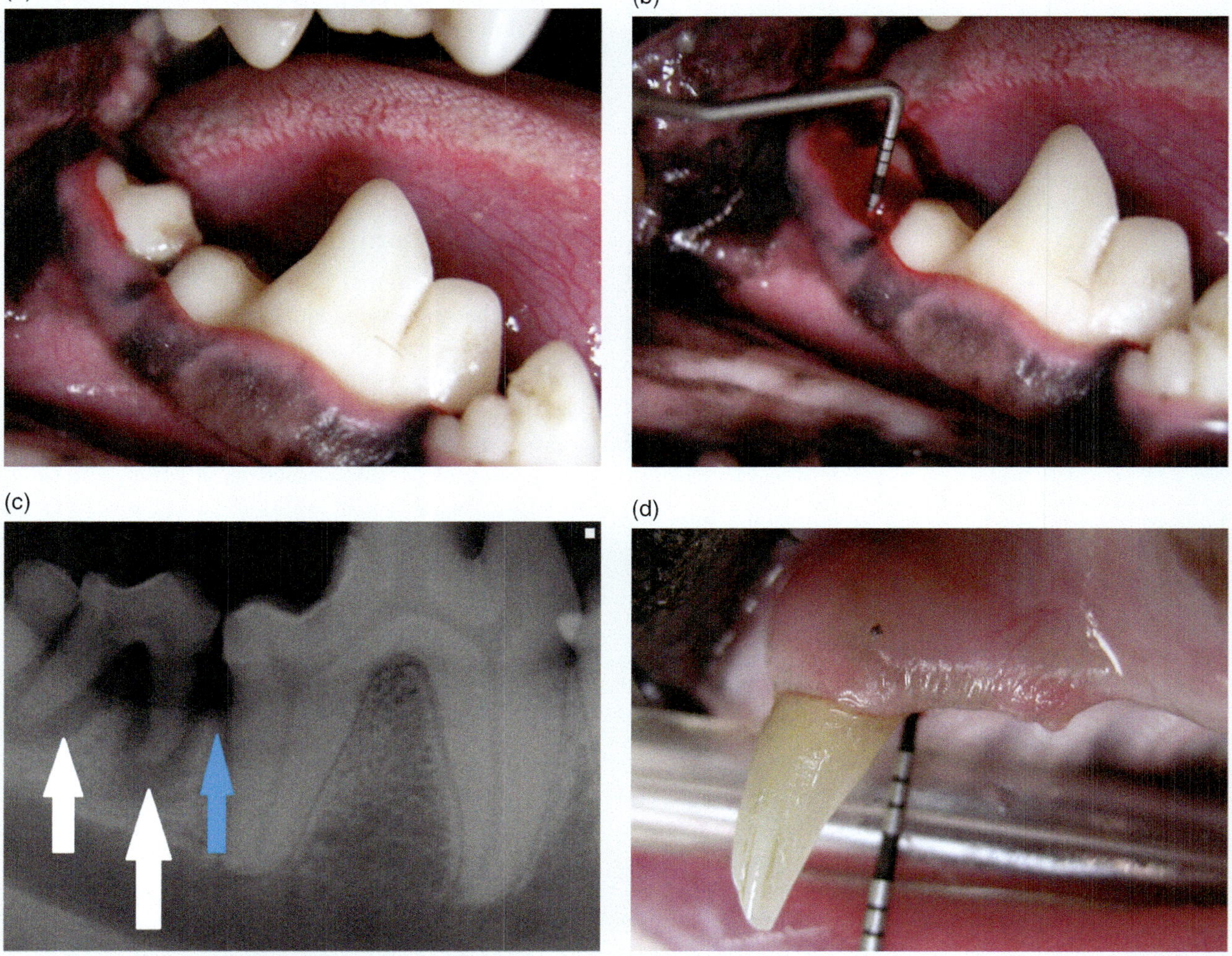

Figure 2.12 (a) Intraoral picture of the mandibular right first and second molars of a dog with fairly normal-appearing dentition/gingiva. (b) When a periodontal probe is carefully introduced into the gingival sulcus, a deep periodontal pocket is identified. The significant hemorrhage is indicative of the high level of inflammation. (c) The dental radiograph of the area reveals the significant alveolar bone loss to 410 (blue arrow). In this case, it is vertical (angular loss) (see chapter 9 for a complete discussion of periodontal radiology). Furthermore, note that the periodontal loss has resulted in a class II perio-endo lesion and a non-vital and infected mandibular second molar (410) (white arrows). (See chapter 6 for a complete discussion of these lesions as well as other significant local consequences of periodontal disease.) (d) Intraoral picture of the maxillary left canine (204) in a cat with significant periodontal loss despite normal-appearing gingiva. This image demonstrates the occurrence of this problem in cats as well. This severe infection in these cases would not be elucidated without a complete oral exam (or radiographs) under general anesthesia. This underscores the importance of a complete dental prophylaxis including periodontal probing on a regular basis, despite a fairly normal conscious oral exam.

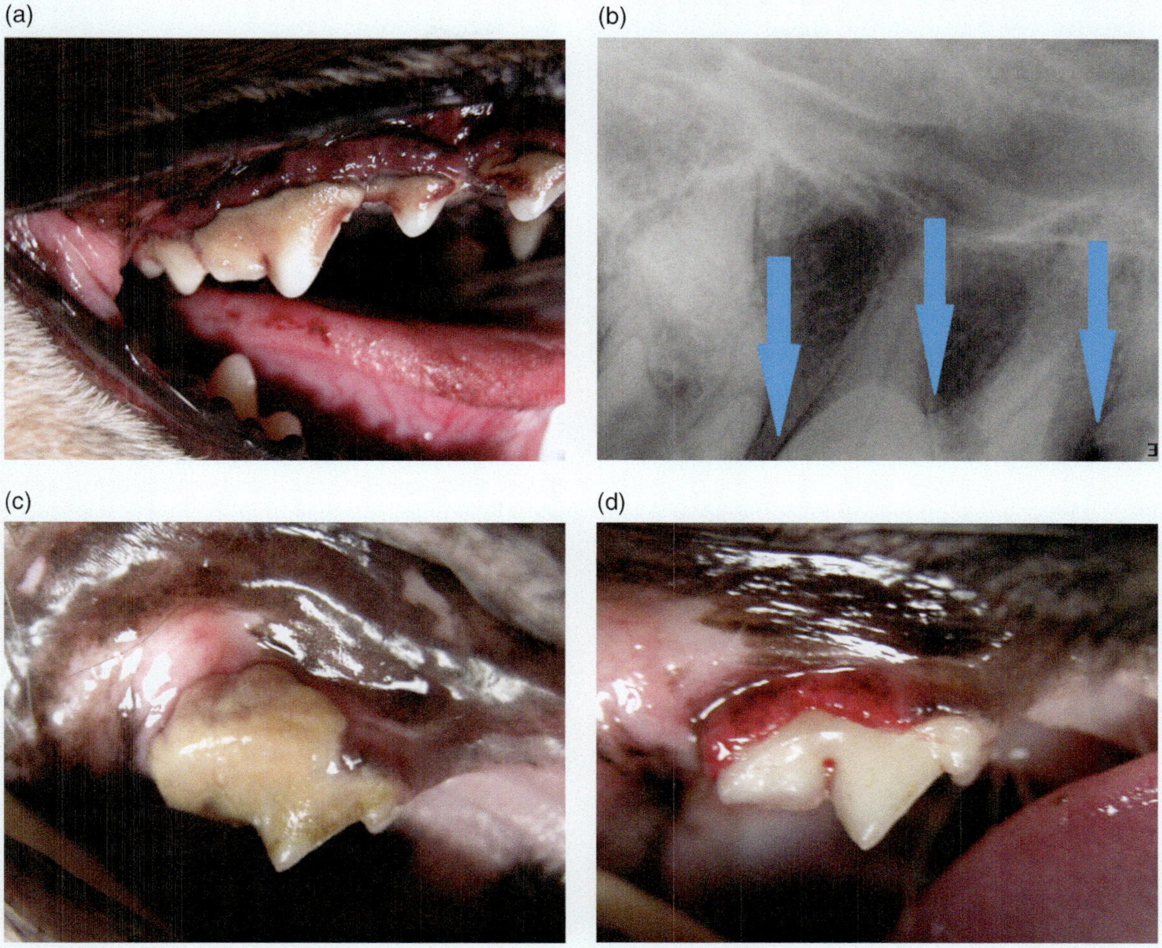

Figure 2.13 (a) Intraoral picture of the right maxillary fourth premolar (108) in a dog with significant calculus accumulation. However, periodontal probing depths were normal. (b) The subsequent intraoral dental radiograph confirms no loss of alveolar bone (blue arrows). (c) Intraoral picture of the right maxillary fourth premolar (108) in a cat with significant calculus accumulation. Periodontal probing depths were normal. (d) After professional scaling only 0.5 mm of gingival recession was noted.

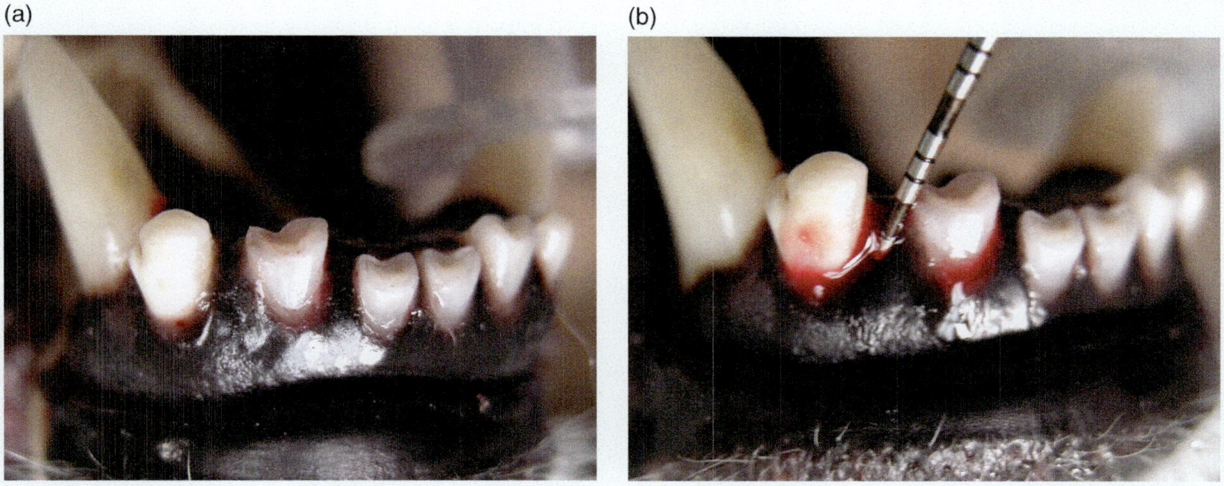

Figure 2.14 (a) Intraoral picture of the right mandibular incisors of a dog with fairly normal-appearing dentition and dark pigmented gingiva. (b) When a periodontal probe is carefully introduced in the gingival sulcus, a deep periodontal pocket is identified. The significant hemorrhage is indicative of the high level of inflammation.

(c) (d)

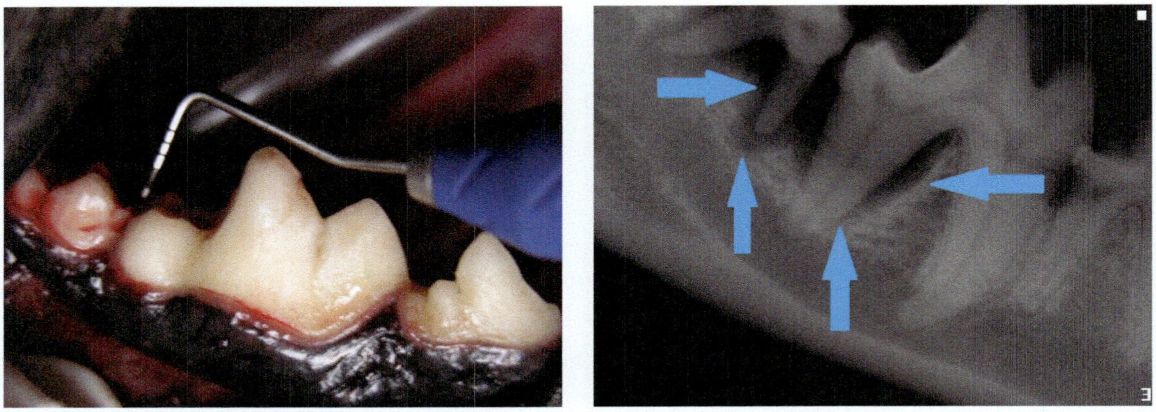

Figure 2.14 (cont'd) (c) Intraoral picture of the right mandibular first and second molars (409 and 410) of a dog with fairly normal-appearing dentition and dark pigmented gingiva. However, when a periodontal probe is carefully introduced into the gingival sulcus, a deep periodontal pocket is identified. (d) The dental radiograph of the area reveals the significant alveolar bone loss (blue arrows). The severe infection evidenced by these images would not be elucidated without a complete oral exam (or radiographs) under general anesthesia. This reinforces the importance of a complete dental prophylaxis including periodontal probing on a regular basis, despite a fairly normal conscious oral exam.

(a) (b)

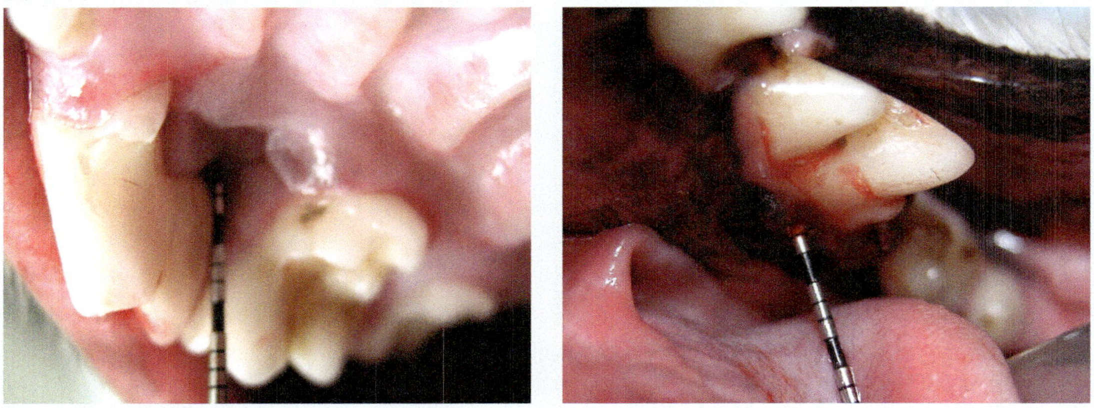

Figure 2.15 Intraoral images of the palatal surface of the right maxillary fourth premolar (a) and right mandibular first molar (b) revealing significant periodontal loss. Again, these lesions cannot be diagnosed without general anesthesia and periodontal probing.

(a) (b)

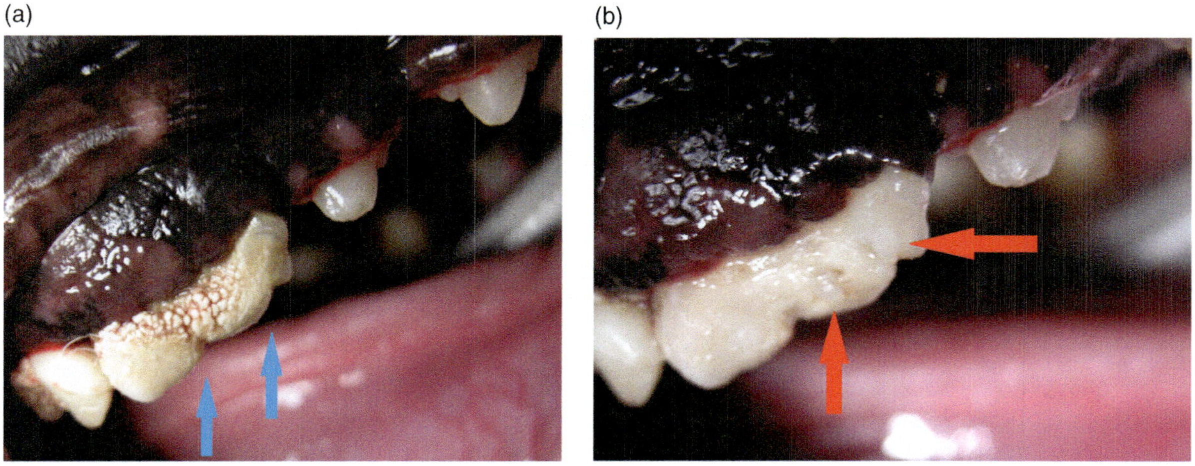

Figure 2.16 Intraoral images of the right maxillary fourth premolar (108) in a dog that received root canal therapy 6 months previously. (a) In this preoperative image note the significant calculus on this tooth (blue arrows) as compared to the relatively clean second and third premolars (106 and 107). (b) After the tooth was scaled, the rough restorative margins (red arrows), which contributed to the quick deposition of calculus, can be appreciated.

(a) (b)

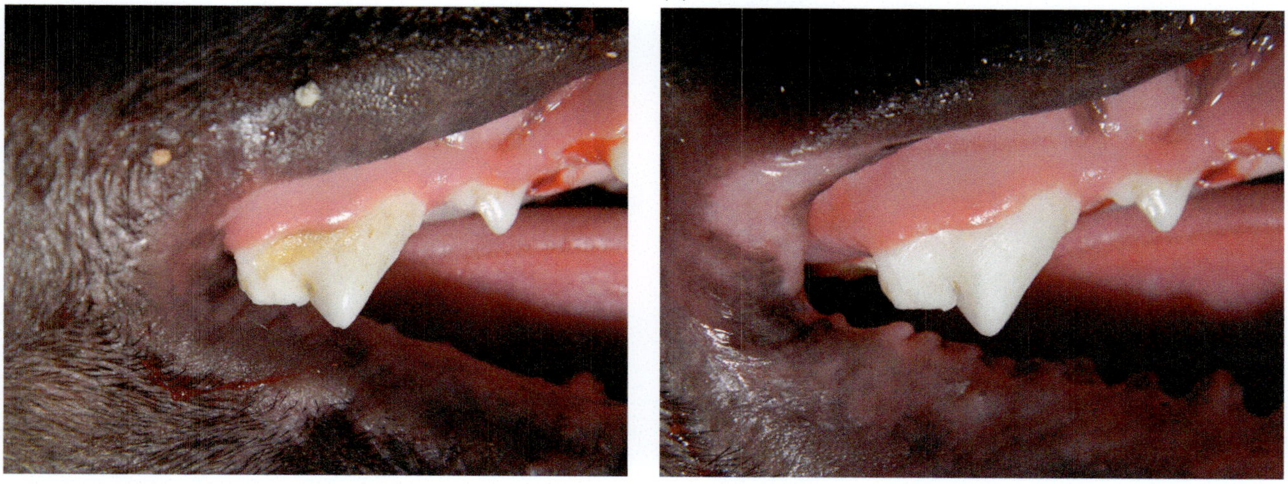

Figure 2.17 (a) Intraoral images of the maxillary right of a dog with significant calculus on the fourth premolar (108) who had been receiving non-anesthetic dentistries every month for the last few years. The teeth were "cleaned" less than 3 weeks previously and the patient was presented for mobile incisors. (b) Once the tooth was professionally scaled, the significant gouges were visible. The patient had 23 teeth extracted due to advanced periodontal disease, demonstrating the inadequacy of non-anesthetic dentistry. (For a further discussion of non-anesthesia dentistry, please see Box 10.2, chapter 10.)

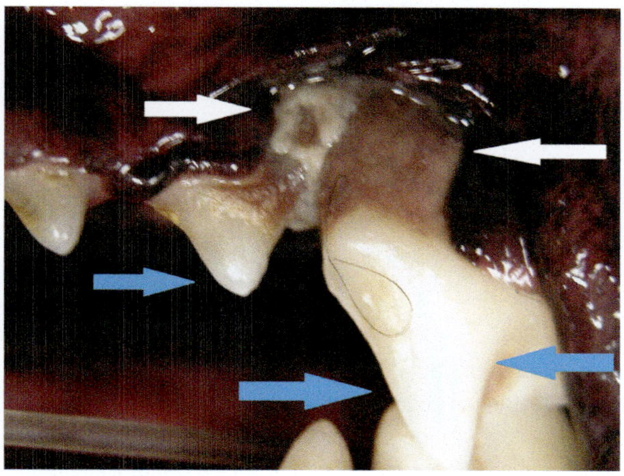

Figure 2.18 Intraoral images of the maxillary left of a dog with significant gingival recession. Note the large accumulation of calculus on the exposed roots (white arrows) while the crowns are relatively clean (blue arrows).

(a)

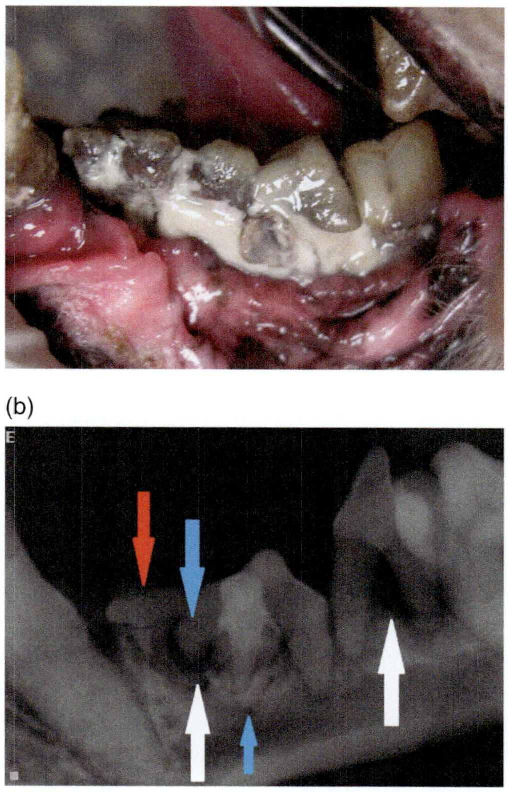

Figure 2.19 (a) Intraoral picture of the mandibular left of a dog with crowded and rotated mandibular premolars with secondary significant calculus accumulation and periodontal disease. (b) The corresponding dental radiograph confirms the severe alveolar bone loss (white arrows) as well as crowded, rotated, and overlapping roots (blue arrows). Incidentally, an embedded mandibular first premolar is noted (red arrow).

of these states predisposes the patient to periodontal disease within 2 weeks of permanent tooth eruption.

Next, direct gingival trauma initiates or worsens periodontal disease (Figure 2.21).[73] This is a common issue in veterinary patients who commonly damage their gingiva secondary to maladaptive behaviors (e.g., cage/fence biting from separation anxiety and chronic chewing secondary to allergic dermatitis). Finally, gingival foreign bodies such as hair result in a rapid onset of periodontal disease (Figure 2.22).

Radiation therapy for head and neck cancers has been shown to exaberate periodontal disease in humans.[74] In addition, oral infections are more problematic for patients

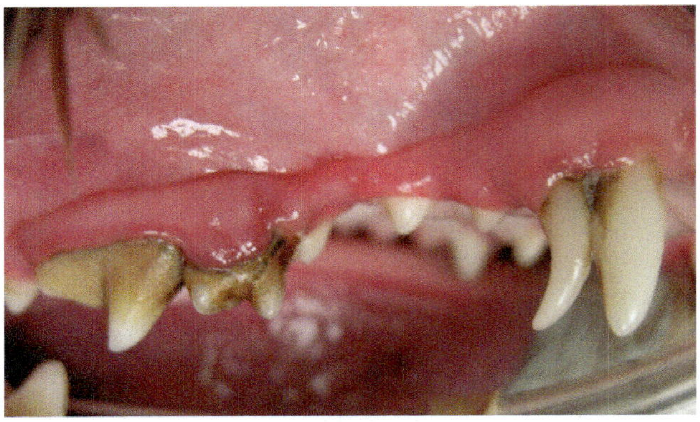

Figure 2.20 Intraoral picture of the maxillary right of a dog with a persistent deciduous canine and third premolar (504 and 507) resulting in crowding. Note the secondary significant calculus accumulation and periodontal inflammation associated with these teeth as compared to the teeth without persistent deciduous dentition.

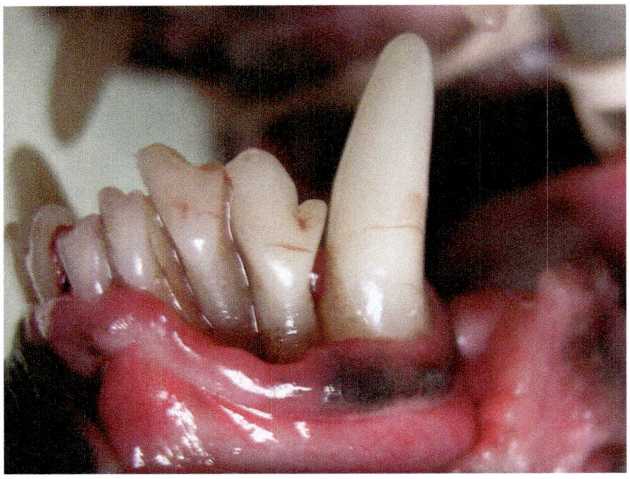

Figure 2.21 Intraoral picture of the rostral mandibular left of a dog with significant gingival recession and bone loss secondary to chronic self-chewing from atopic dermatitis. Note the lack of calculus and gingival inflammation. The remainder of the patient's dentition was relatively normal.

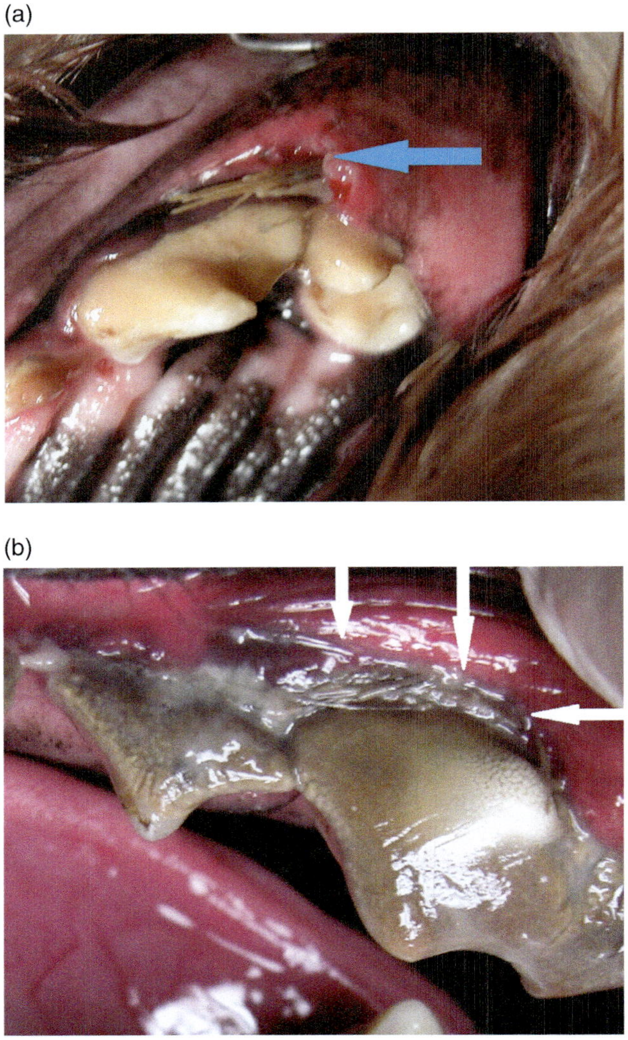

Figure 2.22 (a) Intraoral picture of the maxillary left of a dog with a gingival foreign body (foxtail) (blue arrow) and significant periodontal loss. (b) Intraoral picture of the left maxillary third and fourth premolars of a dog with significant periodontal inflammation and gingival recession secondary to hair entrapment (white arrows).

who have received head and neck radiation therapy.[53] At the same time, there is an increased incidence of surgical complications (e.g., osteonecrosis) in previously irradiated sites. Therefore, the prudent practitioner will treat any oral disease/infection as definitively as possible *prior* to commencing radiation therapy. While this type of therapy is still relatively rare in veterinary medicine, the incidence is rising, and periodontal disease should be considered when embarking on these forms of therapy.

Systemic influences on the progression of periodontal disease

While the presence of certain pathogenic bacteria is required for the initiation and progression of periodontal disease, it does not explain the significant variability of disease among individuals.[10] In reality, it appears that bacterial infection *in combination with* host response determines the progression of disease and that an improper host response (weak or excessive) exacerbates the severity of disease.[10,75] It is critical to recognize that while many disease states may influence the severity of periodontal disease, they do not initiate it.

It is also important to note that periodontal disease is much more common in small and toy breed dogs than medium and large breeds.[76] The complete reasoning behind this is unknown; however, decreased interdental space (crowding), rotation of teeth, decreased oral activity (recreational chewing), increased life span, and relatively short tooth roots all likely play a role in this condition.[70]

(a) (b)

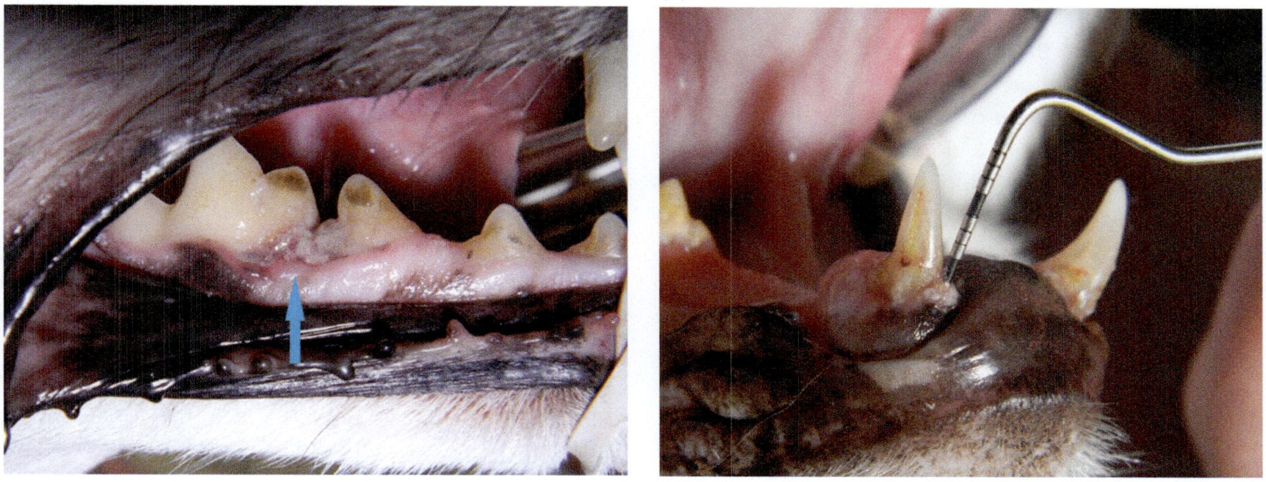

(c)

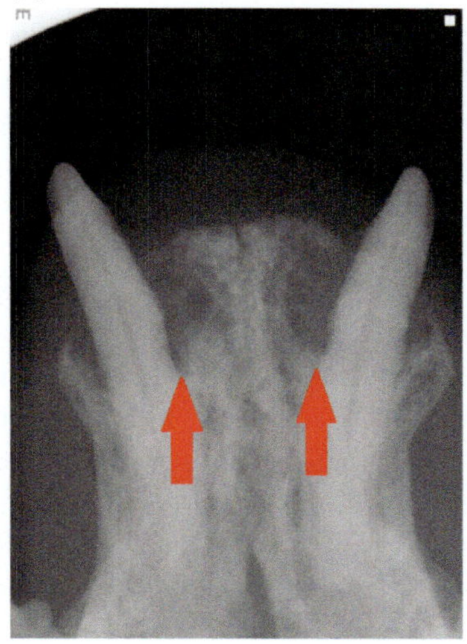

Figure 2.23 (a) Intraoral picture of the mandibular right of a poorly controlled diabetic dog with significant periodontal disease. Note the gingival recession and purulent discharge despite minimal calculus (blue arrow). Following appropriate therapy (including extractions), the patient was well controlled with a much lower insulin dosage. (b) Intraoral picture of the right mandibular canine (404) of a poorly controlled diabetic cat with significant periodontal disease. Note the significant periodontal pocket and purulent discharge despite minimal calculus and gingivitis. (c) The subsequent dental radiograph confirmed the severe alveolar bone loss (red arrows). Following appropriate therapy (including extractions), the patient was well controlled with a much lower insulin dosage.

The most common systemic diseases that affect periodontal health are endocrine diseases, primarily diabetes mellitus.

Diabetes Mellitus

Diabetes has long been known to negatively affect periodontal health, and periodontal health is actually now known as the "sixth complication of diabetes" (Figure 2.23).[10,77–88] The main reason for this is the fact that among other complications, diabetes results in increased susceptibility to infections and decreased wound healing.[89–98]

It has been shown that diabetic humans actually have higher glucose levels in their gingival crevicular fluids,[99] which may affect the bacterial population. Furthermore, patients with diabetes have altered collagen metabolism, which results in reduced collagen synthesis as well as delayed renewal of diseased collagen.[100,101] Finally, a chronic hyperglycemic state results in the production of accumulated glycation end products (AGEs), which are responsible for many of the severe diabetic complications.[102] This includes making the periodontium more susceptible to destruction.[103]

Conversely, periodontal health is better in well-controlled diabetic patients versus patients who are poorly controlled.[104–108]

Corticosteroids

Another important systemic issue that may increase the severity of periodontal loss is excess corticosteroids, either endogenous or exogenous.[10] Excessive amounts of these hormones are known to decrease the immune response through numerous negative effects including suppression of neutrophil activity (such as phagocytois), blocking the acquisition and expression of cell-mediated immunity, affecting the maturation of Langerhans cells, inhibition of dendritic cells, and decreasing the number of circulating lymphocytes.[109–113] A decreased immune response via these mechanisms leads to decreased host defense against infections, which likely includes periodontal pathogens.[114–116] Furthermore, it has been shown that systemic administration of cortisone in experimental animal subjects results in osteoporosis of alveolar bone, degradation of collagen, and increased destruction of periodontal tissues.[117] Additionally, increased endogenous steroid release during stress has been implicated in increased risk of periodontal disease.[10,118,119] Finally, corticosteroids have been shown to cause delayed wound healing.[120] While no studies currently show a relationship between hyperadrenocorticoism and periodontal disease, the immune suppression that is known to occur with this disease state is likely to cause similar issues.

Hematologic derangements, neoplasia, and chemotherapy

Hematologic derangements can negatively affect the periodontal health of human patients. Leukemia reportedly exacerbates periodontal disease by the processes of direct leukemic infiltration, increased gingival bleeding, and increased incidence of oral ulceration and infection secondary to a deranged immune system.[10] In addition, any neutrophil disorder (neutropenia, agranulocytosis, Chediak-Higashi syndrome, and others) or antibody deficiency results in decreased immunity and may exacerbate periodontal disease.[10]

Chemotherapeutic regimens can also have significant negative oral affects in humans.[121–125] These result from consequences such as mucosal ulceration, immune suppression, and xerostomia. Furthermore, proper dental therapy has been shown to markedly decrease the oral complications associated with cancer therapy.[126–128] Therefore, cancer patients and/or those on chemotherapeutic protocols should receive optimum periodontal care.

Additional systemic conditions that have been implicated in the increased severity of periodontal disease include hyperparathyroidism,[129] nutritional deficiencies (mostly vitamin deficiencies), and female sex hormones (especially pregnancy).[10]

Periodontal disease theories

Classically, periodontal disease was thought to arise from an increase in the overall numbers of bacteria. The *non-specific plaque hypothesis* was based on the fact that periodontal disease is generally associated with an increased level of plaque and calculus.[15,130] This theory proposes that low levels of plaque bacteria are controlled by the host response, and moreover research found that the concentration of bacteria in periodontally diseased sites is twice as high as in healthy sites.[131] Recent studies, however, point to a few virulent strains of bacteria as being responsible for the attachment loss seen with periodontal disease.[132–134] The *specific plaque hypothesis* is based on the fact that just a few species of bacteria are seen in virtually all cases of established, chronic periodontal disease.[15] (See chapter 3 for a detailed discussion of the bacteriology of periodontal disease.)

Periodontal inflammation

Once established, bacteria within the subgingival plaque secretes toxins as well as metabolic products that initiate inflammation.[72] Also produced are cytotoxins and bacterial endotoxins that can directly invade tissues, resulting in inflammation to the gingiva and periodontium.[6] Cytokines induce and enhance the production of a destructive family of enzymes, known as MMPs, that break down gingival tissue.[44,135] This inflammation causes damage to the gingival tissues, initially resulting in gingivitis. If left untreated, the inflammation can lead to periodontitis, which is defined as destruction of the attachment between the periodontal tissues and the teeth.[6]

In addition to directly stimulating inflammation, the bacterial metabolic byproducts also elicit an inflammatory response from the animal. White blood cells and other inflammatory mediators migrate out of the periodontal soft tissues and into the periodontal space due to increased vascular permeability and increased space between the crevicular epithelial cells.[136] White blood cells fight the infection by phagocytizing bacteria. However, they may also release enzymes to destroy the bacterial invaders either by design or after their death.[47] When released into the gingival sulcus, these enzymes further inflame the delicate gingival and periodontal tissues. The progression of periodontal disease is determined by the virulence of the bacteria *combined with* the host response.[138] *In fact, it is actually the host response that often damages the periodontal tissues.*[76,135,137] (For a complete discussion of the inflammatory reaction and progression of disease, see chapters 4 and 5.)

Despite this, patients with deficient immune systems typically have more severe periodontal disease than those individuals in good health.[6,136] HIV, diabetes, and stress are significant risk factors for severe periodontitis in humans and could likely be extrapolated to our animal patients.[136] Modulating these host responses may represent the future of periodontal therapy (see chapter 20).

In the progression from gingivitis to periodontitis, the inflammation (produced by the combination of the subgingival bacteria and the host response) damages the soft tissue attachment of the tooth and decreases the bony support via osteoclastic activity.[72] This causes the periodontal attachment of the tooth to move apically (toward the root tip).[6,14] As periodontal disease progresses over time, the attachment loss continues in a non-linear pattern as active stages of destruction are followed by quiescent phases (burst pattern).[138] The end stage of periodontal disease is tooth loss; however, the disease has created significant problems prior to tooth exfoliation (see chapters 6 and 7).

Box 2.3 Key points

- Periodontal disease is initiated by bacteria within the plaque biofilm.
- Plaque starts forming on teeth within seconds of a professional cleaning.
- It is the *subgingival* bacteria that cause the disease.
- "Anesthesia-free" cleanings are insufficient to control disease.
- Systemic diseases that affect the immune system tend to worsen periodontal disease.

References

1. Lindhe J, Hamp S, Löe H. Plaque induced periodontal disease in beagle dogs: A 4-year clinical, roentgenographical and histometrical study. J Perio Res. 10:243–255, 1975.
2. Boyce EN, Ching RJ, Logan EI, Hunt JH, Maseman DC, Gaeddert KL, King CT, Reid EE, Hefferren JJ. Occurrence of gram-negative black-pigmented anaerobes in subgingival plaque during the development of canine periodontal disease. Clin Infect Dis. 20 Suppl 2:S317–9, 1995.
3. Debowes LJ. Problems with the gingiva. In: Small Animal Dental, Oral and Maxillofacial Disease, a Color Handbook (Niemiec BA ed.). London: Manson, 2010, pp. 159–181.
4. Loe H, Theilade E, Jensen SB. Experimental gingivitis in man. J Periodontol. 36:177, 1965.
5. Fiorellini JP, Ishikawa SO, Kim DM. Gingival inflammation. In: Carranza's Clinical Periodontology. St. Louis: Saunders, 2006, pp. 355–361.
6. Wiggs RB, Lobprise HB. Periodontology. In: Veterinary Dentistry, Principles and Practice. Philadelphia: Lippincott-Raven, 1997, pp. 186–231.
7. Carranza FA, Takei HH. Rationale for periodontal treatment. In: Carranza's Clinical Periodontology. St. Louis: Saunders, 2006, pp. 630–635.
8. Van Dyke TE, Serhan CN. Resolution of inflammation: A new paradigm for the pathogenesis of periodontal diseases. J Dent Res. 82:82–90, 2003.
9. Silness J, Loe H. Periodontal disease in pregnancy II. Correlation between oral hygiene and periodontal condition. Acta Odontol Scand. 22:121, 1964.
10. Klokkevold PR, Mealey BL. Influence of systemic disorders and stress on the periodontium. In: Carranza's Clinical Periodontology. St. Louis: Saunders, 2006, pp. 228–250, 284–310.
11. Proceedings of the European Workshop on Mechanical Plaque Control, Chicago, 1998. Quintessence.
12. Merin RL. Results of periodontal treatment. In: Carranza's Clinical Periodontology. St. Louis: Saunders, 2006, pp. 1206–1214.
13. Grove TK. Periodontal disease. Compendium of Cont Educ 4(7), 1982.
14. Novak MJ. Classification of diseases and conditions affecting the periodontium. In: Carranza's Clinical Periodontology. St. Louis: Saunders, 2006, pp. 100–109.
15. Quirynen M, Teughels W, Kinder Haake S, Newman MG. Microbiology of periodontal diseases. In: Carranza's Clinical Periodontology. St. Louis: Saunders, 2006, pp. 134–169.
16. Bowen WH. Nature of plaque. Oral Sci Rev. 9:3, 1976.
17. Socransky SS, Haffajee AD. Dental biofilms: difficult therapeutic targets. Periodontol 2000 2002;28:12–55.
18. DuPont GA. Understanding dental plaque: Biofilm dynamics. J Vet Dent 14(3):91–93, 1997.
19. Pavlica Z. Biofilm: Microbial communities and periodontal disease. 2006 World Congress (WSAVA).
20. Isogai E, Isogai H, Sawada H, et al. Bacterial adherence to gingival epithelial cells of rats with naturally occuing gingivitis. J Periodontol. 57:225, 1986.
21. Perry DA, Schnid MO, Takei HH. Phase I periodontal therapy. In: Carranza's Clinical Periodontology. St. Louis: Saunders, 2006, pp. 722–727.
22. Ramburg P, Axelsson P, Lindhe J. Plaque formation at healthy and inflamed gingival sites in young individuals. J Clin Periodont. 21:51, 1994.
23. Baier RE, Glantz PO. Characterization of oral in vivo films formed on different types of solid surfaces. Acta Odontol Scand. 36(5):289–301, 1978.
24. Ruan MS, Di Paola C, Mandel ID. Quantitative immunochemistry of salivary proteins adsorbed in vitro to enamel and cementum from caries-resistant and caries-susceptible human adults. Arch Oral Biol. 31(9):597–601, 1986.
25. Pratt-Terpstra IH, Weerkamp AH, Busscher HJ. The effects of pellicle formation on streptococcal adhesion to human enamel and artificial substrata with various surface free-energies. J Dent Res. 68(3):463–7, 1989.
26. Rönström A, Edwardsson S, Atiström R. Streptococcus sanguis and streptococcus salivarius in early plaque formation on plastic films. J Periodontal Res. 12(5):331–339, 1977.
27. Scheie AA. Mechanisms of dental plaque formation. Adv Dent Res. 8:246–253, 1994.
28. Kolenbrander PE, London J. Ecological significance of coaggregation among oral bacteria. Adv Microb Ecol. 12:183–217, 1992.
29. Kolenbrander PE, London J. Adhere today, here tomorrow: Oral bacterial adherence. J Bacteriol. 175(11):3247–3252, 1993.
30. Mergenhagen SE, Sandberg AL, Chassy BM, Brennan MJ, Yeung MK, Donkersloot JA, Cisar JO. Molecular basis of bacterial adhesion in the oral cavity. Rev Infect Dis. 9 Suppl 5:S467–474, 1987.
31. Scannapieco FA, Torres GI, Levine MJ. Salivary amylase promotes adhesion of oral streptococci to hydroxyapatite. J Dent Res. 74(7):1360–1366, 1995.
32. Hallberg K, Hammarström KJ, Falsen E, Dahlén G, Gibbons RJ, Hay DI, Strömberg N. Actinomyces naeslundii genospecies 1 and 2 express different binding specificities to N-acetyl-beta-D-galactosamine, whereas Actinomyces odontolyticus expresses a different binding specificity in colonizing the human mouth. Oral Microbiol Immunol. 13(6):327–336, 1998.
33. Nyvad B, Killian M. Microbiology of the early colonization of human enamel and root surfaces in vivo. Scand J Dent Res. 95:369–380, 1987.
34. Kolenbrander PE, Andersen RN, Moore LV. Coaggregation of Fusobacterium nucleatum, Selenomonas flueggei, Selenomonas infelix, Selenomonas noxia, and Selenomonas sputigena with strains from 11 genera of oral bacteria. Infect Immun. 57(10): 3194–3203, 1989.

35. Kolenbrander PE, Ganeshkumar N, Cassels FJ, Hughes CV. Coaggregation: Specific adherence among human oral plaque bacteria. FASEB J. 7(5):406–413, 1993.
36. Schroeder HE, DeBoever J. The structure of microbial dental plaque. In: Dental Plaque. Edinburgh: Livingstone, 1970, p. 49.
37. Loesche WJ, Grossman NS. Periodontal disease as a specific, albeit chronic, infection: Diagnosis and treatment. Clin Microbiol Rev. 14:727–752, 2001.
38. Coghlan A. Slime city. New Scientist 2045:32–36, 1996.
39. Costerton JW, Lewandowski Z, Caldwell DE, Korber DR, Lappin-Scott HM. Microbial biofilms. Annu Rev Microbiol. 49:711–745, 1995.
40. Shearer BJ. Biofilm and the dental office. J Am Dent Assoc. 127:181–189, 1996.
41. Elder MJ, Stapleton F, et al. Biofilm related infections in ophthalmology. Eye 9(1):102–109, 1995.
42. Williams JE. Microbial contamination of dental lines. In: Current and Future Trends in Veterinary Dentistry: Proceedings of the Upjohn Worldwide Companion Animal Veterinary Dental Forum, 1995, pp. 8–11.
43. Costerton JW, Lewandowski Z, Caldwell DE, Korber DR, Lappin-Scott HM. Microbial biofilms. Annu Rev Microbiol. 1995, 49:711–745.
44. Page RC. Periodontal diseases: A new paradigm. J Dent Educ. 62:812–821, 1998.
45. Williams JF, Molinari JA, Andrews N. Microbial contamination of dental unit waterlines: Origins and characteristics. Compendium of Cont Educ in Dentistry 17(6):538, 1996.
46. Niemiec BA. Periodontal disease. Top Companion Anim Med. 23(2):72–80, 2008.
47. Westfelt E, Rylander H, Dahlen G, Lindhe J. The effect of supragingival plaque control on the progression of advanced periodontal disease. J Clin Periodontol. 25(7):536–541, 1998.
48. Harvey CE. Anatomy of the oral cavity in the dog and cat. In: Veterinary Dentistry (Harvey CE ed.). Philadelphia: Saunders, 1985.
49. Hennet PR, Harvey CE. Anaerobes in periodontal disease in the dog: A review. J Vet Dent. 8(2):18–21, 1991.
50. Listgarten MA, Hellden L. Relative distribution of bacteria at clinically healthy and periodontally diseased sites in humans. J Clin Periodontol. 5(2):115–132, 1978.
51. Slots J. Subgingival microflora and periodontal disease. J Clin Periodontol. 6(5):351–382, 1979.
52. Riviere GR, Thompson AJ, Brannan RD, McCoy DE, Simonson LG. Detection of pathogen-related oral spirochetes, Treponema denticola, and Treponema socranskii in dental plaque from dogs. J Vet Dent. 13(4):135–138, 1996.
53. Hinrichs JE. The role of dental calculus and other predisposing factors. In: Carranza's Clinical Periodontology. St. Louis: Saunders, 2006, pp. 170–192.
54. Tibbitts L, Kashiwa H. A histochemical study of early plaque mineralization. Abstract #616, J Dent Res. 19:202, 1970.
55. Clarke DE. The crystalline components of dental calculus in the domestic cat. J Vet Dent. 16(4):165–168, 1999.
56. Mandel I. Biochemical aspects of calculus formation. J Periodontal Res. 4 (Supp):7–8, 1957.
57. Conroy CW, Sturzenberger OP. The rate of calculus formation in adults. J Periodontol. 39(3):142–144, 1968.
58. Volpe AR, Kupczak LJ, King WJ, Goldman HM, Schulman SM In vivo calculus assessment. IV. Parameters of human clinical studies. J Periodontol. 40(2):76–86, 1969.
59. Verstraete FJ, van Aarde RJ, Nieuwoudt BA, et al. The dental pathology of feral cats on Marion Island, part II: Periodontitis, external odontoclastic resorption lesions and mandibular thicking. J Comp Pathol. 115(3):283–297, 1996.
60. Clarke DE, Cameron A. Relationship between diet, dental calculus, and periodontal disease in domestic and feral cats in Australia. Aust Vet J. 76(10):690–693, 1998.
61. Steenkamp G, Gorrel C. Oral and dental conditions in adult African wild dog skulls: A preliminary report. J Vet Dent. 16: 65–68, 1999.
62. Sherman PR, Hutchens LH Jr, Jewson LG. The effectiveness of subgingival scaling and root planing. II. Clinical responses related to residual calculus. J Periodontol. 61(1):9–15, 1990.
63. Jahn CA. Sonic and ultrasonic instrumentation. In: Carranza's Clinical Periodontology. St. Louis: Saunders, 2006, pp. 828–835.
64. Bellows J. Periodontal equipment, materials, and techniques. In: Small Animal Dental Equipment, Materials, and Techniques, a Primer. Ames, IA: Blackwell, 2004, pp. 115–173.
65. Silness J. Fixed prosthodontics and periodontal health. Dent Clin North Am. 24(2):317–329, 1980.
66. Berglundh T, Gotfredsen K, Zitzmann NU, Lang NP, Lindhe J. Spontaneous progression of ligature induced peri-implantitis at implants with different surface roughness: An experimental study in dogs. Clin Oral Implants Res. 18(5):655–661, 2007.
67. Björn AL, Björn H, Grkovic B. Marginal fit of restorations and its relation to peridontal bone level. I. Metal fillings. Odontol Revy. 20(3):311–321, 1969.
68. Jeffcoat MK, Howell TH. Alveolar bone destruction due to overhanging amalgam in periodontal disease. J Periodontol. 51(10):599–602, 1980.
69. Buckley LA. The relationship between malocclusion and periodontal disease. J Periodontol. 43(7):415–417, 1972.
70. Bellows J. Equipping the dental Ppactice. In: Small Animal Dental Equipment, Materials, and Techniques, a Primer. Ames, IA: Blackwell, 2004, pp. 13–55.
71. Hobson P. Extraction of retained primary canine teeth in the dog. J Vet Dent. 22(2):132–137, 2005.
72. Harvey CE, Emily PP. Periodontal disease. In: Small Animal Dentistry. St. Louis: Mosby, 1993, pp. 89–144.
73. Blanton PL, Hurt WC, Largent MD. Oral factitious injuries. J Periodontol. 48(1):33–37, 1977.
74. Epstein JB, Lunn R, Le N, Stevenson-Moore P. Periodontal attachment loss in patients after head and neck radiation therapy. Oral Surg Oral Med Oral Pathol Oral Radiol Endod. 86(6):673–677, 1998.
75. Lang NP, Mombelli A, Attstrom R. Dental plaque and calculus. In: Clinical Periodontology and Implant Dentistry (Lindhe J, Karring T, Lang NP eds.). 3rd ed. Copenhagen: Munksgaard, 2002, pp. 102–134.
76. Hamp SE, Hamp M, Olsson SE, Lindberg R, Schauman P. Radiography of spontaneous periodontitis in dogs. J Periodontal Res. 32(7):589–597, 1997.
77. Loe H. Periodontal disease: The sixth complication of diabetes mellitus. Diabetes Care 16:329–334, 1993.
78. Schlosman M, Knowler WC, Pettitt DJ, Genco RJ. Type 2 diabetes mellitus and periodontal disease. J Am Dent Assoc. 121:532–536, 1990.
79. Collin HL, Uusitupa M, Niskaken L, Kontturi Narhi V, Markkanen H, Koivisto AM, et al. Periodontal findings in elderly patients with non-insulin dependent diabetes mellitus. J Periodontol. 69: 962–966, 1998.
80. Bartolucci EG, Parkes RB. Accelerated periodontal breakdown in uncontrolled diabetes: Pathogenisis and treatment. Oral Surg Oral Med Oral Pathol 52:387, 1981.
81. Emrich LJ, Slossman M, Greco RJ. Periodontal disease in non-insulin dependent diabetes mellitus. J Periodontol. 62:123, 1991.

82. Canpus G, Salem A, Uzzau S, Baldoni E, Tonolo G. Diabetes and periodontal disease: A case-control study. J Periodontol. 76(3):418–425, 2005.
83. Papapanou PN. World workshop in clinical periodontics. Periodontal diseases: Epidemiology. Ann Periodontol. 1:1–36, 1996.
84. Salvi GE, Yalda B, Collins JG, Jones BH, Smith FW, Arnold RR, et al. Inflammatory mediator response as a potential risk marker for periodontal diseases in insulin dependent diabetes mellitus patients. J Periodontol. 88:127–315, 1997.
85. Cianciola LJ, Park BH, Bruck E, Mosovich L, Genco RJ. Prevalence of periodontal disease in insulin dependent diabetes mellitus (juvenile diabetes). J Am Dent Assoc. 104:653–660, 1982.
86. Firatli E. The relation between clinical periodontal status and insulin dependent diabetes mellitus. J Periodontol. 68:136–140, 1997.
87. Tervonen T, Karjalainen K, Knuuttila M, Huumonen S. Alveolar bone loss in type 1 diabetic subjects. J Clin Periodontol. 27:567–571, 2000.
88. Taylor GW, Burt BA, Becker MP, Genco RJ, Shlossman M, Knowler WC, et al. Non-insulin dependent diabetes mellitus and alveolar bone loss progression over 2 years. J Periodontol. 69: 76–83, 1998.
89. Rosenberg CS. Wound healing in the patient with diabetes mellitus. Nurs Clin North Am. 25(1):247–261, 1990.
90. Feldman EC, Nelson RW. Canine diabetes mellitus. In: Canine and Feline Endocrinology and Reproduction. Philadelphia: Saunders, 2004, pp. 486–538.
91. Ferringer T, Miller F 3rd. Cutaneous manifestations of diabetes mellitus. Dermatol Clin. 20(3):483–492, 2002.
92. Delamaire M, Maugendre D, Moreno M, Le Goff MC, Allannic H, Genetet B. Impaired leucocyte functions in diabetic patients. Diabet Med. 14(1):29–34, 1997.
93. Wysocki J, Wierusz-Wysocka B, Wykretowicz A, Wysocki H. The influence of thymus extracts on the chemotaxis of polymorphonuclearneutrophils (PMN) from patients with insulin dependent diabetes mellitus (IDD). Thymus 20(1):63–67, 1992.
94. Blakytny R, Jude E. The molecular biology of chronic wounds and delayed healing in diabetes. Diabet Med. 23(6):594–608, 2006.
95. Schubert S, Heesemann J. [Infections in diabetes mellitus]. Immun Infekt 23(6):200–204, 1995.
96. Velander P, Theopold C, Hirsch T, et. al. Impaired wound healing in an acute diabetic pig model and the effects of local hyperglycemia. Wound Repair Regen. 16(2):288–293, 2008.
97. Hirsch T, Spielmann M, Zuhaili B, et al. Enhanced susceptibility to infections in a diabetic wound healing model. BMC Surg. 8:5, 2008.
98. Lerman O, Galiano R, Armour M, Levine J, Gurtner G. Cellular dysfunction in the diabetic fibroblast: Impairment in migration, vascular endothelial growth factor production, and response to hypoxia. Am J Pathol. 162:303–312, 2003.
99. Ficara AI, Levin MP, Grover MF, et al. A comparison of the glucose and protein content of gingival fluid from diabetics and nondiabetics. J Periodontal Res. 10:171, 1975.
100. Grossi SG, Zambon JJ, Ho AW, et al. Assesment of risk for periodontal diease. I. Risk indicators for attachement loss. J Periodontol. 65:260, 1994.
101. Schnier M, Imberman M, Ramamurthy N, et al. Streptozotocin-induced diabetes and the rat periodontium: Decreased relative collagen production. Coll Relat Res. 8:221, 1998.
102. Brownlee M. Glycation and diabetic complications. Diabetes 43: 836, 1994.
103. Schmidt AM, Weidman E, Lalla E. Advanced glycation endproducts (AGEs) induce oxidant stress in the gingiva, a potential mechanism underlying accelerated periodontal disease associated with diabetes. J Periodontal Res. 31:508, 1996.
104. Tervonen T, Knuuttila M. Relation of diabetes control to periodontal pocketing and alveolar bone level. Oral Surg Oral Med Oral Pathol 61:346–349, 1986.
105. Tsai C, Hayes C, Taylor GW. Glycemic control of type 2 diabetes and severe periodontal disease in US adult population. Community Dent Oral Epidemiol. 30:182–192, 2002.
106. Christgau M, Palitzsch KD, Schmalz G, Kreiner U, Frenzel S. Healing response to non-surgical periodontal therapy in patients with diabetes mellitus: Clinical, microbiological and immunologic results. J Clin Periodontol. 25:112–124, 1998.
107. Stewart JE, Wager KA, Friedlander AH, Zadeh HH. The effect of periodontal treatment on glycemic control in patients with type 2 diabetes mellitus. J Clin Periodontol. 28:306–310, 2001.
108. Westfelt E, Rylander H, Blohme G, Jonasson P, Lindhe J. The effect of periodontal therapy in diabetics. Results after 5 years. J Clin Periodontol. 23:92–100, 1996.
109. Tizard IR. Drugs and other agents that affect the immune system. In: Veterinary Immunology, an Introduction. Philadelphia: Saunders, 2000, pp. 426–433.
110. Boothe DM, Mealey KA. Glucocorticoid therapy in the dog and cat. In: Small Animal Clinical Pharmacology and Theraputics (Boothe DM ed). Philadelphia: Saunders, 2001, pp. 313–319.
111. Auphan N, DiDonato JA, Rosette C, Helmberg A, Karin M. Immunosuppression by glucocorticoids: Inhibition of NF-kappa B activity through induction of I kappa B synthesis. 270(5234):286–290, 1995.
112. Stary G, Klein I, Baurer W, et al. Glucocorticosteroids modify Langerhans cells to produce TGF-b and expand regulatory T cells. J Immunol. 186:103–112, 2011.
113. Vanderheyde N, Verhasselt V, Goldman M, Willems F. Inhibition of human dendritic cell functions by methylprednisolone. Transplantation 67:1342–1347, 1999.
114. Feldman EC, Nelson RW. Glucocorticoid therapy. In: Canine and Feline Endocrinology and Reproduction. Philadelphia: Saunders, 2004, pp. 464–483.
115. Calvert CA, Greene CE, Hardie EM. Cardiovascular infections in dogs: Epizootiology, clinical manifestations, and prognosis. JAVMA 187(6):612–616, 1985.
116. Zen M, Canova M, Campana C. The kaleidoscope of glucorticoid effects on immune system. Autoimmun Rev. 9, 2011.
117. Glickman I, Stone IC, Chawla TN. The effect of cortisone acetate upon the periodontium of white mice. J Periodontol. 24:161, 1953.
118. Genco RJ. Current view of risk factors for periodontal diseases. J Periodontol. 67 (Suppl):1041, 1996.
119. Croucher R, Marcenes WS, Torres MC, Hughes F, Sheiham A. The relationship between life-events and periodontitis. A case-control study. J Clin Periodontol. 24(1):39–43, 1997.
120. Papich MG. Saunders Handbook of Veterinary Drugs. 2nd ed. St. Louis: Saunders, 2007, pp. 551–554.
121. Sonis ST, Sonis AL, Lieberman A. Oral complications in patients receiving treatment for malignancies other than of the head and neck. J Am Dent Assoc. 97(3):468–472, 1978.
122. Jensen SB, Mouridsen HT, Bergmann OJ, Reibel J, Brünner N, Nauntofte B. Oral mucosal lesions, microbial changes, and taste disturbances induced by adjuvant chemotherapy in breast cancer patients. Oral Surg Oral Med Oral Pathol Oral Radiol Endod. 106(2):217–226, 2008.

123. El-Housseiny AA, Saleh SM, El-Masry AA, Allam AA. Assessment of oral complications in children receiving chemotherapy. J Clin Pediatr Dent. 31(4):267–273, 2007.
124. Fayle SA, Curzon ME. Oral complications in pediatric oncology patients. Pediatr Dent. 13(5):289–295, 1991.
125. Fleming P. Dental management of the pediatric oncology patient. Curr Opin Dent. 1(5):577–582, 1991.
126. Sonis S, Jensen SB, Mouridsen HT, Bergmann OJ, Reibel J, Brünner N, Nauntofte B. Kunz A. Impact of improved dental services on the frequency of oral complications of cancer therapy for patients with non-head-and-neck malignancies. Oral Surg Oral Med Oral Pathol. 65(1):19–22, 1988.
127. Levy-Polack MP, Sebelli P, Polack NL. Incidence of oral complications and application of a preventive protocol in children with acute leukemia. Spec Care Dentist. 18(5):189–193, 1998.
128. Cheng KK, Molassiotis A, Chang AM, Wai WC, Cheung SS. Evaluation of an oral care protocol intervention in the prevention of chemotherapy-induced oral mucositis in paediatric cancer patients. Eur J Cancer. 37(16):2056–2063, 2001.
129. Svanmberg G, Lindhe J, Hugoson A, et al. Effect of nutritional hyperparathyroidism on experimental periodontitis in the dog. Scan J Dent Res. 81:155, 1973.
130. Loesche WJ. Chemotherapy of dental plaque infections. Oral Sci Rev. 9:65–107, 1976.
131. Socransky SS, Gibbons RJ, Dale AC, et al. The microbiota of the gingival crevice area of man (I). Total microscopic and viable counts and counts of specific organisms. Arch Oral Biol. 8:275–280, 1963.
132. Newman MG Socransky SS. Predominant cultivable microbiota in periodontal disease. J Periodontal Res. 12(2):120–128, 1977.
133. Isogai H, Kosako Y, Benno Y, Isogai E. Ecology of genus Porphyromonas in canine periodontal disease. Zentralbl Veterinarmed B. 46(7):467–473, 1999.
134. Hardham J, Dreier K, Wong J, Sfintescu C, Evans RT. Pigmented-anaerobic bacteria associated with canine periodontitis. Vet Microbio. 106(1–2):119–128, 2005.
135. Scannapieco FA. Periodontal inflammation: From gingivitis to systemic disease? Comp Cont Educ Dent. 25:16S–25S, 2004.
136. Nisengard RJ, Kinder Haake S, Newman MG, Miyasaki KT. Microbial interactions with the host in periodontal diseases. In: Carranza's Clinical Periodontology. St. Louis: Saunders, 2006, pp. 228–250.
137. Thoden Van Velzen SK, Abraham-Inpijin L, Modrer WDR. Plaque and systemic disease: A reappraisal of the focal infection concept. J Clin Periodontol. 11:209–220, 1984.
138. Goodson JM, Tanner AC, Haffajee AD, et al. Patterns of progression and regression of advanced destructive periodontal disease. J Clin Periodontol. 9:472, 1982.

3

Bacteriology of periodontal disease

Colin E. Harvey

Periodontal disease is caused by accumulation of dental plaque in the space adjacent to the gingiva, as shown in a classic 4-year study in dogs.[14] The causative bacteria develop in the complex biofilm that forms on the exposed surfaces of teeth,[6,22] which in the absence of effective oral hygiene leads to gingival and connective tissue inflammation. This inflammation leads to soft tissue and alveolar bone destruction and eventual loss of teeth, as described in detail elsewhere in this book.

The bacterial content of plaque and gingival fluids in dogs, and to a much lesser extent cats, has been studied for many years.[10–12,21,27,28,30] It should be noted that changes in microbiological methodology and in the names assigned to bacterial species can be confusing when reading reports and textbooks on this topic.

There is a well-studied sequence of development of dental plaque following a professional scaling in both humans and dogs.[3] Following scaling, a glycoprotein pellicle is deposited on the tooth surface from salivary fluid, which acts like flypaper. Bacteria in oral fluid, initially small cocci, become attached to the pellicle and colonies develop. These colonies provide a rough surface that enhances attachment of rod-shaped bacteria. The mixed-species biofilm initially consists of aerobic organisms. However, in the absence of effective oral hygiene, the biofilm grows in complexity and thickness, and by about 24 hours following scaling, the layer closest to the inert, non-vascularized tooth surface is sufficiently anaerobic to support growth of anaerobes and microaerophilic species caught within the biofilm.[3] (See chapter 2 for a complete discussion of the pathogenesis of periodontal disease.)

Proof of an infectious cause of disease results from fulfillment of Koch's postulates: *The microorganism must be found and isolated in pure culture from the site of disease in clinical patients; the cultured organism must cause disease when introduced into a healthy host; and the organism must be reisolated from the inoculated, diseased experimental host and identified as being identical to the original specific causative agent.*

Because the dental plaque biofilm is a complex mix of bacteria, it is impossible to apply Koch's postulates to prove pathogenicity of a particular species.

Culturing and identifying bacteria in gingival fluid samples is notoriously challenging and expensive, given the fastidious nature of many of the species present. Change in the constituents of the biofilm as the gingiva moves from health to disease can be assessed by the checkerboard DNA-DNA hybridization technique.[23–25] Using this technique, and recognizing that periodontopathogens do not develop without a supportive microbial milieu, periodontal microbiologists have identified "clusters" of oral organisms associated with particular disease states in humans.[23,26] Socransky's postulates (Box 3.1) have been adopted as an alternative to Koch's postulates to account for the bacterial complexity at the site of periodontal infection.[24] Specific bacteria are now recognized as human periodontopathogens based on Socransky's postulates. The studies identifying periodontopathogens have provided additional understanding of the complex bacterial biology occurring in the unique periodontal ecological niche.

Many of the bacteria recognized as human periodontopathogens have been isolated from gingival samples in dogs and cats,[1,2,5,8,9,16–18,27,28] and a study using a human DNA-DNA test panel in dog samples has shown that this technique is applicable in dogs.[20] However, assuming that human periodontopathogens are also carnivore periodontopathogens is overly simplistic. For example: *Porphyromonas gingivalis* is a primary human

Veterinary Periodontology, First Edition. Brook A. Niemiec.

Box 3.1 Socransky's postulates—human periodontal microbiology

To be recognized as a periodontopathogen, a bacterial species must meet the following criteria:

- *Association*: The causative agent must be found in active "sites" in higher numbers than in non-active sites.
- *Elimination*: The elimination of the agent must stop the progression of disease.
- *Host response*: The cellular or humoral immune response must validate the specific role of the agent in the disease.
- *Virulence factors*: The agent must possess virulence factors that are relevant for the initiation and progression of the disease.
- *Animal models*: The pathogenicity of the agent in an animal model must provide conclusive evidence that it can cause periodontitis.

Table 3.1 Putative Periodontopathogens in Dogs and Cats, Based on Culture and Epidemiological Evidence.

Organism	Reference
Gram-negative, non-motile anaerobes of the black-pigmented *Bacteroides* group:	
Bacteroides denticanium	8
Porphyromonas cangingivalis	4,8
Porphyromonas canoris	8,15
Porphyromonas cansulci	8,4
Porphyromonas denticanis	8
Porphyromonas endodontalis	8,9
Porphyromonas gingivalis	2,9,20
Porphyromonas gulae	8
Porphyromonas salivosa	2,8
Prevotella intermedia (intermedius)	2,9,20
Tannerella forsythensis (forsythia)	8,20
Other organisms:	
Campylobacter rectus	9,20
Peptostreptococcus anaerobius	9
Peptostreptococcus micros	9
Streptococcus constellatus	9,20
Treponema denticola	20,29

periodontopathogen.[26] Initially, this organism was identified in feline gingival samples[17] and subsequently canine samples, although it was recognized as being catalase positive; 16S rRNA phylogenetic analysis of canine samples has shown this catalase-positive variant of *P. gingivalis* to be a separate species, now classified as *P. gulae*,[7] and it is commonly isolated from diseased canine gingival sites.[8] There are several other *Porphyromonas* spp., which are also catalase positive, that occur in canine or feline samples but that have yet to be reported in studies of human samples.[4,9,13,15] One possible explanation for these differences in periodontopathogenic bacteria between humans and carnivores is the difference in the mean oral pH (6.5–7 in humans, and 7.5–8 in dogs and cats). A list of putative canine and feline periodontopathogens is shown in Table 3.1.

Spirochetes are found in gingival samples from periodontally diseased dogs in large numbers.[12,19,29] However, although they meet the epidemiological criteria for recognition as putative periodontopathogens, little else is known about their pathogenic role in dogs and cats because of the difficulty of culturing these organisms.

Box 3.2 Key points

- Periodontal disease is caused by accumulation of dental plaque in the space adjacent to the gingiva.
- Because dental plaque is a complex mix of bacteria, it is impossible to prove pathogenicity of a particular species.
- Spirochetes are found in gingival samples from periodontally diseased dogs in large numbers.
- Gram-negative non-motile anaerobes of the black-pigmented *Bacteroides* group are thought to be the most common periodontopathogens.

References

1. Allaker RP, de Rosayro R, Young KA, Hardie JM:. Prevalence of *Porphyromonas* and *Prevotella* species in the dental plaque of dogs. Vet Rec. 140:147–148, 1997.
2. Allaker RP, Young KA, Langlois T, de Rosayro R, Hardie JM. Dental plaque flora of the dog with reference to fastidious and anaerobic bacteria associated with bites. J Vet Dent. 14:127–130, 1997.
3. Boyce EN, Ching RJ, Logan EI, Hunt JH, Maseman DC, Gaeddert KL, King CT, Reid EE, Hefferren JJ. Occurrence of gram-negative black-pigmented anaerobes in subgingival plaque during the development of canine periodontal disease. Clin Infect Dis. 20 Suppl 2:S317–319, 1995.
4. Collins MD, Love DN, Karjalainen J, Kanervo A, Forsblom B, Willems A, Stubbs S, Sarkiala E, Bailey GD, Wigney DI, Jousimiessomer H. Phylogenetic analysis of members of the genus *Porphyromonas* and description of *Porphyromonas-cangingivalis* sp-nov and *Porphyromonas-cansulci* sp-nov. Int J System Bact. 44:674, 1994.
5. Elliott DR, Wilson M, Buckley CM, Spratt, DA. Cultivable oral microbiota of domestic dogs. J Clin Microbiol. 43:5470–5476, 2005.
6. Feng Z, Weinberg A. Role of bacteria in health and disease of periodontal tissues. Periodontology 40:50–76, 2006.

7. Fournier D, Mouton C, Lapierre P, Kato T, Okuda K, Menard C. *Porphyromonas gulae* sp. nov., an anaerobic, gram-negative coccobacillus from the gingival sulcus of various animal hosts. Int J Syst Evol Microbiol. 51:1179–1189, 2001.
8. Hardham J, Dreier K, Wong J, Sfintescu C, Evans RT. Pigmented-anaerobic bacteria associated with canine periodontitis. Vet Microbiol. 106:119–128, 2005.
9. Harvey CE, Thornsberry C, Miller B. Subgingival bacteria—comparison of culture results in dogs and cats with gingivitis. J. Vet Dent. 12:147–150, 1995.
10. Hennet PR, Harvey CE. Aerobes in periodontal disease in the dog: A review. J Vet Dent. 8:9–11, 1991.
11. Hennet PR, Harvey CE. Anaerobes in periodontal disease in the dog: A review. J Vet Dent. 8:18–21, 1991.
12. Hennet PR, Harvey CE. Spirochetes in periodontal disease in the dog: A review. J Vet Dent. 8:16–17, 1991.
13. Isogai H, Kosako Y, Benno Y, Isogai E. Ecology of genus *Porphyromonas* in canine periodontal disease. Zentralbl Veterinarmed B. 46:467–473, 1999.
14. Lindhe J, Hamp S, Löe H. Plaque induced periodontal disease in beagle dogs: A 4-year clinical, roentgenographical and histometrical study. J Perio Res. 10:243–255, 1975.
15. Love DN, Karjalainen J, Kanervo A, Forsblom B, Sarkiala E, Bailey GD, Wigney DI, Jousimiessomer H. *Porphyromonas canoris* sp-nov, an asaccharolytic, black-pigmented species from the gingival sulcus of dogs. Int J System Bact. 44:204–208, 1994.
16. Mager DL, Ximenez-Fyvie LA, Haffajee AD, Socransky SS. Distribution of selected bacterial species on intraoral surfaces. J Clin Periodontol. 30:644–654, 2003.
17. Mallonee DH, Harvey CE, Venner M, Hammond BF. Bacteriology of periodontal disease in the cat. Arch Oral Biol. 33:677–683, 1988.
18. Norris JM, Love DN. Associations amongst three feline *Porphyromonas* species from the gingival margin of cats during periodontal health and disease. Vet Microbiol. 65:195–207, 1999.
19. Riviere GR, Thompson AJ, Brannan RD, McCoy DE, Simonson LG. Detection of pathogen-related oral spirochetes, *Treponema denticola*, and *Treponema socranskii* in dental plaque from dogs. J Vet Dent. 13:135–138, 1996.
20. Rober M, Quirynen M, Haffajee AD, Schepers E, Teughels W. Intra-oral microbial profiles of beagle dogs assessed by checkerboard DNA-DNA hybridization using human probes. Proc ECVD, 2006, 2007. Vet Microbiol. 127:79–88, 2008.
21. Sarkiala E, Harvey C. Systemic antimicrobials in the treatment of periodontitis in dogs. Sem Vet Med Surg. 8:197–203, 1993.
22. Soames JV, Davis RM. The structure of sub-gingival plaque in a beagle dog. J Perio Res. 9:333, 1974.
23. Socransky SS, Haffajee AD. Periodontal microbial ecology. Periodontol. 38:135–187, 2005.
24. Socransky SS, Haffajee AD, Smith C, Martin L, Haffajee JA, Uzel NG, Goodson JM. Use of checkerboard DNA-DNA hybridization to study complex microbial ecosystems. Oral Microbiol Immunol. 19:352–362, 2004.
25. Socransky SS, Smith C, Martin L, Paster BJ, Dewhirst FE, Levin AE. "Checkerboard" DNA-DNA hybridization. Biotechniques 17:788–792, 1994.
26. Socransky SS, Tanner AC, Goodson JM, Haffajee AD, Walker CB, Ebersole JL, Sornberger GC. An approach to the definition of periodontal disease syndromes by cluster analysis. J Clin Periodontol. 9:460–471, 1982.
27. Syed SA, Svanberg M, Svanberg G. The predominant cultivable dental plaque flora of beagle dogs with gingivitis. J Periodontal Res. 15:123–136, 1980.
28. Syed SA, Svanberg, M, Svanberg G. The predominant cultivable dental plaque flora of beagle dogs with periodontitis. J Clin Periodontol. 8:45–56, 1981.
29. Valdez M, Haines R, Riviere KH, Riviere GR, Thomas DD. Isolation of oral spirochetes from dogs and cats and provisional identification using polymerase chain reaction (PCR) analysis specific for human plaque *Treponema* spp. J Vet Dent. 17:23–26, 2000.
30. Wunder JA, Briner WW, Calkins GP. Identification of the cultivable bacteria in dental plaque from the beagle dog. J Dent Res. 551097–1102, 1976.

SECTION 2

The progression of disease

4
Gingivitis

Introduction

Gingivitis is defined as any inflammation to the gingival; however, it is classically thought of as the inflammation induced by plaque bacteria.[1,2] In fact, research has shown that inflammation will continue as long as the gingiva is exposed to a bacterial biofilm and will resolve after its removal.[3]

It is important to be familiar with normal gingival features in order to identify abnormal findings. Normal gingival tissues are coral pink in color[4,5] (allowing for normal pigmentation), and have a thin, knife-like edge, and a smooth, regular texture (Figure 4.1).[1,6] The coloration is produced by the vascularity and modified by the overlying keritinazation. There should be no demonstrable plaque or calculus on the dentition. In human dentistry, this lack of inflammation is defined as gingival index (0).[7] The American Veterinary Dental College does not utilize a gingival index per se; rather gingivitis and periodontitis scoring is combined in the periodontal disease classification, where no inflammation is known as PD0.[8]

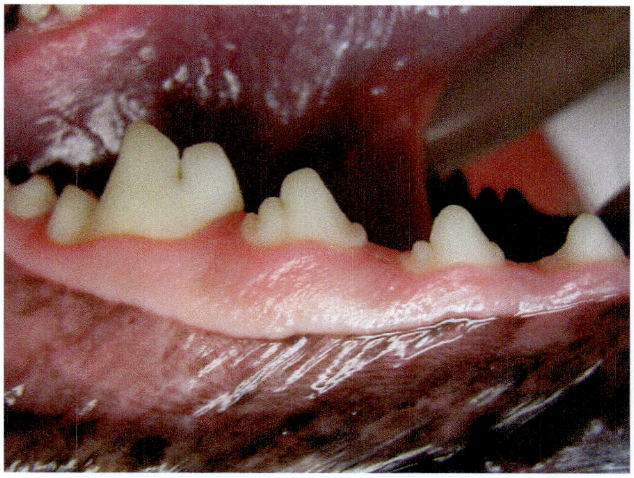

Figure 4.1 Normal gingival tissues. The gingiva is coral pink (except where pigmented). There is no evidence of gingival inflammation or plaque/calculus on the teeth.

Etiology

While multifactorial in nature, gingivitis is initiated by the bacteria in dental plaque.[1,2,9–11] The bacteria and their metabolic byproducts directly create inflammation.[9] However, not only are these products directly injurious, they also elicit an inflammatory response from the host, further damaging the delicate oral tissues.[1] This initial periodontal inflammation is due to an overall increase in the numbers of bacteria, which consists mostly of gram-negative anaerobes.[12] (See chapters 2 and 3 for a more detailed description of the pathogenesis and bacteriology of gingivitis).

Gingival inflammation is hastened by factors that enhance plaque accumulation.[1] These may include crowding[13] (Figure 4.2), roughened teeth (due to fracture [Figure 4.3], enamel hypoplasia [Figure 4.4], or aggressive scaling[14]), or faulty restorations (Figure 4.5).[1,15,16] In addition, diseases (e.g., diabetes and Cushing's) and drugs (e.g., corticosteroids and cancer chemotherapeutic agents) that alter the host inflammatory response may predispose the patient to the development of gingivitis.[17–21]

Gingival defense

There are several players involved in gingival defense. These include gingival crevicular fluid (GCF), saliva, and white blood cells. Gingival crevicular fluid was first studied in the 1950s and was initially considered to be transudate.[24–26] However, it is produced in only very

Veterinary Periodontology, First Edition. Brook A. Niemiec.

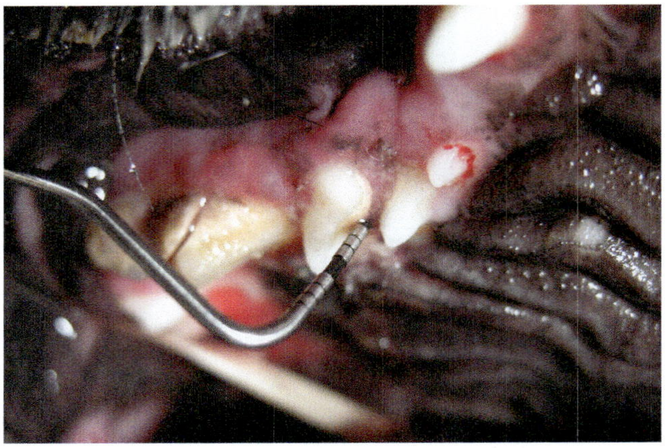

Figure 4.2 Intraoral picture of the maxillary right of a dog with crowding and rotation of the second through fourth premolars, and secondary periodontal disease as evidenced by the depth of the periodontal probe.

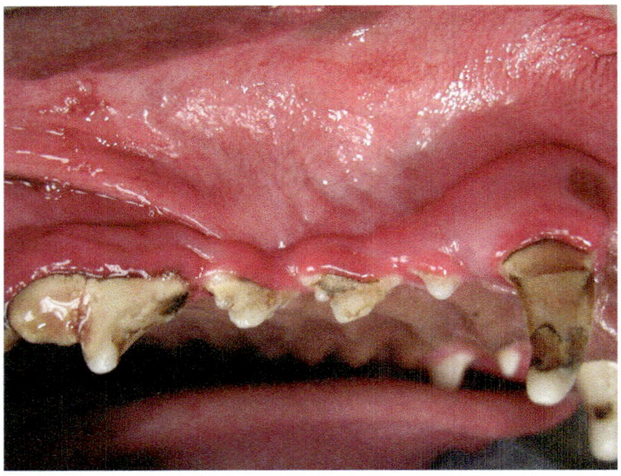

Figure 4.4 Intraoral picture of the maxillary right of an 11-month-old dog with widespread enamel hypocalcification. Note the significant calculus and gingival inflammation.

(a)

(b)

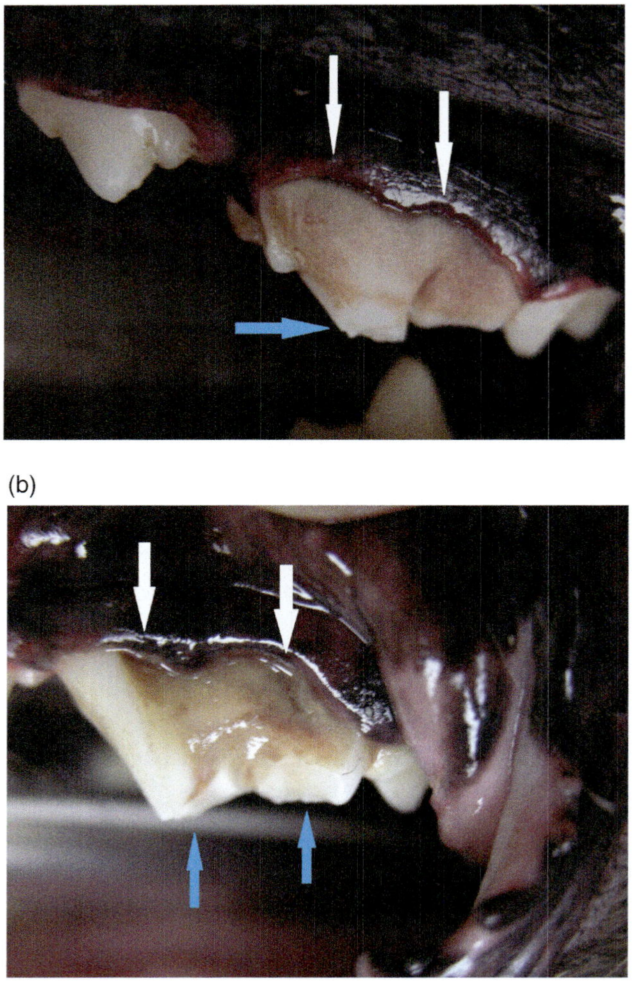

Figure 4.3 (a and b) Intraoral pictures of the left maxillary fourth premolars (208) of two dogs that have an uncomplicated crown fractures (blue arrows). Note the significant calculus present (white arrows).

(a)

(b)

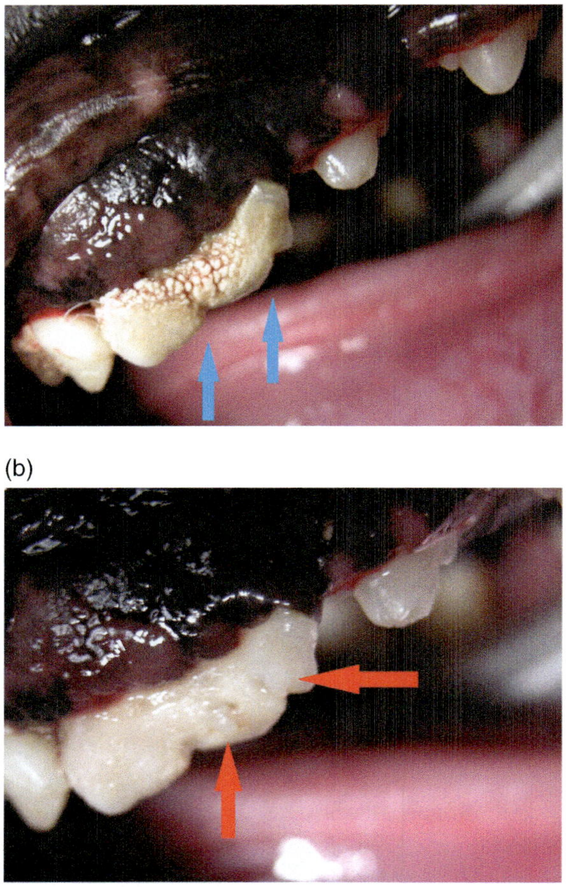

Figure 4.5 Intraoral images of the right maxillary fourth premolar (108) in a dog that received root canal therapy 6 months previous. (a) The preoperative image reveals the significant calculus on this tooth (blue arrows) as compared to the relatively clean second and third premolars (106 and 107). (b) After the tooth was scaled, the rough restorative margins (red arrows), which contributed to the quick deposition of calculus, can be appreciated.

Box 4.1 Key clinical point

Gingivitis is typically associated with calculus on the involved dentition but is primarily elicited by *plaque* and thus can be seen in the absence of calculus (Figure 4.6).[22,23] Alternatively, widespread supragingival calculus may be present with little to no gingivitis (Figure 4.7). It is critical to remember that calculus acts as an irritant as well as a rough surface for plaque attachment, but is in and of itself essentially non-pathogenic.[14,23] Therefore, the degree of gingival inflammation (not the amount of calculus) should be used to judge the need for professional therapy. This is a radical change in thought, but this is a much more accurate measure of disease. (See chapter 2 for a complete discussion of calculus.)

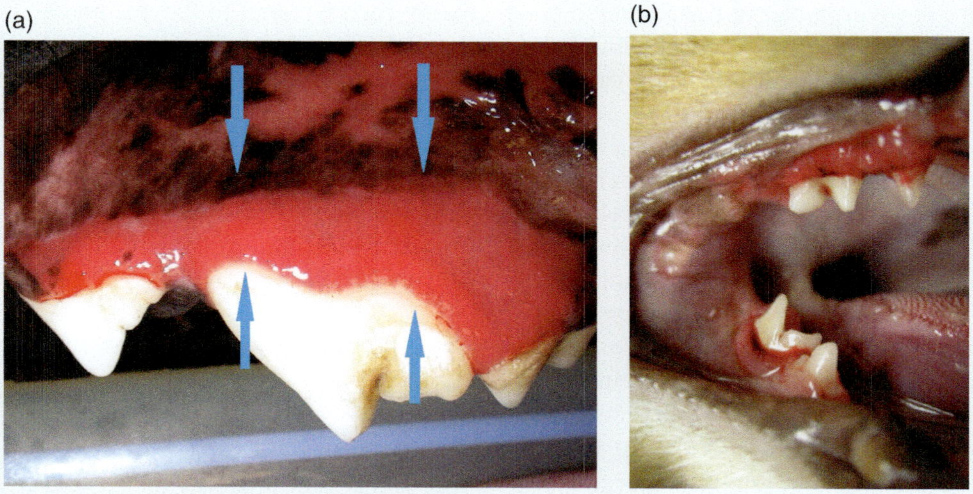

Figure 4.6 (a) Intraoral picture of the left maxillary third and fourth premolars (207 and 208) in a dog with severe gingival inflammation that affects the entire attached gingiva (blue arrows) despite the presence of minimal calculus. (b) Intraoral picture of the maxillary right in a cat with severe hyperplastic gingival inflammation despite the presence of minimal calculus.

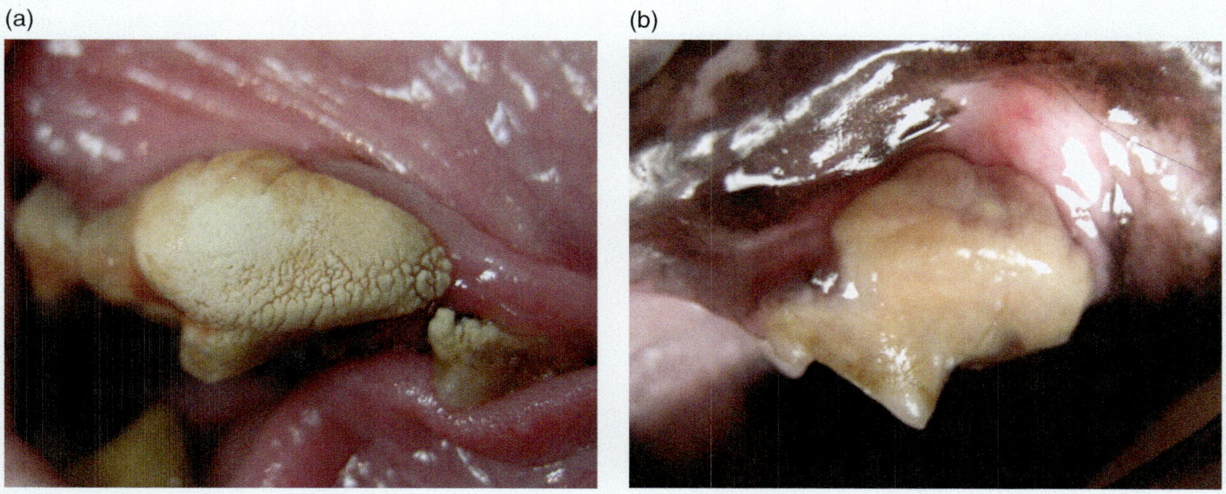

Figure 4.7 Intraoral photographs of a maxillary fourth premolar of a dog (a) and cat (b) with severe dental calculus covering the entire crown as well as extending over the gingiva. Note, however, that there is minimal gingival inflammation. There was no periodontal pocketing or alveolar bone loss on subsequent exam and radiographs.

minute amounts (if any) in normal gingiva increasing with inflammation, and in some cases correlating with the degree of inflammation.[27,28] Therefore, *GCF* is considered an inflammatory exudate, which is produced in reaction to bacterial infection.[29–31] GCF contains numerous products, including enzymes that may be of host or bacterial origin. The most protective constituents of GCF are antibodies, although their exact role is currently unknown.[32] In addition, some antibiotics (such as tetracyclines and metronidazole) are secreted in the GCF, which may prove beneficial as a treatment modality.[33,34]

Saliva plays a protective role, as it maintains the oral tissues in a proper physiologic state. It performs this function by providing an antibacterial action, buffering the bacterial acids, and acting as a mechanical cleaning agent.[29] In this way, saliva exerts a significant influence on plaque and calculus accumulation as well as periodontal disease. Xerostomia (decreased to absent saliva) is a well-known promoter of periodontal disease in humans.[30] This was also evidenced in an animal study where the removal of the salivary glands caused an increase in periodontal disease.[35]

There are numerous antibacterial products in saliva. These products include enzymes such as lysozyme, lactoferrin, lactoperoxidase-thiocynate, and myeloperoxidase, which all have been shown to have antimicrobial properties.[36–39] In addition, saliva contains antiproteases such as the cathepsins and *tissue inhibitors of metalloproteinases* (TIMPs), which inhibit the degradatory effects of proteolytic enzymes.[40,41] Salivary glycoproteins appear to have both protective and promotive functions, as they may inhibit pathogenic alterations and help to move bacteria out of the oral cavity.[29] However, these glycoproteins concurrently facilitate plaque accumulation.[42,43] Saliva also contains a significant amount of antibodies, with IgA being the most prevalent.[29] These antibodies appear to be synthesized locally, as they react with oral bacteria but not with bacteria from the GI tract.[43] Furthermore, these antibodies in saliva may impair the ability of bacteria to attach to the oral surfaces.[43]

Finally, the saliva plays an important role in buffering the salivary pH against bacterial-induced changes via the bicarbonate-carbonic system.[29,44] This keeps the oral environment at a proper physiologic pH for optimum health.

White blood cells (WBCs) also play a role in the defense mechanisms of the gingiva. Leukocytes are present in the saliva but generally enter the oral cavity via the gingival sulcus.[45] The vast majority of leukocytes in the oral cavity are polymorphonuclear leukocytes (PMNs), with a small percentage (approximately 9% in humans) of monocytes.[29] These PMNs are active WBCs with phagocytic and killing abilities,[46,47] and they are actually attracted by plaque bacteria.[48] Therefore, the WBCs represent a significant weapon in the fight against the extension of plaque into the gingival sulcus.[29]

There are a small number of leukocytes present in the gingival sulcus of healthy and even germ-free gingiva.[49,50] The leukocyte numbers are increased with gingivitis, with some indication that the degree of increase is related to the severity of the gingival inflammation. Therefore, leukocyte numbers can be used as a marker of gingival inflammation.[51] The WBCs in the gingival crevicular fluid are known as *orogranulocytes* and the degree of movement into the oral cavity is known as the *orogranulocytic migration rate.*[29]

Features and clinical signs of the stages of gingivitis

The level of gingival inflammation is broken down into several stages. However, these stages are somewhat arbitrary and gingivitis proceeds through them in a fluid fashion, with no clear demarcations.[9] This is especially true when it comes to the line between normal gingiva and the initial stages of gingivitis.[52] The majority of biopsies from "normal" gingiva contain leukocytes, the majority of which are T cells.[53] These cells do not appear to create inflammation but rather are responsible for the daily maintenance of gingival health. Thus, there is a constant stream of WBCs migrating through the junctional epithelium, and then through the sulcus, and finally into the oral cavity.[54]

Stage I (initial gingivitis)

The initial events in gingivitis are actually changes in the gingival vasculature, specifically increased blood flow through dilated capillaries.[9] These capillary changes occur within 7 days (but can start as soon as 48 hours) after plaque has been allowed to accumulate.[55,56] PMNs move through these widened spaces and then migrate through the walls and congregate in the connective tissue, junctional epithelium, and gingival sulcus.[57–59] This low level of inflammation is NOT clinically evident,[9] and therefore is known as subclinical gingivitis.[60]

In addition to changes within the vasculature, the junctional epithelium and the connective tissue matrix become slightly altered.[9] This takes the form of exudation and fibrin deposition in the involved areas.[52]

It is important to note that the host response at this point determines the disease course. An appropriate response causes the lesion to resolve quickly, while an inappropriate one results in the creation of a localized chronic inflammatory state.[9]

Stage II (the early lesion)

This stage occurs approximately 1 week following the initiation of plaque accumulation.[55,61] There is no distinct line between this level and stage I, as it is essentially an *intensification* of the same changes seen in the initial lesion.[61–63] The PMNs that have migrated through the vessel walls will travel through the epithelium and finally emerge into the pocket area.[9] They are then chemotactically drawn to the bacteria and ingest them (phagocytosis),[9] resulting in release of lysozymes[64] by design or after cell death.[23] This local inflammation, and the patient's continued response to it, causes the fibroblasts to begin showing cytotoxic alterations,[65] leading to a decrease in collagen production and an increase in collagen destruction.[63,66] The combination of these processes leads to early tissue changes.

Classically, the first clinical sign of gingivitis was believed to be a color change caused by erythema of the gingival margin, termed "marginal gingivitis" (Figure 4.8).[1,67] This is caused by the proliferation of capillaries as well as formation of capillary loops.[9] This stage of gingivitis may be present with or without demonstrable plaque and calculus. This initial level of gingivitis is classified as gingival index (GI) 1.

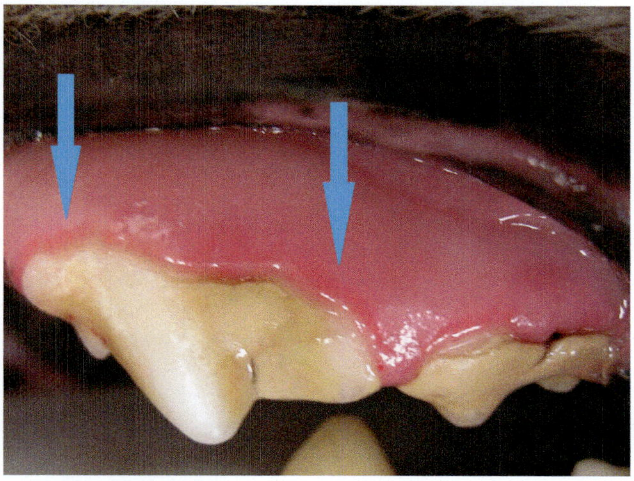

Figure 4.8 Intraoral picture of the left maxillary fourth premolar (208) in a dog with early "marginal gingivitis" (blue arrows).

In addition to being an early marker for gingivitis, bleeding on probing can also be used subjectively as a measure of the severity of inflammation. It has been shown that the degree of bleeding corresponds to the level of inflammation.[4] Furthermore, bleeding on probing is believed to be a sign of active tissue destruction, and in humans has been shown to occur as soon as 2 days after cessation of homecare.[4]

Gingivitis leads to gingival bleeding via dilation and/or engorgement of the capillaries and also thinning or ulceration of the sulcular epithelium. This inflammation and/or thinning of the capillaries results in rupture and bleeding, which can occur secondary to previously innocuous stimuli (such as brushing or chewing).

Chronic inflammation secondary to plaque bacteria is by far the most common cause of gingival bleeding.[70] However, gingival bleeding can also result secondary to uremia,[71] multiple myeloma,[72] and clotting disorders[4] such as thrombocytopenia, hemophilia, and vitamin K antagonism (rodenticide toxicity). In patients with significant or spontaneous gingival bleeding, practitioners

Box 4.2 Key clinical point

While color change is a reliable sign of disease, it is now known that increased gingival bleeding on probing (Figure 4.9) occurs prior to a color change.[4,68] Although it is difficult to perform this on awake patients and therefore is not commonly used as a screening test in practice, clients may notice bleeding during brushing or after chewing hard/rough toys.[1,23,69] If this is discovered, a diagnosis of early gingivitis can be made despite a lack of demonstrable color change. In fact, this is a more objective measure of inflammation than identifying a subtle color change! Practitioners should consider carefully probing or brushing a tractable patient's teeth on conscious exam to demonstrate the level of inflammation to hesitant owners.

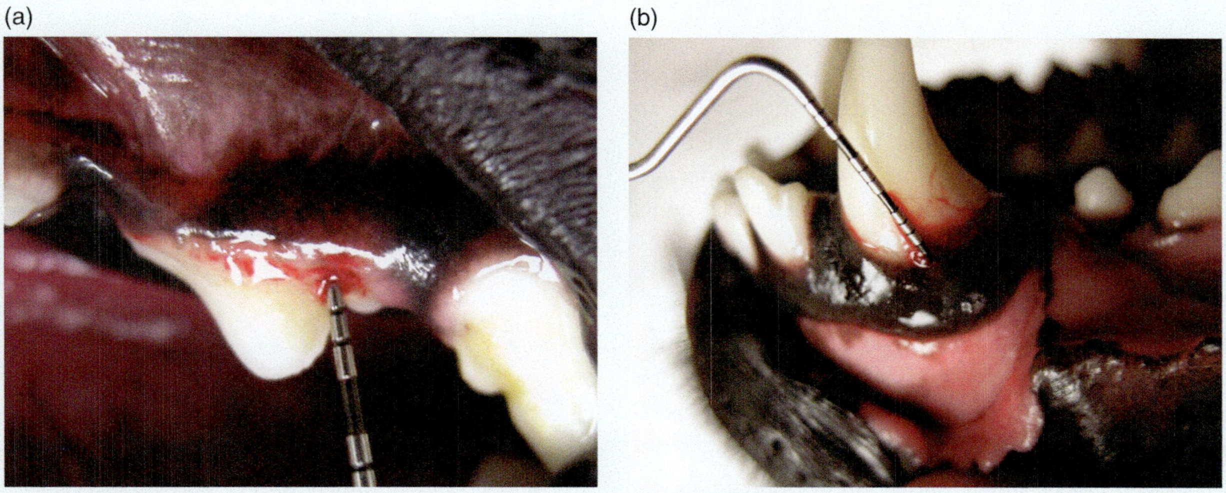

Figure 4.9 Intraoral pictures of the left maxillary third premolar (a) and left mandibular canine (b) in a dog with bleeding induced by probing. Note that the gingiva appears normal and there is minimal calculus.

should consider performing a coagulation profile prior to surgery, especially if the periodontal tissues appear relatively healthy.

Stage III gingivitis (Established)

If left untreated, the established lesion eventually develops. In humans this generally occurs after about 2–3 weeks without homecare.[9] Stage III gingivitis is characterized by a further increase in the level of plasma cells.[58] In addition, B cells are seen in high numbers and are typically of the IgG variety (specifically types 1 and 3).[52] The junctional epithelium shows widened intracellular spaces and often contains lysosomes from PMNs, which can further damage the delicate gingival tissues.[9]

Increased inflammation results in increased collagenolysis in the area. This is caused by the increased production of collagenase (by bacteria and PMNs),[73] as well as numerous other inflammatory/destructive enzymes such as esterases, aminopeptidase,[74] cytochrome oxidase,[75] and B-galactocidase. In fact, an inverse relationship appears to exist between the number of inflammatory cells and the amount of intact collagen.[76]

Increased levels of inflammation also intensify the vascular changes, resulting in engorged and congested vessels, impaired venous return, and sluggish blood flow. In addition, some red blood cells (RBCs) may become extravasated into the connective tissue, where the breakdown products further affect the gingiva.[9]

Clinically, the vascular changes and congestion intensify the color changes to the gingiva,[9] which can be seen as deeper shades of red (Figure 4.10). With increasing chronicity and levels of inflammation, more of the gingiva becomes affected; eventually the entire attached gingiva may be involved (Figure 4.11). Extravasated RBCs and their breakdown products can also further intensify the color changes. In some cases of severe inflammation, a bluish tinge may become superimposed on the reddened gingiva (anoxemia) (Figure 4.12).[77]

In addition to color changes, as the inflammation progresses gingival edema will occur (Figure 4.13).[23] In advanced cases, gingival bleeding may be spontaneous.[23] Finally, although halitosis is more commonly associated with periodontal disease, it can also be noted as a sequela of significant gingivitis.[1,23]

Stage IV gingivitis (Advanced)

This stage of gingivitis is defined as extension into the alveolar bone, causing periodontal breakdown.[63] It is therefore more truly defined as early periodontitis.[63,65] (This is discussed in detail in the next chapter.) Interestingly, not all cases of severe gingivitis will progress into periodontitis, as the patient must be susceptible. However, active periodontitis (periodontal inflammation) is never seen

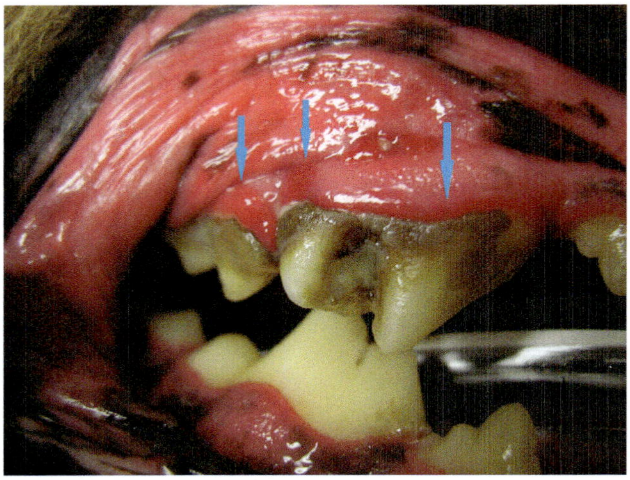

Figure 4.10 Intraoral picture of the right maxillary fourth premolar/first molar in a dog with severe gingival inflammation, as evidenced by the intense erythema (blue arrows).

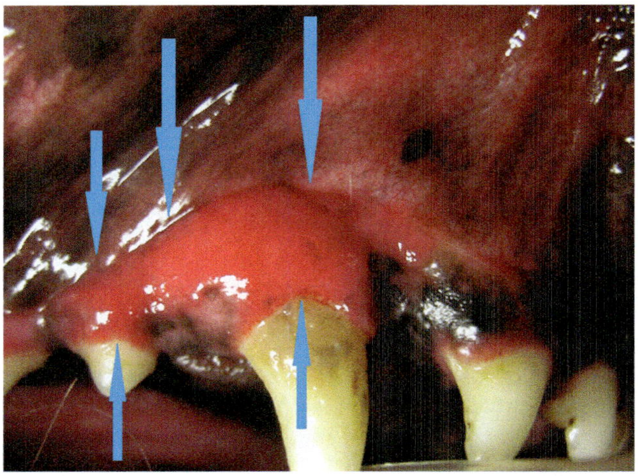

Figure 4.11 Intraoral picture of the right maxillary canine (104) in a dog with severe gingival inflammation that affects the entire attached gingiva (blue arrows) despite the presence of minimal calculus.

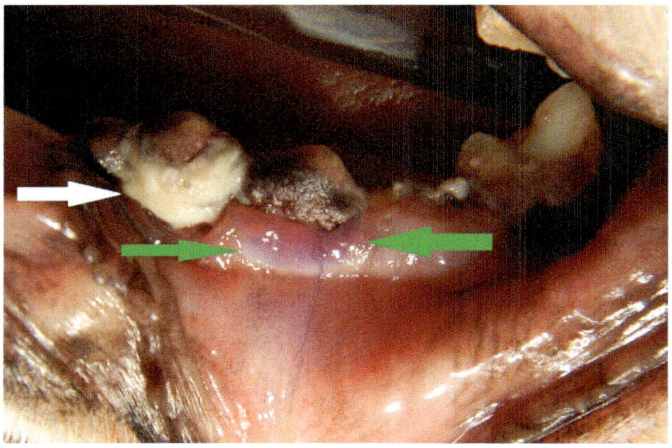

Figure 4.12 Intraoral picture of the mandibular left premolars in a dog with anoxemia of the gingiva over the mandibular third premolar (307) (green arrows). Note the purulent discharge around the first and second premolars (white arrow).

(a) (b)

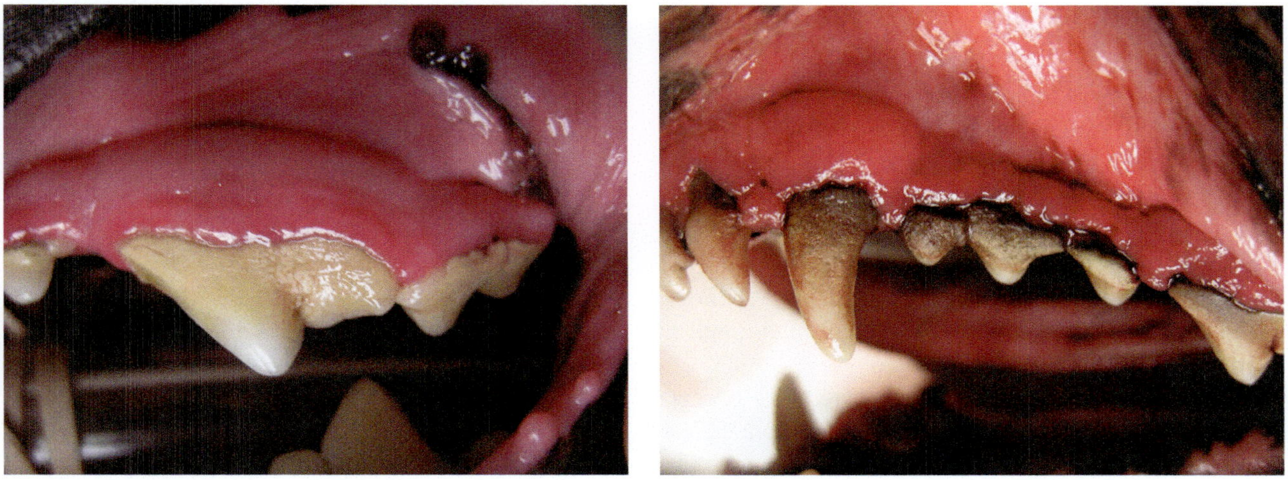

Figure 4.13 (a and b). Intraoral pictures of the maxillary left in two dogs with periodontally induced gingival enlargement.

(a) (b)

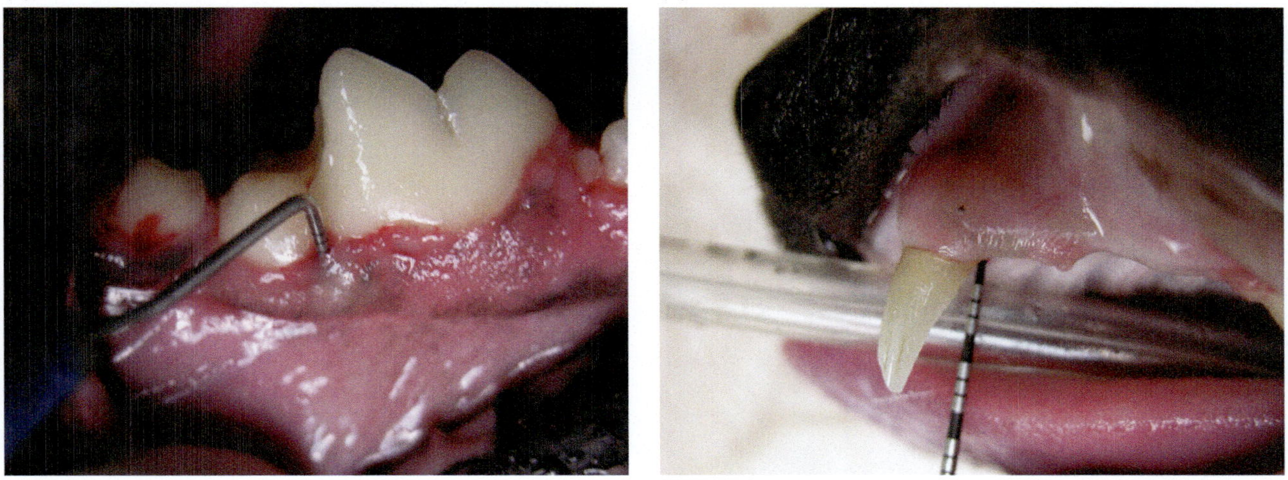

Figure 4.14 Intraoral picture of severe periodontal loss of the right mandibular first molar (409) (a) and the left maxillary canine (204) in a cat (b). Note there is minimal current gingivitis.

without concurrent gingivitis.[9] However, alveolar bone loss may be present from past destruction (Figure 4.14).

Gingivitis scoring index

In the interest of standardizing gingival evaluations, gingival indices have been developed. The AVDC currently does not have an approved/standardized gingivitis index. At this point it is included in the periodontal disease classification as PD1. However, gingival indices are utilized by human dentists and may be valuable to veterinarians as well as we advance in our dental knowledge, since there is a significant difference between gingivitis grades 1 and 4. Therefore, a prudent practitioner will record the degree of gingivitis and utilize the severity to communicate more accurately the level of disease. There are two indices commonly used in human dentistry. The first relies on probing and therefore is more appropriate to the anesthetized exam, whereas the second (modified) version does not rely on probing and therefore should be the preferred method for veterinary patients, as it can be completed on most conscious patients.

- Loe, 1967[78]
- GI 0 = Normal gingiva.
- GI 1 = Mild inflammation: slight color change and edema. No bleeding on probing.
- GI 2 = Moderate inflammation: redness, edema, and glazing. Bleeding on probing.

- GI 3 = severe inflammation: marked redness and edema as well as ulceration. Tendency for spontaneous bleeding.

- Lobene, 1986[79]
- GI 0 = Absence of inflammation (Figure 4.15).
- GI 1 = Mild inflammation. Slight change in color (Figure 4.16). Little change in texture of any portion, but not the entire marginal gingival.
- GI 2 = Mild inflammation as above but involving entire marginal gingiva (Figure 4.17).
- GI 3 = Moderate inflammation. Glazing, redness, edema, and/or hypertrophy of the marginal gingival unit (Figure 4.18).
- GI 4 = Severe inflammation. Marked redness, edema, and/or hypertrophy of the marginal gingiva, spontaneous bleeding, congestion, ulceration (Figure 4.19).

Therapy

The basis of treatment for gingivitis is strict plaque control.[1,3,14,23,80,81] This is classically accomplished via a combination of homecare and professional dental cleanings (prophylaxis) performed under general

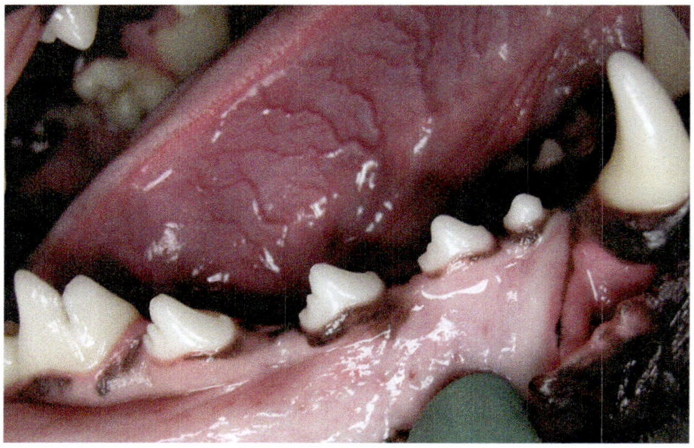

Figure 4.15 Gingival index zero (0), lack of inflammation, normal gingiva.

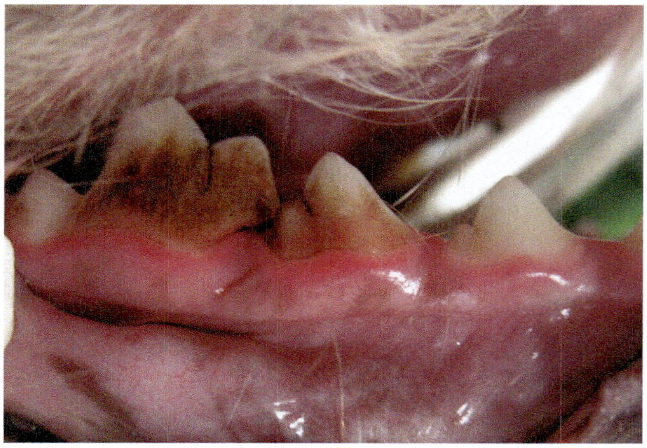

Figure 4.16 Gingival index one (1), mild marginal gingivitis. Involves most but not all of the marginal gingiva.

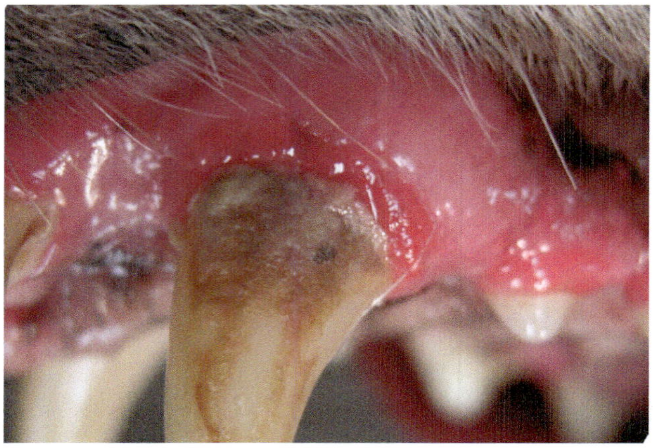

Figure 4.17 Gingival index two (2), mild to moderate inflammation of the entire marginal gingiva.

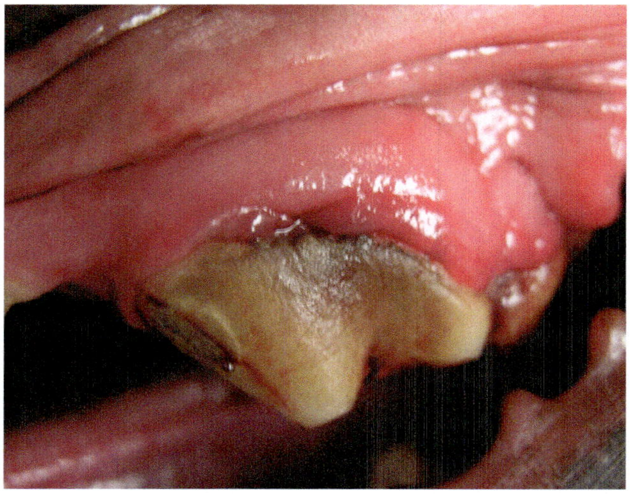

Figure 4.18 Gingival index three (3), moderate inflammation with edema and hemorrhage.

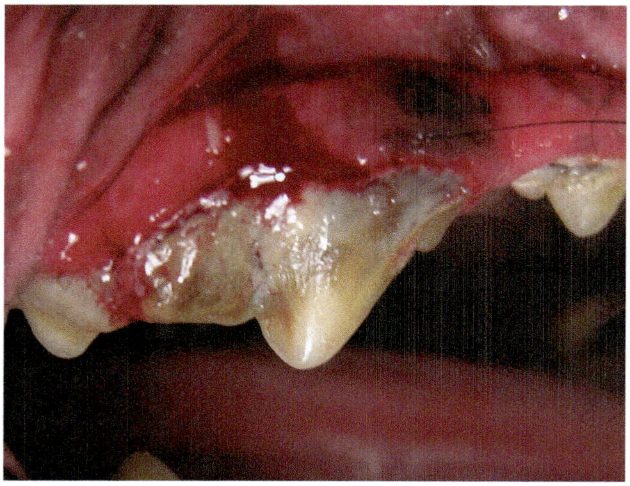

Figure 4.19 Gingival index four (4), severe inflammation with purulent discharge and spontaneous hemorrhage.

anesthesia.[1,14,23] In addition, correction of any predisposing factors such as roughened tooth surfaces or gingival hyperplasia should also be performed.[1,82] In general, if these steps are meticulously and consistently performed, gingivitis should be controlled. It should be noted, however, that without homecare gingival infection and inflammation will quickly recur.[1,4,83] Since there is no attachment loss present with gingivitis, further professional therapy (such as periodontal surgery or extraction) is not necessary. (For further information on complete dental cleaning or homecare, please see chapters 10 and 13, respectively.)

Box 4.3 Key points

- Gingivitis is a local infection secondary to plaque bacteria.
- Gingivitis is reversible and preventable with proper care.
- Calculus, while an indicator, is NOT an accurate marker as to the level of disease.
- Gingival bleeding is the first sign of gingivitis.
- Plaque control via professional cleanings and homecare is the ideal form of therapy.

References

1. Debowes LJ. Problems with the gingiva. In: Small Animal Dental, Oral and Maxillofacial Disease, a Color Handbook (Niemiec BA ed.). London: Manson, 2010, pp. 159–181.
2. Loe H, Theilade E, Jensen SB. Experimental gingivitis in man. J Periodontol 36:177, 1965.
3. Silness J, Loe H. Periodontal disease in pregnancy II. Correlation between oral hygiene and periodontal condition. Acta Odontol Scand. 22:121, 1964.
4. Fiorellini JP, Ishikawa SO, Kim DM. Clinical features of fingivitis. In: Carranza's Clinical Periodontology. St. Louis: Saunders, 2006, pp. 362–372.
5. Fiorellini JP, Kim DM, Ishikawa SO. The gingiva. In: Carranza's Clinical Periodontology. St. Louis: Saunders, 2006, pp. 46–67.
6. Niemiec BA. Periodontal disease. Top Companion Anim Med. 23(2):72–80, 2008.
7. Beck JD, Arbes SJ. Epidemiology of gingival and periodontal diseases. In: Carranza's Clinical Periodontology. St. Louis: Saunders, 2006, pp. 110–131.
8. AVDC Nomenclature Committee. www.AVDC.org. Accessed Jan 1, 2001.
9. Fiorellini JP, Ishikawa SO, Kim DM. Gingival inflammation. In: Carranza's Clinical Periodontology. St. Louis: Saunders, 2006, pp. 355–361.
10. Lindhe J, Hamp S, Löe H. Plaque induced periodontal disease in beagle dogs: A 4-year clinical, roentgenographical and histometrical study. J Perio Res. 10:243–255, 1975.
11. Boyce EN, Ching RJ, Locbgan EI, Hunt JH, Maseman DC, Gaeddert KL, King CT, Reid EE, Hefferren JJ. Occurrence of gram-negative black-pigmented anaerobes in subgingival plaque during the development of canine periodontal disease. Clin Infect Dis. 20 Suppl 2:S317–319, 1995.
12. Quirynen M, Teughels W, Kinder Haake S, Newman MG. Microbiology of periodontal diseases. In: Carranza's Clinical Periodontology. St. Louis: Saunders, 2006, pp. 134–169.
13. Buckley LA. The relationship between malocclusion and periodontal disease. J Periodontol. 43(7):415–417, 1972.
14. Wiggs RB, Lobprise HB. Periodontology. In: Veterinary Dentistry, Principles and Practice. Philadelphia: Lippincott-Raven, 1997, pp. 186–231.
15. Björn AL, Björn H, Grkovic B. Marginal fit of restorations and its relation to periodontal bone level. I. Metal fillings. Odontol Revy. 20(3):311–321, 1969.
16. Jeffcoat MK, Howell TH. Alveolar bone destruction due to overhanging amalgam in periodontal disease. J Periodontol. 51(10):599–602, 1980.
17. Nisengard RJ, Kinder Haake S, Newman MG, Miyasaki KT. Microbial interactions with the host in periodontal diseases. In: Carranza's Clinical Periodontology. St. Louis: Saunders, 2006, pp. 228–250.
18. Emrich LJ, Slossman M, Greco RJ. Periodontal disease in non-insulin dependent diabetes mellitus. J Periodontol. 62:123, 1991.
19. Bartolucci EG, Parkes RB. Accelerated periodontal breakdown in uncontrolled diabetes: Pathogenesis and treatment. Oral Surg Oral Med Oral Pathol 52:387, 1981.
20. Glickman I, Stone IC, Chawla TN. The effect of cortisone acetate upon the periodontium of white mice. J Periodontol. 24:161, 1953.
21. Genco RJ. Current view of risk factors for periodontal diseases. J Periodontol. 67(Suppl):1041, 1996.
22. Hinrichs JE. The role of dental calculus and other predisposing factors. In: Carranza's Clinical Periodontology. St. Louis: Saunders, 2006, pp. 170–192.
23. Niemiec BA. Periodontal disease. Top Companion Anim Med. 23(2):72–80, 2008.
24. Brill N, Krasse B. The passage of tissue fluid into the clinically healthy gingival pocket. Acta Odontol Scand. 16:233–245, 1958.
25. Brill N. The gingival pocket fluid. Studies of its occurrence, composition and effect (thesis). Copenhagen, 1962.
26. Brill N. Effect of chewing on flow of tissue fluid into human gingival pockets. Acta Odontol Scand. 17:277–284, 1959.
27. Shapiro L, Goldman H, Bloom A. Sulcular exudate flow in gingival inflammation. J Periodontol. 50(6):301–304, 1979.
28. Orban JE, Stallard RE. Gingival crevicular fluid: A reliable predictor of gingival health? J Periodontol. 40(4):231–235, 1969.
29. Bulkacz J, Carranza FA. Defense mechanisms of the gingiva. In: Carranza's Clinical Periodontology. St. Louis: Saunders, 2006, pp. 344–354.
30. Loe H, Holm-Pedersen P. Absence and presence of fluid from normal and inflamed gingivae. Periodontics 149:171–177, 1965.
31. Weinstein E, Mandel ID, Salkind A, Oshrain H, Pappas G. Studies of gingival fluid. Periodontics 5:161–166, 1967.
32. Lamster IB, Celenti R, Ebersole J. The relationship of serum IgG antibody titers to periodontal pathogens to indicators of the host response in gingival crevicular fluid. J Clin Periodontol. 17:419, 1990.
33. Eissenberg L, Suchow R, Coles RS, et al. The effects of metronidazole administration on clinical and microbiologic parameters of periodontal disease. Clin Prev Dent. 13:28, 1991.
34. Bader HJ, Goldhaber P. The passage of intravenously administered tetracycline in the gingival sulcus of dogs. J Oral Ther. 2:324, 1966.
35. Gupta OH, Blechman H, Stahl SS. The effects of desalivation on periodontal tissues of the Syrian hamster. Oral Surg. 13: 470, 1960.

36. Iacono VC, Bolot PR, Mackay JB, et al. Lytic sensitivity of Actinobacillus Actionmycetocomans to lysozyme. Infect Immun. 40:773, 1983.
37. Muhlemann HR, Schroeder H. Dynamics of supragingival calculus formation. Avd Oral Biol. 1:175, 1964.
38. Kalmar JP, Arnold RP. Killing of Actinobacillus actinomycetocomans by human lactoferrin. Infect Immun. 56:2552, 1988.
39. Miyasaki KT, Wilson ME, Genco RJ. Killing of Actinobacillus actinomycetocomans by the human peroxide chloride system. Infect Immun. 53:161, 1986.
40. Isemura S, Ando K, Nakashizoka T, et al. Cystatin S: A cysteinproteinase inhibitor of human saliva. J Biochem. 96:1311, 1984.
41. Drouin L, Overall CM, Sodek J. Identification of matrix metalloendoproteinase inhibitor (TIMP) in human parotid and submandibular saliva: Partial purification and characterization. J Periodontal Res. 23:370, 1988.
42. Ellen RP, Gibbons RJ. Protein associated adherence of streptococcus pyogenes to epithelial surfaces: Prerequisite for virulence. Infect Immun. 5:826, 1972.
43. Gibbons RJ, van Houte J, Liljemark WF. Some parameters that affect the adherence of S. Salivarius to oral epithelial surfaces. J Dent Res. 51:424, 1972.
44. Mandel I. Relation of saliva and plaque to caries. J Dent Res. 53(Suppl):246, 1974.
45. Schlott CR, Loe H. The origin and variation in the number of leukocytes in the human saliva. J Periodontal Res. 4(Supp):24, 1969.
46. Passo SA, Tsai CC, McArthur WP, et al. Interaction of inflammatory cells and oral microorganisms. IX. The bacterial effect of human PMN leukocytes on isolated plaque organisms. J Periodontal Res. 15:470, 1980.
47. Renggli HH. Phagocytosis and killing by crevicular neutrophils. In: The Borderland between Caries and Periodontal Disease (Lehner T ed.). New York: Grune and Stratton, 1977.
48. Kahnberg KE, Lindhe J, Helden J. Initial gingivitis induced by topical application of plaque extract: A histrometric study in dogs with normal gingiva. J Periodontal Res. 11:218, 1976.
49. Attstrom R, Egelberg J. Emigration of blood neutrophils and monocytes into the gingival crevices. J Periodontal Res. 5:48, 1970.
50. Rovin S, Costich ER, Gordon HA. The influence of bacteria and irritation in the initiation of periodontal disease in germfree and conventional rats. J Periodontal Res. 1:193, 1966.
51. Skougaard MR, Bay I, Kilnkhammer JM. Correlation between gingivitis and orogranulocytic migratory rate. J Dent Res. 48:716, 1994.
52. Page RC. Gingivitis. J Clin Periodontol. 13:345, 1986.
53. Seymour GJ, Powell RN, Cole KL, et al. Experimental gingivitis in humans: A histochemical and an immunological characterization of the lymphoid cell subpopulations. J Periodontal Res. 18:375, 1983.
54. Ryder MI. Histological ultrastructural characteristics of the periodontal syndrome in the rat. I. General light microscopic observations and ultrastructural observations of initial inflammatory changes. J Periodontal Res. 15:502, 1980.
55. Payne WA, Page RC, Olgolvie AL, et al. Histopathologic features of the initial and early stages of experimental gingivitis in man. J Periodontal Res. 10:51, 1975.
56. Hock J, Nuki K. A vital microscopy study of the morphology of normal and inflamed gingiva. J Periodontal Res. 6:81, 19771.
57. Attstrolm R. Studies on neutrophil polymorphonuclear leukocytes at the dentogingival junction in gingival health and disease. J Periodontal Res. 8(Suppl):1, 1971.
58. Schroeder HE, Graf-de Beer M, Attstrom R. Initial gingivitis in dogs. J Periodontal Res. 10:128, 1975.
59. Attstrom R. The roles of gingival epithelium and phagocytizing leukocytes in gingival defense. J Clin Periodontol. 2:25, 1975.
60. Lindhe J, Socransky SS, Loe H. Experimental gingivitis in the beagle dog. Int Dent J. 23:232, 1973.
61. Page RC. The role of inflammatory mediators in the pathogenesis of periodontal disease. J Periodontal Res. 26:230, 1991.
62. Gavin JB. Ultrastructural features of chronic marginal gingivitis. J Periodontal Res. 5:19, 1970.
63. Lindhe J, Schroeder HE, Page RC, et al. Clinical and stereologic analysis of the course of early gingivitis in dogs Periodontal Res. 9:314, 1974.
64. Lange D, Schroeder HE. Cytochemistry and ultrastructure of gingival sulcus cells. Helv Odontol Acta. 15:65, 1971.
65. Page RC, Simpson DM, Ammons WF. Host tissue response in chronic inflammatory periodontal disease. IV. The periodontal and dental status of a group of aged great apes. J Periodontol 46:144 1975.
66. Flieder DE, Sun CN, Schneider BC. Chemistry of normal and inflamed human gingival tissues. Periodontics 4:302, 1966.
67. Fiorellini JP, Ishikawa SO, Kim DM. Clinical features of gingivitis. In: Carranza's Clinical Periodontology. St. Louis: Saunders, 2006, pp. 362–372.
68. Meitner SW, Zander H, Iker HP, et al. Identification of inflamed gingival surfaces. J Clin Periodontol. 6:93, 1979.
69. Amato R, Canton J, Polson A, et al. Interproximal gingival inflammation related to the conversion of a bleeding to a non-bleeding state. J Periodontol. 57:63, 1986.
70. Milne AM. Gingival bleeding in 848 army recruits: An assessment. Br Dent J. 122:111, 1967.
71. Merril A, Peterson LJ. Gingival bleeding secondary to uremia: Review and report of a case. Oral Surg Oral Med Oral Pathol. 29:530, 1970.
72. Benett JH, Shankar S. Gingival bleeding as the presenting feature of multiple myeloma. Br Dent J. 157:101, 1984.
73. Hancock EB, Cray RJ, O'Leary TJ. The relationship between gingival crevicular fluid and gingival inflammation: A clinical and histologic study. J Periodontol. 50:13, 1979.
74. Quintarelli G. Histochemistry of the gingiva. III. The distribution of amino-peptidase in normal and inflammatory conditions. Arch Oral Biol. 2:271, 1960.
75. Burstone MS. Histochemical study of study of cytochrome oxidase in normal and inflamed gingiva. Oral Surg Oral Med Oral Pathol. 15:123, 1988.
76. Simpson DM, Avery BE. Histopathologic and ultrastructural features of inflamed gingiva in the baboon. J Periodontol. 45: 500, 1974.
77. Hanioka T, Shizukuishi S, Tsunemitsu A. Changes in hemoglobin concentration and oxygen saturation in human gingiva with decreasing inflammation. J Periodontol. 62:366, 1991.
78. Loe H. The gingival index, the plaque index and the retention index systems. J Periodontol. 38(6):Suppl:610–616, 1967.
79. Lobene RR, Weatherford T, Ross NM, Lamm RA, Menaker L. A modified gingival index for use in clinical trials. Clin Prev Dent. 8(1):3–6, 1986.
80. Perry DA. Plaque control for the periodontal patient. In: Carranza's Clinical Periodontology. St. Louis: Saunders, 2006.
81. Hellström MK, Ramberg P, Krok L, Lindhe J. The effect of supragingival plaque control on the subgingival microflora in human periodontitis. J Clin Periodontol. 23(10):934–940, 1996.
82. Perry DA, Schnid MO, Takei HH. Phase I periodontal therapy. In: Carranza's Clinical Periodontology. St. Louis: Saunders, 2006, pp. 722–727.
83. Rober M. Effect of scaling and root planing without dental homecare on the subgingival microbiota. Proceedings of the 16th European Congress of Veterinary Dentistry, 2007, pp. 28–30.

5

Periodontitis

Introduction

Quite often the terms *periodontitis* and *periodontal disease* are used interchangeably, which is not accurate. Partially it is because these terms have not been strictly defined by the American Veterinary Dental College or in any true reference. A poll of veterinary dentists has resulted in the following definitions:

Periodontal disease is a plaque-induced pathology of any part of the tissues that hold the tooth in the mouth, commonly known as the periodontium (gingiva, periodontal ligament, alveolar bone, and cementum). It can spread along the periodontal ligament space toward the root apex, causing loss of alveolar bone as it progresses. It can include current inflammation or evidence of alveolar bone loss without current inflammation.

Periodontal disease may be separated into two clinical conditions:

Gingivitis is an inflammation of the gingiva WITHOUT periodontal tissue inflammation/destruction.

Periodontitis is defined as "an inflammatory disease of the supporting tissues of the teeth caused by specific microorganisms or groups of specific microorganisms, resulting in progressive destruction of the periodontal ligament and alveolar bone with pocket formation, recession, or both."[1] The clinical feature that distinguishes it from gingivitis is the presence of clinically detectable attachment loss. [2,3]

The bacteria that cause this disease are primarily gram-negative anaerobic bacteria, particularly the black-pigmented species.[2] A recent study has identified three species of *Porphyromanas (gulae, salivosa,* and *denticanis)* as present in the vast majority of periodontal pockets in the dog.[4] (For a detailed discussion of periodontal bacteria, see chapter 3.) This inflammation leads to progressive alveolar bone loss due to osteoclastic activity and can ultimately result in tooth exfoliation.[2] (For a complete discussion of the pathogenesis of periodontal disease, see chapter 2).

Periodontal disease is an extremely common problem in small animal veterinary patients.[2,5] In fact, it has been reported that by 2 years of age, 80% of dogs and 70% of cats have some form of periodontal disease.[6] Small and toy breed dogs are particularly susceptible.[7]

Clinical signs

As gingivitis progresses to periodontitis, the oral inflammatory changes (erythema, edema, hemorrhage) intensify (Figure 5.1).

The hallmark clinical feature of established periodontitis is attachment loss.[6] In other words, the periodontal attachment to the tooth migrates apically. As periodontitis progresses, alveolar bone is lost via osteoclastic activity. Periodontal loss is generally considered to be irreversible, meaning that lost bone cannot be regained without advanced regenerative surgeries (see chapter 18).[2,8]

There are two different clinical presentations of attachment loss. In some cases, the apical migration results in gingival recession while the sulcal depth remains the same. Consequently, tooth roots become exposed and the disease process may be easily identified on conscious exam (Figure 5.2). In other cases, the gingiva remains at the same height while the area of attachment moves apically, thus creating a periodontal pocket.[9] This form is typically diagnosed only under general anesthesia with a periodontal probe (Figure 5.3). It is important to note that both presentations of attachment loss can occur in the same patient, as well as the

Veterinary Periodontology, First Edition. Brook A. Niemiec.

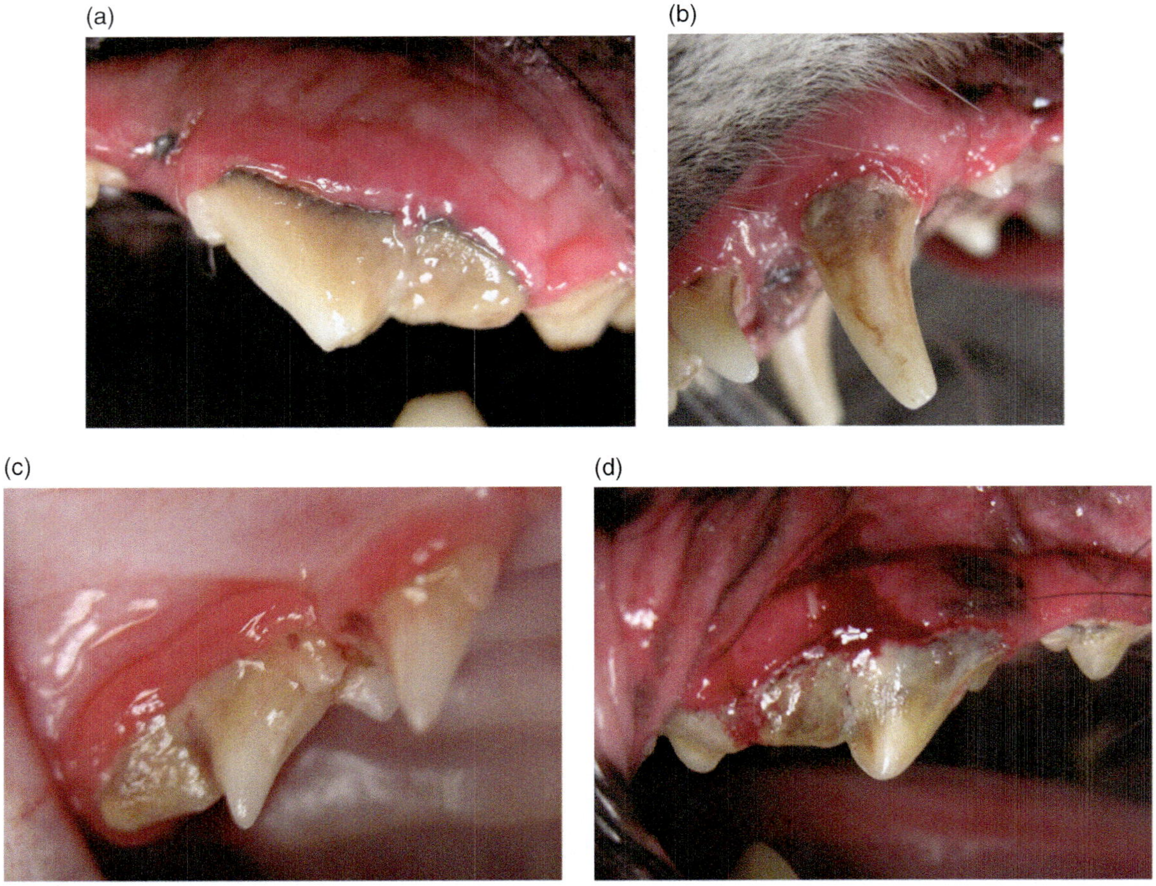

Figure 5.1 Severe gingivitis/early periodontitis: (a and b) Intraoral dental pictures of two dogs with significant gingivitis as evidenced by erythema and edema. (c) Intraoral dental picture of a cat also with significant gingivitis as evidenced by erythema and edema. (d) This culminates in the severe inflammation seen here, where purulent discharge and spontaneous hemorrhage are evident.

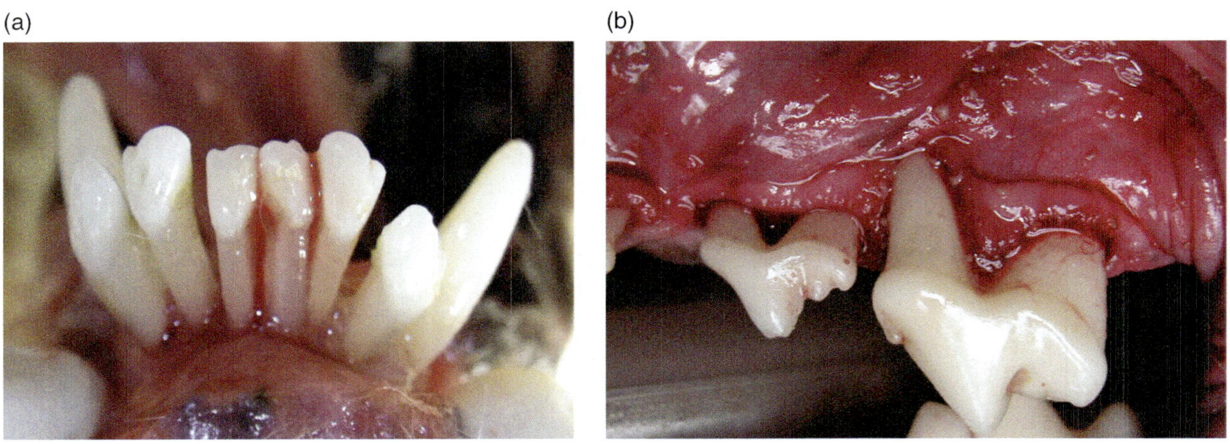

Figure 5.2 (a and b) Gingival recession: Intraoral dental pictures of the (a) mandibular incisors and (b) maxillary left in two dogs with advanced periodontal disease as evidenced by significant gingival recession.

same tooth (Figure 5.4). As attachment loss progresses, alveolar bone loss continues (Figure 5.5), until tooth exfoliation in some cases. After tooth exfoliation occurs, the area typically returns to an uninfected state, but the bone loss is permanent.[6]

Patterns of bone loss

There are two common patterns of alveolar bone loss, horizontal and vertical (or angular).[6,10] The pattern of bone loss is determined by several factors, including

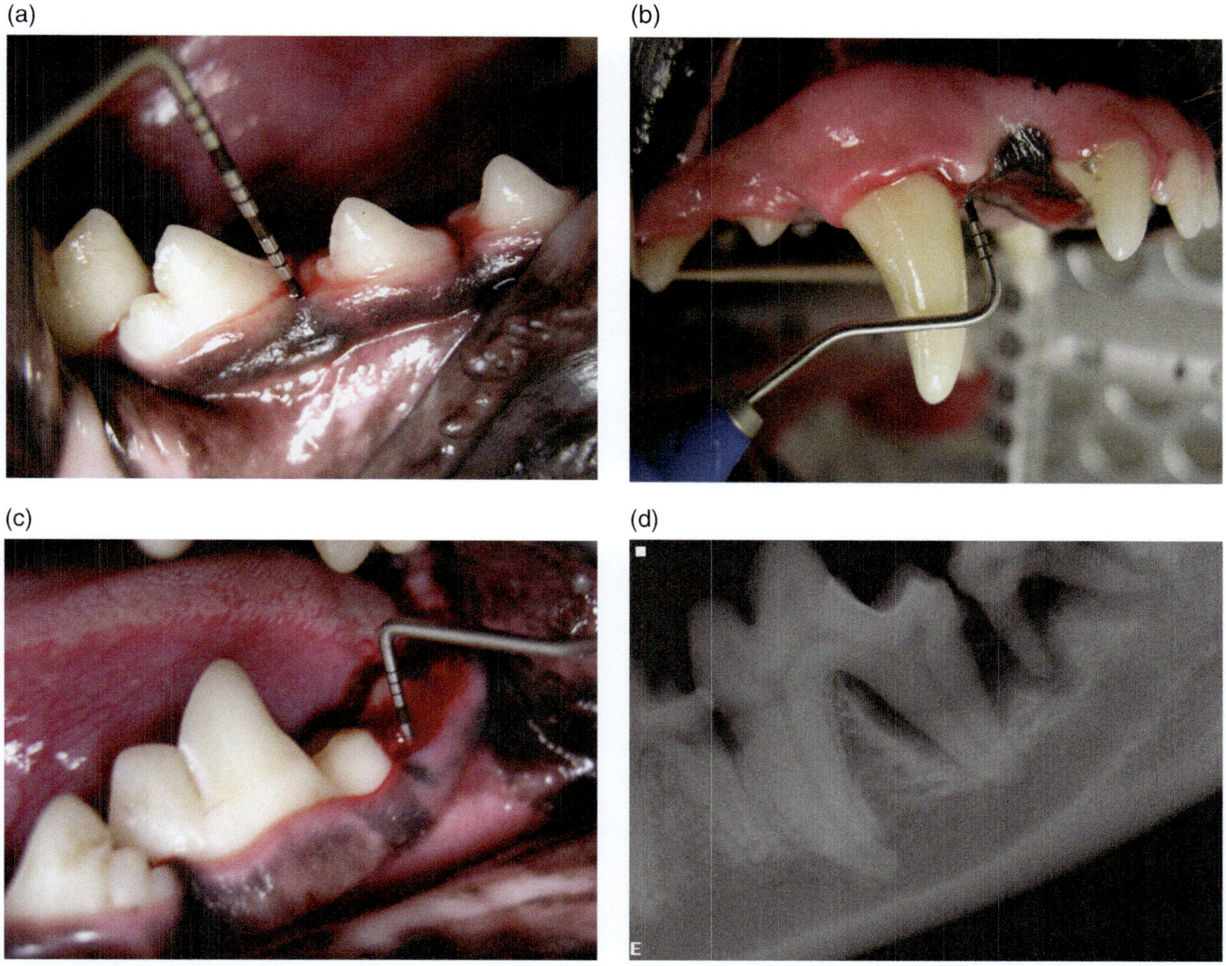

Figure 5.3 Periodontal pocketing: (a and b) Intraoral dental pictures of two dogs with periodontal bone loss as evidenced by the periodontal probe depth, despite fairly normal gingival appearance. (c) Intraoral dental picture of the mandibular left in a dog with normal-appearing gingival tissues. However, probing resulted in severe hemorrhage and revealed a deep periodontal pocket. (d) The severe alveolar bone loss was confirmed via dental radiographs. These cases are not unusual and reinforce the necessity of anesthetized exams on a regular basis regardless of the clinical appearance.

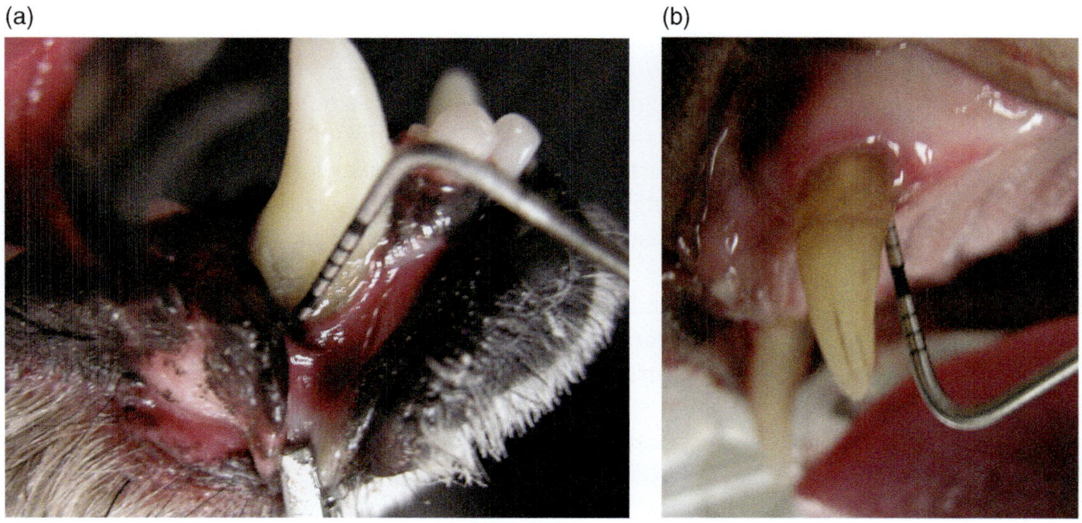

Figure 5.4 Intraoral dental pictures of the right mandibular canine (404) in a dog (a) and left maxillary canine (204) in a cat (b) that show examples of gingival recession and periodontal pockets on the same tooth.

(a) (b) (c) (d)

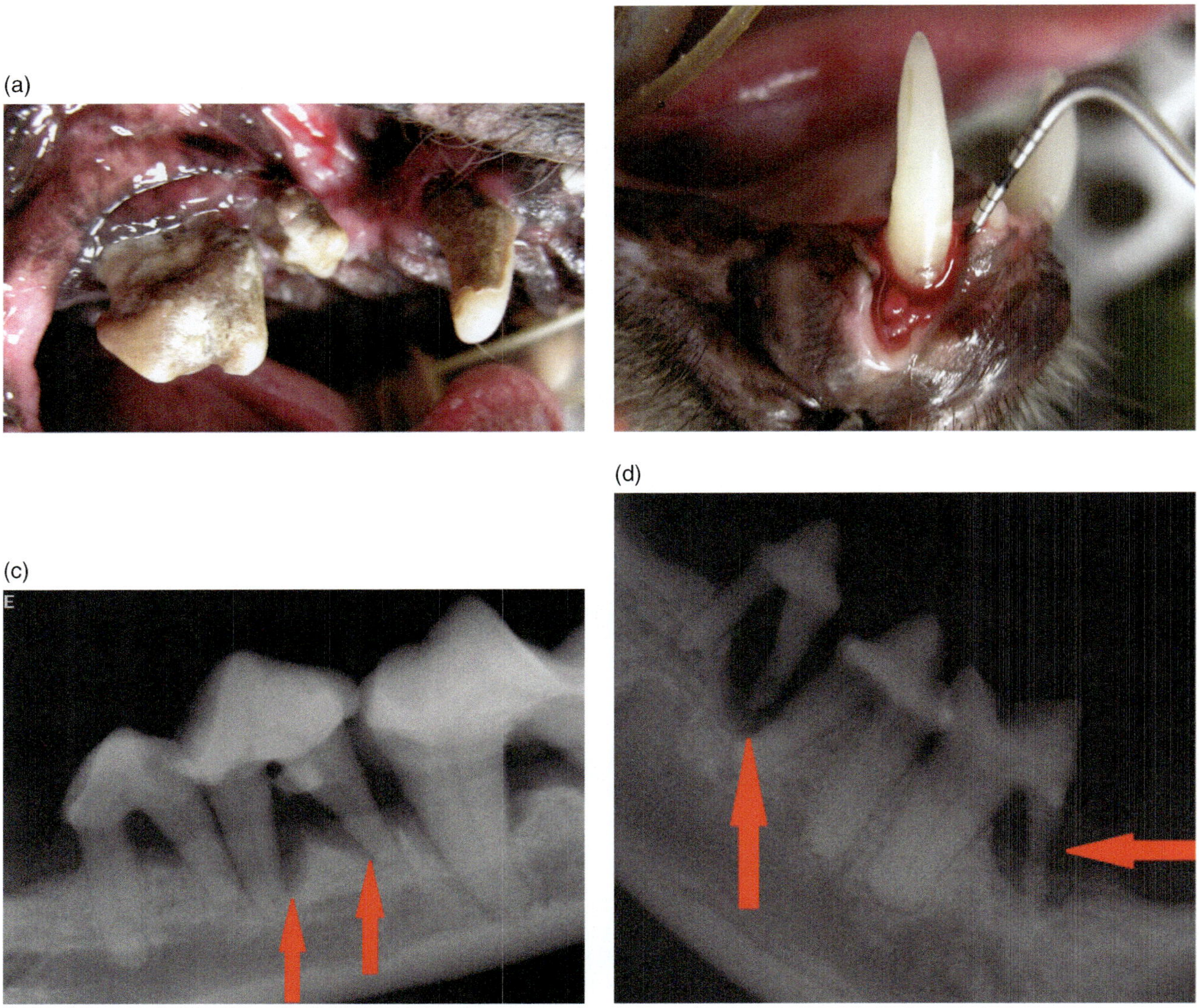

Figure 5.5 (a and b) Intraoral pictures of the maxillary right in a dog (a) and the right mandibular canine (404) in a cat (b) with significant alveolar bone loss. (c and d) Intraoral dental radiographs of the left mandibular fourth premolar (308) of a dog (c) and the left mandibular third premolar and first molar of a cat (d) that reveal severe alveolar bone loss (red arrows).

the thickness of the surrounding bone, the alignment of teeth, and the root anatomy and position, as well as the proximity of other teeth.[11] The most important of these factors is the thickness of the surrounding bone, that is, the interdental septa, lingual, and vestibular plates. For example, vertical (angular) loss rarely occurs in thin plates of bone (like the mandibular incisors), and horizontal loss is unlikely in areas of relatively thick bone (as seen on the palatine surface of the maxillary canines).

Horizontal bone loss (Figure 5.6) is the most common pattern of bone loss in veterinary patients.[11] This is seen when the bony defect is at approximately the same level across the arcade (or a portion of it). This may also be called a 0 (zero) walled pocket (see below). Exceptions to this are the palatine surface of the maxillary canines and the distal root of the mandibular first molars, where vertical (angular) pockets are common.

Vertical (or angular) bone loss (Figure 5.7) is diagnosed when there is an area of bone that is significantly apical to the surrounding bone on a particular tooth.[6,10,11] This is the most common type of bone loss in human patients but is not often seen in veterinary patients, other than in the places mentioned above.

It is important to note that these two patterns may be seen in the same patient as well as on the same tooth (Figure 5.8).

Vertical bone loss is further defined by the number of bony walls surrounding the root.[6,10] A four-walled (or cup) pocket occurs as a defect surrounded by bone

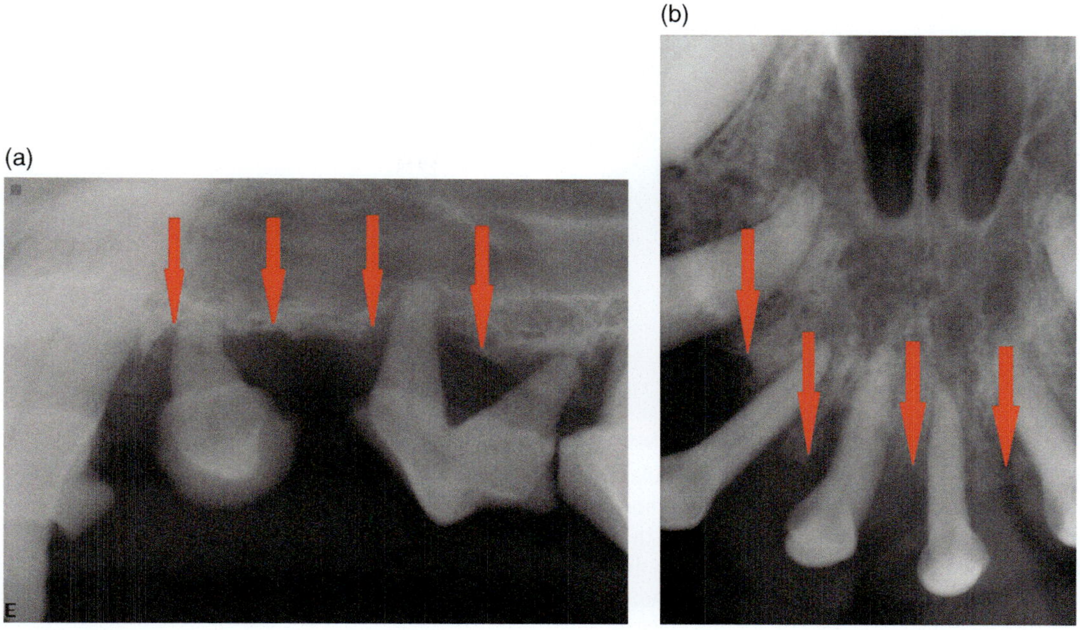

Figure 5.6 Horizontal bone loss: Intraoral dental radiographs of the maxillary left (a) and maxillary incisors (b) of two dogs with periodontally induced alveolar bone loss. Note the bone is at approximately the same level across the arcade (red arrows).

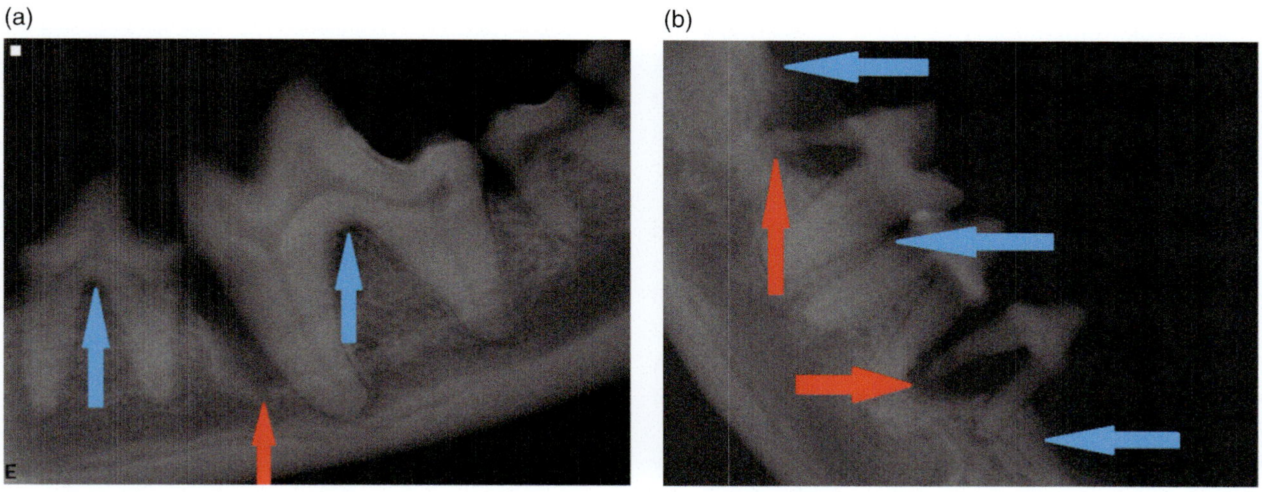

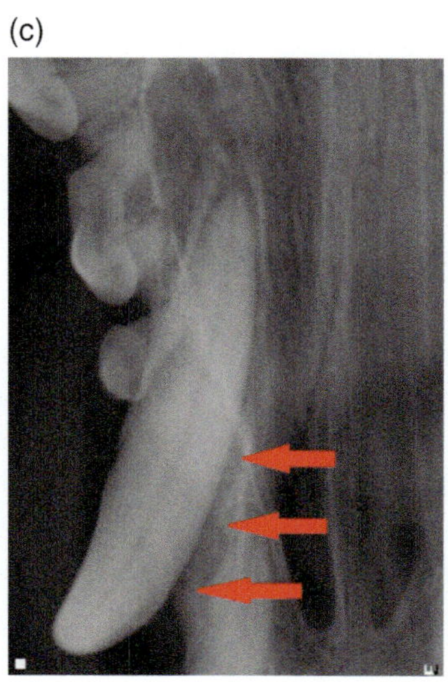

Figure 5.7 Vertical (angular) bone loss: (a and b) Intraoral dental radiographs of the mandibular left of a dog (a) and right of a cat (b) with significant vertical bone loss. This is seen with the nadir of the bone in the deep pockets by the red arrow, as compared to the relatively normal bone height elsewhere (blue arrows). (c) Intraoral dental radiograph of the right maxillary canine (104) of a dog with vertical bone loss on the palatine aspect (red arrows). This is a very common presentation in chrondrodystrophic breeds and is responsive to guided tissue regeneration (see chapter 18). If untreated, this lesion will eventually result in an oronasal fistula.

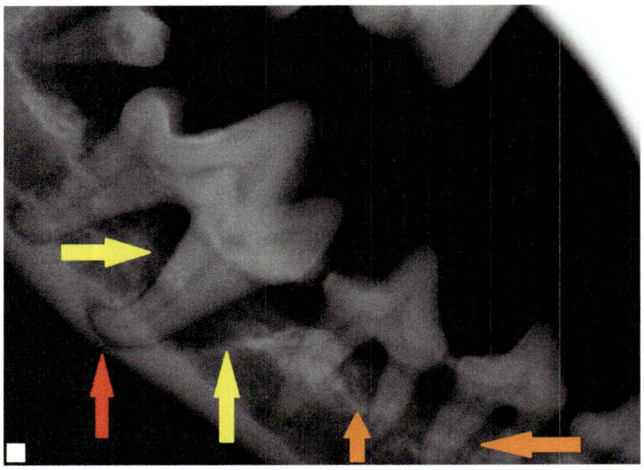

Figure 5.8 Intraoral dental radiograph of the mandibular left of a dog with periodontal disease. Note this patient has horizontal bone loss in the premolars (orange arrows), within the same quadrant of a significant area of angular bone loss on the mandibular first molar (yellow arrows). There is an additional finding of a hook-shaped tip on the mesial root of the first molar as well as a very thin mandibular ventral cortex (red arrow), both of which will complicate extraction.

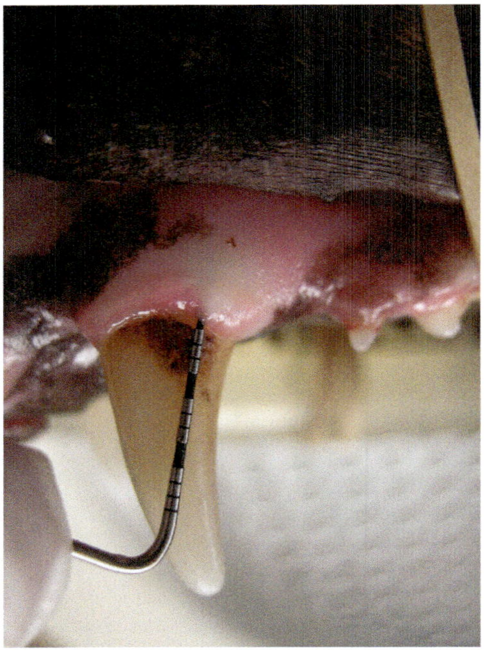

Figure 5.9 Intraoral picture of the left maxillary canine (204) in a dog. In this case, the gingiva is at a normal level, which means the periodontal pocket depth (5 mm) is essentially the same as attachment loss. Note, however, that some periodontal pocketing (up to 3 mm in dogs) is considered "normal."

around its circumference. This lesion has a good prognosis for cure with regenerative osseous surgery.[6] A three-walled pocket has bone surrounding the defect except on the exposed surface of the root. This type of defect also has a good prognosis with regenerative surgery.[10,12] When an additional wall is missing (either vestibular, lingual-palatal, or interdental), a two-walled pocket is created. This type of pocket has a fair prognosis for healing with regenerative surgery.[6,12] A one-walled pocket is created when bone remains only on one aspect of the pocket (either vestibular or lingual-palatal). A zero-walled pocket has no bone between the roots of adjacent teeth (also called horizontal bone loss above). Both zero-walled and one-walled pockets have a very poor prognosis for a positive outcome with periodontal surgery.[6,12] (See chapter 9 for a further discussion of bony defects.)

Staging periodontal disease

There are numerous indices that strive to define the level of periodontal disease present. These are quite often very subjective and therefore difficult to compare between patients and operators. The main clinical determination for degree of periodontal disease is attachment loss. Attachment loss is defined as the distance between the *cementoenamel junction* (CEJ) and the current gingival attachment (Figure 5.9).[13]

Attachment loss is a much more accurate determination of the level of disease than is periodontal pocket depth, since gingival recession and/or enlargement is taken into account. Attachment loss is measured either from the CEJ or from an area of clinically normal gingiva (if available). In cases of gingival recession, attachment loss is the depth of the periodontal pocket *plus* the amount of gingival recession (Figure 5.10). In contrast, in cases of gingival enlargement it is the periodontal pocket depth *minus* the amount of enlargement (Figure 5.11).

Furthermore, the staging of periodontal disease is expressed in a percentage of attachment loss rather than a strict measurement (in millimeters), which is more appropriate because of the tremendous variation in root length between teeth and breeds. For example, 3 mm of attachment loss on the incisor of a Yorkshire Terrier is severe, whereas 5 mm of attachment loss on the canine of a Rottweiler is only mild (Figure 5.12). Attachment loss should be determined by a combination of periodontal probing and dental radiology, as each modality has its benefits and limitations (Figure 5.13).[6,14,15] Below is the American Veterinary Dental College accepted staging of periodontal disease (Box 5.1). It is critical to note that a whole mouth score for periodontal disease is an estimate at best. This is because the severity of periodontal disease relates to a single tooth and virtually all patients have teeth at different stages of periodontal disease. For example, most patients with PD4 teeth will still have

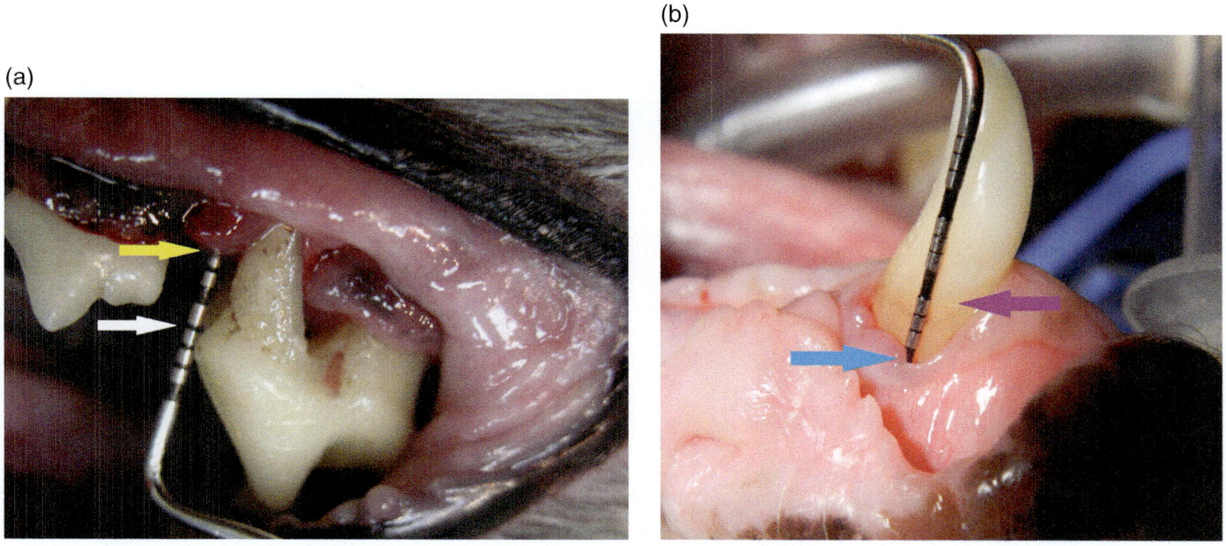

Figure 5.10 Intraoral pictures of canine patients with gingival recession and periodontal pockets. (a) Left maxillary fourth premolar (208) with significant recession and a pocket. In this case the periodontal pocket is 7 mm (yellow arrow), but there is additional recession of 4 mm, which gives an attachment loss of 11 mm (white arrow). (b) Right mandibular canine (404) with only a 5 mm periodontal pocket (blue arrow), which normally would require only closed root planning. However, there is additional recession of 4 mm, resulting in an attachment loss of 9 mm (purple arrow), which is very significant in a small breed dog. This illustrates the importance of attachment loss as a measurement of periodontal health.

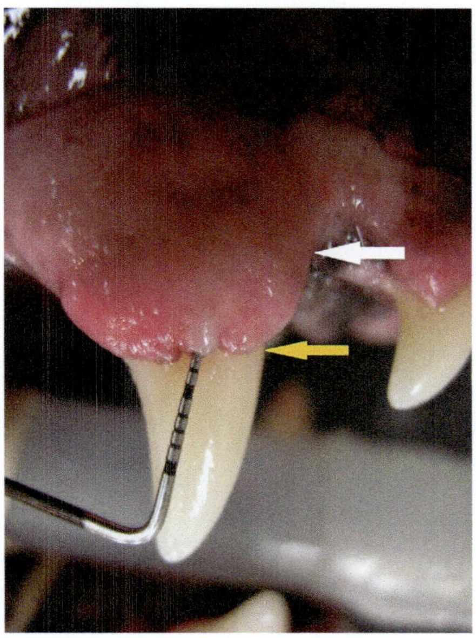

Figure 5.11 Intraoral picture of the right maxillary canine (104) in a dog with gingival enlargement. The probing depth is 7 mm (white arrow), which is significant. However, the measurement to the CEJ is almost the same (yellow arrow). This means that there is actually no attachment loss, regardless of the probing depth.

some teeth that are PD0 (Figure 5.14), and some patients with normal-appearing mouths overall often have one or more significantly diseased teeth (especially distal molars) (Figure 5.15). Therefore, *each* tooth must be evaluated individually.

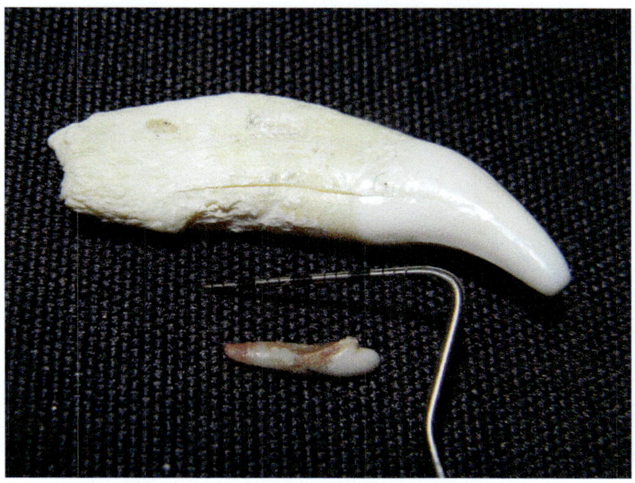

Figure 5.12 An extracted mandibular canine from a Labrador Retriever and a mandibular second incisor from a Yorkshire Terrier. A periodontal probe is added for perspective. Note the amount of alveolar loss (as indicated by the subgingival calculus), which created mobility (and required extraction) of the toy breed's incisor tooth but would have minimal effect on the canine tooth of the large breed dog.

Other clinical signs of diagnostic and/or prognostic importance in periodontal disease

Furcational exposure

The apical movement of the alveolar bone often results in exposure of the area between the roots of multirooted teeth. This area is known as the "furcation," and this

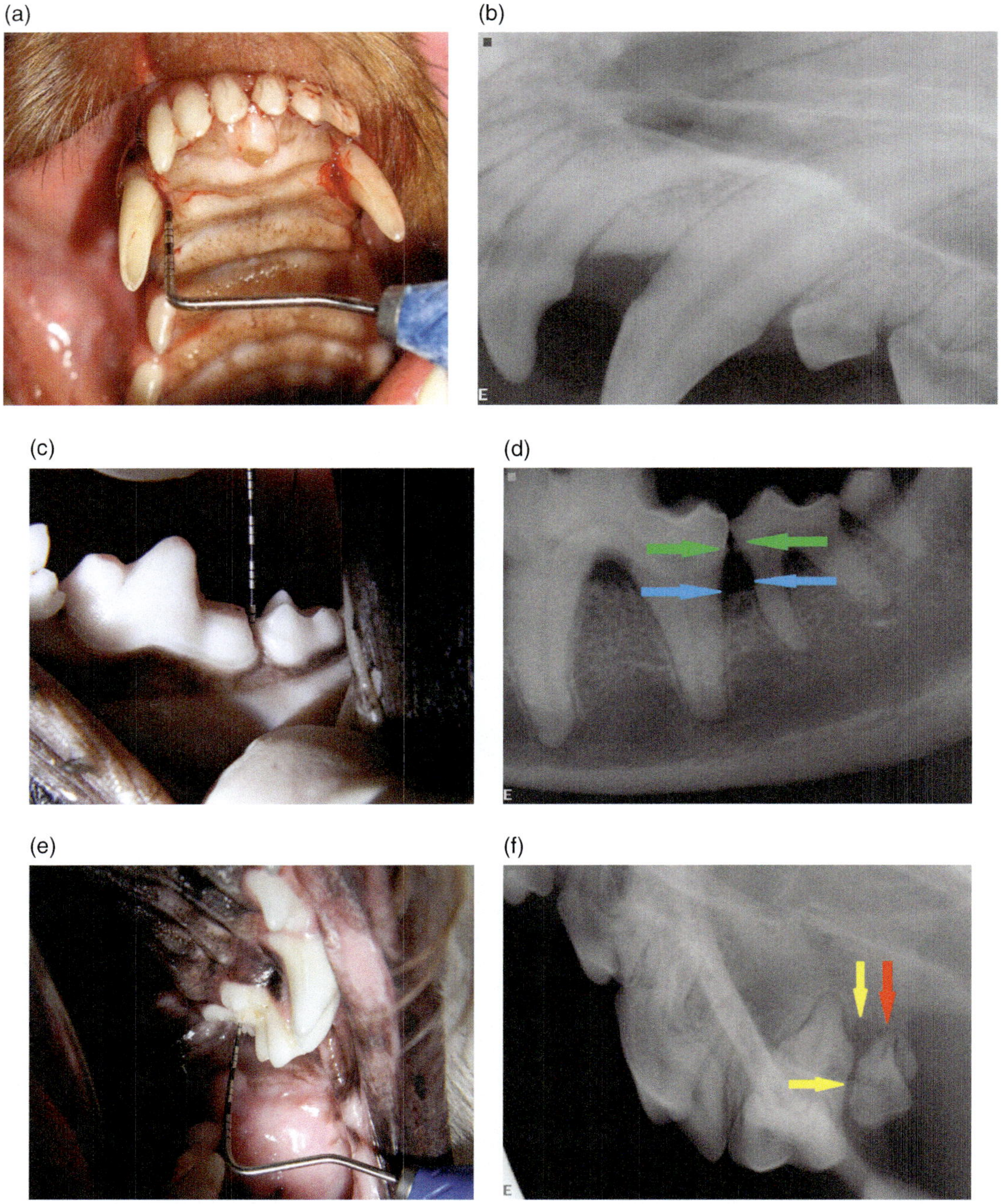

Figure 5.13 (a) Intraoral picture of the right maxillary canine (104) in a dog. The probe reveals a 9 mm periodontal pocket on the palatal surface. (b) The subsequent dental radiograph is relatively normal, as the narrow defect is obscured by the summation of the tooth and buccal plate of bone. This case demonstrates the limitations of dental radiographs in diagnosis of periodontal disease. (c) Intraoral dental picture of the left mandibular first and second molar (309 and 310) in a dog. The gingiva appears normal and there is no probing depth. Note, however, that the probe cannot enter the interproximal space due to the tight contact. Moreover, the lack of probing depth is not accurate and may result in missed pathology. (d) The corresponding intraoral dental radiograph reveals moderate alveolar bone loss (blue arrows) as well as subgingival calculus (green arrows). (e) Intraoral dental picture of the left maxillary first and second molar (209 and 210) in a dog. The gingiva appears normal and there is no probing depth. Note, however, that the probe cannot enter the interproximal space due to the tight contact. Therefore, the lack of probing depth is not accurate and may result in missed pathology. (f) The corresponding intraoral dental radiograph reveals moderate alveolar bone loss (yellow arrows), which has likely caused a class II perio-endo lesion on the second molar (red arrow). These cases demonstrate the limitation of probing in certain situations. It is thus recommended to use both modalities for complete and proper diagnosis.

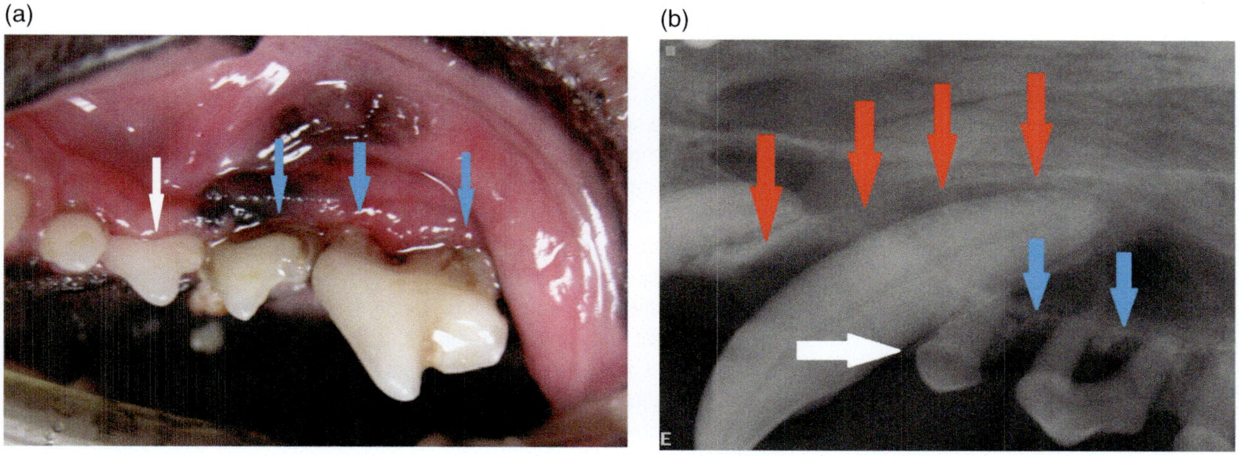

Figure 5.14 (a) Intraoral dental picture of the maxillary left of a dog. Note the significant gingival recession and purulent discharge associated with the third and fourth premolars (207 and 208) (blue arrows), whereas the second premolar (206) is essentially normal (white arrow). (b) Intraoral dental radiograph of the maxillary left, which reveals severe vertical (angular) bone loss to the palatine surface of the maxillary canine (204), resulting in an oronasal fistula (red arrows) as well as severe horizontal bone loss to the second premolar (blue arrows). However, the first premolar (205) is essentially normal (white arrow).

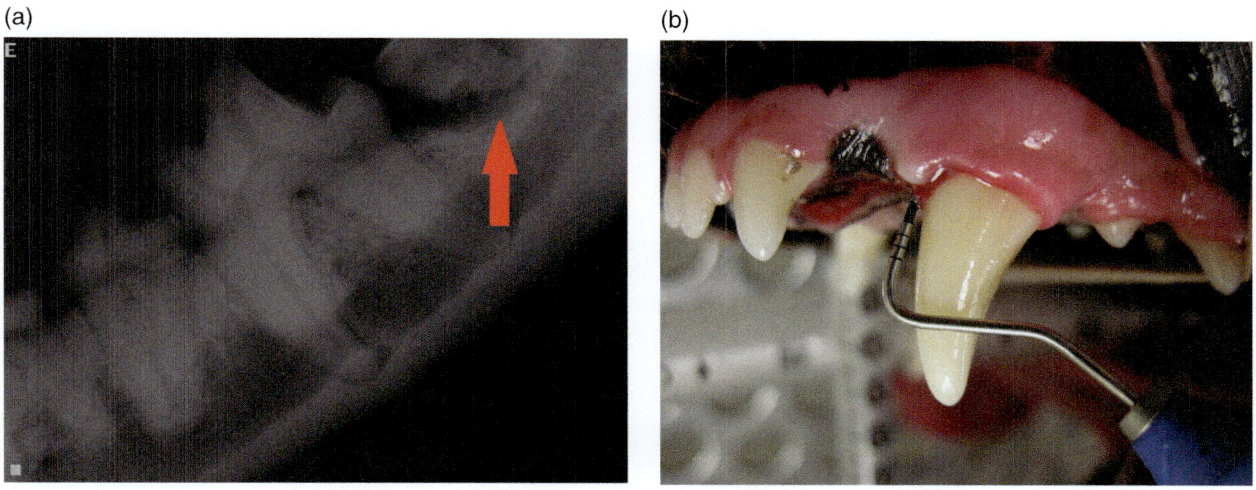

Figure 5.15 (a) Intraoral dental radiograph of the mandibular left of a dog that has a severely diseased second premolar (310) (red arrow), despite the remainder of the arcade having normal bone height. (b) Intraoral dental picture of the maxillary left of a dog, which reveals a severe periodontal pocket on the canine (204), despite the fact that the rest of the teeth in the area are normal. These cases illustrate the fact that all teeth need to be carefully evaluated individually.

condition is called furcational exposure.[6] While furcational exposure occurs late in the disease course in human periodontology, owing to the significant amount of "reserve" crown, it actually occurs fairly early in small animal veterinary patients.[17] This is especially true in cats and small breed dogs, where as little as 1 mm of alveolar bone loss can create this condition (Figure 5.21).

There are several furcation exposure (FE) indices, but the one most commonly used in veterinary dentistry and that is accepted by the AVDC nomenclature committee is as follows:[16]

Note that some dentists (human and veterinary) recognize a fourth stage (F4), where the probe passes all the way through to the other side of the furcation without soft tissue obscuring the communication.[18]

Once the furcation is exposed, it allows for increased plaque, calculus, and food accumulation and therefore increases susceptibility to periodontal disease.[6] Furthermore, it inhibits the homecare efforts of clients. Finally, it is very difficult to effectively clean during the initial scaling procedure, requiring direct visualization offered by periodontal flaps for stage II or III defects.[19]

Box 5.1 Periodontal disease classification[16]

- *Normal (PD0)*: Clinically normal; no gingival inflammation or periodontitis clinically evident (Figures 5.16a and b).
- *Stage 1 (PD1)*: Gingivitis only, without attachment loss. The height and architecture of the alveolar margin are normal (Figure 5.17).
- *Stage 2 (PD2)*: Early periodontitis; less than 25% of attachment loss, or at most there is a stage 1 furcation involvement in multirooted teeth. There are early radiographic signs of periodontitis. The loss of periodontal attachment is less than 25% as measured either by probing of the clinical attachment level or radiographic determination of the distance of the alveolar margin from the cementoenamel junction relative to the length of the root (Figures 5.18a–c).
- *Stage 3 (PD3)*: Moderate periodontitis; 25–50% of attachment loss as measured either by probing of the clinical attachment level or radiographic determination of the distance of the alveolar margin from the cementoenamel junction relative to the length of the root, or there is a stage 2 furcation involvement in multirooted teeth (Figures 5.19a–c).
- *Stage 4 (PD4)*: Advanced periodontitis; more than 50% of attachment loss as measured either by probing of the clinical attachment level or radiographic determination of the distance of the alveolar margin from the cementoenamel junction relative to the length of the root, or there is a stage 3 furcation involvement in multirooted teeth (Figures 5.20a–c).

(a) (b)

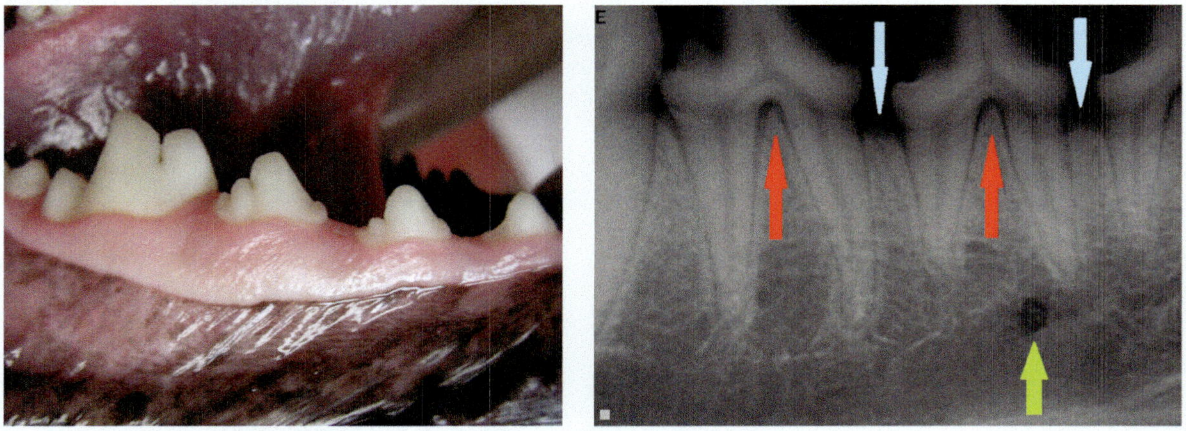

Figure 5.16 (PD0) Normal: (a) Intraoral dental picture of the mandibular right in a dog with normal gingival tissues. Note the gingiva is coral pink in color, with no erythema or edema. Furthermore, there is no plaque or calculus on the teeth. (b) Intraoral dental radiograph of the mandibular right of the patient in Figure 5.16a. This is a normal dental radiograph where the alveolar bone completely fills the furcations (red arrows) and comes to the cementoenamel junctions (blue arrows). The area of lucency (yellow arrow) is the middle mental foramina (a normal anatomical landmark).

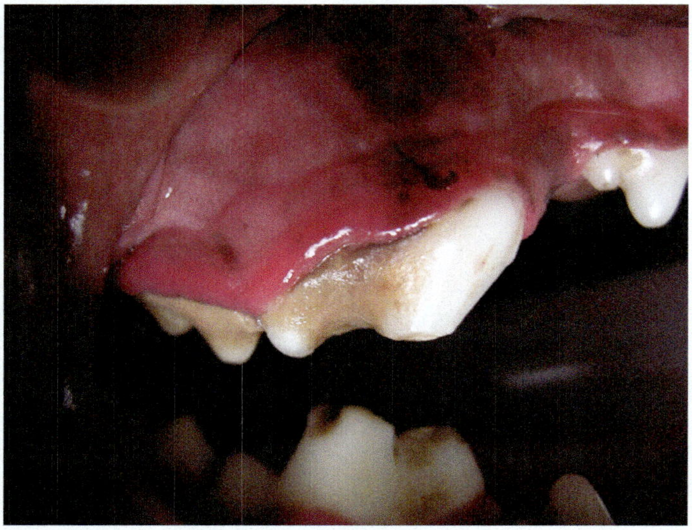

Figure 5.17 (PD1) Gingivitis: Intraoral picture of the right maxillary fourth premolar (108) of a dog with gingivitis. There is no abnormal probing depth and the radiographs are normal.

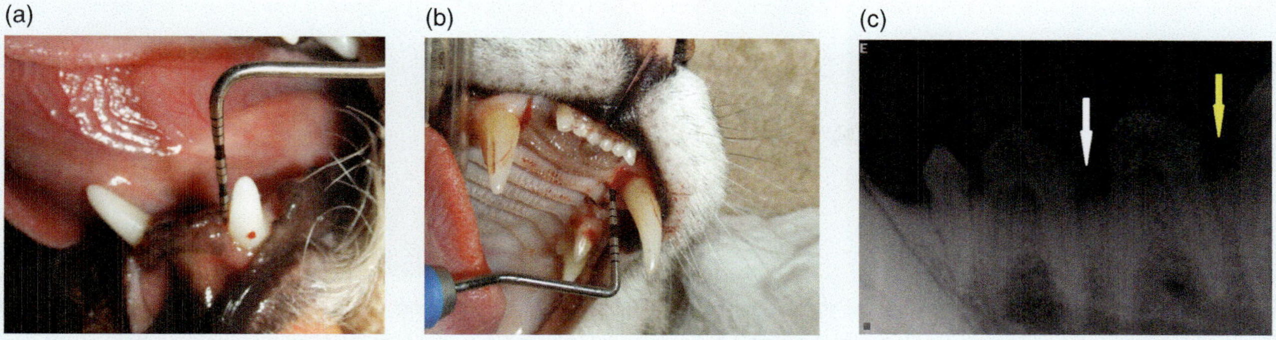

Figure 5.18 (PD2) Mild periodontitis: (a) Intraoral picture of the left mandibular canine (304) of a dog with a 6 mm periodontal pocket on the lingual surface. (b) Intraoral picture of the left maxillary canine (204) of a cat with a 4 mm periodontal pocket on the palatal surface. (c) Intraoral dental radiograph of the mandibular left premolars of a dog. There is approximately 10% alveolar bone loss between the second and third premolars (306–307) (white arrow). There is also a smaller amount between the third and fourth (307–308) (yellow arrow).

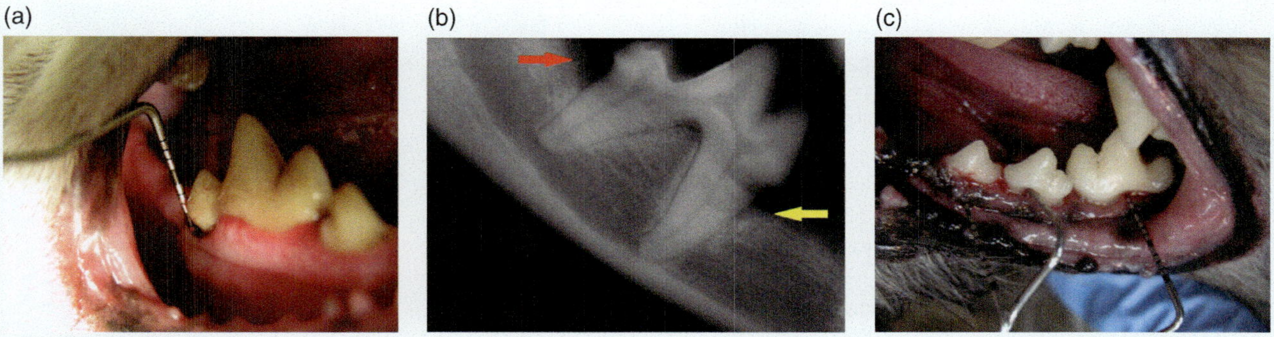

Figure 5.19 (PD3) Moderate periodontitis: (a) Intraoral dental picture of the right mandibular first molar (409) of a dog with a 4 mm periodontal pocket and 2 mm of gingival recession. This is 6 mm of attachment loss. (b) Dental radiograph that reveals approximately 33% bone loss to the distal root (red arrow) and a lesser amount mesially (yellow arrow). (c) Intraoral dental picture of the mandibular left of a dog with the third and fourth premolars and first molar (307–309) all having class II furcation exposure (halfway through).

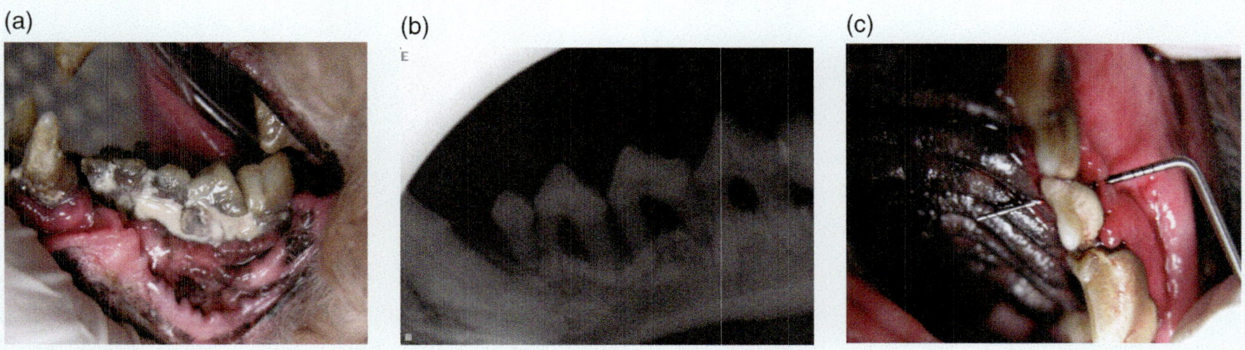

Figure 5.20 (PD4) Severe periodontitis: (a) Intraoral picture of the mandibular left of a dog with severe periodontal disease. Note the gingival recession and purulent discharge. (b) Corresponding intraoral dental radiograph confirming severe alveolar bone loss (> 50%). (c) Intraoral dental picture of the left maxillary third premolar (207) in a dog. This tooth has grade III furcation exposure (through and through).

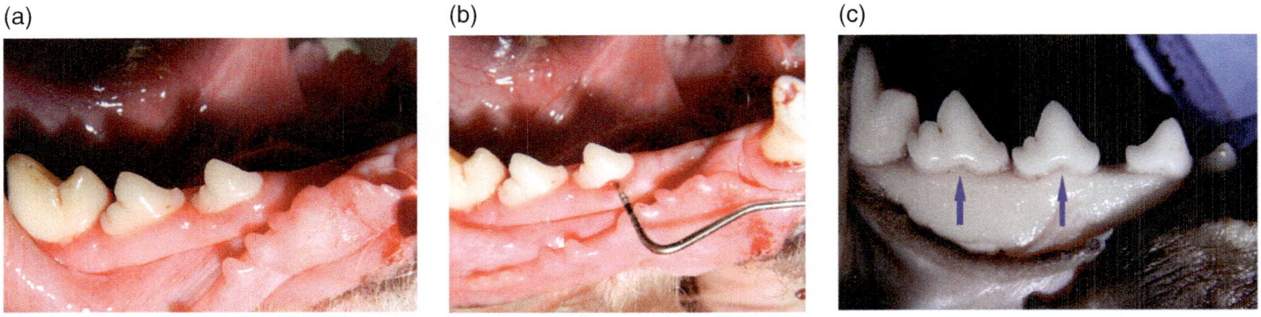

Figure 5.21 (a and b) Intraoral pictures of the mandibular right third premolar (407) in a dog. (a) The gingiva appears to be healthy with no inflammation or attachment loss. (b) However, the probe passes through the furcation (level III), even though there is less than 2 mm of pocketing. (c) Cadaver picture of the mandible of a large breed dog with the soft tissue retracted in order to reveal how coronal the furcation is even in large breed canines.

Box 5.2 Furcation involvement/exposure

- *Stage 0 (F0)*: No furcational exposure (Figure 5.22).
- *Stage 1 (F1)*: Exists when a periodontal probe extends less than halfway under the crown in any direction of a multirooted tooth with attachment loss (Figures 5.23a and b).
- *Stage 2 (F2)*: Exists when a periodontal probe extends greater than halfway under the crown of a multirooted tooth with attachment loss, but not through and through (Figures 5.24a–d).
- *Stage 3 (F3)*: Exists when a periodontal probe extends under the crown of a multirooted tooth, through and through, from one side of the furcation out the other (Figures 5.25a and b).

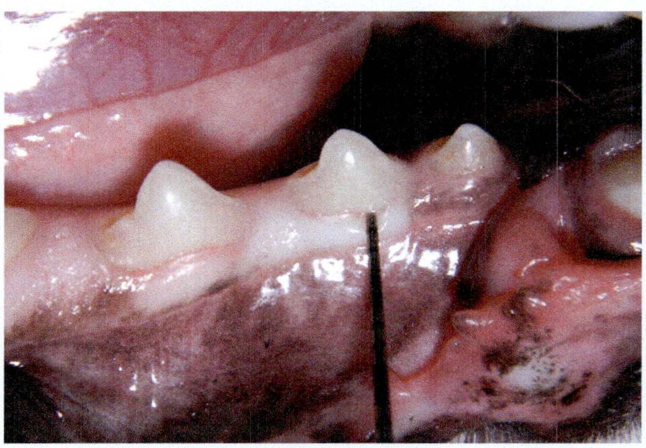

Figure 5.22 (F0) Intraoral picture of the mandibular right of a dog with normal periodontal tissues. Note that the probe does not enter the soft tissue at all.

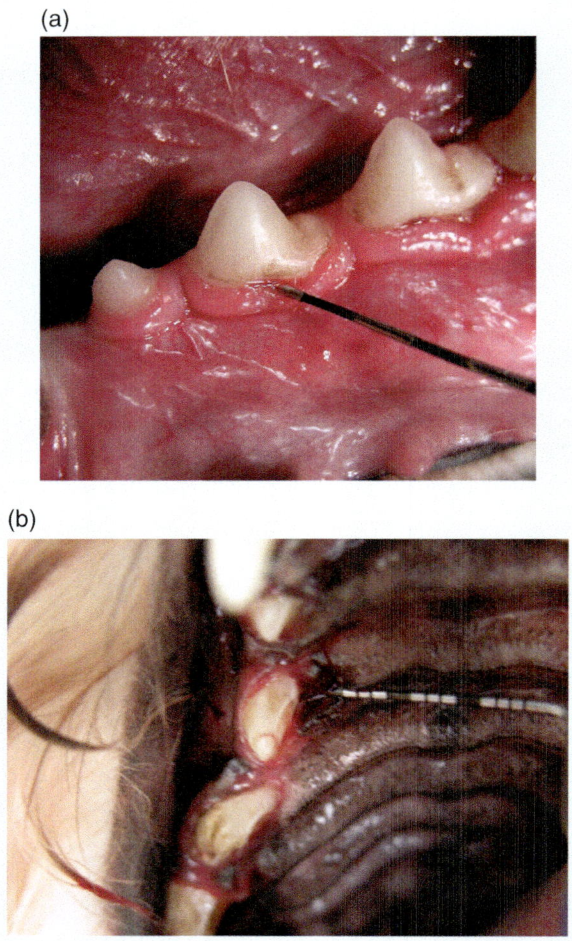

Figure 5.23 (F1) (a) Intraoral pictures of the left mandibular and (b) right maxillary second premolar in dogs with early furcational exposure. Notice that the probe barely enters the furcation. Also note the furcation can be exposed on the buccal (a) as well as palatal/lingual (b) sides of the teeth.

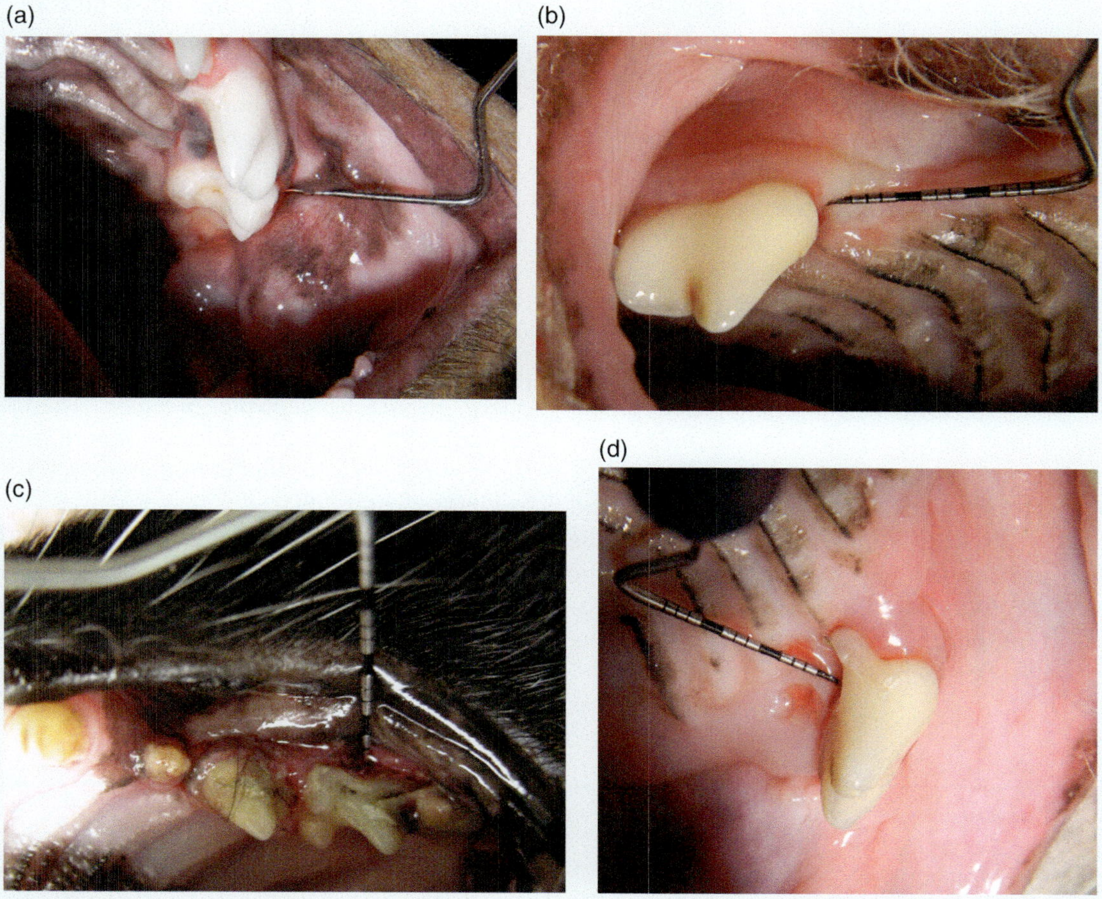

Figure 5.24 (F2) Intraoral pictures of class II furcational defects in several patients. (a) Reveals the furcation exposure from the buccal surface of the left maxillary first molar (209) in a dog. (b) Demonstrates the furcation exposure from mesial surface (between the mesio-buccal and mesio-palatine roots) of right maxillary fourth premolar (108) in a dog. (c) Picture of class II furcational exposure from the buccal surface of the left maxillary fourth premolar (208) of a cat. (d) Shows the furcation exposure from the palatal aspect of a maxillary left fourth premolar (208) of a dog. These pictures (as well as those in Figure 5.23 above) demonstrate the importance of careful evaluation of all sides of the teeth.

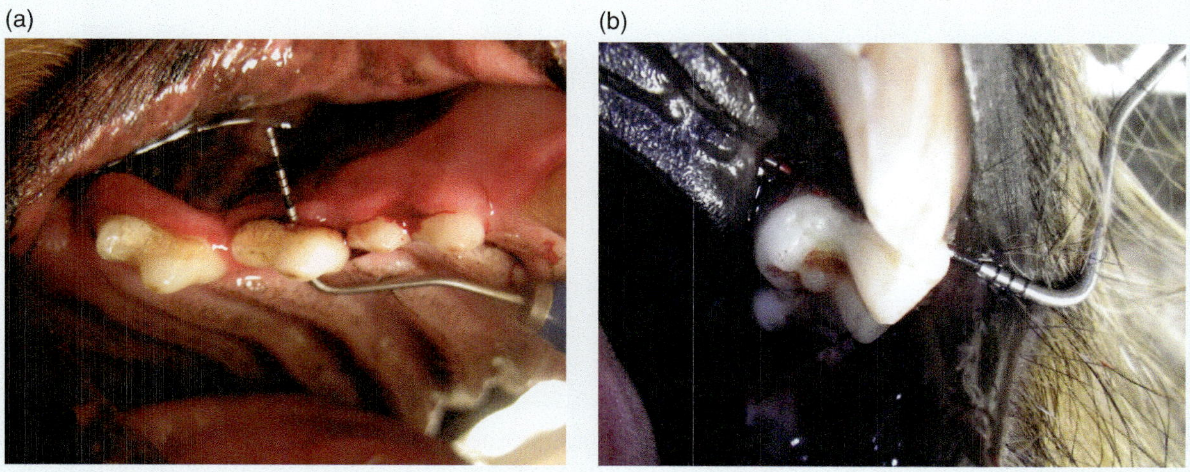

Figure 5.25 (F3) Intraoral pictures of through and through furcation exposure in a dog. (a) Very common presentation of a maxillary premolar. (b) More unusual presentation of a maxillary first molar.

To further complicate this issue, the teeth that most commonly develop furcational defects are the more distal teeth, which are also the most difficult to maintain with homecare.[20] Therefore, teeth (especially three-rooted maxillary molar teeth) with furcational exposure are often best treated with extraction. However, mesial premolar teeth with gingival recession (which creates a more open furcation for cleaning) can often be salvaged if the client is committed to homecare.[6] (See chapter 19 for more treatment options for furcational exposure.)

Mobility

The apical migration of the alveolar bony attachment eventually leads to mobility in the affected teeth.[6] Additional minor causes of mobility include inflammatory changes extending from the gingiva as well as the periapex (periapical lesion), occlussal trauma, and pregnancy (at least in humans).[21,22] Although the inflammatory changes and trauma can often be corrected,[23] and tooth mobility associated with pregnancy is self-limiting, stabilizing the tooth by increasing the amount of bony attachment is rarely achieved.

The amount of bone loss required for pathologic mobility to occur depends on a host of variables, including the length of the root and quality of the supporting alveolar bone. For example, mandibular bone is denser than maxillary bone, and distal bone is harder than rostral.[24] This can be extrapolated to show that more bone loss (or at least a higher percentage) is necessary to create mobility in distal mandibular teeth than rostral mandibular or maxillary teeth. This is most notable in the area of the mandibular first incisors, where the placement of the teeth near or within the fibrous symphyisis results in hypermobility with minimal, and occasionally no, alveolar bone loss (especially in bracheocephalic breeds).[6] Therefore, it is important to interpret the degree of periodontal loss in light of radiographic and periodontal probing depth, in addition to mobility.

There are numerous mobility indices, but the definition and nomenclature accepted by the American Veterinary Dental College is as follows:[16]

Tooth mobility is not only evidence of the degree of periodontal disease, it is also an important prognostic

Box 5.3 Key clinical point

Additional causes of tooth mobility are pathologic processes of the jaw, such as neoplasia (most common), osteomyelitis, root fractures, and hyperparathyroidism "rubber jaw."[21] Practitioners should keep these processes in mind when mobile teeth are encountered, especially where the level of mobility does not correspond to the level of the periodontal disease in either the affected area or of the mouth in general. Dental radiographs will help distinguish between periodontal disease and neoplasia (Figure 5.26), but histopathology should be performed in any questionable cases.

(a) E (b)

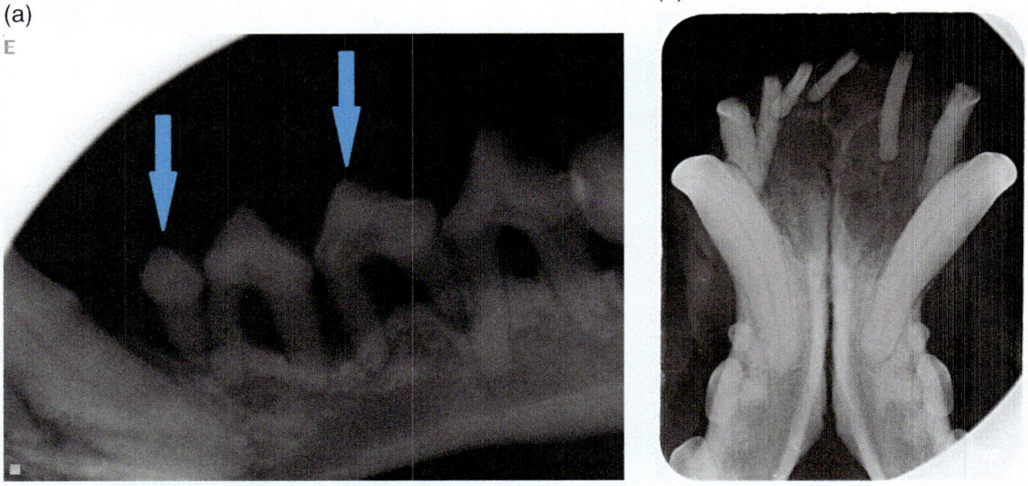

Figure 5.26 Intraoral dental radiographs of mobile teeth. (a) Classic, severe periodontally induced alveolar bone loss on the mandibular left of a dog. Notice that all teeth, but especially the first and third premolars (blue arrows), have minimal support remaining. This has resulted in mobility. The fact that the bone loss is complete (as opposed to mottled [below]) and that the teeth are in the correct position is indicative of a periodontal process. (b) A case of mobility induced by the bony destruction caused by a neoplastic process (squamous cell carcinoma) of the rostral mandible of a dog. Note that the loss is not regular and the teeth are being moved.

indicator. The ability to decrease mobility is inversely proportional to the level of alveolar bone loss. In addition, some studies show that mobile teeth may respond less favorably to therapeutic measures than similar non-mobile teeth.[25] Additional treatment modalities for mobile teeth are discussed in chapter 18.

Box 5.4 Tooth mobility

- *Stage 0 (M0)*: Normal physiologic mobility of up to 0.2 mm.
- *Stage 1 (M1)*: The mobility is increased in any direction other than axial over a distance of more than 0.2 mm and up to 0.5 mm.
- *Stage 2 (M2)*: The mobility is increased in any direction other than axial over a distance of more than 0.5 mm and up to 1.0 mm.
- *Stage 3 (M3)*: The mobility is increased in any direction other than axial over a distance exceeding 1.0 mm or any axial movement.

Other clinical signs

Halitosis is a very common finding in small animal veterinary patients. It can occur secondary to a number of disease states including ketoacidosis, uremia, chronic liver disease, sinusitis, chronic bronchitis, GI disease, ischemic necrosis, necrotic oral tumors, or an infected oral foreign body (e.g., wood or food).[18,26] However in the vast majority of cases, halitosis is caused by periodontal disease.[27–29] In fact, halitosis is typically a sign of advanced periodontal disease, which means there is significant infection within the body. Therefore, clients should be counseled that "doggy breath" is NOT normal and is an indication for professional therapy. The typical "rotten egg" odor from periodontal disease is the result of increased production of volatile sulfur compounds (VSCs).[26] These VSCs are almost exclusively produced by tissue destruction and putrefaction of amino acids by gram-negative bacteria.[26,27,30] Finally, the degree of halitosis is positively correlated to the level of periodontal inflammation.[31,32]

Furthermore, it is known that these VSCs exacerbate the existing periodontal inflammation by several methods.[26] First, by increasing vascular permeability, the underlying connective tissue is exposed to toxic bacterial byproducts. In addition, one common VSC (methyl mercaptan) directly enhances the effects of collagenase as well as other proinflammatory products.[33,34] Finally, this same product impedes wound healing and negatively affects human fibroblasts.[35] Therefore, control of halitosis should be part of the treatment plan for any periodontal patient.

Halitosis measurement can be performed subjectively on a scale from 0 to 3,[36] or objectively measured using a commercially available sulfide monitor.[18,37]

Additional clinical signs of periodontal disease include oral pain, periodontal abscesses (Figure 5.27), nasal discharge (from an oronasal fistula) (Figure 5.28), and even mandibular fractures (Figure 5.29).[2] These conditions are covered in detail in chapters 6 and 8. These conditions are severe and very late ramifications of periodontal disease and should not be relied upon to diagnose the disease. Conversely, it is critical to keep

(a)

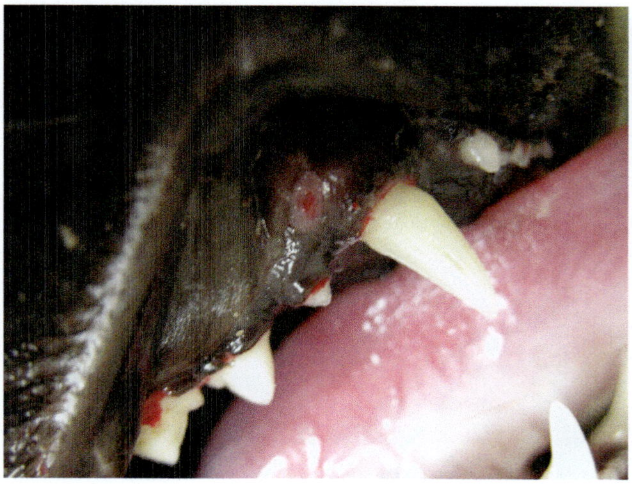

(b)

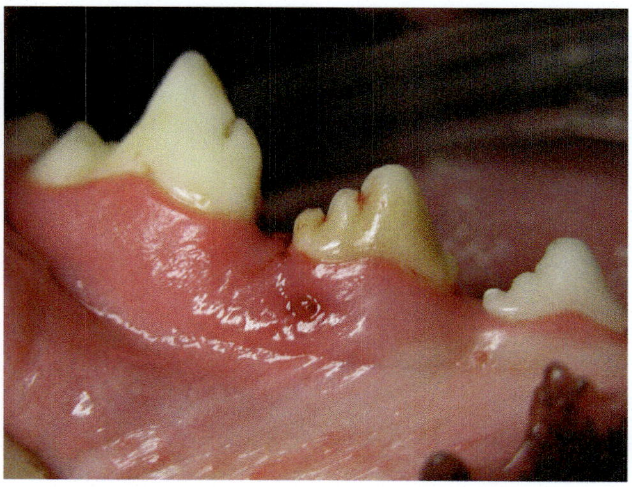

Figure 5.27 Intraoral pictures of periodontal abscesses. (a) On the right maxillary canine (104) of a cat. (b) The right mandibular second premolar (406) in a dog. Note that the draining tracts are coronal to the gingival margin, which is typical of a periodontal rather than endodontic origin. Dental radiographs should be exposed to confirm the diagnosis prior to therapy. (See chapter 8.)

periodontal disease on the rule-out list when these conditions are encountered.

A final clinical sign of advanced periodontal disease is missing teeth that have been exfoliated or extracted due to the advanced state of disease.[2,38] While these teeth are no longer creating infection for the patient, they should be taken into account when assessing the level of periodontal burden by which the patient has been historically affected. In addition, dental radiographs should be exposed to ensure that these teeth are truly missing, as they could have retained roots or be impacted.

Finally, significant widespread periodontal disease can cause generalized lethargy.[2] This happens because the patient is using so much energy fighting off the significant oral infection. This lethargy or "low-energy state" is commonly misinterpreted by clients as "getting older." It can be and most often is reversed with proper periodontal therapy, anecdotally resulting in a marked increase in energy and activity.[2] This author gets common remarks from owners that "my dog is acting like a puppy again."

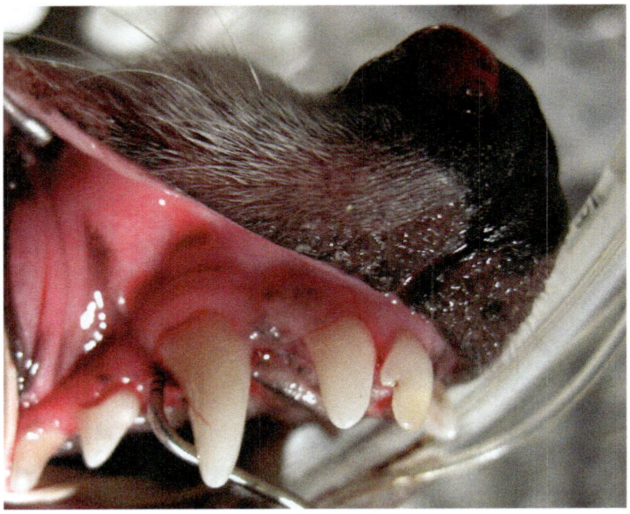

Figure 5.28 Intraoral picture of the maxillary right of a dog with an oronasal fistula of the maxillary canine (104). Note the probe is over 13 mm deep on the palatine surface of the tooth and there is nasal hemorrhage induced by the probing. Notice that the teeth/gums appear outwardly very healthy. This case further demonstrates the value of an anesthetized oral exam regardless of outward appearance. (See chapter 6 for a complete discussion of oronasal fistulas.)

Treatment

At the time of this writing, the basic treatment for periodontal disease is meticulous removal of plaque and calculus and consistent plaque control (homecare).[6,28] However, once attachment loss is present, it requires more than routine scaling and polishing to clear the infection from the root surfaces.[2,39] Depending on the level of attachment loss, as well as other confounding factors (furcational exposure, mobility, inaccessible areas, etc.), additional therapy is required. The most common form of therapy is closed root planing, which is also known as non-surgical root debridement (see chapter 11), which may be employed when periodontal pockets are less than 6 mm and without evidence of other confounding conditions listed above.[2] Closed root planing may be followed by a perioceutic application (see chapter 12).

(a) (b)

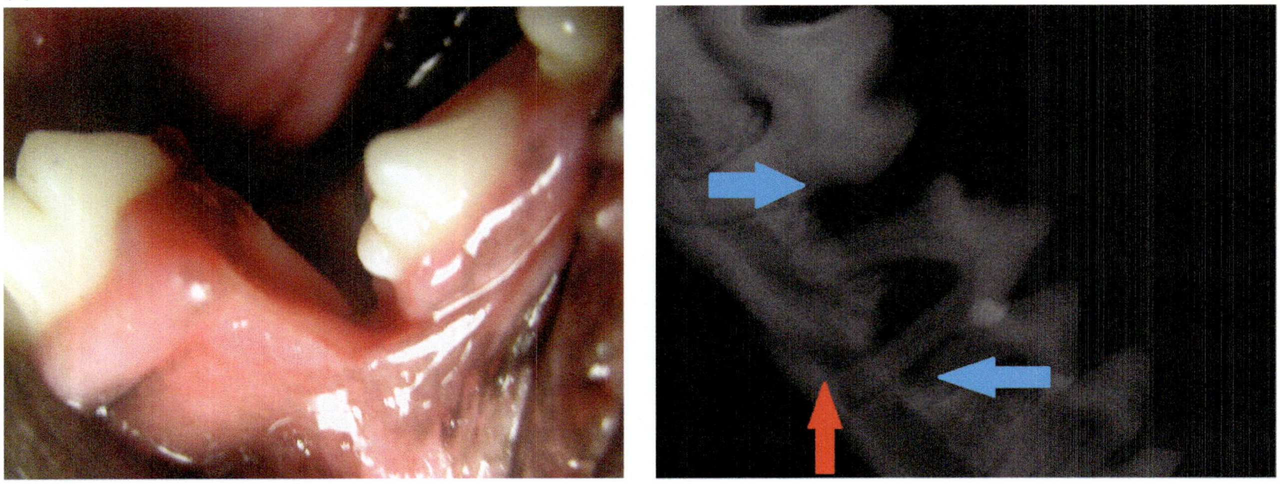

Figure 5.29 (a) Intraoral dental picture of the right mandibular first molar of a dog with a pathologic fracture. (b) Intraoral dental radiograph of the mandibular right of a dog with a pathologic mandibular fracture at the level of the fourth premolar (408) (red arrow). Note the significant alveolar loss (blue arrows), which caused marked bone weakening and resulted in a jaw fracture from mild trauma (dog fight). (See chapter 6 for a complete discussion of pathologic fractures.)

Once the pockets extend beyond 5–6 mm, or other problems are present (particularly furcation level II or III), then direct visualization is *required* to properly clean the teeth.[40–42] There are some experts, however, who support the use of ultrasonic scalers in these deep pockets, which is discussed in chapter 11. Direct visualization of the root surface is achieved via periodontal flap surgery. After the flap is raised, the root is cleaned via surgical root debridement and the flap is sutured closed. Additional therapies (barrier membranes and bone augmentation) may be performed prior to flap closure if indicated (see chapters 16–18).

The client must be instructed on the necessity of consistent homecare prior to the performance of advanced periodontal therapy. If the client is unwilling or unable to perform this task and/or unable/willing to return for regular professional cleanings, then tooth salvage via periodontal surgery may not be in the patient's best interest.

New and future directions of periodontal therapy include laser therapy, bone morphogenetic proteins, stem cell therapy, and host modulation. Some of these modalities, which will be available in the near future, are discussed in chapters 18 and 20.

Depending on the level of disease, the client's wishes, and the health status of the patient, a treatment plan is devised. In scenarios where the periodontal disease is severe, the client is unwilling/unable to perform homecare due to time or the patient's temperament, or the patient is geriatric or at a higher anesthesia risk, extraction may be the best alternative. Although extreme, extraction is the true cure of periodontal disease and allows the body to permanently clear the infection.[6,43]

Box 5.5 Key points

- The hallmark clinical sign of periodontal disease is attachment loss.
- Attachment loss is best expressed as a percentage rather than straight measurements due to the great variability in tooth size in veterinary patients.
- Halitosis is not normal; it is a sign of established oral disease.
- Furcation exposure occurs early in the course of the disease in animal patients and typically requires advanced surgical therapy.
- General anesthesia, periodontal probing, and dental radiography are necessary for the proper diagnosis and therapy of periodontal disease.

References

1. Armitage GC. Development of a classification system for periodontal diseases and conditions. Ann Periodontol. 4(1):1–6. 1999.
2. Debowes LJ. Problems with the gingiva. In: Small Animal Dental, Oral and Maxillofacial Disease, a Color Handbook (Niemiec BA ed.). London: Manson, 2010, pp. 159–181.
3. Novak MJ. Classification of disease and conditions affecting the periodontium. In: Carranza's Clinical Periodontology. St. Louis: Saunders, 2006, pp. 100–109.
4. Hardham J, Dreier K, Wong J, Sfintescu C. Pigmented-anaerobic bacteria associated with canine periodontitis. Veterinary Microbiology 106(1–2):119–128, 2005.
5. Wiggs RB, Lobprise HB (1997). Oral exam and diagnosis. In: Veterinary Dentistry, Principles and Practice. Philadelphia: Lippincott-Raven, 1997, pp. 87–103.
6. Wiggs RB, Lobprise HB. Periodontology. In: Veterinary Dentistry, Principles and Practice. Philadelphia: Lippincott-Raven, 1997, pp. 186–231.
7. Hoffmann TH, Gaengler P. Clinical and pathomorphological investigation of spontaneously occurring periodontal disease in dogs. J Small Anim Pract. 37:471–479, 1996.
8. Shoukry M, Ali B, Naby MA, Soliman A. Repair of experimental plaque-induced periodontal disease in dogs. J Vet Dent. 24(3):152–165, 2007.
9. West-Hyde L, Floyd M. Dentistry. In: Textbook of Veterinary Internal Medicine (Ettinger SJ, Feldman EC eds.). 4th ed. Philadelphia: Saunders, 1995, pp. 1097–1123.
10. Bellows J. Periodontal equipment, materials, and techniques. In: Small Animal Dental Equipment, Materials, and Techniques, a Primer. Ames, IA: Blackwell, 2004, pp. 115–173.
11. Carranza FA, Takei HH. Bone loss and patterns of bone destruction. In: Carranza's Clinical Periodontology. St. Louis: Saunders, 2006, pp. 452–466.
12. Sims TN, Ammons W. Resective osseous surgery. In: Carranza's Clinical Periodontology. St. Louis: Saunders, 2006, pp. 950–967.
13. Beck JD, Arbes SJ. Epidemiology of gingival and periodontal diseases. In: Carranza's Clinical Periodontology. St. Louis: Saunders, 2006, pp. 110–131.
14. Niemiec BA. Case based dental radiology. Top Companion Anim Med. 24(1):4–19, 2009.
15. Tetradis S, Carranza FA, Fazio RC, Takei HH. Radiographic aids in the diagnosis of periodontal disease. In: Carranza's Clinical Periodontology. St. Louis: Saunders, 2006, pp. 561–578.
16. AVDC Nomenclature Committee. www.avdc.org.
17. Page RC, Schroeder HE. Spontaneous chronic periodontitis in adult dogs. A clinical and histologic survey. J Periodontol. 52:60–73, 1981.
18. Huffman LJ. Oral examination. In: Small Animal Dental, Oral and Maxillofacial Disease, a Color Handbook (Niemiec BA ed.). London: Manson, 2010, pp. 39–61.
19. Carranza FA, Takei HH. Phase II periodontal therapy. In: Carranza's Clinical Periodontology. St. Louis: Saunders, 2006, pp. 881–886.
20. Capik I. Periodontal health vs. different preventative means in toy breeds—clinical study. Proceedings of the 16th European Congress of Veterinary Dentistry, 2007, pp. 31–34.
21. Carranza FA, Takei HH. Clinical diagnosis. In: Carranza's Clinical Periodontology. St. Louis: Saunders, 2006, pp. 540–560.
22. Novak KF, Goodman SF, Takei HH. Determination of prognosis. In: Carranza's Clinical Periodontology. St. Louis: Saunders, 2006, pp. 614–625.
23. Morris ML. The diagnosis, prognosis, and treatment of loose tooth. Oral Surg Oral Med Oral Pathol. 6(9):1037–1046, 1953.

24. Huja SS, Fernandez SA, Hill KJ, Gulati P. Indentation modulus of the alveolar process in dogs. J Dent Res. 86:237–241, 2007.
25. Fleszar TJ, Knowles JW, Morrison EC, Burgett FG, Nissle RR, Ramfjord SP. Tooth mobility and periodontal therapy. J Clin Periodontol. 7(6):495–505, 1980.
26. Quirynen M, van Steenberghe D. Oral malodor. In: Carranza's Clinical Periodontology. St. Louis: Saunders, 2006, pp. 330–342.
27. Persson S, Claesson R, Carlsson J. The capacity of subgingival microbiotas to produce volatile sulfur compounds in human serum. Oral Microbiol Immunol. 4(3):169–172, 1989.
28. Yaegaki K, Sanada K. Biochemical and clinical factors influencing oral malodor in periodontal patients. J Periodontol. 63(9):783–789, 1992.
29. Lee CH, Kho HS, Chung SC, Lee SW, Kim YK. The relationship between volatile sulfur compounds and major halitosis-inducing factors. J Periodontol. 74(1):32–37, 2003.
30. Tonzetich J. Production and origin of oral malodor: A review of mechanisms and methods of analysis. J Periodontol. 48(1):13–20, 1977.
31. Yaegaki K, Sanada K. Volatile sulfur compounds in mouth air from clinically healthy subjects and patients with periodontal disease. J Periodontal Res. 27:233–238, 1992.
32. Persson S. Hydrogen sulfide and methyl mercaptan in periodontal pockets. Oral Microbiol Immunol. 7(6):378–379, 1992.
33. Ratkay LG, Tonzetich J, Waterfeild JD. The effect of methylmercaptan on the enzymatic and immunological activity leading to periodontal tissue destruction. In: Bad Breath, a Multidisciplinary Approach (vanSteenberghe D, Rosenberg M eds.). Leuven, Belgium: Leuven Universiy Press, 1996.
34. Lancero H, Niu J, Johnson PW. Exposure of periodontal ligament cells to methyl mercaptan reduces intracellular pH and inhibits cell migration. J Dent Res. 75(12):1994–2002, 1996.
35. Brunette DM, Ouyang Y, Glass-Brudzinski J, et al. Effects of methyl mercaptan on human gingival fibroblast shape, cytoskeleton and protein synthesis and the inhibition of its effects by Zn++. In: Bad Breath, a Multidisciplinary Approach (vanSteenberghe D, Rosenberg M eds.). Leuven, Belgium: Leuven Universiy Press, 1996.
36. Jensen L, Setser C, Simone A, Smith M, Suelzer M. Assessment of oral malodor in dogs. J Vet Dent. 11(2):71–74, 1994.
37. Davot JL, Delille B, Hennet P. Oral malodor in dogs: Measurement using a sulfide monitor. J Vet Dent. 12(3):101–103, 1995.
38. Pavlica Z, Petelin M, Juntes P, et al. Periodontal disease burden and pathological changes in the organs of dogs. J Vet Dent. 25(2):97–108, 2008.
39. Holmstrom SE, Frost PF, Eisner ER. Periodontal therapy and surgery. In: Veterinary Dental Techniques for the Small Animal Practitioner. 3rd ed. Philadelphia: Saunders, 2004, pp. 233–290.
40. Caffesse RG, Sweeney PL, Smith BA. Scaling and root planing with and without periodontal flap surgery. J Clin Periodontol. 13(3):205–210, 1986.
41. Perry DA, Schmid MO, Takei HH. Phase I periodontal therapy. In: Carranza's Clinical Periodontology. St. Louis: Saunders, 2006, pp. 722–727.
42. Zetner K, Rothmueller G. Treatment of periodontal pockets with doxycycline in beagles. Vet Ther. 3(4):441–452, 2002.
43. Danser MM, van Winklehoff AJ, de Graff J, et al. Short term effect of full mouth extraction on periodontal pathogens colonizing the oral mucous membranes. J Clin Periodontol. 21:484, 1994.

6

Local and regional consequences of periodontal disease

Introduction

In addition to tooth loss, there are many other potential serious local consequences of periodontal disease. These maladies are generally caused by the significant bone loss that occurs with chronic periodontal disease. It is important to note, however, that these problems may present in young patients, especially in small and toy breed dogs. These conditions include oronasal fistula, osteomyelitis, ocular damage, class II perio-endo lesion, pathologic mandibular fracture, and oral neoplasia.

Oronasal fistulas

Oronasal fistulas (ONFs) are the most common of the local consequences of periodontal disease. This problem is generally seen in older, small breed dogs (especially chondrodystrophic breeds such as Dachshunds and Basset Hounds), but they can occur in any breed as well as felines.[1,2] ONFs are typically created by the apical progression of periodontal disease on the palatal surface of the maxillary canines[1,3] (however, any maxillary tooth is a candidate).[2] This will eventually result in the destruction of the maxillary bone causing a communication between the oral and nasal cavities, thus leading to a chronic infection (sinusitis).[2]

Clinical signs of an ONF include chronic nasal discharge (Figure 6.1), sneezing, and occasionally anorexia and halitosis.[2,4] Occasionally, a large fistula may be noted on conscious exam (especially one that has resulted from an extraction) (Figure 6.2), but definitive diagnosis of an oronasal fistula typically requires general anesthesia.[2] The diagnosis is made by introducing a periodontal probe into the periodontal space on the palatal surface of the tooth (Figures 6.3 through 6.6). Interestingly, ONFs can occur even when the remainder of the patient's periodontal tissues are relatively healthy, including other surfaces of the affected tooth (Figure 6.7).[5] Appropriate treatment of an ONF requires extraction of the tooth and closure of the defect with a mucogingival flap.[1,6,7] Alternatively, if a deep periodontal pocket is discovered prior to development of a fistula (Figure 6.8), periodontal surgery with guided tissue regeneration can be performed to save the tooth[2,5,8] (see chapter 18).

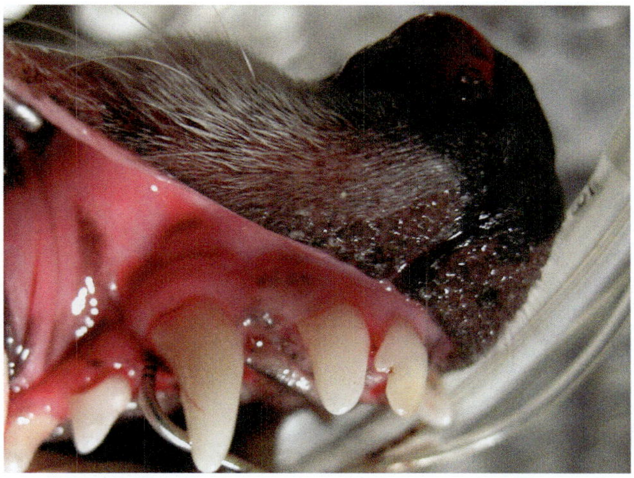

Figure 6.1 Intraoral picture of the maxillary right of a dog with an oronasal fistula of the maxillary canine (104). Note that the probe is over 13 mm deep on the palatine surface of the tooth and there is nasal hemorrhage induced by the probing. Importantly, however, note that the buccal surface of the teeth appears normal. This highlights the importance of an anesthetized oral exam in all patients, regardless of outward appearance.

Class II perio-endo lesion

These infections are another potential consequence of periodontal disease that can be seen in multirooted

Veterinary Periodontology, First Edition. Brook A. Niemiec.

(a)

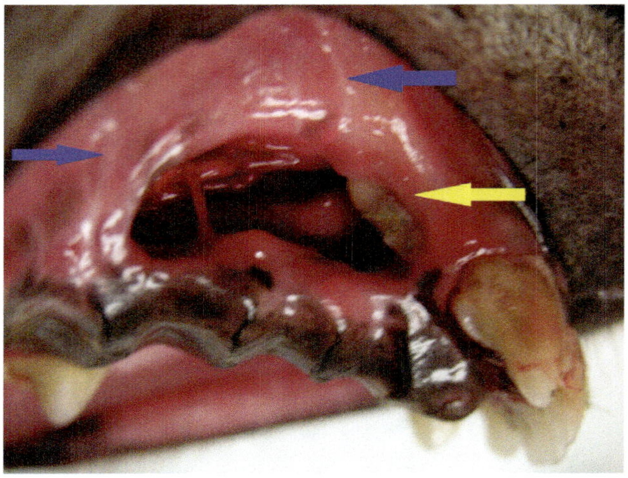

(b)

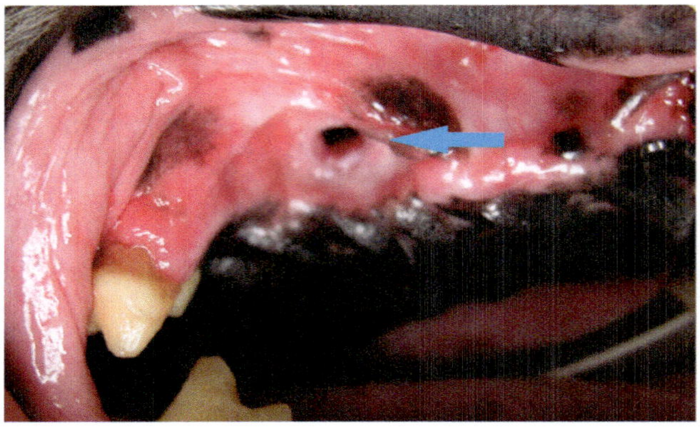

Figure 6.2 (a) Intraoral picture of the maxillary right of a dog with a large oronasal fistula from the extraction of the canine (104). This condition is easily diagnosed on conscious oral exam. Note the scar tissue on the flap (blue arrows), which is the result of four previous surgical attempts to close the fistula. Proper surgical correction of oronasal fistulas is challenging, and thus hands-on instruction is recommended (see appendix 4 for a list of classes). Additionally, there is calculus on the exposed root of the maxillary third incisor (yellow arrow), indicating the chronicity of the condition. This tooth requires extraction as part of the treatment plan. (b) Intraoral picture of the maxillary right of a dog with a large oronasal fistula from the extraction of the fourth premolar (108) (blue arrow). This case demonstrates that care must be taken to properly close all extraction sites.

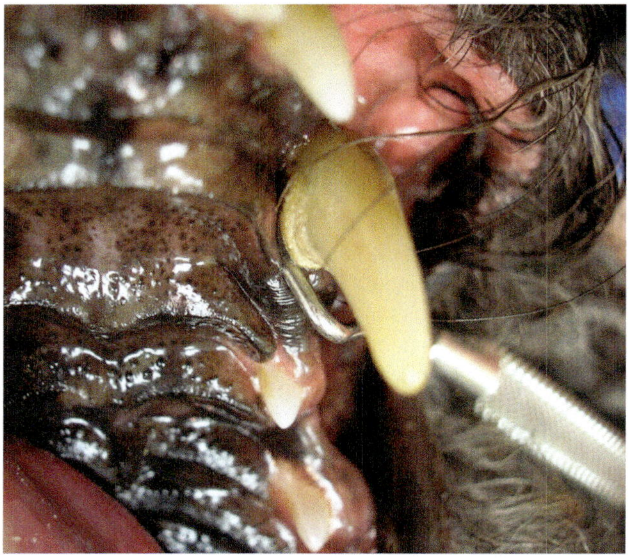

Figure 6.3 Intraoral picture of the maxillary left of a dog with an oronasal fistula of the canine (204). Note that the probe did not reach the bottom of a pocket on the palatine surface of the tooth. Importantly, however, note the lack of gingivitis in this area as well as the surrounding teeth. This again highlights the importance of an anesthetized oral exam in all patients, regardless of outward appearance.

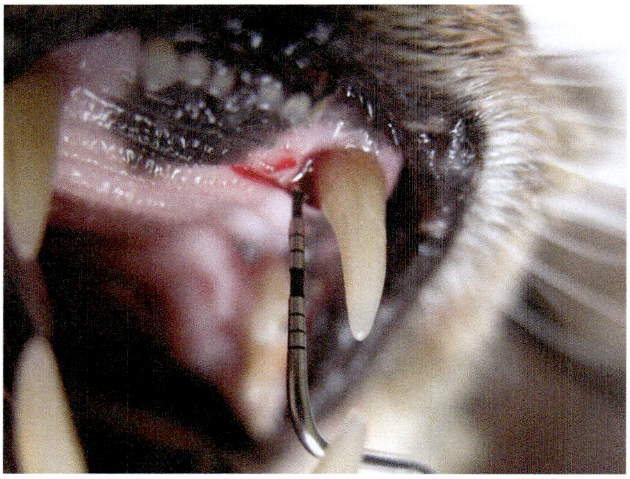

Figure 6.4 Intraoral picture of the maxillary left of a cat with an oronasal fistula of the canine (204). Note the probe is not that deep, but the addition of the gingival recession was sufficient for the creation of an ONF. Note also the lack of gingival inflammation, yet there is bleeding induced by probing. This highlights the importance of an anesthetized oral exam in all patients, regardless of outward appearance.

teeth.[5,9–11] This condition occurs when the periodontal loss progresses apically and gains access to the endodontic system through what used to be the blood supply, thereby causing endodontic disease via bacterial contamination.[10–12] Due to the relative rarity of non-apical ramifications (blood supply other than at the apex) in veterinary patients,[13] these infections typically occur via the apex. The endodontic infection subsequently spreads though the tooth via the common pulp chamber and causes periapical ramifications on the other root(s)

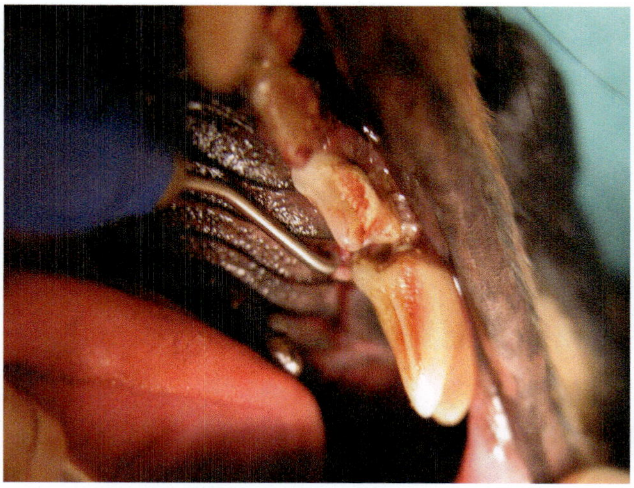

Figure 6.5 Intraoral picture of the maxillary left of a dog with an oronasal fistula of the fourth premolar (208). Note that the probe did not reach the bottom of a pocket on the palatine surface of the tooth.

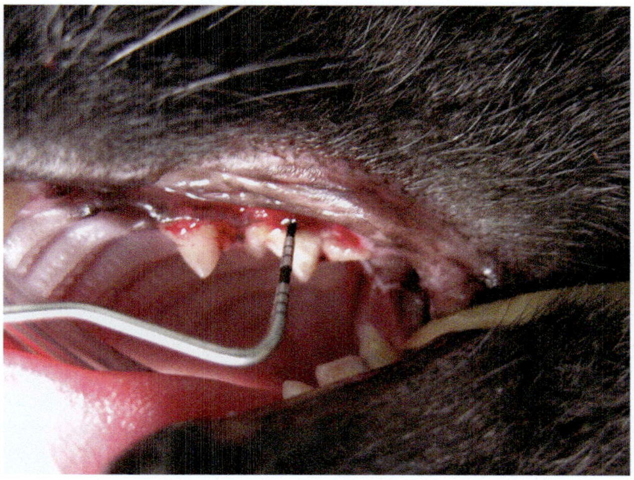

Figure 6.6 Intraoral picture of the left maxillary premolar (208) of a cat with an oronasal fistula.

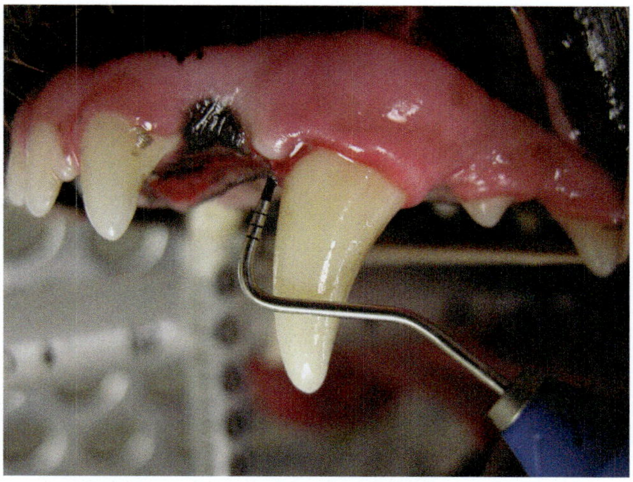

Figure 6.7 Intraoral picture of the maxillary left of a dog with an oronasal fistula of the canine (204). Note the probe is over 9 mm deep on the palatine surface of the tooth; however, the buccal surface of the teeth appears normal. This highlights the importance of an anesthetized oral exam in all patients, regardless of outward appearance.

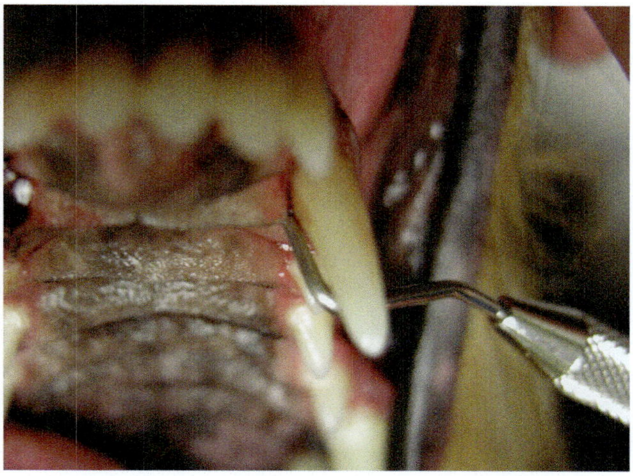

Figure 6.8 Intraoral picture of the maxillary left of a dog with a deep periodontal pocket on the palatal surface of the canine (204). Note the probe is over 9 mm deep on the palatine surface of the tooth but has not entered the nasal cavity yet. This case is likely a good candidate for periodontal flap surgery and guided tissue regeneration. See Chapters 16 and 18.

(Figure 6.9).[11,12] However, the infected tooth may be held in position by the large surface area of the other roots(s).[11]

The most common site for class II perio-endo lesions in small animal patients is the distal root of the mandibular first molar (Figure 6.10), but any multirooted tooth is a candidate.[5] This problem occurs most commonly in older small and toy breed dogs, but this author has treated a case in a Labrador Retriever and also in several patients as young as 3 years of age.

Pathologic fracture

One of the most significant local consequences of periodontal disease is a pathologic jaw fracture.[4,14] These fractures typically occur in the mandible (especially the area of the canines and first molars) due to chronic periodontal loss that weakens the bone in affected areas (Figures 6.11 and 6.12).[5] Again, this condition is more common in small breed dogs,[14] owing mostly to the fact that their teeth (especially the mandibular first molar) are larger in proportion to their mandible in comparison to large breed dogs (Figure 6.13).[15] Therefore, small breed dogs have a very minimal amount of bone apical to the tooth root, putting this area at high risk of fracture when apical

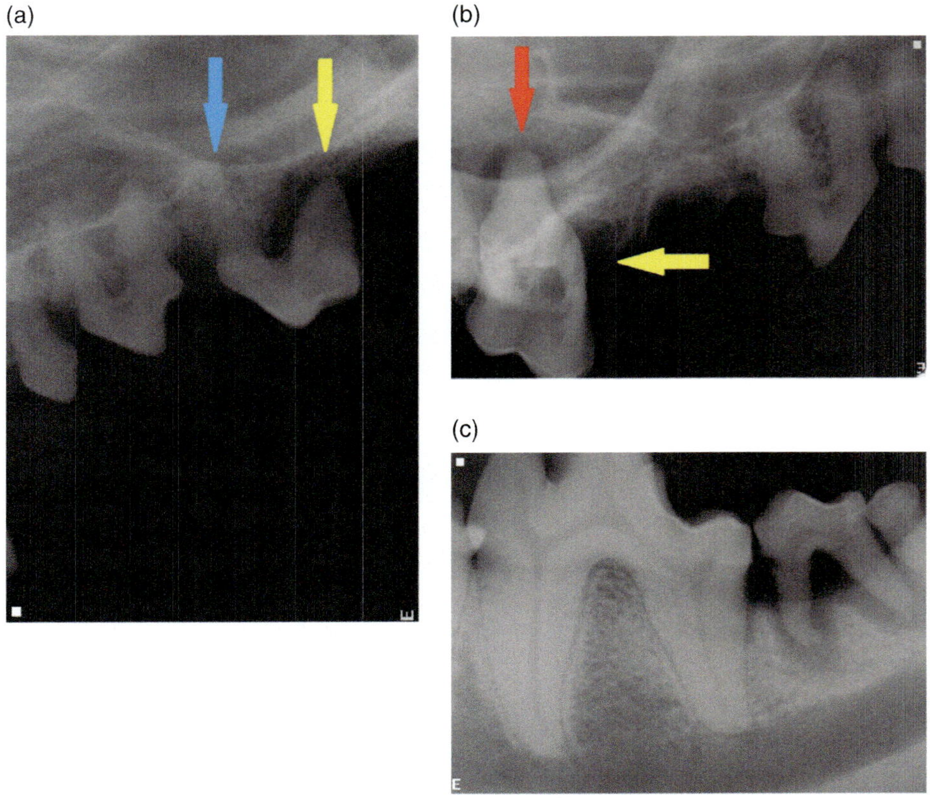

Figure 6.9 Intraoral dental radiographs of class II perio-endo lesions on various teeth. (a) Left maxillary third premolar (207). Note that the endodontic system is exposed and affected (yellow arrow), yet no radiographically identifiable lucency to the mesial root is present at this point (blue arrow). (b) Right maxillary first molar (109) where the periodontal bone loss has caused exposure of the mesial buccal root (yellow arrow). Bacteria entered the endodontic system via the apex of this root and spread to the palatal root, resulting in periapical disease, which is evidenced by the rarefaction (red arrow). Note, this patient was treated for a "carnassial abscess" by the extraction of 108 without radiographs. When the procedure failed, it was referred for radiographs, which documented the cause of the abscess. 108 was likely not the cause of the infection in the first place, and the extraction was unnecessary. This case highlights the need for intraoral dental radiographs in all abscess cases. (c) Severe class II perio-endo lesion of a left mandibular second molar (310). The mesial root was coated in calculus, while the distal root was clean other than granulation tissue.

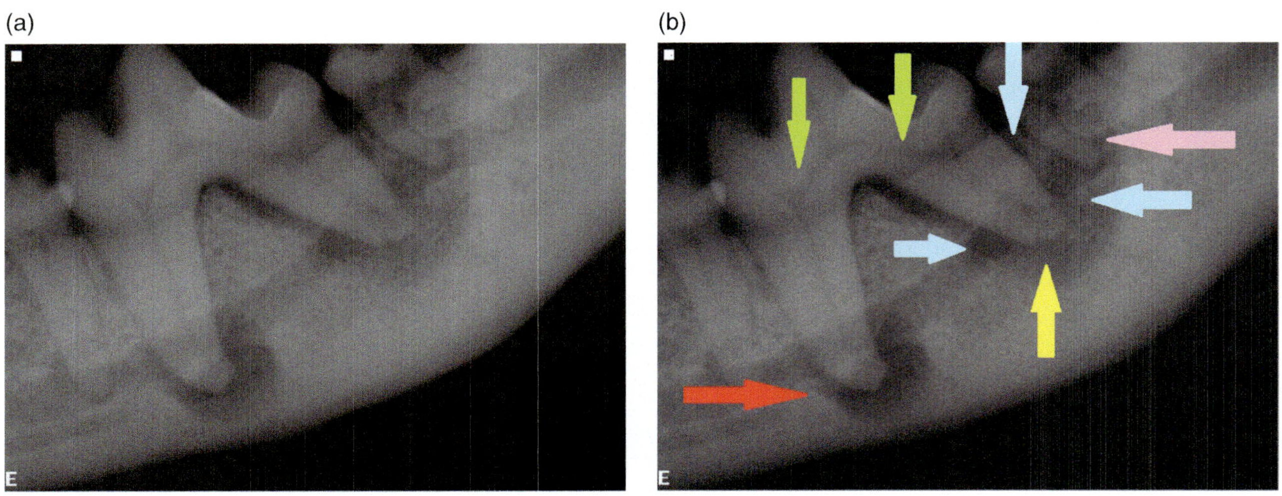

Figure 6.10 (a and b) Intraoral dental radiographs of the mandibular left of a dog revealing the classic appearance and location of a class II perio-endo lesion. The mandibular first molar (309) is affected. These are identical images; (a) is without identifiers to allow for easier viewing. The periodontal disease progressed apically all the way down the distal root (blue arrows) to enter the endodontic system via the apical foramina (yellow arrow). The infection then spread via the common pulp chamber (green arrows), to create infection and rarefaction at the apex of the mesial root (red arrow). Note the mesial root is periodontally healthy (except at the apex) and the mesial area of the furcation is not affected. This patient is a candidate for tooth resection/root canal of the mesial root (after extraction of the distal). See Figure 16.19 and Chapter 19. Finally, note the apex of the mesial root of the second molar (310) appears to be involved (pink arrow).

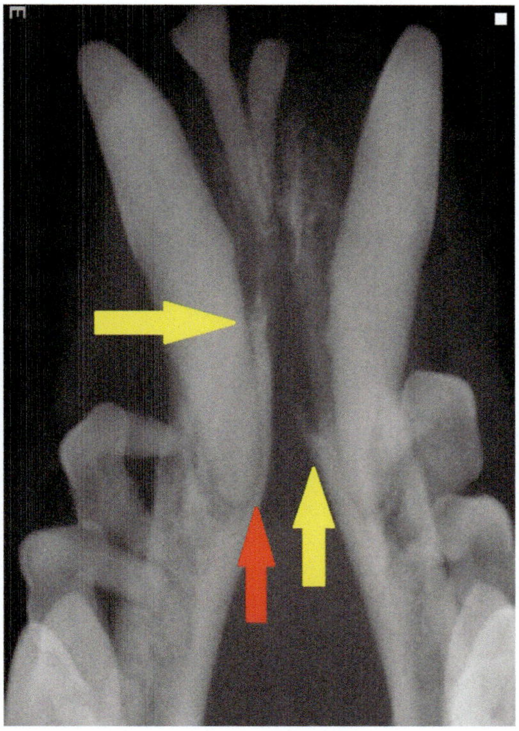

Figure 6.11 Intraoral dental radiograph of the mandibular canines in a dog with advanced periodontal disease. Note the significant amount of bone destruction that has resulted in marked weakening of the alveolar bone (yellow arrows). There is a high risk of fracture of the mandible in these areas. Further note that there is minimal bone around the apex of these teeth (red arrow), which makes extraction of these teeth challenging even in healthy patients.

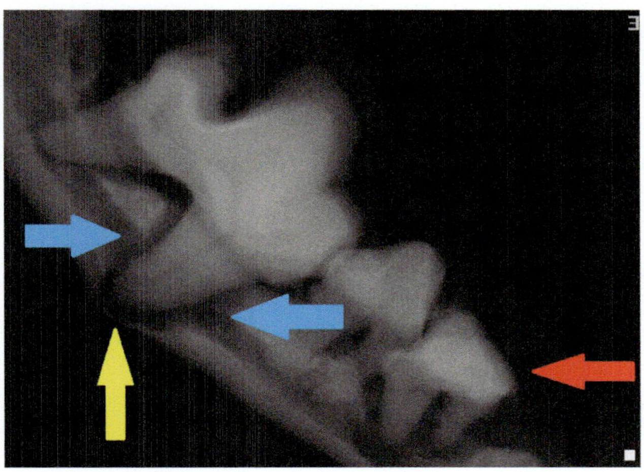

Figure 6.12 Intraoral dental radiograph of the mandibular right in a dog with advanced periodontal disease. Note the significant amount of bone destruction (blue arrows) that has resulted in marked weakening of the alveolar bone in the area of the mesial root of the first molar (409) (yellow arrow). This measured as 0.3 mm of bone. There is a high risk of fracture of the mandible in this area. Further note that the third premolar is completely denuded of bone and is actually being held in only by a "calculus bridge" to the fourth premolar (red arrow). (Reprinted from the "Importance of Dental Radiographs" client educational poster, www.vetdentalrad.com, 2006.)

(a) (b)

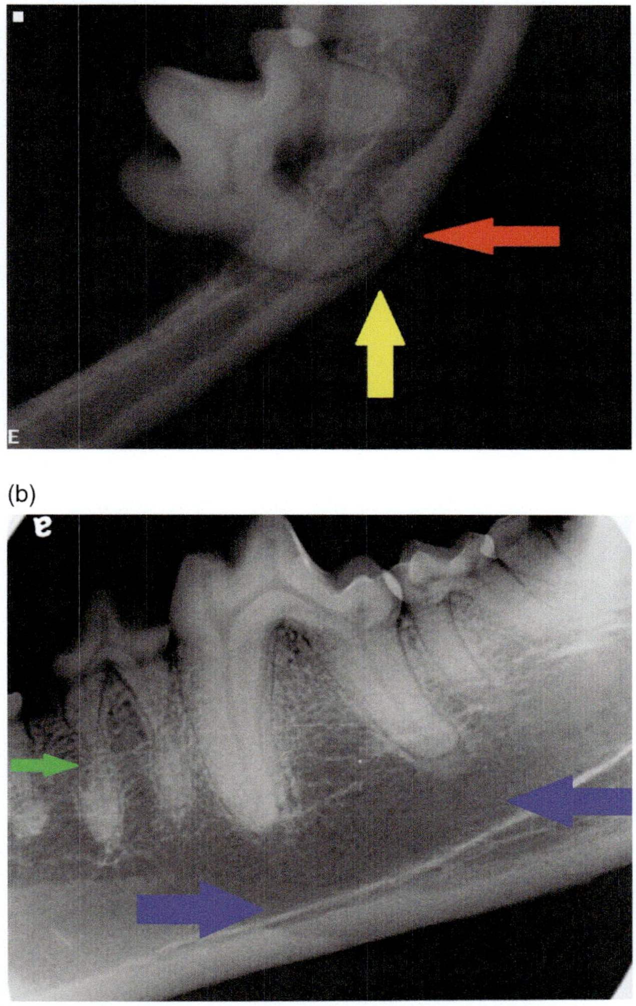

Figure 6.13 Comparison of small/toy and large breed dog mandible. Dental radiographs of the left mandible of (a) a Yorkshire Terrier and (b) a Labrador Retriever. Note the minimal amount (less than 1 mm) of alveolar bone on the ventral cortex of the Yorkshire Terrier at the mesial root of the first molar (yellow arrow). This arrangement predisposes to pathologic mandibular fracture. In contrast, the same area in the Labrador has significant bone ventral to the apex (blue arrows), which would support the jaw even if the alveolar loss continued to the apex. There is an incidental finding of tooth resorption in Figure 6.13b (green arrow). Finally, the mesial root of the Yorkshire Terrier has a significant curve "hook" at the apex (red arrow), which would further complicate the extraction process.

bone loss occurs.[15] In addition, they tend to have more severe periodontal disease than medium to large breed dogs.[16] Finally, small and toy breed dogs tend to enjoy a longer life span than larger breeds, allowing for more advanced periodontal disease in geriatric years.

Pathologic jaw fractures typically occur as a result of mild trauma, and oftentimes during dental

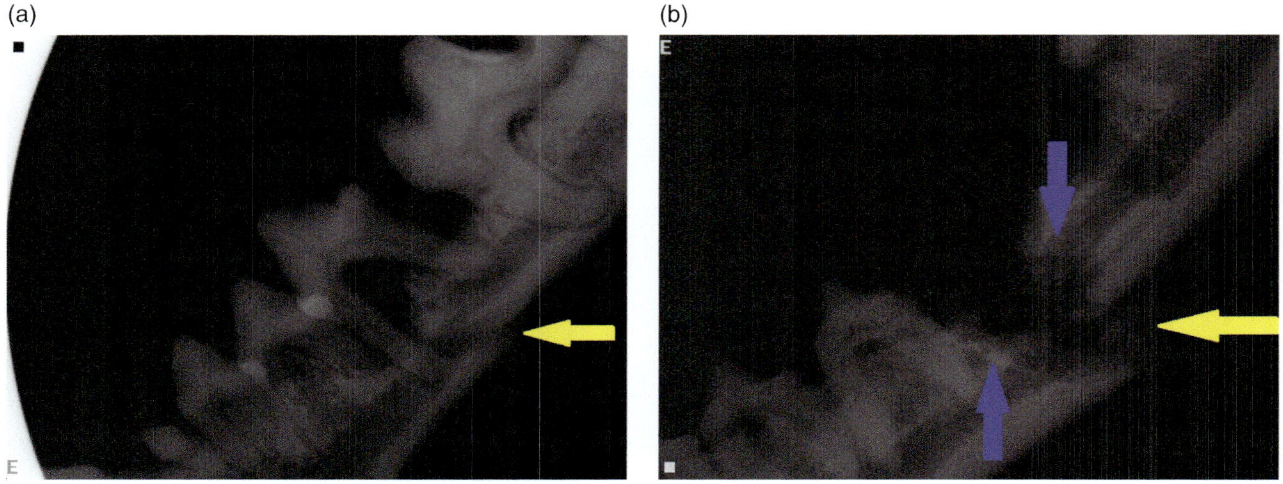

Figure 6.14 (a) Intraoral dental radiograph of the mandibular left of a dog. The mandible was fractured during an extraction attempt of the fourth premolar (308) (yellow arrow). Note that the tooth was not sectioned, which likely contributed to the iatrogenic fracture. (b) Postoperative dental radiograph of the mandibular left of a dog. The mandible was fractured (yellow arrow) during the extraction of the first molar (309). The bone was weakened due to the periodontal disease that is evidenced by the ragged bone in the alveolus of the mesial root (blue arrows).

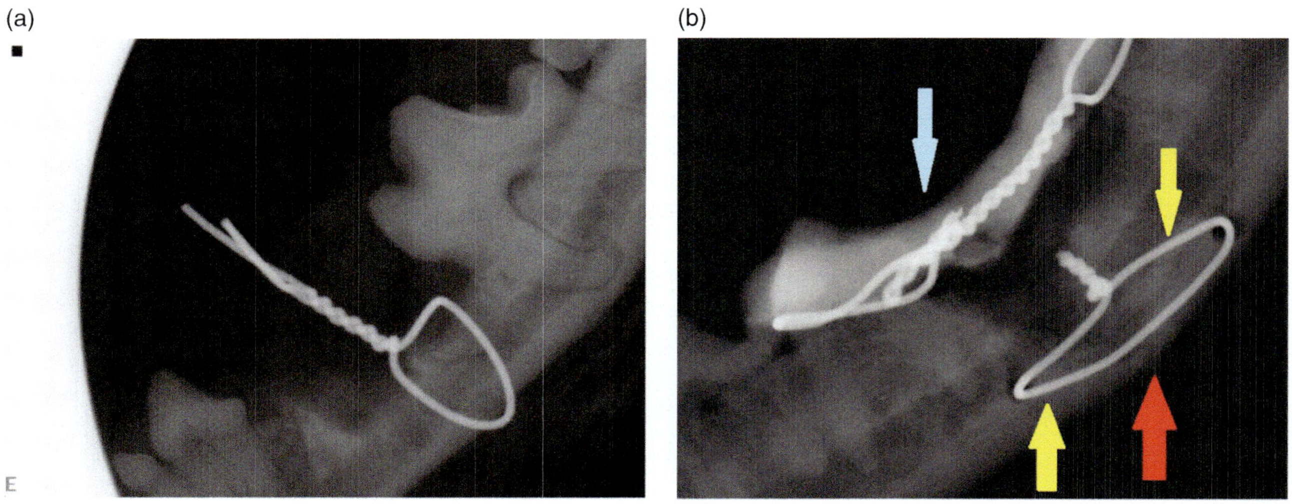

Figure 6.15 (a) Postoperative dental radiograph of the patient in Figure 6.14a. The diseased teeth were extracted, the fracture reduced, and a circummandibular wire used as fixation. Note the reduction is excellent without directly invading the bone. (b) Postoperative dental radiograph of the patient in Figure 6.14b. Due to the large defect, two forms of stabilization were necessary. These consisted of an interosseous wire in the ventral cortex (yellow arrow) and an intraoral acrylic splint (supported with interdental wire) (blue arrow). Note that despite the large bony defect, the reduction is excellent (red arrow). Finally, note that once the diseased teeth were removed, this relatively non-invasive fixation was sufficient for healing, as compared to bone plates and KE apparatus (see Figure 6.16a).

extraction procedures (Figure 6.14). However, some dogs have suffered fractures while simply eating. This is typically considered a disease of older patients, but this author has treated several cases in dogs less than 3 years of age.

Pathologic fractures carry a guarded prognosis for several reasons.[17] Adequate healing is difficult to obtain due to lack of remaining bone, low oxygen tension in the area, and difficulty in rigidly fixating the caudal mandible.[1,5] There are numerous options for fixation, but the use of wires, pins, or plates is generally required (Figure 6.15). Regardless of the method of fixation, the periodontally diseased root(s) *must* be extracted for healing to occur (Figures 6.16 and 6.17).[5,17]

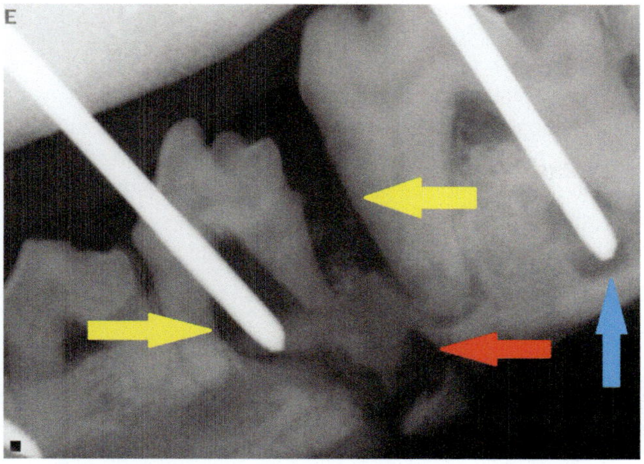

Figure 6.16 Intraoral dental radiograph of the mandibular left in a patient with a bilateral mandibular fracture. This is a recheck radiograph of the *third* KE apparatus placed at a referral surgical facility. Note the significant alveolar bone loss (yellow arrows) as well as the bony sequestra (red arrow) in the surgical area. This fracture would have likely responded to therapy had the diseased tooth/roots been extracted. Finally, note the significant amount of bony damage caused by the distal pin (blue arrow). Veterinary dentists feel that invasive means of fixation for mandibular fractures are typically excessive.

Ocular damage

Another local consequence of severe periodontal disease results from inflammation close to the orbit, which can potentially lead to ocular inflammation, naso-lacrimal disease, retrobulbar abscesses, and possibly *blindness*.[5,20,21] The proximity of the tooth root apices of the maxillary molars and fourth premolars places the delicate optic tissues in jeopardy (Figure 6.20).[21,22] In cats (especially brachycephalic breeds), the apices of the maxillary canine teeth lie in this area and can create similar issues.[5,20] Finally, severe iatrogenic eye trauma can occur during extraction attempts of maxillary molars if care is not taken, which may result in loss of the eye.[22]

Oral cancer

Recent studies in human dentistry have linked chronic periodontal disease to an increased risk of oral cancer (Figure 6.21).[5,23–26] The association in this case is likely due to the chronic inflammatory state that exists with periodontitis. Since neoplasia typically requires a promoter to propagate, it is typically controlled in patients with healthy gingival tissues.[27] The significant inflammation associated with periodontal disease acts as a confounder to the body's defenders, much in the same way that smoking increases the incidence of lung cancer.[28]

Osteomyelitis

Alveolar osteomyelitis is defined as an area of dead, infected bone.[29] Periodontal disease and other dental infections are the most common cause of mandibular or maxillary osteomylitis.[5,17,29] Furthermore, once an area of bone is necrotic, it does not respond effectively to antibiotic therapy.[17,30] This is because the pockets of dead bone and the associated microorganisms are protected from the antibiotics.[31] Therefore, definitive therapy generally requires aggressive surgical debridement of all necrotic tissue.[31–34]

In some cases, the bacterial infection may also result in a septicemia. In one case treated by this author, the

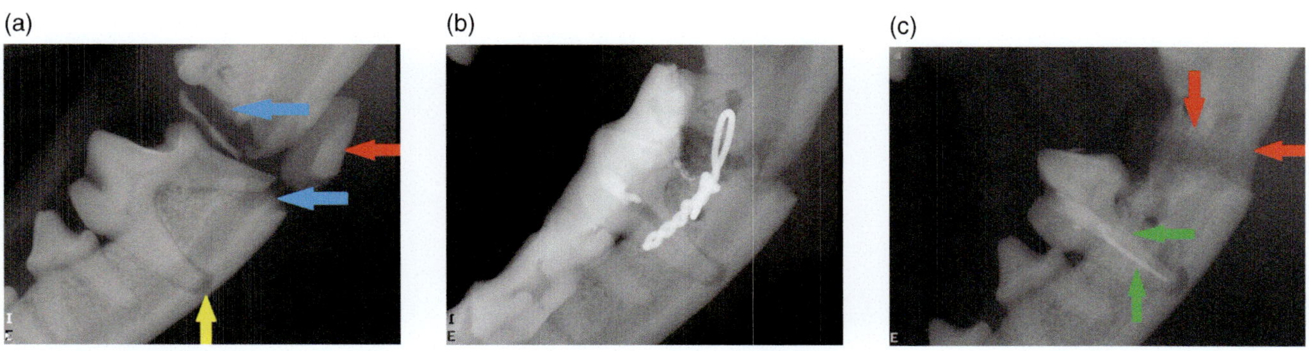

Figure 6.17 Successfully managed pathologic left mandibular fracture. (a) Preoperative dental radiograph revealing a pathologic fracture at the distal aspect of the distal root of the first molar (309) (blue arrows). Also note the small area of periapical rarefaction on the mesial root (yellow arrow). Finally, there are free bone pieces (red arrow). (b) Postoperative image of a case where the tooth has been sectioned and the distal root extracted; the endodontic system of the mesial root cleaned, medicated, and temporarily sealed; and the facture reduced and fixed with an interosseous wire and intraoral acrylic splint. Note that despite the large bony defect, the reduction is adequate. (c) Recheck dental radiograph following splint removal and root canal obturation. Note the excellent reduction and healing (red arrows) and good endodontic obturation (green arrows). The periapical lucency responded to endodontic therapy and was healed at the 6-month recheck.

Box 6.1 Key clinical point

Awareness of the risk of pathologic fractures can help the practitioner to avoid problems in at-risk patients during dental procedures (Figure 6.18). If one root of an affected multirooted tooth is periodontally healthy, there is an even greater chance of mandibular fracture due to the increased force needed to extract the healthy root.[5,11] An alternate form of treatment for these cases is to section the tooth, extract the periodontally diseased root, and perform root canal therapy on the periodontally healthy root (Figure 6.19).[11,12,18,19] In cases where severe alveolar bone loss is noted (especially if the mandibular canine or first molar is affected), it is recommended to inform the owners of the possibility of an iatrogenic jaw fracture prior to attempting extraction of the offending tooth.[5]

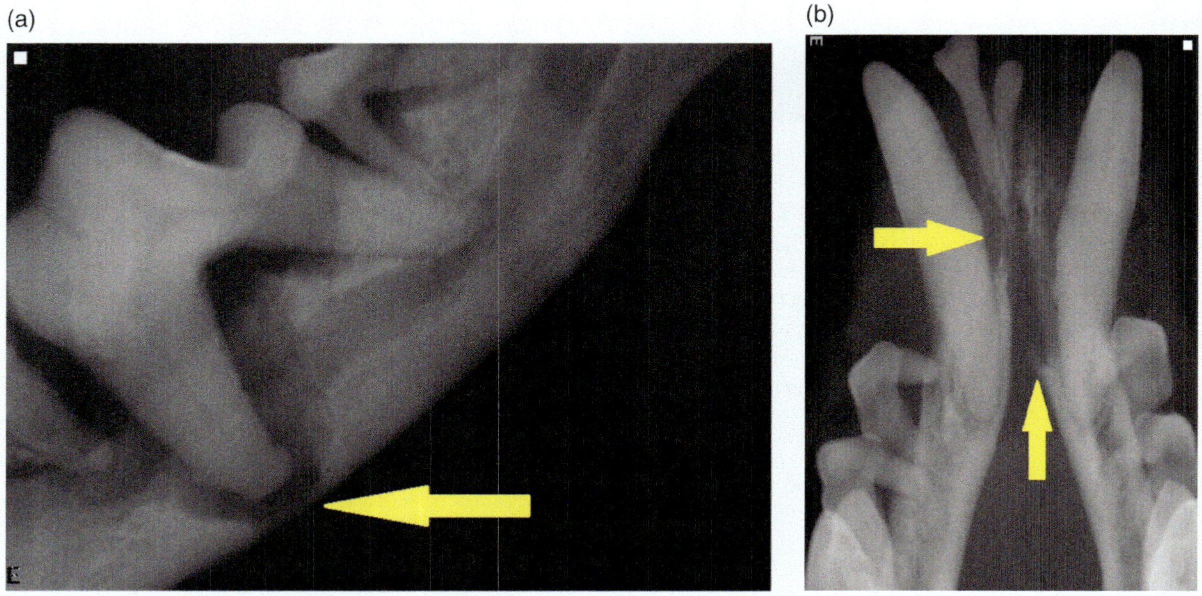

Figure 6.18 Intraoral dental radiographs of canine patients with significant periodontally induced alveolar bone destruction. (a) Left mandibular first molar of a small breed dog with advanced loss on the mesial root. There is less than 1 mm of bone remaining (yellow arrow). (b) Mandibular canine region of a dog, revealing the minimal bony support at the apex of the canine teeth. Both of these areas are at high risk for iatrogenic mandibular fracture during an extraction attempt. Extreme care and patience must be exercised for a positive outcome. Moreover, referral to a veterinary dentist would allow the best opportunity for a successful extraction.

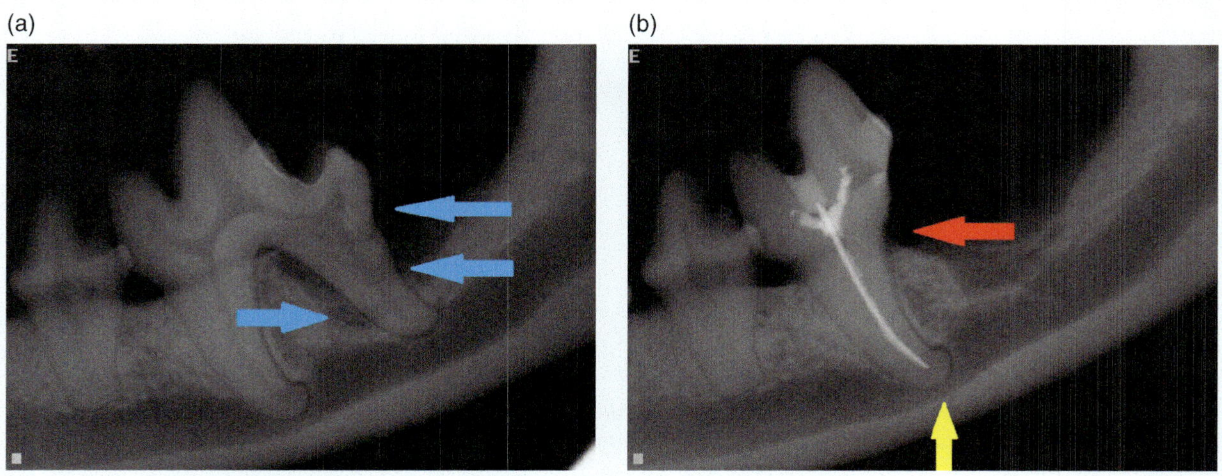

Figure 6.19 (a) Intraoral dental radiograph of a patient with advanced alveolar bone loss on the distal root of the left mandibular first molar (309). Note, there is severe disease to the distal root (blue arrows), while the mesial root is periodontally normal. (b) The 2-year recheck radiograph of the patient who was treated with extraction of the distal root and root canal therapy of the mesial root. Note the relative stability of the periodontal health of the mesial root (red arrow) and lack of periapical rarefaction (yellow arrow) indicating successful therapy.

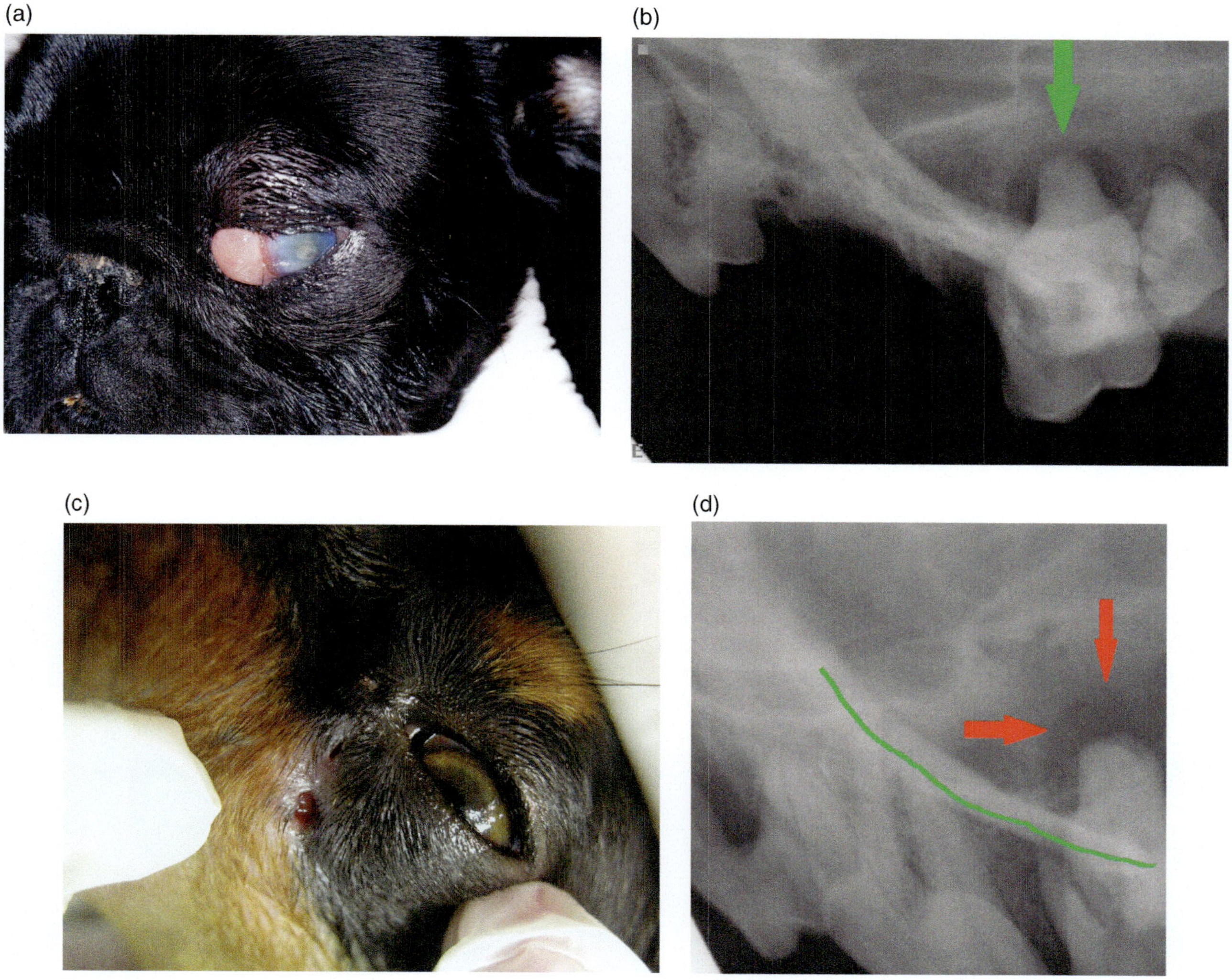

Figure 6.20 (a) Picture of a Pug with a chronic, severe ocular infection and retrobulbar abscess of the left eye. This eventually led to enucleation of the eye. (b) Subsequent dental radiographs (due to continued problems) revealed periapical lucency to the maxillary first molar (209) (green arrow), which caused the facial swelling and likely the ocular infection. (c) Picture of a patient who had a severe and chronic draining abscess below the left eye. (d) Intraoral dental radiograph of the patient in Figure 6.20C, confirming the periapical rarefaction from the first molar (209) (red arrows) at the orbit as outlined by the zygomatic arch (green line). (Figure 6.20 reprinted with permission from Emergency Veterinary Dentistry, Practical Veterinary Publishing, 2012.)

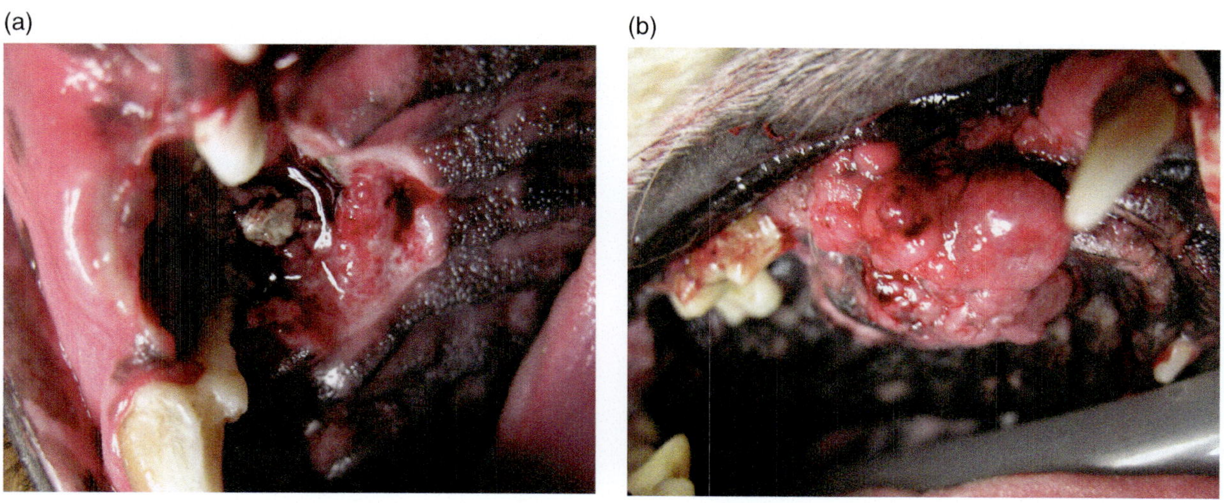

Figure 6.21 (a and b) Intraoral pictures of the maxillary right of two different dogs with significant periodontal disease and oral neoplasia.

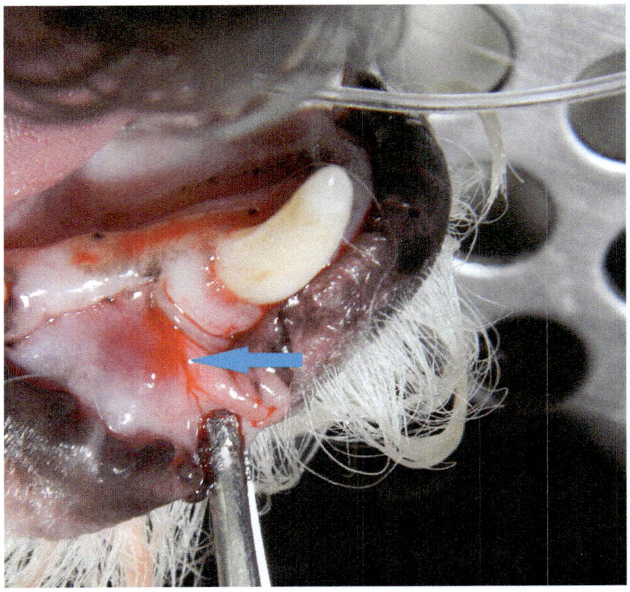

Figure 6.22 Intraoral picture of the small inflammatory/fistulating tract on the mandibular right of a dog with chronic systemic disease. Note that several premolars are missing, but that the area is not inflamed and the canine tooth appears relatively normal.

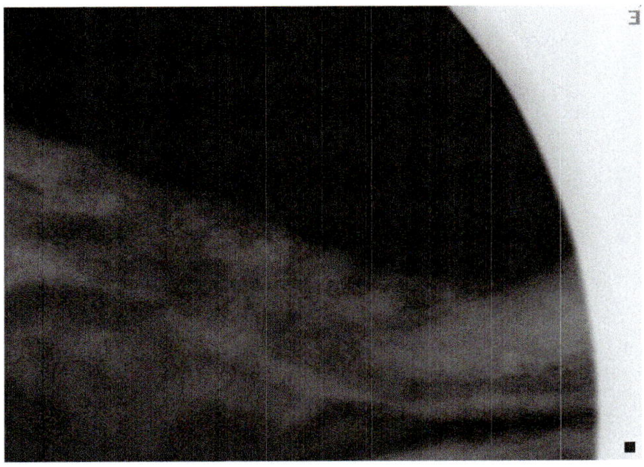

Figure 6.23 Intraoral dental radiograph of the patient in Figure 6.22. Note the significant bony destruction as well as periosteal reaction. Histopathology confirmed the diagnosis of osteomyelitis. Subsequent rostral mandibulectomy proved curative.

(a) (b)

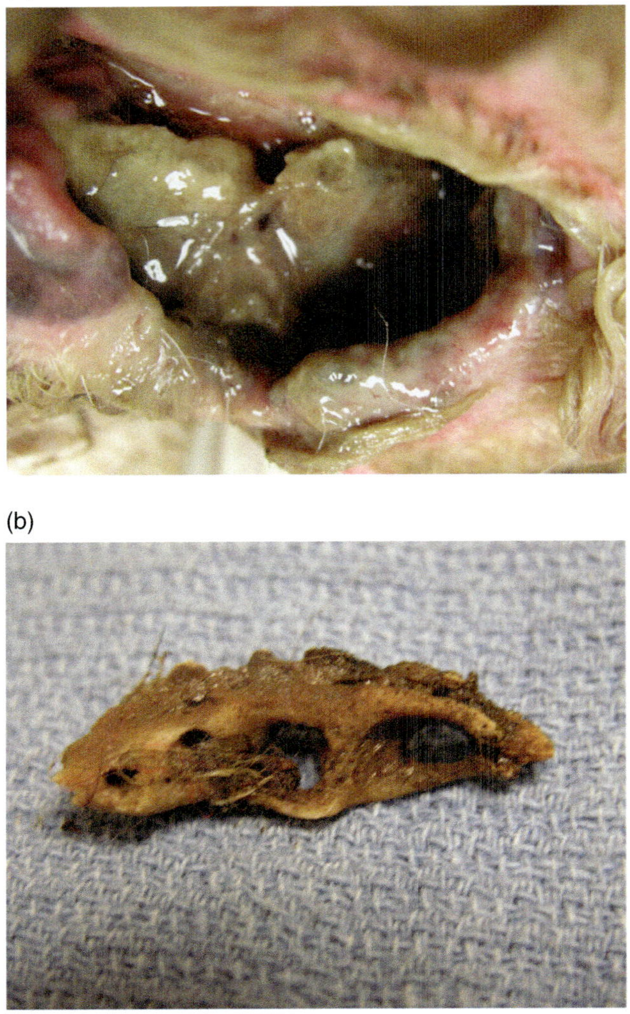

Figure 6.24 (a) Intraoral dental picture of a patient with severe osteomyelitis of the left hemi-mandible. (b) Piece of necrotic bone from the patient in Figure 6.24a. Note that the alveoli are not healed, indicating the bone has been non-vital since the extractions performed 8 months previous.

patient had white blood cell counts of > 50,000 on several occasions, which responded transiently to antibiotics.[35] However, each time the antibiotics were discontinued the infection recurred. On presentation, the patient had halitosis but no obvious dental disease other than a small fistulous tract (Figure 6.22). An intraoral dental radiograph revealed bony proliferation with significantly mottled bone in the area (Figure 6.23), indicative of bony reaction and suspect for osteomyelitis.[31,36] The radiographic appearance prompted aggressive surgical debridement of the necrotic bone. Histopathology was consistent with osteomylitis and following surgery and a course of antibiotics, the patient did not relapse.

In another case treated by this author, the patient presented with an entire hemi-mandible that was necrotic secondary to osteomylitis (Figure 6.24). In this case, the dental radiograph (Figure 6.25) revealed bony proliferation was classic for osteomyelitis,[17] and the patient required a complete mandibulectomy.

Conclusion

Chronic periodontal disease in veterinary patients can have disastrous consequences within the oral cavity. Furthermore, many of these disease processes will not have obvious clinical signs until very late in the disease

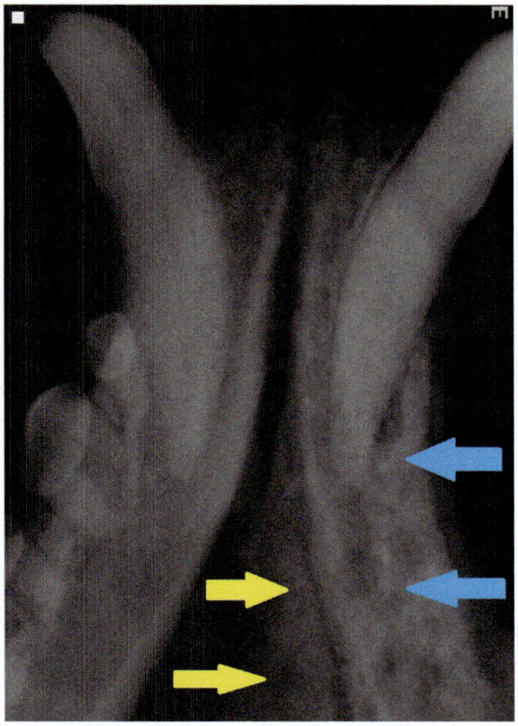

Figure 6.25 Intraoral dental radiograph of the patient in Figure 6.24. Note the significant bony destruction (blue arrows) and periosteal reaction (yellow arrows) on the left side, compared with the normal mandible on the right. A left-sided mandibulectomy proved curative.

course, if ever. Obtaining a definitive diagnosis often requires careful evaluation under general anesthesia. Finally, it is important to note that all of these conditions can be prevented with standard, routine periodontal care. These problems (as well as the systemic issues covered in the next chapter) should be discussed with ALL clients, especially owners of small and toy breed dogs. In fact, a homecare discussion should take place at the initial visit to the practice (e.g., a well puppy exam); don't wait until periodontal disease is established. Appropriate client education should increase compliance with oral health care recommendations and help to avoid these significant disastrous consequences.

Box 6.2 Key points

- Periodontal disease has numerous severe local effects:
  - Oronasal fistulas
  - Class II perio-endo abscesses
  - Pathologic mandibular fracture
  - Eye damage and possible blindness
  - Increased risk of oral cancer
  - Osteomyelitis
- Small and toy breed dogs are most prone; however, any breed as well as cats can suffer from these maladies.
- These are typically, but not exclusively, seen in older patients.
- Use these examples to improve compliance with treatment options.

References

1. Holmstrom SE, Frost P, Eisner ER. Exodontics. In: Veterinary Dental Techniques. 2nd ed. Philadelphia: Saunders, 1998, pp. 215–254.
2. Niemiec BA. Pathologies of the oral mucosa. In: Small Animal Dental, Oral and Maxillofacial Disease, a Color Handbook (Niemiec BA ed.). London: Manson, 2010, pp. 183–198.
3. Marretta SM, Smith MM. Single mucoperiosteal flap for oronasal fistula repair. J Vet Dent. 22(3):200–205, 2005.
4. Debowes LJ. Problems with the gingiva. In: Small Animal Dental, Oral and Maxillofacial Disease, a Color Handbook (Niemiec BA ed.). London: Manson, 2010, pp. 159–181.
5. Niemiec BA. Periodontal disease. Top Companion Anim Med. 23(2):72–80, 2008.
6. Harvey CE, Emily PP. Oral surgery. In: Small Animal Dentistry. St. Louis: Mosby, 1993, pp. 312–377.
7. Marretta SM, Smith MM. Single mucoperiosteal flap for oronasal fistula repair. J Vet Dent, 22(3):200–205, 2005.
8. Wiggs RB, Lobprise HB. Periodontology. In: Veterinary Dentistry, Principles and Practice. Philadelphia: Lippincott-Raven, 1997, pp. 186–231.
9. Wiggs RB, Lobprise HB. Basic endodontic therapy. In: Veterinary Dentistry, Principles and Practice. Philadelphia: Lippincott-Raven, 1997, pp. 280–324.
10. Debowes LJ. Problems with the dental hard tissues. In: Small Animal Dental, Oral and Maxillofacial Disease, a Color Handbook (Niemiec BA ed.). London: Manson, 2010, pp. 159–181.
11. DuPont GG. Problems with the gingiva. In: Small Animal Dental, Oral and Maxillofacial Disease, a Color Handbook (Niemiec BA ed.). London: Manson, 2010, pp. 127–157.
12. Wang HL, Glickman GN. Endodontic and periodontic interrelationships. In: Pathways of the Pulp. St. Louis: Mosby, 2002, pp. 651–664.
13. Gioso MA, Knobl T, Venturini MA, Correa HL. Non-apical root canal ramifications in the teeth of dogs. J Vet Dent. 14(3):89–90, 1997.
14. Mulligan TW, Aller S, Williams CE. Trauma. In: Atlas of Canine and Feline Dental Radiography. Trenton, NJ: Veterinary Learning Systems, 1998, pp. 176–183.
15. Gioso MA, Shofer F, Barros PS, Harvery CE. Mandible and mandibular first molar tooth measurements in dogs: Relationship of radiographic height to body weight. J Vet Dent. 18(2):65–68.
16. Bellows J. Equipping the dental practice. In: Small Animal Dental Equipment, Materials, and Techniques, a Primer. Ames, IA: Blackwell, 2004, pp. 13–55.
17. Taney KG, Smith MM. Problems with muscles, bones, and joints. In: Small Animal Dental, Oral and Maxillofacial Disease, a Color Handbook (Niemiec BA ed.). London: Manson, 2010, pp. 199–204.
18. Wiggs RB, Lobprise HB. Advanced endodontic therapy. In: Veterinary Dentistry, Principles and Practice. Philadelphia: Lippincott-Raven, 1997, pp. 325–350.
19. Niemiec BA. Treatment of mandibular first molar teeth with endodontic-periodontal lesions in a dog. J Vet Dent. 18(1):21–26, 2001.
20. Anthony JMG, Sammeyer LS, Laycock AR. Vet Opthamol. 13:106–109, 2010.

21. Ramsey DT, Marretta SM, Hamor RE, et al. Ophthalmic manifestations and complications of dental disease in dogs and cats. J Am Anim Hosp Assoc. 32(3):215–224, 1996.
22. Smith MM, et al. Orbital penetration associated with tooth extraction. J Vet Dent. 20(1):8–17, 2003.
23. Rosenquist K. Risk factors in oral and oropharengeal squamous cell carcinoma: A population-based case-control study in southern Sweden. Swed Dent J Suppl. 179:1–66, 2005.
24. Rosenquist K, Wennerberg J, Schildt EB, et al. Oral status, oral infections and some lifestyle factors for oral and oropharengeal squamous cell carcinoma. A population-based case-controlled study in southern Sweden. Acta Otolaryngol. 125(12):1327–1336, 2005.
25. Zheng TZ, Boyle P, Hu HF, et al. Dentition, oral hygiene, and risk of oral cancer: A case-control study in Beijing, People's Republic of China. Cancer Causes Control. 1:235–241, 1990.
26. Graham S, Dayal H, Rohrer T, et al. Dentition, diet, tobacco, and alcohol in the epidemiology of oral cancer. J Natl Cancer Inst. 59:1611–1618, 1977.
27. Trosko JE. Commentary: Is the concept of "tumor promotion" a useful paradigm? Mol Carcinog. 30:131–137, 2001.
28. Jerbi G, et al. Melanoma arising in burn scars: Report of three observations and literature review. Arch Dermatol. 135:1551–1553, 1999.
29. Wiggs RB, Lobprise HB. Veterinary Dentistry, Principles and Practice. Philadelphia: Lippincott-Raven, 1997, pp. 128, 163.
30. Bubenik LJ, Smith MM. Orthopaedic infections. In: Textbook of Small Animal Surgery (Slatter DH ed.). 3rd ed. Philadelpia: Saunders, 2003, pp. 1862–1875.
31. Neville BW, Damm DD, Allen CM, Bouquot JE. Pulpal and periapical disease. In: Oral and Maxillofacial Pathology. 2nd ed. Philadelphia: Saunders, 2002, pp. 107–137.
32. Lu JD, Wang XD, Shen GF. Diagnosis and treatment of osteopetrosis complicated by osteomyelitis in maxilla and mandible: Report of two cases. Shanghai Kou Yi Xue. 16(5): 551–554, 2007.
33. Prasad KC, Prasad SC, Mouli N, Agarwal S. Osteomyelitis of the head and neck. Acta Otolaryngol. 127(2):194–205, 2007.
34. Verstraete FM. In: Textbook of Small Animal Surgery (Slatter DH ed.). 3rd ed. Philadelpia: Saunders, 2003.
35. Niemiec BA. Osteomyelitis secondary to periodontal disease. Proceedings of the American Veterinary Dental Forum. Albuquerque, NM, 2000.
36. Mulligan, T Aller, S, and Williams, C. Atlas of Canine and Feline Dental Radiography. Trenton, NJ: Veterinary Learning Systems, 1998, pp. 176–183.

7

Systemic manifestations of periodontal disease

Introduction

Infections of the teeth and the periodontium have long been thought to have a negative effect throughout the body. It was reported that Hippocrates cured a patient of arthritis by extracting an infected tooth.[1] This theory was first proposed by a British physician, William Hunter, in 1900.[2] Following this, Frank Billings introduced the concept of focal infections to American physicians.[3] Since then, the role of oral infections in regard to systemic health has been accepted as well as rejected, depending on the current state of research.[4,5] Recent research, however, utilizing the evidence-based approach has accepted several systemic ramifications of periodontal disease. While true cause-and-effect studies may be minimal, the correlations and connections are numerous and convincing. These conditions have been well documented in both human and animal studies. While the majority of studies have involved human patients, we can expect correlations to generally hold true for our animal patients. (In fact, there are many medical beliefs held for humans that have been extrapolated from animal studies in the same fashion.)

Prevalence of periodontal disease

Periodontal disease is the number one diagnosed medical problem in small animal veterinary patients.[6,7] In fact, by 2 years of age, 80% of dogs and 70% of cats have some form of periodontal disease.[8] Small and toy breed dogs are particularly susceptible.[9] Furthermore, it has been shown that even the most complete periodontal treatment (ranging from a thorough dental prophylaxis to periodontal surgery) cannot reliably eradicate infection.[10] Finally, this high level of dental expertise is currently rare within general practices.

Even after the teeth are completely cleaned during a dental prophylaxis, bacteria start colonizing the tooth surfaces within *seconds*,[11] and mature plaque forms on the tooth surfaces *within 24 hours*, growing rapidly for the first 4 days.[8,12] In humans, Cessation of homecare for as little as 1 week can result in gingivitis in some patients, and after 3 weeks leads to gingivitis in all patients.[13] Furthermore, some authors report that gingivitis (at least histologic if not clinical) may occur after only a few days of missed homecare.[14,15] Finally, one veterinary study found that pockets were reinfected within 2 weeks of a dental cleaning if homecare was not performed.[16]

These findings prove that professional cleanings alone are grossly insufficient for periodontal disease control. They also illustrate that the periodontium is often continually inflamed, in turn allowing for almost consistent systemic infections. Based on this information, it can be inferred that the majority of veterinary patients are infected at least 50 weeks a year *if annual cleanings are performed* (which is often not the case). This is certainly not an acceptable level of disease control. Therefore, we should strive to educate our clients on the importance of consistent and effective homecare as well as professional care.

Pathogenesis of systemic effects

White blood cells and other inflammatory mediators migrate out of the periodontal soft tissues and into the periodontal space due to increased vascular permeability and increased space between the crevicular epithelial cells.[17] The bacteria within the gingival sulcus therefore gain ready access to the bloodstream via the inflamed sulcular epithelium. The inflammatory response of the gingival and periodontal tissues allows the body's

Veterinary Periodontology, First Edition. Brook A. Niemiec.

defenses to attack the invaders but also allows these bacteria to gain access to the body.[5,8,18,19] In fact, the subgingival microbiota in animals with active periodontitis provides a *significant and consistent* gram-negative challenge to the host.[19] Not only are the bacteria themselves allowed access but also their inflammatory mediators such as lipopolysaccharide (LPS). These bacteria and their byproducts can have severe deleterious effects throughout the body.[20,21] In addition to the bacteria themselves and their toxic byproducts, distant effects can also occur secondary to the activation of the patient's own inflammatory mediators such as cytokines (e.g., IL-1 and 6, PGE2, and TNF).[5,22–25] These mediators have been linked to numerous systemic problems such as cardiovascular, hepatic, and renal insults.[22,26,27] It is reported that human patients with periodontal disease are 4 times more likely to have multiple (three or more) systemic maladies than those in good periodontal health.[28] It is also critical to note that even low grade gingivitis (i.e., no periodontal loss) is sufficient to create systemic consequences.

The subgingival area provides a large surface area for bacterial exposure. In humans, it has been estimated that the surface area of the sulcal epithelium in patients with active disease is equal to the size of the palm of the hand and is even larger with deepening pockets.[29] The greater proportional size of the oral cavity and tooth roots of animal patients (particularly dogs and especially small and toy breeds)[30] creates a significant increase in the surface area for bacterial ingress. This fact, combined with the increased incidence of periodontal disease in these species,[31] means periodontal infections likely represent a more severe issue in our patients than in the vast majority of humans. Furthermore, it appears that these changes intensify with increasing periodontal disease burden.[22] These oral inflammatory repercussions are even more of a problem in toy and small breed dogs.[32,33]

A purulent infection equal to the size of the palm of your hand on a visible portion of your body or a proportionally sized infection on the flank of a dog or cat would cause significant concern for the average person, resulting in an immediate visit to the clinic and prompt definitive therapy. Periodontal disease should be viewed with the same degree of respect since it is a significant gram-negative and anaerobic infection capable of severe inflammation and potential systemic spread of these dangerous microorganisms. However, since the oral cavity is rarely scrutinized by owners or veterinarians, and no more than a cursory evaluation can be performed without general anesthesia, periodontal disease is drastically underdiagnosed. Furthermore, the lack of any outward clinical signs (in animals *and* humans) often results in significantly delayed therapy. Therefore, periodontal disease has been called "The Silent Killer."[10] Ignoring the periodontal health of our pets and patients can be likened to ostriches putting their head in the sand to avoid a lion. The lion (just like periodontal disease) is still lurking regardless of it being recognized.

Furthermore, we know that periodontal therapy (from homecare to professional scaling) results in transient bacteremia. However, daily activities such as chewing can also create these inflammatory states.[34] As a matter of fact, daily activities such as mastication and tooth brushing in humans result in *more* bacteremia than does a professional cleaning.[35–37]

> **Box 7.1** Key clinical point
>
> Avoiding professional cleanings in patients who are particularly susceptible to the negative effects of bacteremias (such as pets with diabetes mellitus, renal or hepatic disease, or heart murmurs/low-grade heart disease) is ***not*** good medicine. As a matter of fact, there is significant evidence supporting the fact that these patients should be even more strongly encouraged to undergo professional dental therapy, because of the health benefits it will provide.[38–42]

Affected organs/systems

Liver and kidneys

The hepatic and renal systems are responsible for filtering the blood. When oral bacteremias occur, the bacteria may settle in these organs. Once within the parenchyma, bacteria may go on to create microabscesses or cause other inflammatory changes in these organs. The bacterial invasion of the liver has been shown to increase parenchymal inflammation and portal fibrosis.[26] Furthermore, bacteremias have been shown to cause cholestasis in dogs,[43,44] and one study showed a significant relationship between the periodontal disease burden and increased inflammation in the hepatic parenchyma.[22]

Periodontopathogenic bacteria appear to have an affinity for endothelium. Renal filtration places them in direct contact with endothelium and therefore significantly increases the likelihood of the glomerular capillary walls being affected.[45–48] Chronic infectious and inflammatory diseases have been shown to contribute to the formation of immune complexes in the kidney, resulting in glomerulonephritis.[31] Once these immune complexes are formed, they appear to self-propagate the inflammation by stimulating the production of other bioactive mediators such as cytokines, growth factors, and nitric acid.[49] They may also stimulate increased intra- and extracellular matrix filaments and proteins, causing further parenchymal changes.[50,51] These changes can lead to chronic inflammation and secondary scarring of the organ, resulting in decreased function over time.[22,25,26,52,53]

Finally, and perhaps most importantly, there is evidence to suggest that periodontal therapy improves renal function. Studies have shown that periodontal therapy improves glomerular filtration rate in healthy as well as predialysis renal patients.[39,54] It is possible that periodontal therapy may provide benefits to other organs as well, but more research is needed in this area. In any case, this is significant evidence to support the importance of providing proper dental care to patients with mild to moderate organ dysfunction.

Heart

Periodontal disease has been linked to significant changes in the cardio-pulmonary system. Several studies have suggested that oral bacteria can adhere to previously damaged heart valves (i.e., valvular dysplasia), leading to endocarditis.[55,56] There are also veterinary studies that have noted a significant increase in the incidence of atrio-ventricular valve changes with periodontal disease.[22,57] In fact, one report showed the risk of endocarditis at approximately six-fold higher for dogs with stage 3 periodontal disease, compared with the risk for dogs without periodontal disease.[57] Vegetative endocarditis can result in intermittent infections and potentially thromboembolic disease with disastrous sequela.[55,56,58] These types of vegetative lesions have been cultured, and the results found many of the same bacteria that inhabit the oral cavity.[57,59,60] One study that evaluated the bacterial component of atheromatous plaques found that 44% of the plaques were positive for a periodontal pathogen.[61] This condition was classically blamed on dental procedures, but recent studies report that even normal activities such as eating are sufficient to create a bacteremia.[34–36] Furthermore, it was found that the majority of endocarditis cases in humans and dogs were not associated with a recent dental procedure.[62,63]

Hypertrophic cardiomyopathy is a fairly common occurrence in older feline patients. Periodontal disease may affect this disease process, as it has been shown to be associated with left ventricular hypertrophy.[27] These negative changes are even more common in patients with hypertension.[64,65] One veterinary study has also revealed a possible link between periodontal disease and cardiomyopathies in dogs.[57] Furthermore, it has been demonstrated in humans that the endothelial function of the heart muscle is negatively affected by periodontal disease.[66] Finally, this same study reported an improvement in endothelial function following periodontal therapy.

While ischemic heart disease is not a common problem in veterinary patients, numerous studies have linked periodontal disease and oral bacteremias to myocardial infarctions and other histological changes in humans.[27,45,57,67–71] The incidence of cardiac disease increases with the severity and scope of the periodontal infection,[45] and the endothelial function of the heart muscle is negatively affected by periodontal disease.[66] Finally, periodontal disease is reported to be associated with hypertension in humans.[73]

Ischemic heart disease in humans is precipitated by the process of atherogenesis and thrombogenesis. These conditions are enhanced by increased blood viscosity,[74] which in turn is promoted by systemic infections such as periodontal disease.[75] Fibrinogen is likely to be the most important factor in inciting this hypercoagulable state, and elevations of fibrinogen along with other coagulation factors are seen secondary to periodontal disease.[75] A correlation between periodontal disease and thrombogenesis was found in a study that linked periodontal disease with increased aggregation of platelets via platelet aggregation-associated protein (PAAP) expressed by some periodontal pathogens.[76] In fact, the simple infusion of these bacteria resulted in alterations of physical parameters (such as heart rate, blood pressure, and ECG) consistent with a myocardial infarction.[77] An additional link between periodontal and cardiac disease was provided by studies evaluating the increased level of C-reactive protein[78] as well as other inflammatory markers in association with periodontal disease and its increased incidence in patients with myocardial infarctions.[79–83] These studies provide evidence for the level of systemic inflammation caused by periodontal disease. These findings were further supported by a study that found a direct correlation between decreased tooth brushing frequency and increased incidence of cardiovascular events.[84] Moreover, they found that human patients who brushed their teeth less than twice daily had a 70% increase in the risk rate of heart disease.[84] Finally, there are studies that found periodontal infections to directly cause atherosclerosis in pigs and mice.[85,86]

Lungs

We often do not think about periodontal disease affecting the lungs, but several studies have linked this disease to an increased incidence of chronic respiratory disease (COPD) as well as pneumonia.[28,87–91] Chronic infection of the lungs is thought to occur from the constant inhalation of high numbers of oral bacteria. This type of infection ultimately results in areas of scarring within the lungs (similar to that caused by chronic smoking), leading to bronchitis and emphysema.[19]

While there is no current evidence that periodontal disease affects the incidence of acute respiratory diseases in healthy patients, oral infections are known to exacerbate chronic respiratory diseases.[91] Furthermore, proper oral care has been shown to decrease the incidence of acute exacerbations of chronic respiratory disease,[92] and controlling oral bacteria decreases opportunistic respiratory infections.[93–95]

Hospital-acquired (nosocomial) respiratory infections are also a significant problem (especially in severely ill and ventilator patients),[19,96] resulting in 20–50% mortality in human patients.[97] The oral cavity is the typical reservoir for pulmonary pathogens, and decontamination of the oropharynx has been shown to decrease these types of infections.[98–100] Moreover, the utilization of oral antiseptics such as chlorhexidine gluconate, as well as the mechanical action of tooth brushing, has the ability to decrease nosocomial infections.[101] Therefore, ECC and ICU staff should take oral health status into consideration when formulating treatment plans for severely ill patients, especially those who are immune suppressed or on ventilators.

While typically seen with critically ill and especially long-term ventilator patients, even relatively healthy patients are at risk for intubation-induced pneumonia. This is due to several factors, including introduction of oropharyngeal bacteria into the trachea, bypassing the natural protection of the trachea, loss of macrophages, and possible mucosal damage/inflammation.[102–105] While the incidence of pneumonia is positively related to the duration of intubation, it can occur with even short surgical procedures.[104,106] Therefore, it is recommended to decrease the level of oral pathogens via oral antiseptic rinsing (e.g., chlorhexidine) whenever intubation is planned.[107,108]

Brain

Ischemic cerebral infarctions (or strokes) are often proceeded by a systemic infection.[109] In addition, those with a prestroke infection suffer more significant neurologic deficits than those without.[110] Poor dental health will contribute to strokes in the same fashion it does with myocardial disease (i.e., increased thrombotic events, C-reactive protein, and blood viscosity).[111] In fact, poor dental health was shown to have a very strong influence on cerebral ischemic events, even more so than smoking.[45,112,113] Therefore, proper periodontal care should decrease the incidence and severity of this disease process. While the incidence of cerebral infarction in animal patients is unknown, it does occur and therefore it is helpful to know that good dental health may aid in its prevention.

Other deleterious effects

Diabetes mellitus

Numerous studies have established a strong link between diabetes and increased periodontal disease, as well as between periodontal disease and an increase in insulin resistance.[28,114–118] This makes sense, as any acute infection (bacterial or viral) will increase insulin resistance and worsen glycemic control, even in non-diabetic patients.[119–121] This means that periodontal disease lends to not only poor diabetic control but, maybe more importantly, to the increased severity of diabetic complications (wound healing, microvascular disease) as well as cardiac and renal disease.[122–128] In contrast, proper therapy of periodontal disease (professional periodontal therapy, selected extractions, and homecare) may actually improve glycemic control and decrease insulin requirements.[82,112,129–133] These gains appear to be enhanced by the addition of systemic antibiotic therapy with doxycycline for 2 weeks following the dental scaling and root planing.[134] This may be due to the fact that systemic antibiotics help clear residual bacteria from the periodontium. Finally, periodontal health is improved in patients with good diabetic control.[127,135] While there are no published veterinary studies to this effect, there is significant anecdotal evidence that supports periodontal therapy as a means to improve glycemic control. In fact, this author has several feline patients who no longer needed insulin therapy after dental treatment.

It is also reported that diabetes is actually a risk factor for periodontal disease.[136–142] This is explained by the fact that diabetes weakens the immune system, thereby increasing susceptibility to the disease process.[143–146] Periodontal disease and diabetes are therefore viewed as having a bidirectional interrelationship, wherein each one worsens the other.[147–150]

Malignancies

As stated in the last chapter, periodontal disease has been implicated as a risk factor for oral neoplasia. Additionally, recent studies are proposing a link between periodontal disease and distant neoplasia such as gastrointestinal,[151,152] kidney, pancreatic,[153–155] and hematological cancers.[156] While these reports are far from definitive due to the large number of confounding factors,[157] it makes sense to address and control periodontal inflammation when possible.

Adverse pregnancy effects

Oral bacteremias can cross the placental membrane,[158–160] allowing the bacteria to directly affect the fetus. Several studies have found periodontal infections to be

Box 7.2 Early mortality

A strikingly significant indicator of the degree to which periodontal disease affects overall health is demonstrated in mortality studies. When all other risk factors are ruled out, periodontal disease has been shown to be a significant predictor of early mortality in human beings.[175–177] In fact, one study reported that severe periodontal disease is a higher risk factor than smoking![178]

associated with an increased incidence of adverse pregnancy effects, such as pre-ecclampsia and low birth weight.[161–163] In contrast, proper dental care can help to reduce the rate of preterm births.[164–166] While not a concern for the majority of veterinary patients, this information may be critical for veterinary theriogenologists and their clients, especially breeders of small and toy breed dogs. In any event, it provides further evidence of the significance of periodontal disease as it relates to overall health.

Chronic inflammation

It has been proven that periodontal disease can elicit an increase in inflammatory lipids as well as an overall lipidemic state.[5,23,25,166,167] This is described as a state of overall body inflammation leading to chronic disease processes and an abnormal immune response.[169–172] Furthermore, periodontal therapy can decrease the level of circulating inflammatory products and improve endothelial function.[67,173,174]

Conclusion

While some of the aforementioned studies are not definitive,[19,101] we surely know that periodontal disease is an infectious process that requires affected patients to deal with dangerous bacteria on a daily basis, leading to a state of chronic disease.[179,180] Therefore, we must learn to view periodontal disease as not merely a dental problem that causes bad breath and tooth loss, but as an initiator of more severe systemic consequences. As one human text states, "Periodontitis is a gram-negative infection resulting in severe inflammation, with potential intravascular dissemination of microorganisms throughout the body."[19] This is echoed by an additional author who states: "Periodontal disease is clearly an important and potentially life threatening condition, often underestimated by health professionals and the general public."[181] Only by thinking in these terms can we fully appreciate the scope of this disease process and discuss the problem with clients, so they may understand and appreciate the depth of the problems this disease can cause for their pets. Effectively sharing this information will significantly increase client compliance with homecare and dental prophylaxis, as well as approval of advanced dental procedures for their pets. Consequently, the most important weapon in the fight against periodontal disease in the veterinary field is simple client education.

Box 7.3 Key points

- Periodontal disease has been associated with numerous systemic maladies including cardiopulmonary disease, renal and hepatic malfunction, neoplasia, and diabetes mellitus.
- Systemic changes may be at least somewhat reversible with periodontal therapy.
- Humans with poor periodontal health have a decreased life span.
- While typically thought to be associated with severe periodontal disease, gingivitis is sufficient to cause harmful systemic effects.
- There is significant evidence supporting the fact that patients with any systemic disease benefit from proper dental therapy.

References

1. Francke OC. William Hunter's oral sepsis and American odontology. Bull Hist Dent. 21(2):73–79, 1973.
2. Neuman HN. Focal infection. J Dent Res. 75:1912, 1996.
3. Billings F. Chronic focal infections and their etiologic relations to arthritis and nephritis. Arch Int Med. 9:484–498, 1912.
4. Scannapieco FA. Systemic effects of periodontal disease. Dent Clin North Am. 49:533–550, 2005.
5. Scannapieco FA. Periodontal inflammation: From gingivitis to systemic disease? Comp Cont Educ Dent. 25:16S–25S, 2004.
6. National Companion Animal Study. University of Minnesota Center for Companion Animal Health. Uplinks, p. 3, 1996.
7. Lund EM, Armstrong PJ, et al. Health status and population characteristics of dogs and cats examined at private veterinary practices in the United States. JAVMA 214:1336–1341, 1999.
8. Wiggs RB, Lobprise HB. Periodontology. In: Veterinary Dentistry, Principles and Practice. Philadelphia: Lippincott-Raven, 1997, pp. 186–231.
9. Hoffmann TH, Gaengler P. Clinical and pathomorphological investigation of spontaneously occurring periodontal disease in dogs. J Small Anim Pract. 37:471–479, 1996.
10. Mealey BL, Klokkevold PR. Periodontal Medicine: Impact of periodontal infection on systemic health. In: Carranza's Clinical Periodontology. St. Louis: Saunders, 2006, pp. 170–192.
11. Ronstrom A, Edwardsson S, Atistrom R. Streptococcus sanguis and Streptococcus salvarius in early plaque formation on plastic films. J Periodontal Res. 12:331, 1977.
12. Quirynen M, Teughels W, Kinder Haake S, Newman MG. Microbiology of periodontal diseases. In: Carranza's Clinical Periodontology. St. Louis: Saunders, 2006, pp. 134–169.
13. Loe H, Theilade E, Jensen SB. Experimental gingivitis in man. J Periodontol. 36:177–187, 1965.

14. Debowes LJ. Problems with the gingiva. In: Small Animal Dental, Oral and Maxillofacial Disease, a Color Handbook (Niemiec BA ed.). London: Manson, 2010, pp. 159–181.
15. Payne WA, Page RC, Olgolvie AL, et al. Histopathologic features of the initial and early stages of experimental gingivitis in man. J Periodontal Res. 10:51, 1975.
16. Rober M. Effect of scaling and root planing without dental homecare on the subgingival microbiotia. Proceedings of the 16th European Congress of Veterinary Dentistry, 2007, pp. 28–30.
17. Nisengard RJ, Kinder Haake S, Newman MG, Miyasaki KT. Microbial interactions with the host in periodontal diseases. In: Carranza's Clinical Periodontology. St. Louis: Saunders, 2006, pp. 228–250.
18. Niemiec BA. Periodontal disease. Top Companion Anim Med. 23(2):72–80, 2008.
19. Mealey BL, Klokkevold PR. Periodontal medicine: Impact of periodontal infection on systemic health. In: Carranza's Clinical Periodontology. St. Louis: Saunders, 2006, pp. 312–329.
20. Takai T. Fc receptors and their role in immune regulation and autoimmunity. J Clin Immunol. 25:1–18, 2005.
21. American Academy of Periodontology. Mouth body connection. Available at: http://www.perio.org/consumer/mbc.top2.htm. Accessed June 17, 2006.
22. Pavlica Z, Petelin M, Juntes P, et al. Periodontal disease burden and pathological changes in the organs of dogs. J Vet Dent. 25(2):97–108, 2008.
23. Lah TT, Babnik J, et al. Cysteine proteinases and inhibitors in inflammation: Their role in periodontal disease. J Periodontol. 64:485–491, 1993.
24. Renvert S, Wirkstrom M, et al. Histological and microbiological aspects of ligature induced periodontitis in beagle dogs. J Clin Periodontol. 23:310–319, 1996.
25. Rawlinson JE, Reiter AM, Harvey CE. Tracking systemic parameters in dogs with periodontal disease. Proceedings of the 19th Annual Veterinary Dental Forum, Orlando, 2005, p. 429.
26. Debowes LJ, Mosier D, Logan E, Harvey CE, Lowry S, Richardson DC. Association of periodontal disease and histologic lesions in multiple organs from 45 dogs. J Vet Dent. 13(2)57–60, 1996.
27. Franek E, Blach A, et al. Association between chronic periodontal disease and left ventricular hypertrophy in kidney transplant recipients. Transplantation 80:3–5, 2005.
28. Al-Emadi A, Bissada N, Farah C, Siegel B, Al-Zaharani M. Systemic diseases among patients with and without alveolar bone loss. Quintessence Int. 37(10):761–765, 2006.
29. Page RC. The pathobiology of periodontal diseases may affect systemic diseases: Inversion of a paradigm. Ann Periodontol. 3:108, 1998.
30. Gioso MA, Shofer F, Barros PS, Harvey CE. Mandible and mandibular first molar tooth measurements in dogs: Relationship of radiographic height to body weight. J Vet Dent. 18(2):65–68, 2001.
31. Hoffmann TH, Gaengler P. Clinical and pathomorphological investigation of spontaneously occurring periodontal disease in dogs. J Small Anim Pract. 37:471–479, 1996.
32. Harvey CE, Shofer FS, Laster L. Association of age and body weight with periodontal disease in North American Dogs. J Vet Dent. 11:94–105, 1994.
33. Hoffman TH, Gaengler P. Epidemiology of periodontal disease in poodles. J Small Animal Pract. 37:309–316, 1996.
34. Geerts SO, Nys M, De MP, et al. Systemic release of endotoxins induced by gentle mastication: Association with periodontitis severity. J Periodontol. 73:73, 2002.
35. Guntheroth WG. How important are dental procedures as a cause of infective endocarditis? Am J Cardiol. 54:797, 1984.
36. Hartzell JD, Torres D, Kim P, Wortmann G. Incidence of bacteremia after routine tooth brushing. Am J Med Sci. 329:178–180, 2005.
37. Glass RT, Martin ME, Peter LJ. Transmission of disease in dogs by toothbrushing. Quintessence Int. 20(11):819–824, 1989.
38. Dajani AS, Taubert KA, Wilson W, et al. Prevention of bacterial endocarditis: Recommendations by the American Heart Association. JAMA 27:1794, 1997.
39. Artese HP, Sousa CO, Luiz RR, Sansone C, Torres MC. Effect of non-surgical periodontal treatment on chronic kidney disease patients. Braz Oral Res. 24(4):449–454, 2010.
40. Miller LS, Manwell MA, Newbold D, et al. The relationship between reduction in periodontal inflammation and diabetes control: A control of 9 cases. J Periodontol. 63:843, 1992.
41. Promsudthi A, Pimapansri S, Deerochanawong C, Kanchanavasita W. The effect of periodontal therapy on uncontrolled type 2 diabetes mellitus in older subjects. Oral Disease 11:293–298, 2005.
42. Taylor B, Tofler G, Morel-Kopp MC. The effect of initial treatment of periodontitis on systemic markers of inflammation and cardiovascular risk: A randomized controlled trial. Eur J Oral Sci. 118(4):350–356, 2010.
43. Taboada J, Meyer DJ. Cholestasis associated with extrahepatic bacterial infection in five dogs. J Vet Intern Med. 3:216–220, 1989.
44. Center SA. Hepatobilliary infections. In: Infectious Diseases of the Dog and Cat (Green CE ed.). Philadelphia: Saunders, 1990, pp. 146–156.
45. Arbes SJ Jr, Slade GD, Beck JD. Association between extent of periodontal disease and self-reported history of heart attack: An analysis of NHANES III data. J Dent Res. 78:1777, 1999.
46. Khlgatain M, Nassar H, et al. Fimbria-dependant activation of cell adhesion molecule expression in Porphyromonas gingivalis infected endothelial cells. Infect Immun. 70:257–267, 2002.
47. Nassar H, Chou HH, et al. Role for fimbrie and lysine-specific cysteine proteinase gingipain K in expression of interleukin-8 and monocyte chemoattractant protein in Porphyromonas gingivalis infected endothelial cells. Infect Immune. 70:268–276, 2002.
48. Ortiz A, Gomez-Chiarri M, et al. The role of platelet-activating factor (PAF) in experimental glomerular injury. Lipids. 26:1310–1315, 1991.
49. Baylis C. Effects of administered thromboxane on the intact, normal rat kidney. Ren Physiol. 10:110–121, 1987.
50. MacDougal DF, Cook T, et al. Canine chronic renal disease: Prevalence and types of glomerulonephritis in the dog. Kidney Int. 29:1144–1151, 1986.
51. Sedor JR, Konieczkowski M, et al. Cytokines, mesangial cell activation and glomerular injury. Kidney Int. 39(Suppl):65S–70S, 1993.
52. Fournier D, Mouton C, et al. Porphyromonas gulae sp. Nov., an anaerobic, gram-coccobacillus gingival sulcus of various animal hosts. Int J Syst Evol Microbiol. 51:1179–1189, 2001.
53. Cullinan MP, Ford PJ, Seymore GJ. Periodontal diease and systemic health: Current status. Aust Dent J. 54(Supp 1):SS62–S69, 2009.
54. Graziani F, Cei S, La Ferla F, Vano M, Gabriele M, Tonetti M. Effects of non-surgical periodontal therapy on the glomerular filtration rate of the kidney: An exploratory trial. J Clin Periodontol. 37(7):638–643, 2010.
55. O'Grady MR. Acquired valvular heart disease. In: Textbook of Veterinary Internal Medicine (Ettinger SJ, Feldman EC eds.). 4th ed. Philadelphia: Saunders, 1995, pp. 944–958.

56. Abbott JA. Aquired valvular disease. In: Manual of Canine and Feline Cardiology (Tilley LP ed.). 4th ed. St. Louis: Elsevier, 2008, pp. 110–138.
57. Glickman LT, Glickman NW, Moore GE, Goldstein GS, Lewis HB. Evaluation of the risk of endocarditis and other cardiovascular events on the basis of the severity of periodontal disease in dogs. JAVMA 234(4):486–494, 2009.
58. MacDonald KA, Chomel BB, Kittleson MD, et al. A prospective study of canine infective endocarditis in northern California (1999–2001): Emergence of Bartonella as a prevalent etiologic agent. J Vet Intern Med. 18(1):56–64, 2004.
59. Calvert CA, Greene CE, Hardie EM. Cardiovascular infections in dogs: Epizootiology, clinical manifestations, and prognosis. JAVMA 187:612–616, 1985.
60. Takahasi T, Fujisawa T, Yamamoto K, Kijima M, Takahashi T. Taxonomic evidence that serovar 7 of Erysipelothrix strains isolated from dogs with endocarditis are Erysipelothrix tonsillarum. J Vet Med B Infect Dis Vet Public Health. 47(4):311–313, 2000.
61. Haraszthy VI, Zambon JJ, Trevisan M, Zeid M, Genco RJ. Identification of periodontal pathogens in atheromatous plaques. J Periodontol. 71:1554–1560, 2000.
62. Drangsholt MT. A new causal model of dental diseases associated with endocarditis. Ann Periodontol. 3:184–196, 1998.
63. Peddle GD, Drobatz KJ, Harvey CE, Adams A, Sleeper MM. Association of periodontal disease, oral procedures, and other clinical findings with bacterial endocarditis in dogs. JAVMA 234:1, 100–107, 2009.
64. Angeli F, Verdecchia P, Pellegrino C, et al. Association between periodontal disease and left ventricle mass in essential hypertension. Hypertension 41(3):488–492, 2003.
65. Franek E, Klamczynska E, Ganowicz E, et al. Association of chronic periodontitis with left ventricular mass and central blood pressure in treated patients with essential hypertension. Am J Hypertens. 22(2):203–207, 2008.
66. Mercanoglu F, Oflaz H, Oz O, et al. Endothelial dysfunction in patients with chronic periodontitis and its improvement after initial periodontal therapy. J Periodontol. 75(12):1694–1700, 2004.
67. Southerland JH, Taylor GW, Moss K, Beck JD, Offenbacher S. Commonality in chronic inflammatory diseases: Periodontitis, diabetes, and coronary artery disease. Periodontol. 40:130–143, 2006.
68. Mattila KJ, Nieminen MS, Valtonen VV, et al. Association between dental health and acute myocardial infarction. Br Med J. 298:779, 1989.
69. Loos BG, Craandijk J, Hoek FJ, Wertheim-Van Dillen PM, van der Velden U. Elevation of systemic markers related to cardiovascular diseases in the peripheral blood of periodontitis patients. J Periodontol. 71(10):1528–34, 2000.
70. Janket S, Baird AE, Chuang S, Jones JA. Meta-analysis of periodontal disease and risk of coronary heart disease and stroke. Oral Surg Oral Med Oral Pathol Oral Radiol Endod. 95:559, 2003.
71. Joshipura KJ, Rirum EB, et al. Association of periodontal disease and coronary heart disease. J Dent Res. 75:1631–1636, 1996.
72. Geerts SO, Legrand V, Charpentier J, Albert A, Rompen EH. Further evidence of the association between periodontal conditions and coronary artery disease. J Periodontol. 75(9):1274–1280, 2004.
73. Tsakos G, Sabbah W, Hingorani AD. Is periodontal inflammation associated with raised blood pressure? Evidence from a National US survey. J Hypertens. 2010 Aug. 17. [Epub ahead of print.]
74. Lowe GD, Lee AJ, Rumley A, et al. Blood viscosity and of cardiovascular events: The Edinburgh artery study. Heamotol. 96:168, 1997.
75. Kweider M, Lowe GD, Murray GD, et al. Dental disease, fibrinogen and white cell counts: Links with myocardial infarction? Scott Med J. 38:73–74, 1993.
76. Herzberg MC, Meyer MW. Dental plaque, platelets, and cardiovascular diseases. Ann Periodontol. 3:151, 1998.
77. Meyer MW, Gong K, Herzberg MC. Streptococcus sanguis-induced platelet clotting in rabbits and hemodynamic and cardiopulmonary consequences. Infect Immun. 66(12):5906–5914, 1998.
78. Noack B, Genco RJ, et al. Periodontal infections contribute to elevated systemic C-reactive protein level. J Periodontol. 72: 1221–1227, 2001.
79. Ridker PM, Rifai N, Rose L, et al. Comparison of C-reactive protein and low density lipoprotein cholesterol levels in the prediction of first cardiac events. New England J Med. 347:1557, 2002.
80. Wu T, Trevisan M, Genco RJ, et al. Examination of the relation between periodontal health status and cardiovascular risk factors: Serum total and high density lipoprotein cholesterol, C-reactive protein, and plasma fibrinogen. Am J Epidemiol. 151:273, 2000.
81. D'Aiuto F, Parkar M, et al. Periodontitis and systemic inflammation: Control of the local infection in association with a reduction in serum inflammatory markers. J Dent Res. 83:156–160, 2004.
82. Debowes LJ. C-reactive protien and periodontal disease. Proceedings of the 22nd Annual Dental Forum, 2008.
83. Joshipura KJ, Wand HC, Merchant AT, Rimm EB. Periodontal disease and biomarkers related to cardiovascular disease. J Dent Res. 83:151–155, 2004.
84. de Oliveira C, Watt R, and Hamer M. Toothbrushing, inflammation, and risk of cardiovascular disease: Results from Scottish Health Survey. BMJ DOI:10.1136/bmj.c2451, 2010.
85. Brodala N, Merricks EP, et al. Porphyromonas gingivalis bacteremia induces coronary and aortic atherosclerosis in normocholesterolemic and hypercholesterolemic pigs. Arteroscler Thromb Vasc Biol. 25:1446–1451, 2005.
86. Lalla E, Lamster IB. et al. Oral infection with a periodontal pathogen accelerates early atherosclerosis in apolipoprotein E-null mice. Arteroscler Thromb Vasc Biol. 23:1405–1411, 2003.
87. Garcia R. Epidemiologic associations between periodontal diseases and respiratory diseases. In: The Periodontal-Systemic Connection: A State-of-the-Science Symposium, Bethesda MD, April 18–20, 2001.
88. Limeback H. Implications of oral infections on systemic diseases in the institutionalized elderly with a special focus on pneumonia. Ann Periodontol. 3(1):262–275, 1998.
89. Hayes C, Sparrow D, Cohen M, et al. The association between alveolar bone loss and pulmonary function: The VA Dental Longitudinal Study. Ann Periodontol. 3:257, 1998.
90. Deo V, Bhongade ML, Ansari S, Chavan RS. Periodontitis as a potential risk factor for chronic obstructive pulmonary disease: A retrospective study. Indian J Dent Res. 20(4):466–470, 2009.
91. Scannapieco FA, Papandonatos GD, Dunford RG. Associations between oral conditions and respiratory disease in a national sample survey population. Ann Periodontol. 3(1):251–256, 1998.
92. Nagatake T, Ahmed K, Oishi K. Prevention of respiratory infections by povidone-iodine gargle. Dermatology 204 Suppl 1:32–36, 2002.
93. Kawana R, Nagasawa S, Endo T, Fukuroi Y, Takahashi Y. Strategy of control of nosocomial infections: Application of disinfectants such as povidone-iodine. Dermatology 204 Suppl 1:28–31, 2002.

94. Adachi M, Ishihara K, Abe S, Okuda K. Professional oral health care by dental hygienists reduced respiratory infections in elderly persons requiring nursing care. Int J Dent Hyg. 5(2): 69–74, 2007.
95. Adachi M, Ishihara K, Abe S, Okuda K, Ishikawa T. Effect of professional oral health care on the elderly living in nursing homes. Oral Surg Oral Med Oral Pathol Oral Radiol Endod. 94(2):191–195, 2002.
96. National Nosocomial Infections Surveillance System. National Nosocomial Infections Surveillance (NNIS) System Report, data summary from January 1990–May 1999, issued June 1999. Am J Infect Control 27:520–532, 1999.
97. Craven DE, Steger KE, Barber TW. Preventing nosocomial pneumonia: State of the art and perspectives for the 1990s. Am J Med. 91:44, 1991.
98. Stoutenbeek CP, van Saene HK, Miranda D, et al. The effect of oropharangeal decontamination using topical non-absorbable antibiotics on the incidence of nosocomial respiratory tract in multiple trauma patients. J Trauma 27:357, 1987.
99. Okuda K, Kimizuka R, Abe S, Kato T, Ishihara K. Involvement of periodontopathic anaerobes in aspiration pneumonia. J Periodontol. 76(11 Suppl): 21542160, 2005.
100. Pugin J, Auckenthaler R, Lew DP, Suter PM. Oropharyngeal decontamination decreases incidence of ventilator-associated pneumonia. A randomized, placebo-controlled, double-blind clinical trial. JAMA 265(20):2704–2710, 1991.
101. Scannapieco FA, Bush RB, Paju S. Associations between periodontal disease and risk for nosocomial bacterial pneumonia and chronic obstructive pulmonary disease: A systematic review. Ann Periodont. 8:54, 2003.
102. Craven DE, Steger KA. Nosocomial pneumonia in the intubated patient. New concepts on pathogenesis and prevention. Infect Dis Clin North Am. 3(4):843–866, 1989.
103. Levine SA, Niederman MS. The impact of tracheal intubation on host defenses and risks for nosocomial pneumonia. Clin Chest Med. 12(3):523–543, 1991.
104. Kotani N, Lin CY, Wang JS. Loss of alveolar macrophages during anesthesia and operation in humans. Anesth Analg. 81(6): 1255–1262, 1995.
105. Kotani N, Hashimoto H, Sessler DI, et al. Intraoperative modulation of alveolar macrophage function during isoflurane and propofol anesthesia. Anesthesiology 89(5):1125–1132, 1998.
106. Hall JC, Tarala RA, Hall JL, Mander J. A multivariate analysis of the risk of pulmonary complications after laparotomy. Chest 99(4):923–927, 1991.
107. Okuda M, Kaneko Y, Ichinohe T, Ishihara K, Okuda K. Reduction of potential respiratory pathogens by oral hygienic treatment in patients undergoing endotracheal anesthesia. J Anesth. 17(2): 84–91, 2003.
108. Ogata J, Minami K, Miyamoto H, et al. Gargling with povidone-iodine reduces the transport of bacteria during oral intubation. Can J Anaesth. 51(9):932–936, 2004.
109. Syrjanen J, Valtonen VV, Livanainen M, et al. Preceding infection as an important risk factor for ischemic brain infarction in young and middle age patients. Br Med J. 296:1156, 1988.
110. Grau AJ, Buggle F, Heindl S, et al. Recent infection as a risk factor for cerebrovascular ischemia. Stroke 26:373, 1995.
111. Mealey BL. Influence of periodontal infections on systemic health. Periodontol 2000 21:197–209, 1999.
112. Syrjanen J, Peltola J, Valtonen V, et al. Dental infections in association with cerebral infarction in young and middle-aged men. J Intern Med. 225:197, 1989.
113. Grau AJ, Bruggle F, Ziegler C, et al. Association between acute cerebrovasular ischemia and chronic and recurrent infection. Stroke 28:1724, 1997.
114. Nesbitt MJ, Reynolds MA, Shiau H. Association of periodontitis and metabolic syndrome in the Baltimore Longitudinal Study of Aging. Aging Clin Exp Res. 22(3):238–242, 2010.
115. Benguigui C, Bongard V, Ruidavets JB, Chamontin B, Sixou M, Ferrières J, Amar J. Metabolic syndrome, insulin resistance, and periodontitis: A cross-sectional study in a middle-aged French population. J Clin Periodontol. 37(7): 601–608, 2010.
116. Nagata T. Relationship between diabetes and periodontal disease. Clin Calcium 19(9):1291–1298, 2009.
117. Nishimura F, Soga Y, Iwamoto Y, Kudo C, Murayama Y. Periodontal disease as part of the insulin resistance syndrome in diabetic patients. J Int Acad Periodontol. 7(1):16–20, 2005.
118. Ekuni D, Tomofuji T, Irie K, et al. Effects of periodontitis on aortic insulin resistance in an obese rat model. Lab Invest. 90(3):348–359, 2010.
119. Yri-Jarvinen H, Sammalkorphi K, Koivisto VA, et al. Severity, duration, and mechanism of insulin resistance during acute infections. J Clin Endocrinol Metab. 69:317, 1989.
120. Grossi SG, Mealey BL, Rose LF. Effect of periodontal infection on systemic health and well being. In: Periodontics: Medicine, Surgery, and Implants (Rose LF, Mealey BL, Genco RJ, Cohen DW eds.). St Louis: Elsevier, 2004.
121. Zadik Y, Bechor R, Galor S, Levin L. Periodontal disease might be associated even with impaired fasting glucose. Br Dent J. 208(10):E20, 2010.
122. Iacopino AM. Periodontitis and diabetes interrelationships: Role of inflammation. Ann Periodontol. 6(1):125–137, 2001.
123. Grossi, S. Clinical considerations in the treatment of a diabetic patient with periodontal disease. In: The Periodontal-Systemic Connection: A State-of-the-Science Symposium, Bethesda MD, April 18–20, 2001.
124. Taylor GW, Burt BA, Becker MP, et al. Severe periodontitis and risk for poor glycemic control in patients with non-insulin dependent diabetes mellitus. J Periodontol 67:1085, 1996.
125. Thorstensson H, Kuylensteirna J, Hugoson A. Medical status and complications in relation to periodontal disease experience in insulin dependent diabetics. J Clin Periodontol. 23:194, 1996.
126. Tsai C, Hayes C, Taylor GW. Glycemic control of type 2 diabetes and severe periodontal disease in US adult population. Community Dent Oral Epidemiol. 30:182–192, 2002.
127. Southerland JH, Taylor GW, Moss K, Beck JD, Offenbacher S. Commonality in chronic inflammatory diseases: Periodontitis, diabetes, and coronary artery disease. Periodontol. 40:130–143, 2006.
128. Saremi A, Nelson RG, Tulloch-Reid M, Hanson RL, Sievers ML, Taylor GW, et al. Periodontal disease and mortality in type 2 diabetes. Diabetes Care 28:27–32, 2005.
129. Mine K, Nejat A, Elif U, Faik Murat E. The effect of improved periodontal health on metabolic control in type 2 diabetes mellitus. J Clin Periodontol. 32:266–272, 2005.
130. Miller LS, Manwell MA, Newbold D, et al. The relationship between reduction in periodontal inflammation and diabetes control: A control of 9 cases. J Periodontol. 63:843, 1992.
131. Skaleric U, Schara R, Medvescek M, Hanlon A, Doherty F, Lessem J. Periodontal treatment by Arestin and its effects on glycemic control in type 1 diabetes patients. J Int Acad Periodontol. 6(4 Suppl):160–165, 2004.

132. Promsudthi A, Pimapansri S, Deerochanawong C, Kanchanavasita W. The effect of periodontal therapy on uncontrolled type 2 diabetes mellitus in older subjects. Oral Disease 11:293–298, 2005.
133. Stewart JE, Wager KA, Friedlander AH, Zadeh HH. The effect of periodontal treatment on glycemic control in patients with type 2 diabetes mellitus. J Clin Periodontol. 28:306–310, 2001.
134. Grossi SG, Skrepcinski FB, DeCaro T, et al. Treatment of periodontal disease in diabetics reduces glycated hemoglobin. J Periodontol. 68:713, 1997.
135. Tervonen T, Knuuttila M. Relation of diabetes control to periodontal pocketing and alveolar bone level. Oral Surg Oral Med Oral Pathol. 61:346–349, 1986.
136. American Association of Periodontology. Position paper: Epidemiology of periodontal diseases. J Periodontol. 70(8): 935–949, 1999.
137. Canpus G, Salem A, Uzzau S, Baldoni E, Tonolo G. Diabetes and periodontal disease: A case-control study. J Periodontol. 76(3): 418–425, 2005.
138. King GL. The role of inflammatory cytokines in diabetes and its complications. J Periodontol. 79(8 Suppl):1527–1534, 2008.
139. Papapanou PN. World workshop in clinical periodontics. Periodontal diseases: Epidemiology. Ann Periodontol. 1:1–36, 1996.
140. Moore PA, Weyant RJ, Mongelluzzo MB, Myers DE, Rossie K, Guggenheimer J, et al. Type 1 diabetes mellitus and oral health: Assessment of tooth loss and edentulism. J Public Health Dent. 58:135, 1998.
141. Tervonen T, Karjalainen K, Knuuttila M, Huumonen S. Alveolar bone loss in type 1 diabetic subjects. J Clin Periodontol. 27: 567–571, 2000.
142. Taylor GW, Burt BA, Becker MP, Genco RJ, Shlossman M, Knowler WC, et al. Non-insulin dependent diabetes mellitus and alveolar bone loss progression over 2 years. J Periodontol. 69: 76–83, 1998.
143. Hirsch T, Spielmann M, Zuhaili B, et al. Enhanced susceptibility to infections in a diabetic wound healing model. BMC Surg. 8:5, 2008.
144. Delamaire M, Maugendre D, Moreno M, Le Goff MC, Allannic H, Genetet B. Impaired leucocyte functions in diabetic patients. Diabet Med. 14(1):29–34, 1997.
145. Schubert S, Heesemann J. [Infections in diabetes mellitus]. Immun Infekt. 23(6):200–204, 1995.
146. Feldman EC, Nelson RW. Canine diabetes mellitus. In: Canine and Feline Endocrinology and Reproduction. Philadelphia: Saunders, 2004, pp. 486–538.
147. Taylor GW. Bidirectional interrelationships between diabetes and periodontal diseases: An epidemiologic perspective. Ann Periodontol. 6(1):99–12, 2001.
148. Grossi SG, Genco RJ. Periodontal disease and diabetes mellitus, a two-way relationship. Ann Periodontol. 3:51–61, 1998.
149. Mealey BL, Ocampo GL. Diabetes mellitus and periodontal disease. Periodontology 2000 44:127–153, 2007.
150. Loe H. Periodontal disease: The sixth complication of diabetes mellitus. Diabetes Care 16:329–334, 1993.
151. Watabe K, Nishi M, Miyake H, Hirata K. Lifestyle and gastric cancer: A case-control study. Oncol Rep. 5:1191–1194, 1998.
152. Abnet CC, Qiao YL, Mark SD, Dong ZW, Taylor PR, Dawsey SM. Prospective study of tooth loss and incident esophageal and gastric cancers in China. Cancer Causes Control. 12:847–854, 2001.
153. Stolzenberg-Solomon RZ, Dodd KW, Blaser MJ, Virtamo J, Taylor PR, Albanes D. Tooth loss, pancreatic cancer, and Helicobacter pylori. Am J Clin Nutr. 78:176–181, 2003.
154. Michaud DS, Joshipura K, Giovannucci E, Fuchs CS. A prospective study of periodontal disease and pancreatic cancer in US male health professionals. J Natl Cancer Inst. 99: 171–175, 2007.
155. Hujoel PP, Drangsholt M, Spiekerman C, Weiss NS. An exploration of the periodontitis-cancer association. Ann Epidemiol. 13:312–316, 2003.
156. Michaud DS, Liu Y, Meyer M, Giovannucci E, Joshipura K. Periodontal disease, tooth loss, and cancer risk in male health professionals: A prospective cohort study. Lancet Oncol. 9(6):550–558, 2008.
157. Meyer MS, Joshipura K, Giovannucci E, Michaud DS. A review of the relationship between tooth loss, periodontal disease, and cancer. Cancer Causes Control. 19(9):895–907, 2008.
158. Katz J, Chegini N, Shiverick KT, Lamont RJ. Localization of P. gingivalis in preterm delivery placenta. J Dent Res. 88(6): 575–578, 2009.
159. Bélanger M, Reyes L, von Deneen K, Reinhard MK, Progulske-Fox A, Brown MB. Colonization of maternal and fetal tissues by Porphyromonas gingivalis is strain-dependent in a rodent animal model. Am J Obstet Gynecol. 199(1):86.e1–7, 2008.
160. Lin D, Smith MA, Elter J, Champagne C, Downey CL, Beck J, Offenbacher S. Porphyromonas gingivalis infection in pregnant mice is associated with placental dissemination, an increase in the placental Th1/Th2 cytokine ratio, and fetal growth restriction. Infect Immun. 71(9):5163–5168, 2003.
161. Jeffcoat MK, Guers NC, Reddy MS, et al. Periodontal infection and pre-term birth: Results of a prospective study. J Am Dent Assoc. 132:875, 2002.
162. Lopez NJ, Smith PC, Gutiererrez J. Higher risk of preterm birth and low birth rate in women with periodontal disease. J Dent Res. 81:58, 2002.
163. Offenbacher S, Katz V, Fertik G, et al. Periodontal infection as a possible risk factor for preterm low birth weight. J Periodontol. 67:1103–1113, 1996.
164. Lopez NJ, Da Silva I, Ipinza J, Gutierrez J. Periodontal therapy reduces the rate of preterm low birth weight in women with pregnancy-associated gingivitis. J Periodontol. 76:2144–2153, 2005.
165. Lopez NJ, Smith PC, Gutierrez J. Periodontal therapy may reduce the risk of preterm low birth weight in women with periodontal disease: A randomized controlled trial. J Periodontol. 73(8): 911–924, 2002.
166. Mitchell-Lewis D, Engebretson SP, Chen J, Lamster IB, Papapanou PN. Periodontal infections and pre-term birth: Early findings from a cohort of young minority women in New York. Eur J Oral Sci. 109:34–39, 2001.
167. Nibali L, D'Aiuto F, Griffiths G, Patel K, Suvan J, Tonetti MS. Severe periodontitis is associated with systemic inflammation and a dysmetabolic status: A case-control study. J Clin Periodontol. 34(11):931–937, 2007.
168. Renvert S, Wirkstrom M, et al. Histological and microbiological aspects of ligature induced periodontitis in beagle dogs. J Clin Periodontol. 23:310–319, 1996.
169. Moutsopoulos NM, Madianos PN. Low grade inflammation in chronic infectious diseases: Paradigm of periodontal infections. Ann NY Acad Sci. 1088:251–264, 2006.
170. Iacopino AM, Cutler CW. Pathophysiological relationships between periodontitis and systemic disease: Recent concepts involving serum lipids. J Periodontol. 71(8):1375–1384, 2000.

171. Ebersole JL, Cappelli D, Mott G, Kesavalu L, Holt SC, Singer RE. Systemic manifestations of periodontitis in the non-human primate. J Periodontal Res. 34(7):358–362, 1999.
172. Salvi GE, Brown CE, Fujihashi K, et al. Inflammatory mediators of the terminal dentition in adult and early onset periodontitis. J Periodontal Res. 33:212–225, 1998.
173. Correa FO, Gonçalves D, Figueredo CM, Bastos AS, Gustafsson A, Orrico SR. Effect of periodontal treatment on metabolic control, systemic inflammation and cytokines in patients with type 2 diabetes. J Clin Periodontol. 37(1):53–58, 2010.
174. Duarte PM, da Rocha M, Sampaio E, et al. Serum levels of cytokines in subjects with generalized chronic and aggressive periodontitis before and after non-surgical periodontal therapy: A pilot study. J Periodontol. 81(7):1056–1063, 2010.
175. Jansson L, Lavstedt S, Frithiof L. Relationship between oral health and mortality rate. J Clin Periodontol. 29:1029, 2002.
176. Avlund K, Schultz-Larsen K, Krustrup U. Effect of inflammation in the periodontium in early old age on mortality at 21-year follow-up. J Am Geriatr Soc. 57(7):1206–1212, 2009.
177. Holm-Pedersen P, Schultz-Larsen K, Christiansen N, Avlund K. Tooth loss and subsequent disability and mortality in old age. J Am Geriatr Soc. 56(3):429–435, 2008.
178. Garcia RI, Krall EA, Vokonas PS. Periodontal disease and mortality from all causes in the VA dental longitudinal Study. Ann Periodontol. 3:339, 1998.
179. Harvey CE, Emily PP. Periodontal disease. In: Small Animal Dentistry. St. Louis: Mosby, 1993, pp. 89–144.
180. Holmstrom SE, Frost P, Eisner ER. Dental prophylaxis. In: Veterinary Dental Techniques. 2nd ed. Philadelphia: Saunders, 1998, pp. 133–166.
181. Sculley D, Langley-Evans S. Salivary antioxidants and periodontal disease status. Proceedings of the Nutrition Society, 2002, 137–143.

8

Unusual forms of periodontal disease

Periodontal abscesses

Periodontal abscesses are localized purulent inflammation of the periodontal tissues.[1] There are three distinct groups: gingival, periodontal, and pericoronal. These lesions can be further classified as acute, chronic, or acute on chronic.[2]

Etiology

There are numerous causes for gingival and periodontal abscesses, including foreign body entrapment (e.g., foxtail) (Figure 8.1), trauma, endodontic perforation, tooth fracture, and bacterial plaque infection.[3-5] However, the most common cause of gingival and periodontal abscesses (at least in human periodontology) is incomplete subgingival scaling.[2,6] In these cases, the marginal gingival area has been cleaned, which allows reattachment, while calculus remains apically (Figure 8.2). This traps the bacteria and their produced gasses, creating the abscess.[3] Another common cause for periodontal abscesses is acute exacerbation of existing periodontal pockets, which is generally seen in cases of untreated moderate to severe periodontal disease.[3,7] Additional factors that may predispose patients to a periodontal abscess include more significant infection, lack of spontaneous drainage, a weakened or suppressed immune system,[8] systemic antimicrobial therapy,[9] periodontal surgery,[6] and diabetes mellitus. In fact, uncontrolled diabetes mellitus has been found to be a significant contributor to periodontal abscess formation in humans.[10]

Pericoronal abscesses result from inflammation of the soft tissue operculum during eruption. This generally occurs from trauma or food impaction but can be caused by bacterial plaque.[6]

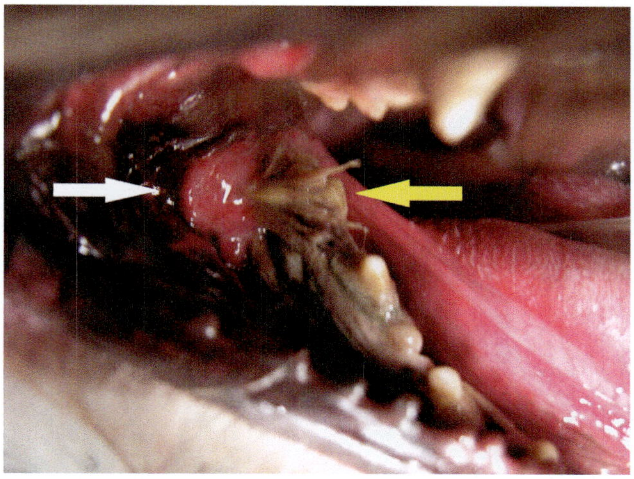

Figure 8.1 Intraoral picture of the mandibular right in a dog. The foreign body (foxtail) (yellow arrow) has created a periodontal abscess (white arrow).

Clinical appearance

The gingival type of periodontal abscess affects only the gingiva and typically presents as a localized, acute inflammatory lesion. They usually appear as a red, smooth, and possibly flocculent swelling (Figure 8.3).[6]

The periodontal type is an extension of a periodontal pocket and involves the periodontal ligament and alveolar bone that may result in their destruction.[6]

Acute periodontal abscesses of any type are typically painful, although this may not be demonstrated by veterinary patients. They usually appear as red, edematous swellings of the gingival tissues, with possible pain on percussion of the tooth.[2,11] Fistulation may also be present, which is usually coronal to the mucogingival line (Figure 8.4).[2] In addition, the tooth is often mobile

Veterinary Periodontology, First Edition. Brook A. Niemiec.

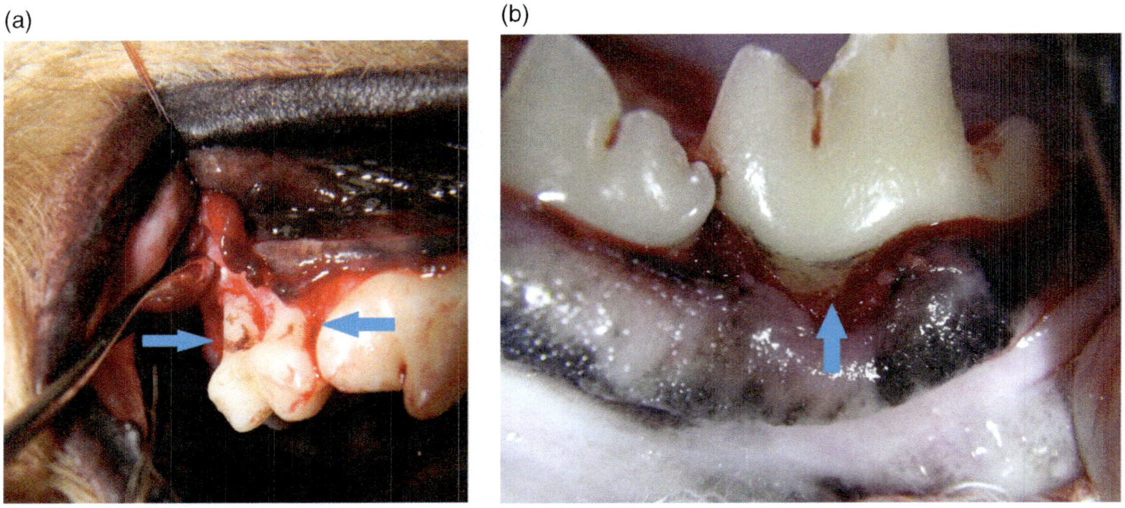

Figure 8.2 (a and b) Intraoral dental pictures of patients with subgingival calculus remaining after dental cleanings at general practices. Note how clean the crowns are, but when the gingiva is reflected, there is significant subgingival calculus (blue arrows). This condition can lead to the development of periodontal abscesses.

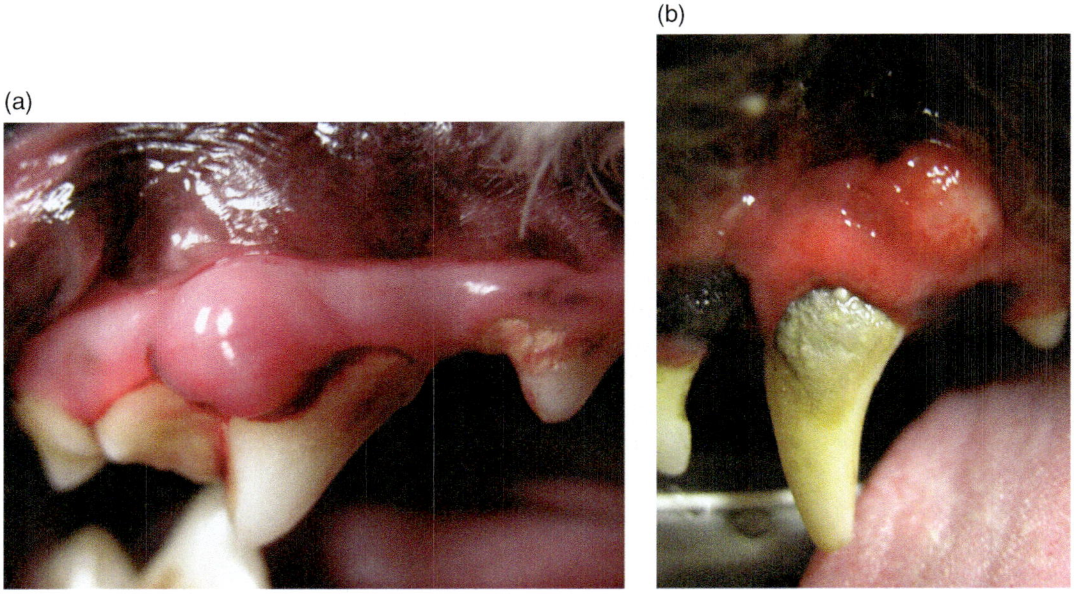

Figure 8.3 Gingival abscesses in two canine patients. Note the red, flocculent swelling on the right maxillary fourth premolar (108) (a) and left maxillary canine (204) (b). These were confirmed as gingival abscesses.

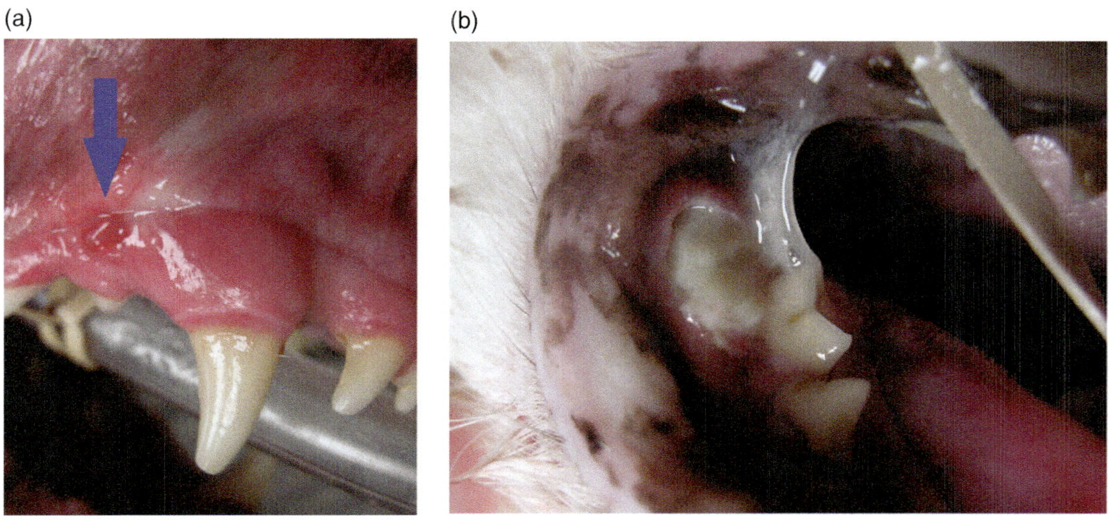

Figure 8.4 (a) Intraoral picture of a periodontal abscess with a draining tract on the right maxillary first premolar (105) (blue arrow). (b) Intraoral picture of a cat with a large fistula with significant purulent discharge over the right mandibular first molar (409).

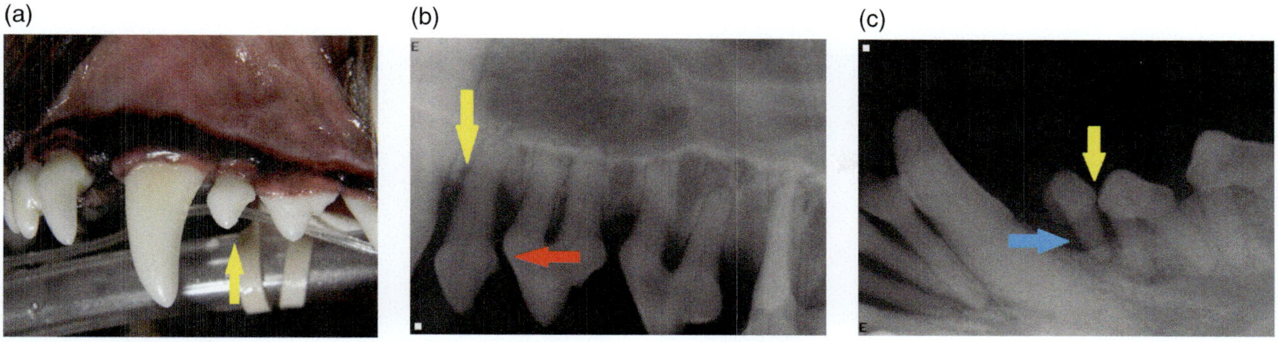

Figure 8.5 (a) Intraoral dental picture of the left maxillary first premolar (205) in a dog with a periodontal abscess in which the tooth is slightly elevated from the alveolus (yellow arrow). The dental radiograph (b) confirms the alveolar bone loss (yellow arrow) and more coronal CEJ (red arrow). (c) Intraoral dental radiograph of the mandibular left a dog with a periodontal abscess on the right mandibular first premolar. Note the significant alveolar bone loss (blue arrow) and the tooth is slightly higher than the second premolar (yellow arrow).

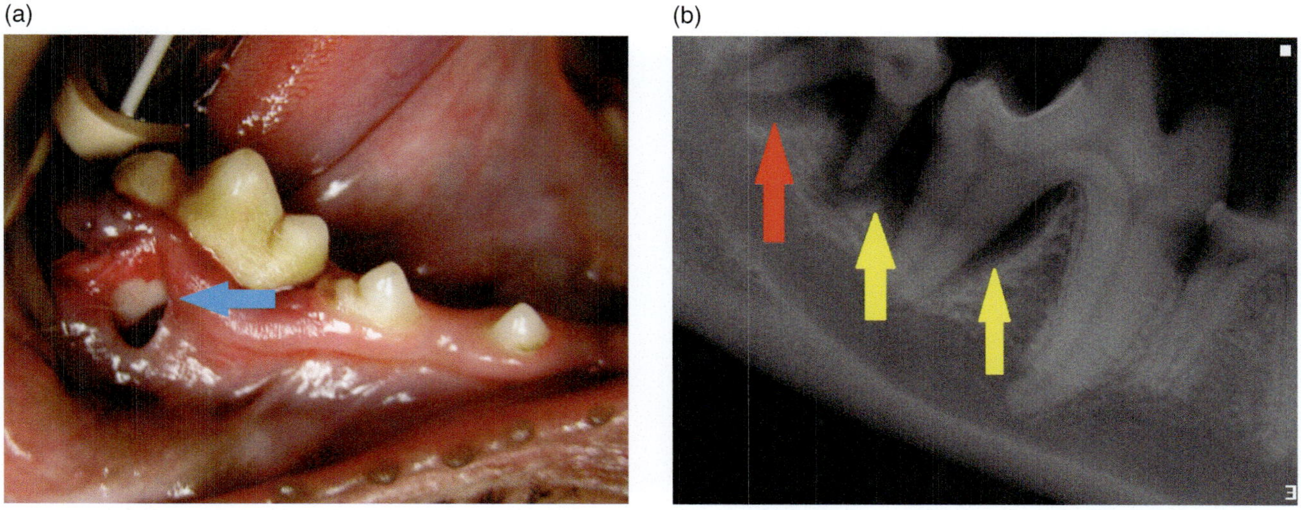

Figure 8.6 (a) Intraoral dental picture of a patient with a periodontal abscess of the right mandibular first molar (409) that has fistulated (blue arrow). (b) Corresponding dental radiograph revealing severe alveolar bone loss (yellow arrows). Note that the second molar (410) also has a class II perio-endo lesion (red arrow).

and may be elevated from the alveolus (Figure 8.5).[6] Systemic signs of infection (fever, malaise, regional lymphadenopathy) may also occur.[2,10,11] *Chronic* periodontal abscesses form after the acute infection has been controlled but not completely eliminated.[2,6] The infection may be controlled in a number of ways, including drainage, immune reaction of the host, or professional therapy.[6] Chronic abscesses are generally asymptomatic[12] but may cause oral pain, which could stimulate a bruxism-type behavior.[2] Chronic lesions may also have a fistulous tract associated with a deep periodontal pocket (Figure 8.6).[6] *Acute on chronic* cases develop due to an acute exacerbation of a chronic state. The clinical appearance of a pericoronal abscess is gingival swelling/inflammation associated with the crown of an erupting tooth.[10]

Diagnosis

The main differential diagnosis for a periodontal abscess is an abscess of endodontic origin. There are several clinical signs that help differentiate these two conditions.[6] First, periodontal abscesses are associated with a periodontal pocket, whereas endodontic abscesses are generally associated with a tooth that has signs of endodontic compromise. This compromise can present as a fracture (complicated or uncomplicated) or intrinsic staining. Furthermore, periodontal abscesses typically fistulate coronal to the mucogingival junction (see Figure 8.4), whereas endodontic abscesses are usually apical to this point (Figure 8.7).[6] Radiographically, periodontal abscesses are often associated with angular bone loss (Figure 8.8), whereas endodontic abscesses are

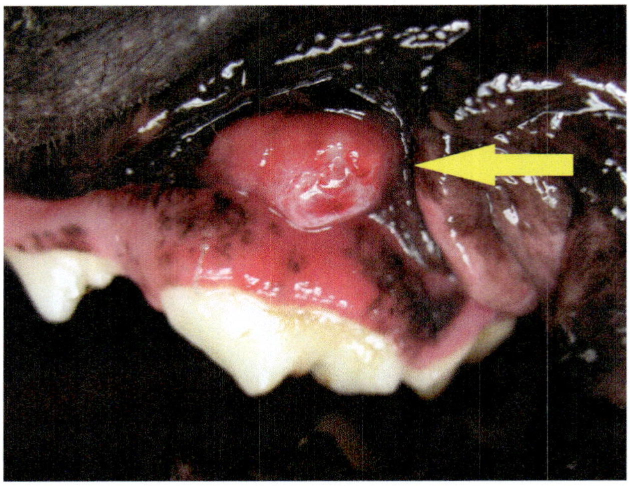

Figure 8.7 Intraoral picture of a patient with a fistulation apical to the mucogingival junction of the left maxillary fourth premolar (208) (yellow arrow). This is the classic appearance of an abscess of endodontic origin.

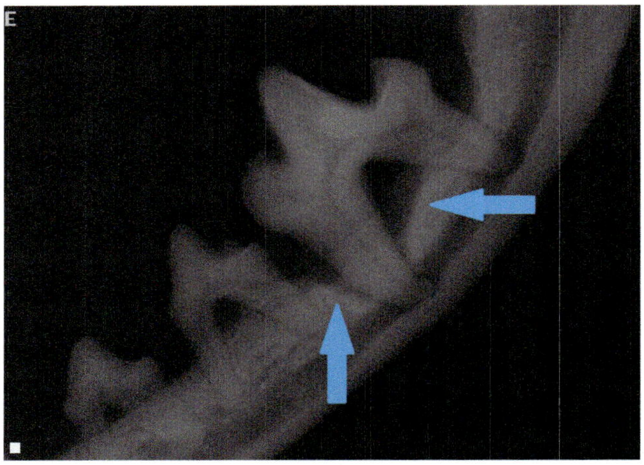

Figure 8.8 Intraoral dental radiograph of the left mandibular first molar (309) in a dog with advanced periodontal (angular) alveolar bone loss (blue arrows). This indicates that an abscess in this area is of periodontal as opposed to endodontic origin.

diagnosed by the presence of periapical rarefaction (Figure 8.9).[2,5,13] Note that the periapical rarefaction is the result of a chronic apical granuloma, not the acute abscess. (See chapter 9 for a discussion of radiography in periodontal disease.)

Treatment

Gingival abscesses are treated[6] by removal of the inciting cause (foreign body or subgingival calculus). Subgingival calculus and infection are removed by thorough scaling and root planing. If this does not resolve the infection, gingival surgery may be indicated.

The treatment of periodontal abscesses is a two-step process. The first step is controlling the acute infection and the second step is managing the chronic condition. The goals of the acute phase are to alleviate the pain, establish drainage, and control the spread of infection. Drainage can be established either through the periodontal pocket or an external incision. If the abscess is small and uncomplicated, drainage can be established by gentle separation of the periodontal ligament and gentle digital pressure. Standard scaling/root planing (SRP) can then be performed closed. Larger lesions require a surgical approach, often through an external incision, which in human dentistry is delayed until the acute symptoms subside. These cases should also be treated with broad spectrum antibiotics and analgesics. If the abscess is accompanied by significant periodontal disease, extraction of the tooth is likely the best form of therapy. The chronic form is managed as any chronic periodontal pocket, with appropriate professional care

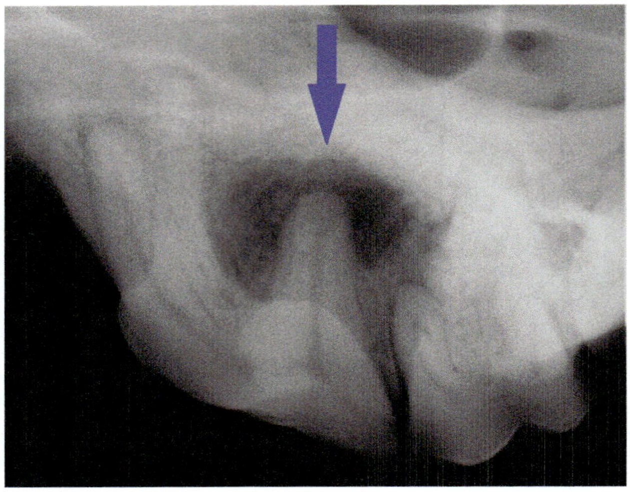

Figure 8.9 Intraoral dental radiograph of the maxillary left fourth premolar (208) in a dog revealing periapical rarefaction (blue arrow). This indicates that an abscess in this area is associated with endodontic as opposed to periodontal disease.

Box 8.1 Key points

- Gingival or periodontal abscesses are typically initiated by chronic periodontal disease but can be caused by a foreign body.
- Gingival or periodontal abscesses most often present after suboptimal scaling.
- It is important to differentiate periodontal abscesses from endodontic disease.
- Effective therapy must establish drainage and treat the periodontal disease.
- Extraction of the diseased tooth is the most definitive form of therapy.

(prophylaxis, SRP, periodontal surgery) combined with meticulous homecare or extraction of the offending tooth. For all types of oral abscesses, antibiotic therapy alone is insufficient.

Pericoronal abscesses are drained by gently lifting the soft tissue operculum and debriding/lavaging the area. In cases where this is insufficient for therapy, the operculum can be excised (operculectomy) or the tooth extracted.

Feline caudal stomatitis (previously called gingivostomatitis)

This is a very misunderstood oral inflammatory disease process in felines. Recently, the nomenclature was changed to divide the disease process into two types (1 and 2). The two types are differentiated by the involvement of the back of the oral cavity/oropharyngeal area. Type 1 is defined as inflammation present anywhere in the mouth other than the caudal area. If the caudal area of the oral cavity is involved (with or without inflammation to the rest of the oral mucosa), it is considered type 2 or caudal stomatitis.[14] This section will focus on type 2 as it is much more challenging to treat.

Caudal stomatitis is a severe inflammatory reaction of the oral tissues of cats. It is a *clinical diagnosis* of inflammation and proliferation of the gingiva and oral mucosa.[15] Specifically, it is inflammation associated with the caudal mouth (mucocitis),[16] which is the delineating factor between caudal stomatitis and periodontal disease.[5,15] Caudal mucocitis is defined as inflammation of mucosa of the caudal oral cavity, bordered medially by the palatoglossal folds and fauces, dorsally by the hard and soft palate, and rostrally by alveolar and buccal mucosa. The fauces are the archway between pharyngeal and oral cavities, formed by the tongue, anterior tonsillar pillars, and the soft palate.[17]

Etiology

The etiology of this disease process is currently unknown.[14] Multiple etiologies may exist that, either singularly or combined, create the inflammation.[14] Possible causative agents include an inflammatory response to plaque bacteria, viruses, *Bartonella henselae* infection, or altered immune status (FeLV or FIV).[15,18,19]

Upper respiratory viruses such as feline calicivirus (FCV) and herpes virus-1 have commonly been linked to caudal stomatitis.[20] This is due to several factors, including the fact that cats with chronic caudal stomatitis are more likely to be currently shedding virus than cats without this oral inflammation.[18] However, herpes virus has been shown in several studies to be an unlikely player in this disease process,[21,22] whereas calicivirus (all biotypes[23]) was found to be the only real correlated etiologic agent.[21] Finally, FCV is reported to cause *acute* caudal stomatitis, but it has not been proven to cause *chronic* caudal stomatitis.[5,24] Based on these studies, it is felt that calicivirus is a factor in the disease process in some cases, but not the true cause.

FeLV and FIV may also play a role in the development of caudal stomatitis. This is thought to be associated with the lower levels of salivary IgA seen in oral inflammatory diseases, as FIV is known to decrease serum IgA levels.[5,25] However, since the majority of cats with caudal stomatitis test negative for these viruses and there is no difference in the level of FIV infection between cats affected with this condition and normal cats,[26] these viruses are clearly not the cause.[27] However, it has been anecdotally noted by this author, as well as others, that retrovirus-positive patients tend to have more severe inflammation.[14]

Bartonella henselae infection has been suggested as a possible eitiology, partly due to the fact that stomatitis is one of its clinical signs.[19] However, this theory has been recently disproven,[21,26] and this author has not found testing or treatment for this disease process to be of benefit in cases of caudal stomatitis.

Bacteria have long been associated with caudal stomatitis and recently *Pasteurella multocida* has been found in greater numbers in cats with this condition in comparison with normal patients.[28] Thus, it has been theorized that *Pasteurella* may represent an etiologic agent. However, this bacteria is also quite common in the feline oral cavity and is increased in most oral diseases. Therefore, a link cannot be established at this time. Finally, it has been suggested that cats with caudal stomatitis have an exaggerated inflammatory response to generalized bacterial plaque.[5,27,29] This theory has been suggested mainly because in many cases of chronic oral inflammatory disease, no other etiology has been identified. Therefore, bacteria should be viewed as a contributor rather than a causative agent of disease. In short, this caudal stomatitis does not seem to be a distinct disease entity. Rather, it appears to be an excessive, inflammatory immune response to a heretofore unknown agent.[14,27]

Clinical signs

In cases of caudal stomatitis, the history typically includes halitosis, dysphagia, pawing at the mouth, reluctance to eat, anorexia (complete or partial), crying out in pain when eating or yawning, weight loss, decreased grooming (which results in an unkempt appearance) (Figure 8.10), and drooling (pseudoptyalism) (Figure 8.11).[5,27,30,31]

The affected gingiva and oral mucosa have varying amounts of inflammation, proliferation, and ulceration (Figure 8.12). The mucosa is generally bright red with cobblestone architecture.[27] The inflammation is often bilaterally symmetrical (Figure 8.13) with friable oral tissues that

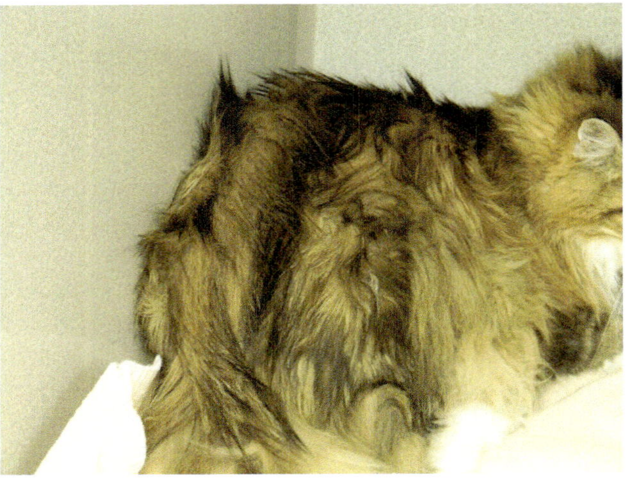

Figure 8.10 Unkempt appearance of a feline patient due to lack of self-grooming. Patients with caudal stomatitis often stop grooming due to oral pain.

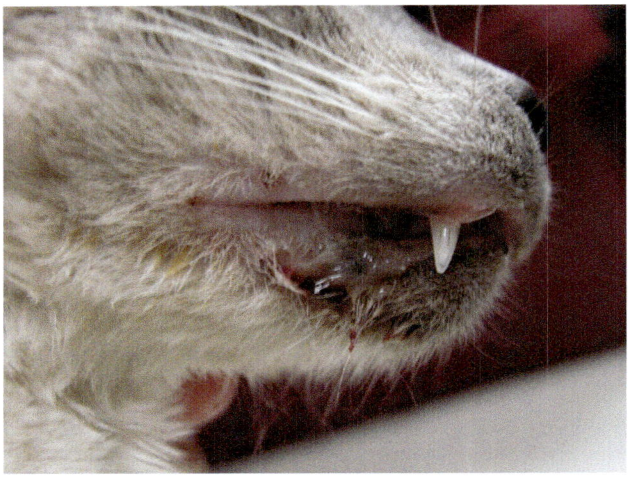

Figure 8.11 Picture of the mandible of a cat with severe caudal stomatitis. The purulent psuedoptalism is a classic outward clinical sign of caudal stomatitis.

bleed easily (Figure 8.14).[30] Gingivostomatitis and periodontal disease can both present with severe gingival inflammation. *The clinical sign that differentiates these two conditions is the presence of caudal inflammation (distal to the teeth) in cases of caudal stomatitis* (Figure 8.15).[5,15,30] This presentation was previously called "faucitis" but is now known as caudal mucositis. In contrast, in cases of typical periodontal disease the inflammation is associated with the gingiva surrounding the teeth and does not extend distally to any significant effect (Figure 8.16).

Diagnostics

Caudal stomatitis is a clinical syndrome and does not indicate a specific etiology or diagnosis.[30] Diagnosis is made by visual inspection of the oral cavity.[15] Diagnostic

(a)

(b)

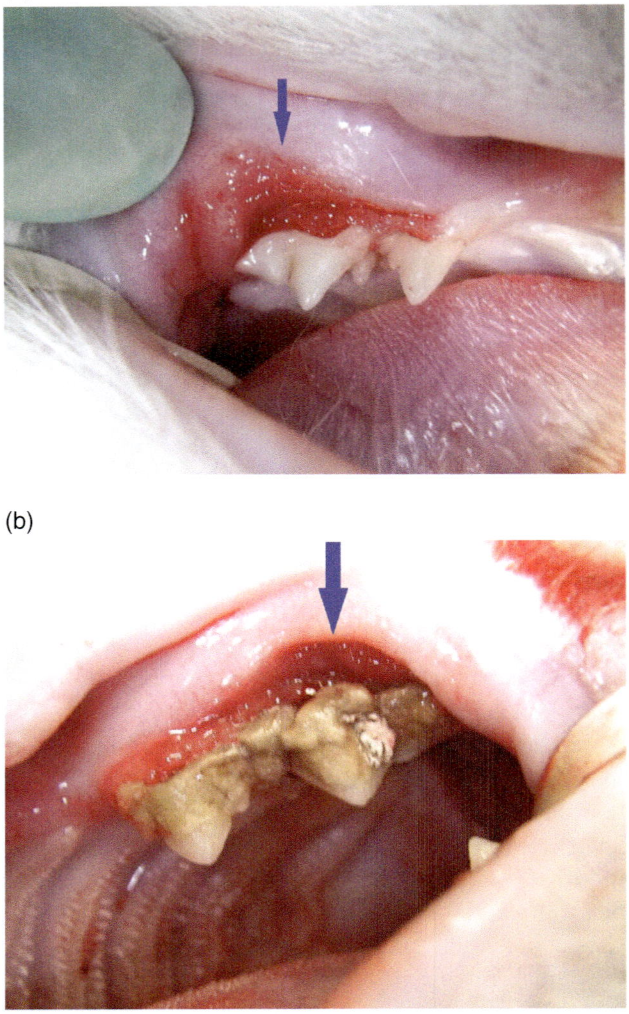

Figure 8.12 (a and b) Intraoral pictures of two feline patients with severe stomatitis. Note the severe inflammation of the attached gingiva as well as the associated buccal mucosa (blue arrows). Note that in Figure 8.12a) there is minimal dental calculus.

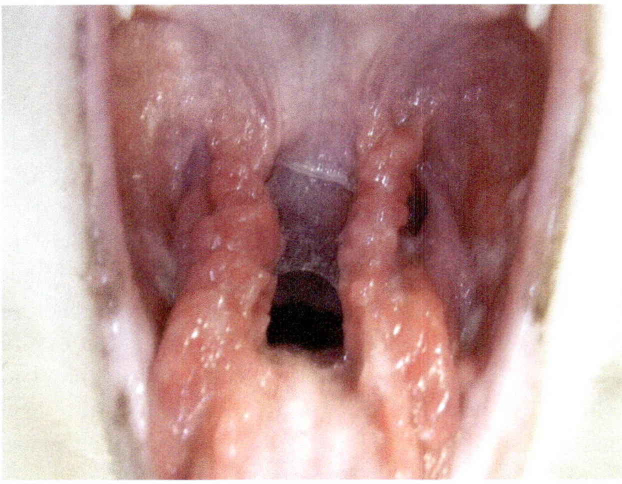

Figure 8.13 Intraoral picture of a feline patient with significant bilateral caudal mucositis.

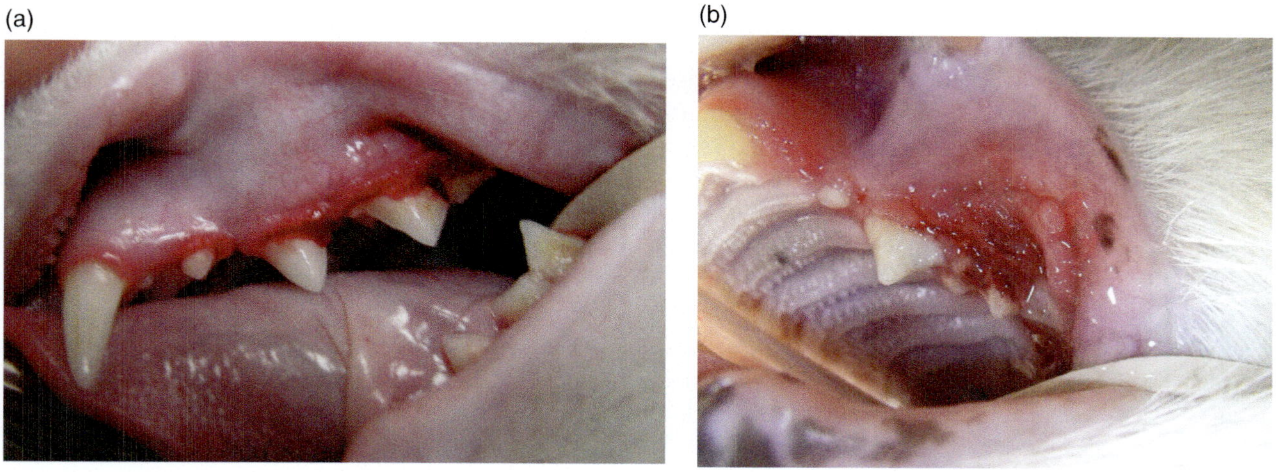

Figure 8.14 (a and b) Intraoral pictures of the maxillary left in two cats with severe caudal stomatitis. These patients have severe oral inflammation and spontaneous hemorrhage.

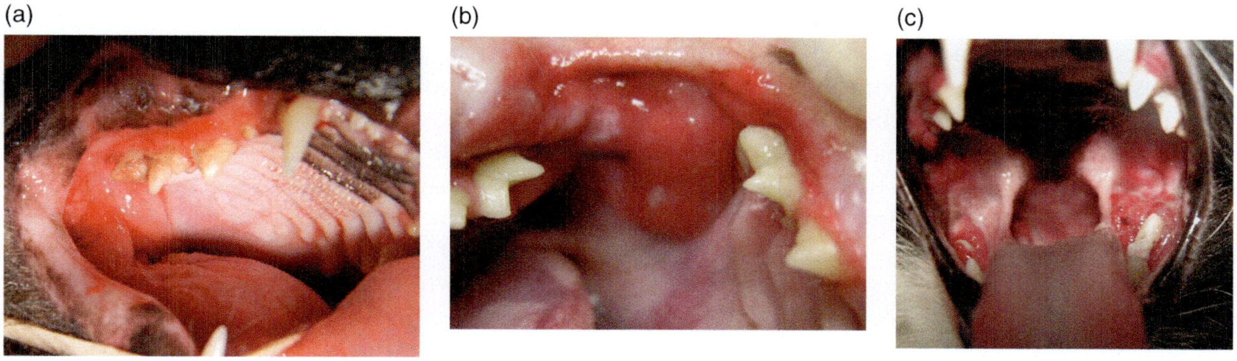

Figure 8.15 (a–c) Caudal mucositis in three feline patients. This is suggestive of caudal stomatitis as opposed to periodontal disease.

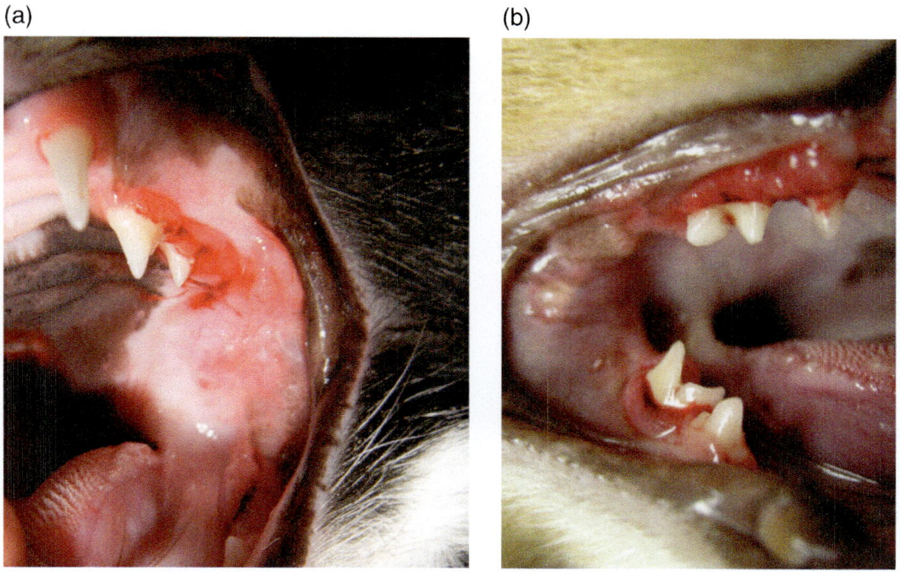

Figure 8.16 (a and b) Intraoral pictures of two patients with significant gingival/periodontal inflammation but no caudal inflammation. This is indicative of periodontal disease as opposed to caudal stomatitis.

tests to further define the disease should minimally include dental radiographs (to evaluate for the presence of retained root tips, periodontal or endodontic disease, or bony changes suggestive of neoplasia), a minimum data base (CBC, chemistry panel, t4, U/A) to evaluate for underlying and/or concurrent systemic health problems, and evaluation of FeLV/FIV status.[14,30] The only common biochemical abnormality is a polyclonal gammopathy.[27]

A biopsy should be taken and submitted for histopathology, especially if the inflammation is asymmetrical or otherwise atypical, or if radiographic findings are suspicious for neoplasia.[5,15] Histopathology typically finds a dominance of plasma cells with some lymphocytes.[32] Serum testing for *B. henselae* may also be considered.

Management

The goal of therapy for this disease process is to completely eradicate the oral inflammation.[27] However, maintaining a state of decreased inflammation is sometimes the best that can be achieved.[5] Several treatments have been suggested, including extraction of all premolars and molars, full mouth extraction, laser treatment to remove inflammatory tissue, chronic immune-suppressive treatment (i.e., cyclosporine, corticosteroids, Imuran), anti-inflammatory treatment (corticosteroids or NSAIDs), interferon, and antibiotics.

Surgical therapy

Controlling inflammation is the key to management of this disease process. Therefore, any tooth affected with inflammation from any cause (periodontal, endodontic, tooth resorption, or alveolar mucocitis) should be extracted.[14] Any remaining teeth must receive strict homecare and routine professional cleanings to keep inflammation at bay. However, since the majority of patients have widespread inflammation that makes homecare challenging, the most successful long-term treatment for cats with chronic gingivostomatitis is the COMPLETE extraction of all premolars and molars as well as careful smoothing of the alveolar bone.[15,30] An additional step taken by many veterinary dentists is to perform careful removal of all periodontal ligament remnants (with a curette or coarse diamond bur), which has anecdotally improved success rates.[5] The reasoning behind extraction therapy is to remove plaque retentive surfaces and therefore virtually eliminate the periodontopathogens from the area, thus decreasing inflammation. Extraction of the canine and incisor teeth is indicated when the inflammation extends to include the gingiva surrounding them (which is the majority of cases).[5,29] Therefore, this author will typically perform FULL mouth extractions in cases of significant oral inflammation, while some veterinary dentists prefer to leave the canines and incisors if at all possible.[5] Postoperative dental radiographs must be exposed to document complete extraction of all tooth roots.[5,29,30]

The vast majority of cats have an excellent response to this treatment, requiring no chronic medical treatment (Figure 8.17).[5,30,33] If the canines and incisors are not extracted, owners must provide meticulous homecare for these teeth. Antibiotic administration (14 days) following extractions is recommended to help resolve the oral infection, and topical rinses such as 0.12% chlorhexidine may also be beneficial during healing.[5] Finally, it has been shown that feeding a recovery food postoperative may be beneficial.[34]

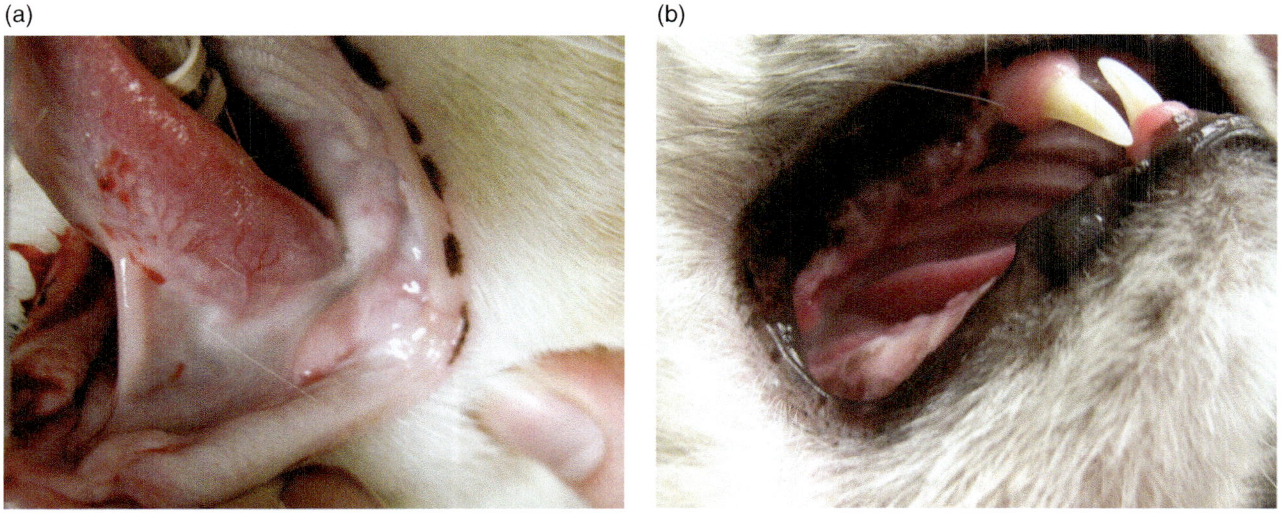

Figure 8.17 Pictures of two feline patients who have received full (a) and caudal (b) mouth extractions. Note the complete resolution of inflammation in both cases.

Regardless of the quality of the extractions, some cats have only partial improvement and require long-term medical management, albeit at much lower doses than prior to surgery. If extraction therapy does not prove to be effective, it is usually due to incomplete extractions (i.e., leaving roots behind), as it is essential to remove all tooth roots (Figures 8.18 and 8.19).[5,30] In rare cases, properly performed extractions may have only a minimal therapeutic effect, and in these cases the patients will require long-term medical management. Fortunately, this is the minority of patients.[30] The patients who have the least response to extraction therapy are typically those that have had long-standing, chronic inflammation that has been treated with repeated high doses of glucocorticoids.[5,30] It is important to note that generally, *the earlier the teeth are extracted the better the outcome.*

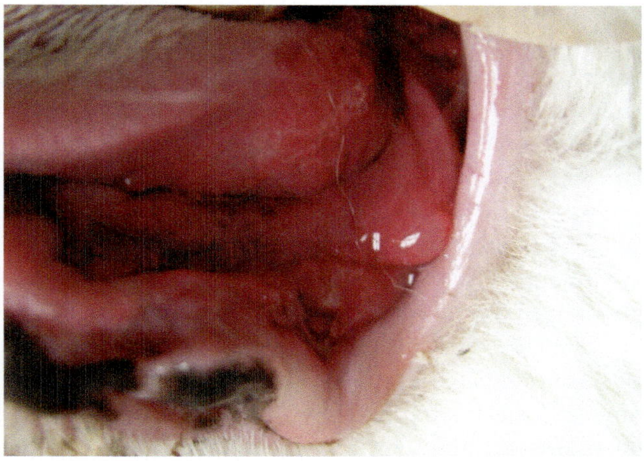

Figure 8.18 Recheck picture of the mandibular left of a cat who had received "full mouth extractions" at a practice without dental radiology. Note the lack of teeth but continued severe oral inflammation.

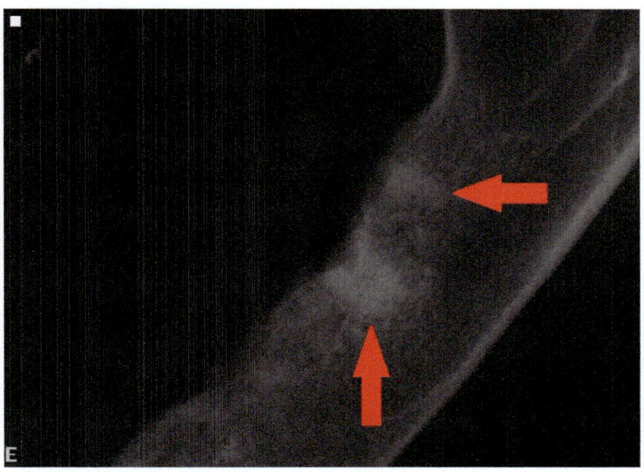

Figure 8.19 Intraoral dental radiograph of the mandibular left of the patient in 8.18 confirming the retained roots (red arrows). Extraction of these retained roots (as well as many others) resulted in complete resolution of inflammation with retained roots (red arrows) from a previous full mouth extraction surgery.

Laser therapy

The use of surgical lasers to control inflammation associated with caudal stomatitis has been anecdotally reported for years. However, there are no current published reports showing laser ablation of the inflamed gingiva has significant beneficial results. One recent case report revealed improvement after surgical laser therapy.[35] However, the improvement did not occur following several laser treatments; resolution occurred only *after* full mouth extractions were eventually performed concurrent to laser ablation. Therefore, laser therapy alone did not have an obvious benefit. Furthermore, the patient appeared to have a significant (although transitory) negative response (pain) after the laser treatments. Finally, this author has treated numerous patients where laser therapy has been used elsewhere with no response. Consequently, it is not currently a recommended form of therapy.

Medical therapy

In cases where owners are reluctant to have multiple extractions performed early in the course of treatment, medical management may be attempted to reduce bacterial load and inflammation. The majority of the products utilized are oral medications, which require daily to twice daily administration. This is difficult to achieve in cats in general, and the oral pain and inflammation only serves to complicate matters. Finally, many of the products have significant side effects (which will be discussed in more detail below). Moreover, clients should be informed that medical therapy is almost invariably a lifelong process with numerous disadvantages. In addition, there are no medical protocols that have been shown to be completely effective; rather they just temporarily reduce the clinical signs.[29] Therefore, clients should be counseled that delaying extraction therapy often results in a decreased response, possibly yet again necessitating long-term medical therapy.

Prior to the initiation of medical therapy, a complete dental prophylaxis should be performed to decrease the amount of oral bacteria and inflammation.[5] At this time, any diseased teeth and/or retained roots should be extracted (as above).[30]

Antibiotics

Systemic antibiotics *may* result in some improvement in the amount of oral inflammation. However, this is generally temporary at best, and most patients will relapse even during the course of antibiotic therapy.[5,29] Amoxicillin-clavulanic acid,[A] clindamycin,[B] metronidazole, and azithromycin[C] are the best antibiotic choices for the oral cavity.[30] Rinsing with a 0.12% chlorhexidine gluconate solution[D] may also be beneficial in some cases.[5]

Anti-inflammatories

Corticosteroids are by far the most commonly used and effective drugs for immune modulation. Steroid administration results in clinical improvement far more often than antibiotic therapy.[5] In addition, glucocorticoids are often used concurrently with antibiotics. Long-term use of corticosteroids may have detrimental effects such as the induction of diabetes mellitus and opportunistic infections.[29,36] Use the lowest effective dose and monitor biochemical values on a regular basis. Injectable treatment (methylprednisone 10–20 mg SC) is usually recommended initially, due to the degree of oral pain.[5,27] This typically results in clinical improvement within 24–48 hours and lasts for 3–6 weeks. However, these intervals tend to progressively shorten the longer the injections are continued, until in some cases no response occurs! For these many reasons, *chronic corticosteroid therapy should only be performed as a last resort when an owner will not allow extractions.*[14]

Another possible option for anti-inflammatory therapy is NSAIDs.[5] These medications are best used on a short-term basis to reduce the inflammation and improve the patient's situation while preparing for extraction surgery.[5] The long-term use of NSAIDs to control the inflammation is a high-risk choice for cats. If this treatment plan is selected, the patient must have good renal function prior to initiating therapy, remain well hydrated, and have routine biochemical testing (including urinalysis) to ensure the kidneys are not being compromised. Meloxicam[5] is approved in cats for a one-time postop injection.[37] If used chronically, it is best to prescribe the lowest possible dose on an every other to every third day schedule.[37] It is important to discuss the risks in detail with the clients and obtain consent for the *off-label* use of these medications. This author does not recommend long-term NSAID use in cats, due to the degree of risk and the potentially fatal effects that can occur.

Cyclosporine

Cyclosporine A has been purported as an immunosuppressive drug for cats with caudal stomatitis.[5] Some have promoted it as an alternative to extractions in order to avoid the use of glucocorticoids. However, this author prefers to withhold its use to those cases where additional medical management is necessary postextraction.

There is scant information that supports its use other than one unpublished veterinary study, which showed efficacy in cases refractory to extractions.[38] However, it may provide an alternative to long-term steroid therapy. It must be used with caution in cats with hepatic or renal disease. In addition, it must be noted that there are reports of fatal opportunistic infections associated the use of cyclosporine.[39–41]

The bioavailability of the three available forms of cyclosporine is quite variable, and therefore dosing depends on which form is used.[29] Recently, a veterinary product has been released for atopy[F] and may be of use in cats. Serum cyclosporine levels should be evaluated within 24–48 hours of beginning therapy and then monitored weekly for a month, and monthly thereafter, to maintain concentrations within the therapeutic range and avoid toxic levels.[5] The recommended range varies between 250 and 1,000 ng/ml.[42] In addition to monitoring cyclosporine levels, standard biochemical tests should be routinely performed as surveillance for deleterious side effects.[29]

Feline interferon

There is currently significant interest in the use of feline interferon[43,G] for caudal stomatitis. It is reported to not only provide an antiviral effect but to also provide an immunomodulatory effect and bring about a return to normal local immune response. Several studies have shown efficacy in resistant cases,[44–46] but as of yet, no evidence exists to show that it works as a primary treatment. There are several options for therapy including intralesional injection and/or oral versus injectable systemic treatment.[14,29] The preferred method at this point is to inject 5 MU intralesional (often at the time of extractions) and then follow this up with the remainder of the vial (5 MU) diluted into 100 cc of sterile saline and administered per os by the owner at a dose of 1 ml once daily for 100 days.[29] Note that this product in not currently available in the United States.

Other medications

Lactoferrin (topically @ 40 mg/kg),[47,48] gold salts (1–2 mg weekly for 8 weeks and then monthly),[27] levamisole (2–5 mg/kg PO 3 times weekly),[27] doxycycline (2 mg/kg BID, with decreasing doses if effective),[29] and coenzyme Q10 (30–60 mg daily)[5] have also been used with occasional success. However, none of these therapies are recommended at this time.

Conclusions

It must be noted that even intense efforts at plaque control in addition to medical therapy (antibiotics and anti-inflammatories) rarely result in an acceptable response.[29] Therefore, at the time of this writing, surgical extraction therapy is the preferred treatment and should be performed as soon as possible. Medical therapy should be reserved for those cases where clients will not

Box 8.2 Key points

- Caudal stomatitis is defined as significant inflammation to the oral mucosa typically centered on the caudal oropharynx.
- Caudal stomatitis is a *clinical* diagnosis.
- Surgical therapy with partial to full mouth extractions is the treatment of choice for this condition.
- Medical therapy requires lifelong management, with numerous deleterious side effects, and is often frustrating.

allow (or cannot afford) extraction therapy. This author's approach with resistant cases (where retained roots are ruled out) is as follows: (1) feline interferon, (2) cyclosporine, (3) corticosteroids.

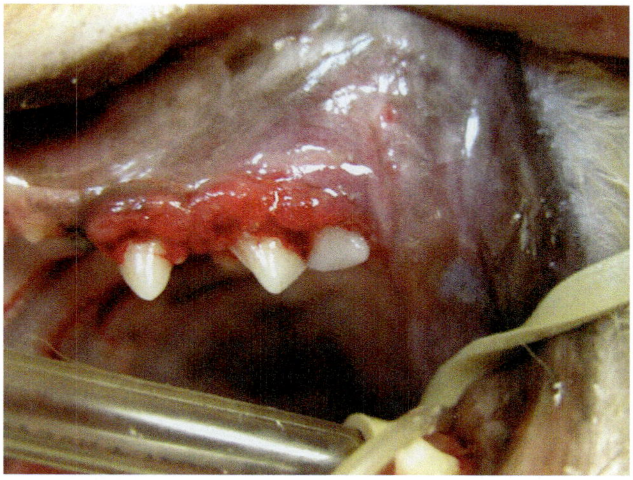

Figure 8.20 Intraoral picture of the maxillary left of a 9-month-old feline patient with severe hyperplastic gingivitis. Note the lack of dental calculus and caudal mucositis. This is the classic appearance of juvenile gingivitis.

Feline juvenile (puberty) gingivitis/periodontitis

Definition

Juvenile periodontal disease is inflammation that occurs soon after permanent tooth eruption.[27] This syndrome can be described in two categories, *feline hyperplastic gingivitis* (where the inflammation is confined to the gingiva), and *juvenile onset periodontitis*.[49]

Etiology

As of this writing, the etiology of this condition is unknown. However, in humans there is a period of increased susceptibility to gingivitis during the pubertal period (puberty gingivitis).[49,50] A genetic predisposition toward feline juvenile onset periodontitis has been reported in Siamese, Somali, and Maine Coon cats.[27]

Clinical features

Hyperplastic gingivitis appears as gingival enlargement and significant inflammation (Figure 8.20), which is confined to the gingiva and begins during the eruptive period of the permanent dentition. Bleeding during mastication and on oral exam is a common finding.[49] While occasionally seen in dogs, this condition has a much higher incidence in cats.[27] It is generally a non-painful condition for the patient, and halitosis is a common complaint. If left untreated, it typically proceeds quickly to periodontal disease, which may result in early exfoliation of the teeth.[49] This disease is commonly mistaken for caudal stomatitis. The distinguishing clinical sign is the lack of caudal inflammation in this disease process (Figure 8.21).

As the patient matures, susceptibility appears to subside at approximately 2 years of age,[27] which is the same type of pattern followed in the human disease.[50] Ergo, if this process is treated aggressively early on, the patient may enjoy normal periodontal health in the future.

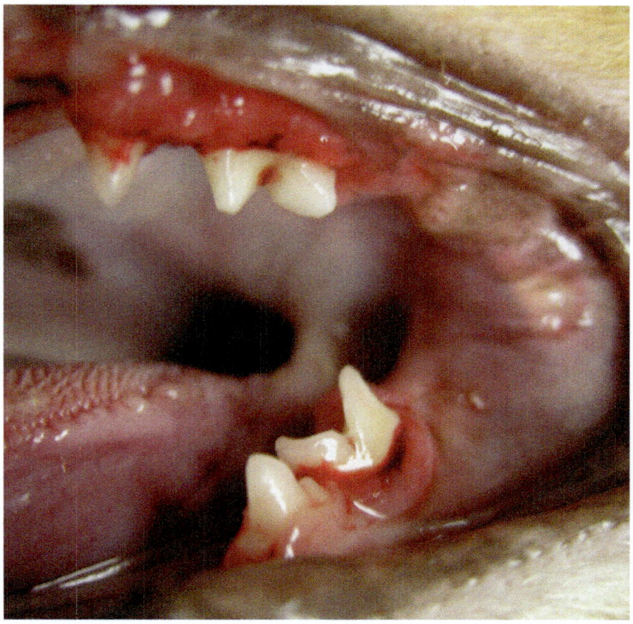

Figure 8.21 Intraoral picture of the left of the patient in Figure 8.20. Note the lack of dental calculus and caudal mucositis. This is the classic appearance of juvenile gingivitis, *not* "stomatitis."

In contrast, *juvenile periodontitis* does not involve enlargement of the gingiva and usually leads to the rapid proliferation of plaque and calculus and subsequent inflammation (Figure 8.22). This in turn results in significant early bone loss, periodontal pocket formation, and furcation exposure (Figure 8.23).[27] This is generally the worst in and around the mandibular first molars (Figure 8.24). Treatment and effective management of these cases is often exceedingly difficult.[49]

(a) (b)

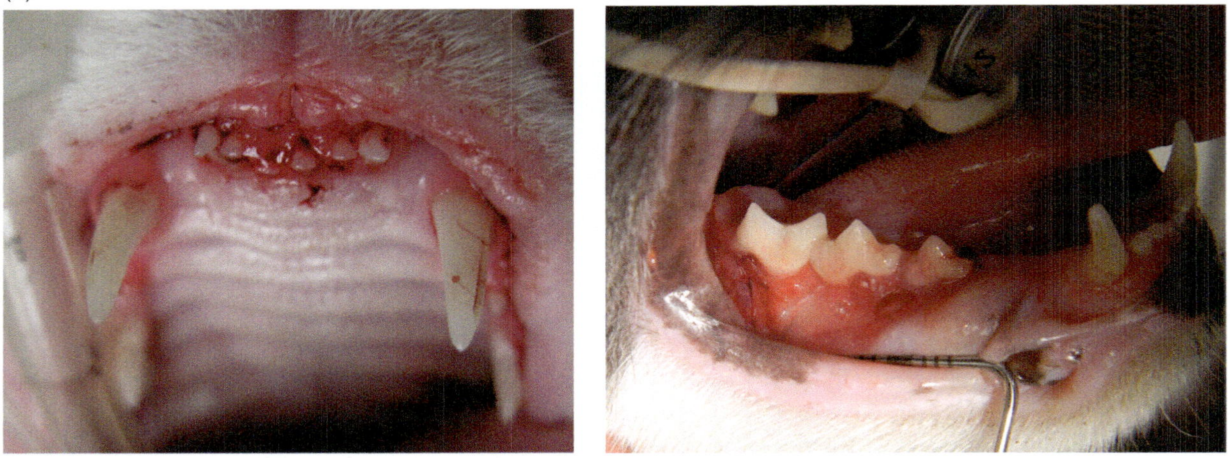

Figure 8.22 Intraoral dental pictures of the maxillary incisors (a) and mandibular right (b) of two different juvenile feline patients with significant juvenile periodontitis. Note the severe oral inflammation and gingival recession with minimal dental calculus.

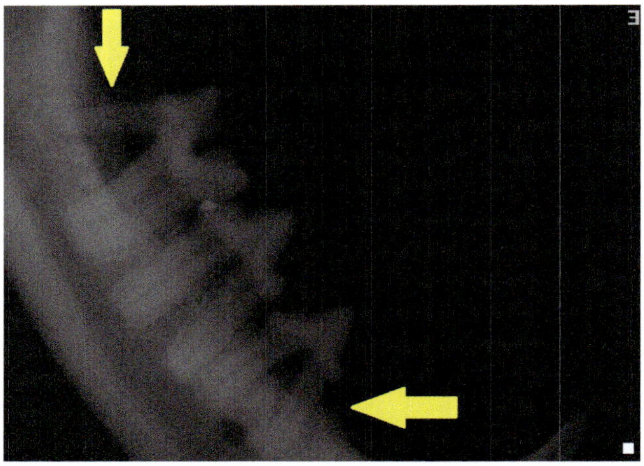

Figure 8.23 Intraoral dental radiograph of the mandibular right of a young feline patient with severe periodontal loss resulting in class III furcation exposure of the third premolar (407) and first molar (409) (yellow arrows).

Diagnostics

Histopathology (via incisional biopsy) should be considered to rule out other causes of gingival inflammation.[49] Culture and sensitivity testing is generally unrewarding but may be of value in non-responsive cases. Dental radiographs should be performed to evaluate the quality of the alveolar bone and also for early tooth resorption. Finally, *Bartonella* testing may be beneficial in some cases, especially in patients who do not respond to traditional management practices.

Management

In the management of both of these conditions, early (9 months of age) and frequent (q 6–9 months) dental prophylaxis (even if only minimal plaque is present)

(a)

(b)

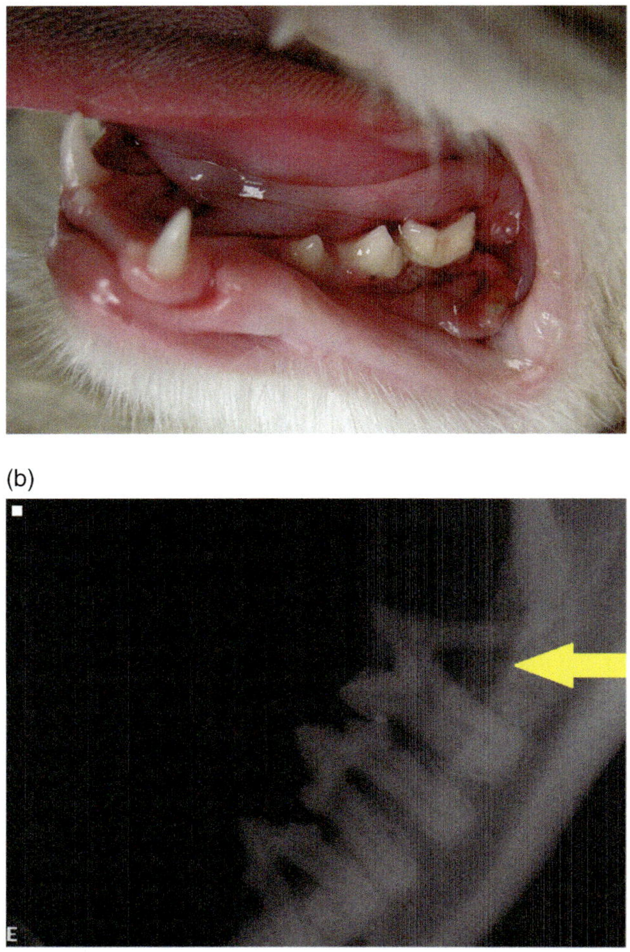

Figure 8.24 (a) Intraoral dental picture of the mandibular left of a feline patient with severe juvenile periodontitis. The entire caudal arcade is involved, but inflammation is worst over the mandibular first molar. (b) Corresponding intraoral dental radiograph confirming the severe alveolar loss, which is worst around the first molar (309) (yellow arrow).

along with strict homecare is critical to decrease inflammation.[49] Ideally, homecare consists of daily brushing, as it is the gold standard of plaque control. Other homecare alternatives include chlorhexadine rinses[H] as well as plaque control diets[I] and treats. Finally, this author has had success with a tasteless, commercially available zinc ascorbate gel.[J] In cases where gingival hyperplasia is present, early gingivectomy is recommended to remove psedopockets, decrease inflammation, and facilitate plaque control (both professional and homecare).[27] Finally, extraction of any significantly diseased teeth is warranted to decrease the degree of inflammation.[49]

Box 8.3 Key points

- Juvenile periodontal disease involves severe periodontal inflammation that occurs during and immediately after eruption of the permanent dentition.
- Treatment and management of this condition includes early (and regular) professional plaque control (dental prophylaxis), gingivectomy (if indicated), and strict homecare.
- With proper therapy, susceptibility may subside at about 2 years of age.

Notes

A. Clavamox, Pfizer Animal Health.
B. Antirobe, Pfizer Animal Health.
C. Zithromax, Pfizer Animal Health.
D. CET Oral Hygiene Rinse, Virbac Animal Health.
E. Metacam, Boehringer Ingelheim Vetmedica, Inc.
F. Atopica, Novartis Animal Health, Inc.
G. Vibragen, Virbac Animal Health.
H. CET Oral Hygiene Rinse, Virbac Animal Health.
I. t/d canine and feline, Hill's Pet Nutrition.
J. Maxiguard oral cleansing gel, Addisons biologics.

References

1. Melnick PR, Takei HH. Treatment of periodontal abscess. In: Carranza's Clinical Periodontology. St. Louis: Saunders, 2006, pp. 714–721.
2. Wiggs RB, Lobprise HB. Periodontology. In: Veterinary Dentistry, Principles and Practice. Philadelphia: Lippincott-Raven, 1997, pp. 186–231.
3. Carranza FA, Carmago PM. The periodontal pocket. In: Carranza's Clinical Periodontology. St. Louis: Saunders, 2006, pp. 434–451.
4. Meng HX. Periodontal abscess. Ann Periodontol. 4:79–83, 1999.
5. Debowes LJ. Problems with the gingiva. In: Small Animal Dental, Oral and Maxillofacial Disease, a Color Handbook (Niemiec BA ed.). London: Manson, 2010, pp. 159–181.
6. Melnick PR, Takei HH. Treatment of periodontal abscess. In: Carranza's Clinical Periodontology. St. Louis: Saunders, 2006, pp. 714–721.
7. Becker W, Berg L, Becker BE. The long term evaluation of periodontal treatment and maintenance in 95 patients. Int J Periodontics Restorative Dent. 4(2):54–71, 1984.
8. Epstein S, Scopp IW. Antibiotics and the intraoral abscess. J Periodontol. 48(4):236–238, 1977.
9. Topoll H, Lange D, Muller R. Multiple periodontal abscesses after systemic antibiotic therapy. J Clin Periodontol. 17(4):268–272, 1990.
10. Meng HX. Periodontal abscess. Ann Periodontol. 4:79–83, 1999.
11. Herrera D, Roldán S, González I, Sanz M. The periodontal abscess (I). Clinical and microbiological findings. J Clin Periodontol. 27(6):387–394, 2000.
12. Dahlén G. Microbiology and treatment of dental abscesses and periodontal-endodontic lesions. Periodontol 2000. 28:206–239, 2002.
13. Mulligan TM, Aller MS, Williams CE. Interpretation of periodontal disease. In: Atlas of Canine and Feline Dental Radiography. Trenton, NJ: Veterinary Learning Systems, 1998, pp. 104–123.
14. Camy G, Fahrenkrug P, Gracis M, et al. Proposed guidelines on the management of feline chronic gingivostomatitis (FCGS) syndrome: A consensus statement, September 2010.
15. Lyon KF. Gingivostomatitis. Vet Clin North Am Small Anim Pract. 35(4):891–911, 2005.
16. AVDC Accepted Nomenclature. WWW AVDC.org, accessed Jan. 1, 2011.
17. Zwemer TJ. In: Boucher's Clinical Dental Terminology: A Glossary of Accepted Terms in Disciplines of Dentistry. Philadelphia: Mosby, 1993, p. 116.
18. Lommer MJ, Verstraete FJM. Concurrent oral shedding of feline calicivirus and feline herpesvirus 1 in cats with chronic gingivostomatitis. Oral Microbiology and Immunology 18:131–134, 2003.
19. Hardy WD, Zuckerman E, Corbishley J. Serological evidence that *Bartonella* cause gingivitis and stomatitis in cats. In Proceedings, 16th Annual Veterinary Dental Forum, October 3–6, 2002, pp. 79–82.
20. Thompson RR, Wilcox GE, Clark WT, Jansen KL. Association of calicivirus infection with chronic gingivitis and pharyngitis in cats. J Small Anim Pract. 25(4):207–210, 1984.
21. Dowers KL, Hawley JR, Brewer MM, Morris AK, Radecki SV, Lappin MR. Association of Bartonella species, feline calicivirus, and feline herpesvirus 1 infection with gingivostomatitis in cats. J Feline Med Surg. 12(4):314–321, 2010.
22. Lee M, Bosward KL, Norris JM. Immunohistological evaluation of feline herpesvirus-1 infection in feline eosinophilic dermatoses or stomatitis. J Feline Med Surg. 12(2):72–79, 2010.
23. Poulet H, Brunet S, Soulier M, Leroy V, Goutebroze S, Chappuis G. Comparison between acute oral/respiratory and chronic stomatitis/gingivitis isolates of feline calicivirus: Pathogenicity, antigenic profile and cross-neutralisation studies. Arch Virol. 145(2):243–261, 2000.
24. Reubel GH, Hoffmann DE, Pederson NC. Acute and chronic faucitis of domestic cats: A feline calicivirus-induced disease. Vet Clin North Am Small Anim Pract. 22(6):1347–1360, 1992.
25. Harley R, Gruffydd-Jones TJ, Day MJ. Determination of salivary and serum immunoglobulin concentrations in the cat. Vet Immunol Immunopath. 65:99–112, 1998.
26. Quimby JM, Elston T, Hawley J, Brewer M, Miller A, Lappin MR. Evaluation of the association of Bartonella species, feline herpesvirus 1, feline calicivirus, feline leukemia virus and feline immunodeficiency virus with chronic feline gingivostomatitis. J Feline Med Surg. 10(1):66–72, 2008.
27. Wiggs RB, Lobprise HB. Domestic feline oral and dental disease. In: Veterinary Dentistry, Principles and Practice. Philadelphia: Lippincott-Raven, 1997, pp. 482–517.

28. Dolieslager SM, Riggio MP, Lennon A, Lappin DF, Johnston N, Taylor D, Bennett D. Identification of bacteria associated with feline chronic gingivostomatitis using culture-dependent and culture-independent methods. Vet Microbiol. Aug. 17, 2010.
29. Bellows J. Treatment of oropharyngeal inflammation. In: Feline Dentistry: Oral Assessment, Treatment, and Preventative Care. Ames, IA: Wiley-Blackwell, pp. 242–268, 2010.
30. Niemiec BA. Oral pathology. Top Companion Anim Med. 23(2):59–71, 2008.
31. Niemiec BA. Ptyalism. In: Textbook of Veterinary Internal Medicine (Ettinger SJ, Feldman EC eds.). 7th ed. New York: Elsevier, 2012.
32. Frost P, Williams CA. Feline dental disease. Vet Clin North Am Small Anim Pract. 16:851–873, 1986.
33. Hennet P. Chronic gingiva-stomatitis in cats: Long term follow up on 30 cases treated by dental extractions. J Vet Dent. 14(1):15–21, 1997.
34. Theyse LFH, et al. Partial extraction in cats with gingivitis-stomatitis-pharengitis-complex—beneficial effects of a recovery food. Symposium Proceedings of Hill's European Symposium on Oral Care, 2003.
35. Lewis JR, Tsugawa AJ, Reiter AM. Use of CO_2 laser as an adjunctive treatment for caudal stomatitis in a cat. J Vet Dent. 24(4):240–249, 2007.
36. Niemiec BA. Problems of the oral mucosa In: Small Animal Dental, Oral and Maxillofacial Disease, a Color Handbook (Niemiec BA ed.). London: Manson, 2010, pp. 183–198.
37. Plumb DC. Plumb's Veterinary Drug Handbook. 6th ed. Ames, IA: Blackwell, 2008, pp. 574–575.
38. Lommer MJ. Use of cyclosporine for the treatment of refractory feline gingivostomatitis. Proceedings of the 22nd Annual Dental Forum, 2008.
39. Last RD, Suzuki Y, Manning T, Lindsay D, Galipeau L, Whitbred TJ. A case of fatal systemic toxoplasmosis in a cat being treated with cyclosporine A for feline atopy. Vet Dermatol. 15(3):194–198, 2004.
40. Beatty J, Barra V. Acute toxoplasmosis in two cats on cyclosporine therapy. Aust Vet J. 81(6):339, 2003.
41. Davis E. Systemic cyclosporine administration and life threatening infections. An emerging problem in veterinary medicine. Proceedings of the American Veterinary Dental Forum, 2007.
42. Plumb DC. Plumb's Veterinary Drug Handbook. 5th ed. Ames, IA: Blackwell, 2005.
43. Southerden P, Gorrel C. Treatment of a case of refractory feline chronic gingivostomatitis with recombinant interferon omega. J Small Anim Pract. 48(2):104–106, 2007.
44. Hennet P, Camay G. Comparitive efficacy of a recombinant feline interferonomega in refractory cases of calici-virus positive cats with caudal stomatitis: A randomized multicentric, controlled, double blind study in 39 cats. Proceedings European Congress of Veterinary Dentistry, 2010.
45. Southererden P, Gorrel C. Treatment of a case of refractory feline chronic gingivostomatitis with feline recombinant interferon omega. J Small Anim Pract. 47:1–3, 2006.
46. Mihaljevic S. Felne gingivitis-somatitis FORI complex: First clinical data on the use of interferon. Procedings of the BTP Congress, Nuremberg, 2002.
47. Sato R, Inanami O, Tanaka Y, Takase M, Naito Y. Oral administration of bovine lactoferrin for treatment of intractable stomatitis in feline immunodeficiency virus (FIV)-positive and FIV-negative cats. Am J Vet Res. 57(10):1443–1446, 1996.
48. Addie DD, Radford A, Yam PS, Taylor DJ. Cessation of feline calicivirus shedding coincident with resolution of chronic gingivostomatitis in a cat. J Small Anim Pract. 44(4):172–176, 2003.
49. Niemiec BA. Pathology in the pediatric patient. In: Small Animal Dental, Oral and Maxillofacial Disease, a Color Handbook (Niemiec BA ed.). London: Manson, 2010, pp. 189–226.
50. Neville BW, Damm DD, Allen CM, Bouquot JE. Periodontal diseases. In: Oral and Maxillofacial Pathology. 2nd ed. Philadelphia: Saunders, 2002, pp. 137–162.

SECTION 3

Initial therapy of periodontal disease

9

Dental radiology for periodontal disease

Jerzy Gawor

More is missed by not looking than by not knowing.
Thomas McCrae, 1870–1935

The value of periodontal radiography

Periodontal disease is the number one health problem in small animal patients, and therefore appropriate diagnosis has become very important.[1] The periodontium is the three-dimensional group of tissues, structures, and substances that represent different levels of x-ray beam penetration (Figure 9.1). A clinical evaluation of the periodontium is always performed first, followed by the radiographic study. These two examinations are complementary,[2] and therefore the gold standard of veterinary oral health care includes thorough clinical assessment of all teeth (periodontal probing) as well as full mouth radiography.[3]

Radiographic examination is an important part of clinical assessment; moreover, the examination is not complete without radiography. For periodontal disease, endodontic problems, fractures, caries, resorptive lesions, bone pathology and proliferative conditions radiography is mandatory[4,5] (Figures 9.2 and 9.3).

The value of radiographic evaluation in veterinary patients was proven in studies that found 27.8% of clinically important lesions in dogs and 41.7% in cats would be missed without full mouth radiography[5,6] (Figures 9.4 and 9.5).

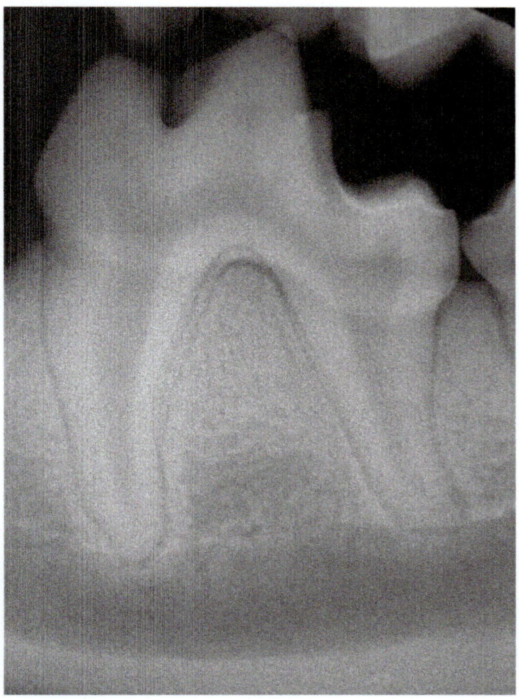

Figure 9.1 The periodontium is the three-dimensional group of different tissues, structures, and substances that represent different levels of x-ray beam penetration.

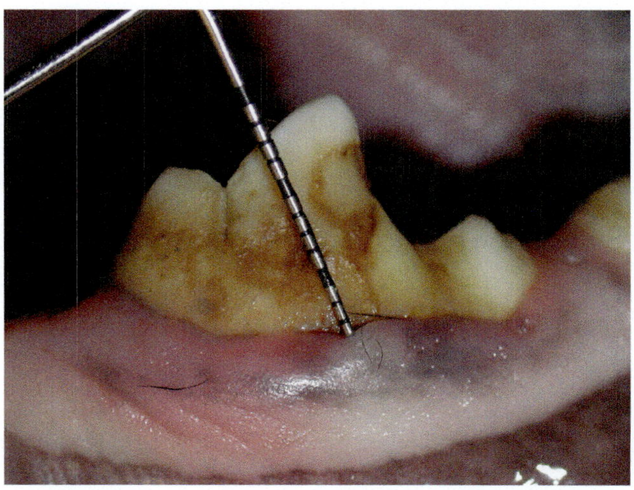

Figure 9.2 Apart from enamel and dentinal hypoplasia, periodontal examination of the left mandibular first molar (309) tooth does not reveal any pathology.

Veterinary Periodontology, First Edition. Brook A. Niemiec.

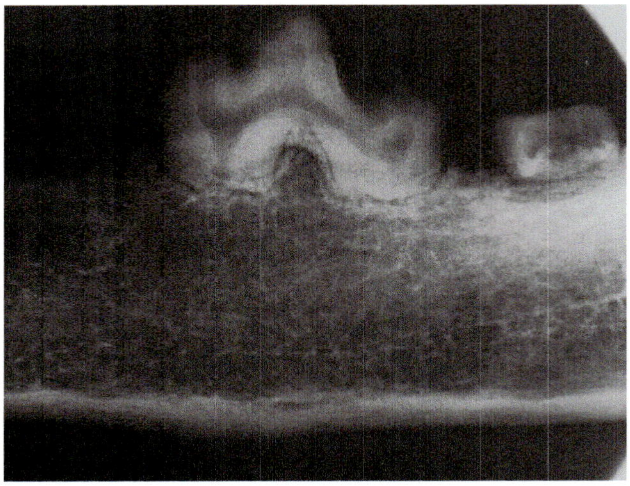

Figure 9.3 Radiograph of the tooth from Figure 9.2; reduced periodontal structures present due to the undeveloped roots.

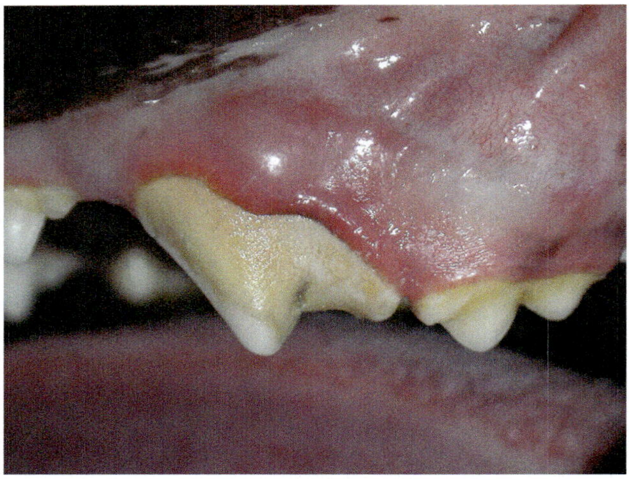

Figure 9.4 Intraoral dental picture of the left maxillary fourth premolar (208) which is covered by calculus and plaque; the gingiva is slightly inflamed. Periodontal probing revealed a pathologic pocket at the buccal aspect of 208. Adjacent teeth are normal.

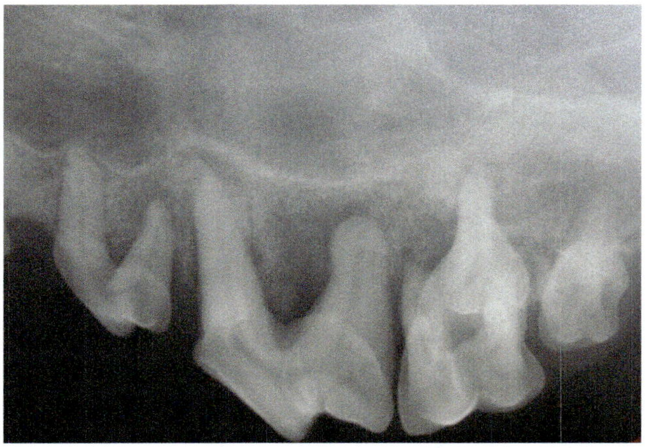

Figure 9.5 Radiograph of the 208 from Figure 9.4. The radiograph reveals significant pathology affecting entire periodontal tissue of 207 through 210.

It has been shown that older patients benefit more from radiography[7] and that periodontal disease is more common in older animals.[8] Therefore, full mouth radiography is an obligatory part of the diagnostic plan in older animals or in those more prone to periodontal disease (small and toy breed dogs) as well as other predisposed breeds (e.g., Greyhounds)[5,6] (Figures 9.6 and 9.7). Another study revealed that the clinical and

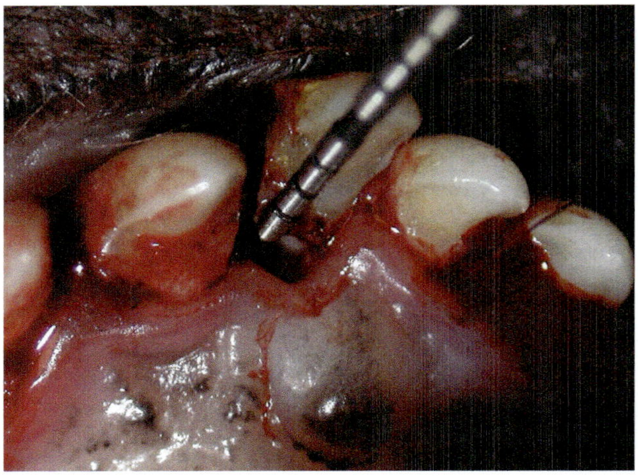

Figure 9.6 10-year-old Yorkshire Terrier. Clinical evaulation of the maxillary incisors. PD2 (<25% attachment loss) in 103 and 203. PD3 (25–50% attachment loss) in 102 and 202, PD4 (more than 50% of the attachment loss) in 101 and 201. Mobility grade 3 in 101.

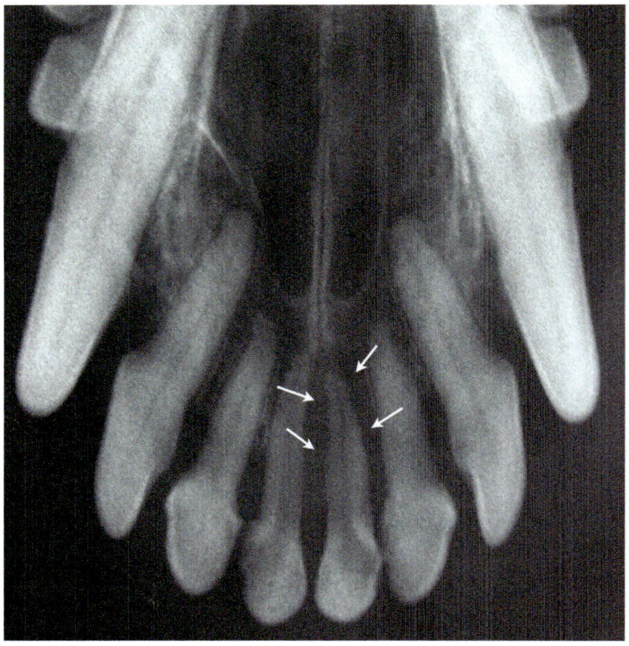

Figure 9.7 Patient from Figure 9.6. Radiograph of the maxillary incisors. Bone loss of the alveolar socket in 101 marked by the white arrows.

radiographic examination may differ and this difference is increased when utilizing histometric measurements. The disparity reported in published studies was between 14% and 60%[9,10] (Figures 9.8 and 9.9). In addition, the clinical appearance of the evaluated area does not correlate completely with the radiographic one and vice versa[11] (Figures 9.10 and 9.11).

The major limitations of radiographic evaluation of the alveolar bone are:

1. Dental radiographs will not show changes until more than 30–60% bone resorption has occurred.[12,13]
2. There are certain situations where clinical examination is necessary for proper diagnosis; for example, if the bone loss occurs on the lingual or buccal/palatal site of the alveolar bone only[14] (Figure 9.12).
3. The early stage of periodontal disease (gingivitis) is not radiographically evident, and therefore clinical evidence of disease preceeds radiographic changes.
4. The first grade of furcation involvement is not evident radiographically.

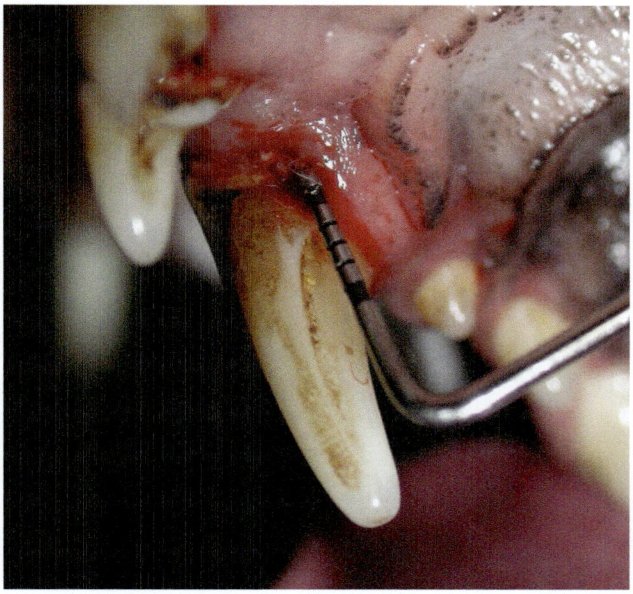

Figure 9.8 Periodontal probing revealed 9 mm perio-pocket from the mesio-palatal aspect of the right maxillary canine 104.

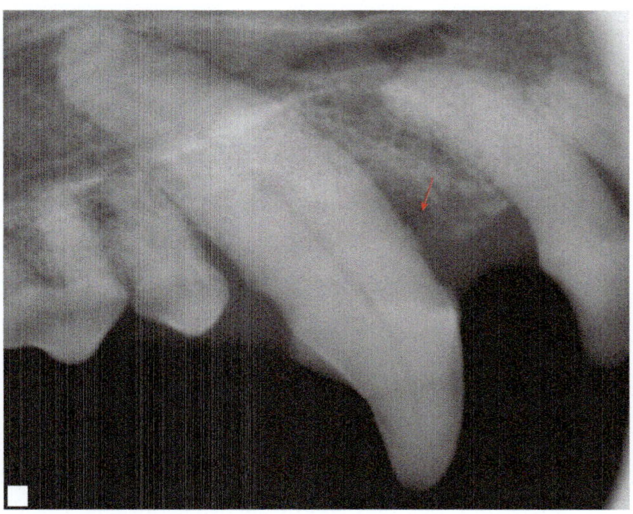

Figure 9.9 Radiograph of 104 from Figure 9.8. Distance from CEJ to the pocket bottom is 11 mm (arrow).

Appropriate evaluation of the radiographs depends on the quality of exposure, which requires correct positioning and conditions. Underexposed, burnout, and malpositioned radiographs are non-diagnostic[14] (Figures 9.13 and 9.14). In general, dental radiographs for periodontal assessment should be made slightly underexposed.[15]

Quality of the x-ray depends on the resolution as well. Erikssen provided the results of microfocal radiography in evaluation of the delicate feline periodontal

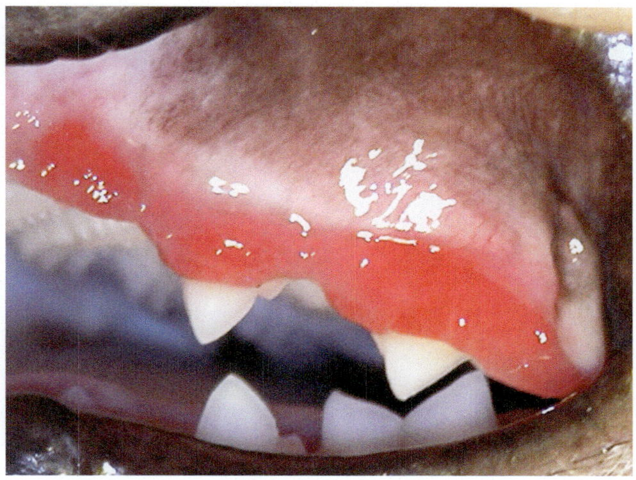

Figure 9.10 A 10-month-old female, Maine Coon cat with juvenile gingivitis.

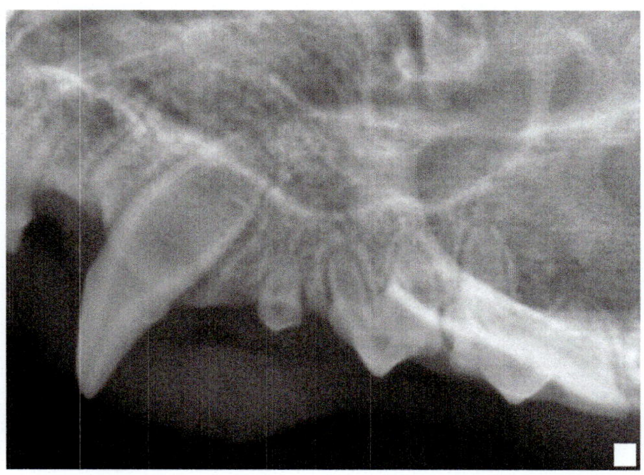

Figure 9.11 Radiograph of the area presented in Figure 9.10. No radiographic evidence of the severe gum disease.

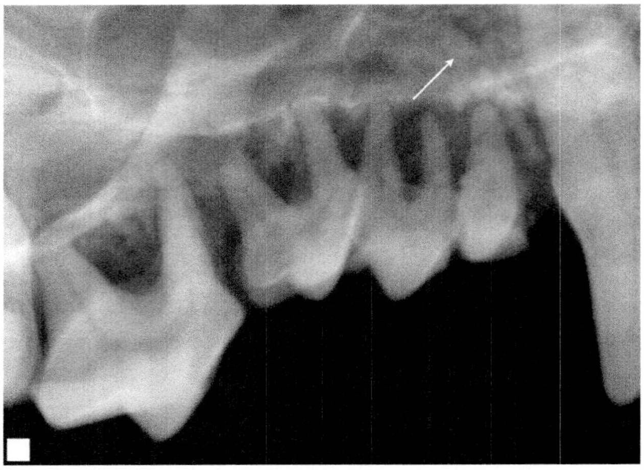

Figure 9.12 Radiograph of the right maxilla with horizontal bone loss in all four premolars and canine. Clinical examination can define which site of the alveolar bone is more affected. Root remnant of 504 is visible (white arrow).

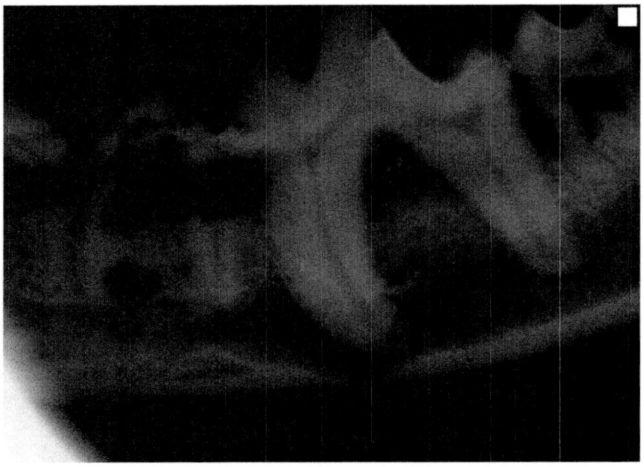

Figure 9.13 Radiograph of the left mandible (teeth 307–310) is overexposed and non-diagnostic.

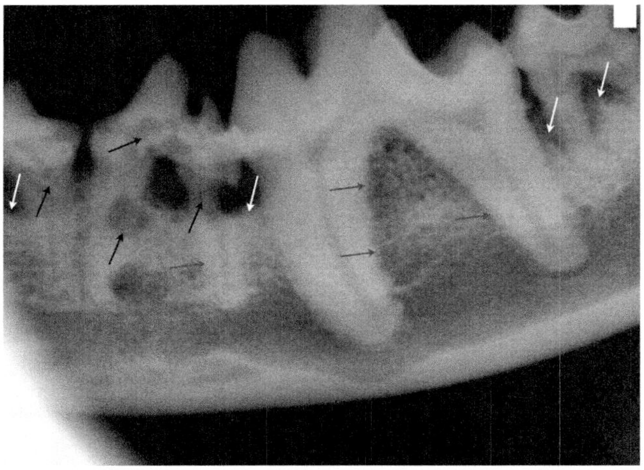

Figure 9.14 The same projection with reduced exposure. Visible: bone loss, resorption, and ankylosis. White arrows indicate bone loss, black arrows resorption, and red arrows show ankylosis.

structures.[16] Though valuable findings were provided, this method is not currently practical for general and wide application in veterinary medicine.

Before any radiographs are taken it is useful to clean the teeth, as the dental calculus is radiodense and can obscure pathological lesions on a radiograph.[17]

The best radiographic technique for avoiding image distortion is the direct lateral view (parallel technique).[18] This technique requires parallel positioning of the film to the object (tooth/root). However, the anatomy of dogs and cats does not allow this projection for all teeth.[18,19] In addition, placement of the tube head perpendicular to the film is necessary to achieve diagnostic images. The importance of correct positioning of the x-ray beam is demonstrated in Figures 9.15, 9.16,

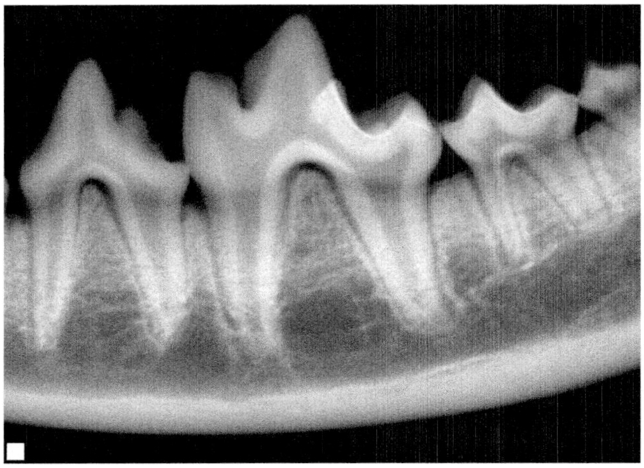

Figure 9.15 Radiograph of the left mandible (teeth 308–311). Lateral projection with x-ray beam perpendicular to the object and film.

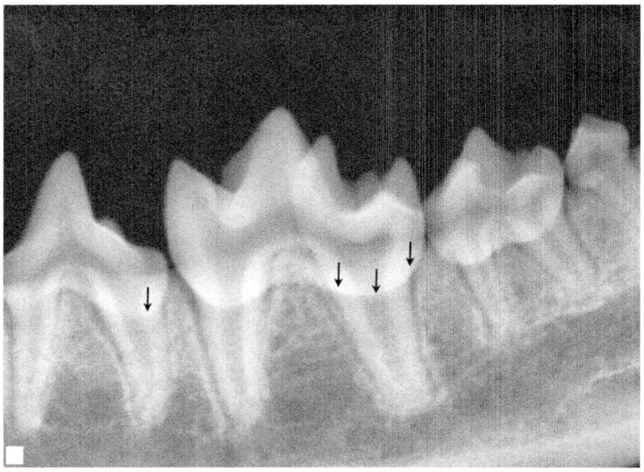

Figure 9.16 The same area as in Figure 9.15, with the same position of film. The x-ray beam is focused on the same object but the beam is shifted dorsally (x-ray beam is non-perpendicular to the film and object). Foreshortened image, teeth crowns overlap roots (black arrows).

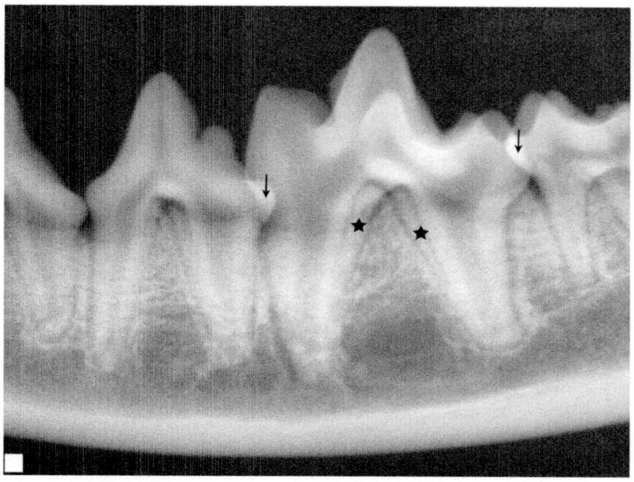

Figure 9.17 The same area as in Figure 9.15, with the same position of film. The x-ray beam is focused on the same object but shifted mesially (x-ray beam is not pependicular to the film and object). Interproximal crown surfaces (black arrows) and radicular grooves (black stars) overlap one another.

and 9.17. In human radiology, four criteria to determine adequate angulation of periapical radiographs are (1) the radiograph should show the tips of molar cusps with little or none of the occlusal surface showing, (2) enamel caps and pulp chambers should be distinct, (3) interproximal spaces should be open, and (4) proximal contacts should not overlap unless teeth are out of line anatomically.[20]

Some efforts had been made to evaluate different radiographic views for periodontal attachment evaluation of the canine teeth in dogs.[21] It is also mentioned that radiographs produced with the bisecting angle technique may appear to indicate greater destruction of the alveolar bone than is actually present.[17]

The periodontal hard tissues consist of cementum and alveolar bone. The periodontal aspect of radiography is focused on

1. The continuity of lamina dura.
2. The width of periodontal ligament space.
3. The shape, height, and density of alveolar bone process.

The alveolar process of the maxilla and mandible fills the furcation (the interradicular space) and interalveolar space.[22] Both parts may be affected by periodontitis[23] (Figure 9.18).

The radiographic appearance of healthy human periodontal tissues is as follows:

1. There is a continuous visible and linear lamina dura.
2. The angle between lamina dura of the alveolar sockets is sharp.
3. There is a minimum 2 mm distance between the edge of the alveolus and the CEJ.[24]

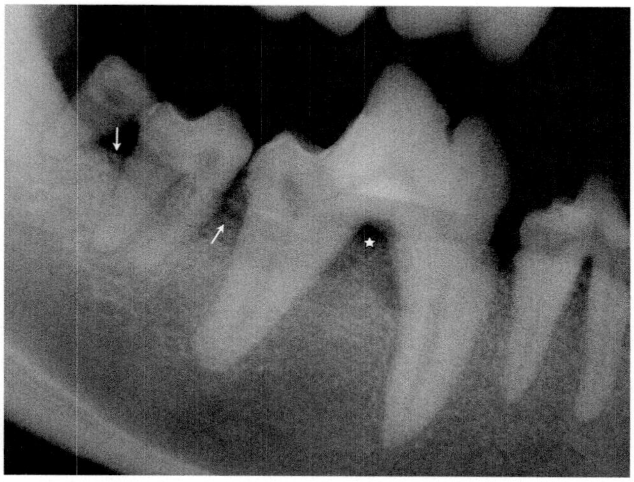

Figure 9.18 Radiograph of the right mandible (teeth 408–411). The interradicular space (star) and interalveolar space (arrows) of the alveolar bone may be affected by periodontitis.

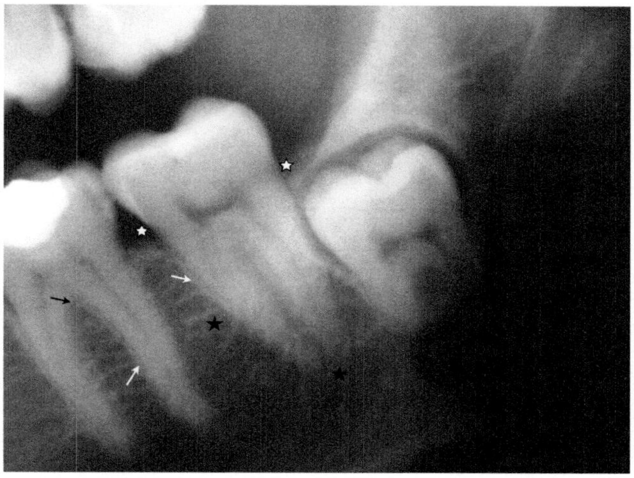

Figure 9.19 Radiograph of the left mandible of a 42-year-old male human patient. Human healthy periodontium radiography requires continuous visible and linear lamina dura (white arrows). The angle between lamina dura of the alveolar sockets is sharp (black arrow). Another standard is the minimum 2 mm distance between the edge of the alveolus and the CEJ (white stars). The spongious bone appearance in the periapical area should be the same as in the interalveolar region (black stars). Also note the impacted molar.

4. The spongious bone appearance in the periapical area should be the same as in the interalveolar region[24] (Figure 9.19).

The furcation is an important and delicate area to evaluate. When furcational bone loss is evident, it is reasonable to make an additional image with a decreased exposure to confirm the bone loss, as opposed to an overexposed film[15] (Figures 9.20 and 9.21).

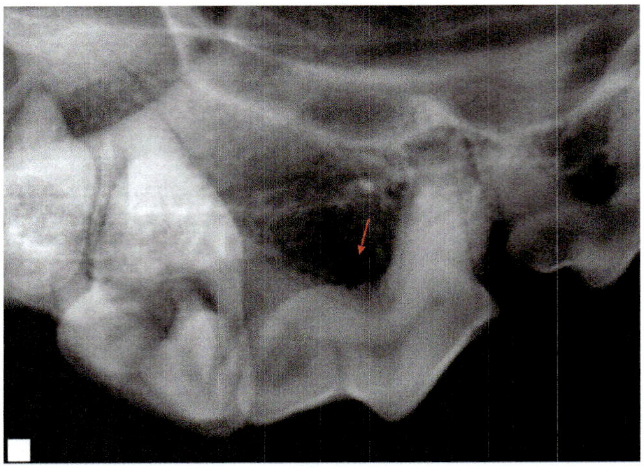

Figure 9.20 Radiograph of the right maxilla (teeth 107–110). Due to overexposure the furcation area of the 108 shows radiolucency (red arrow).

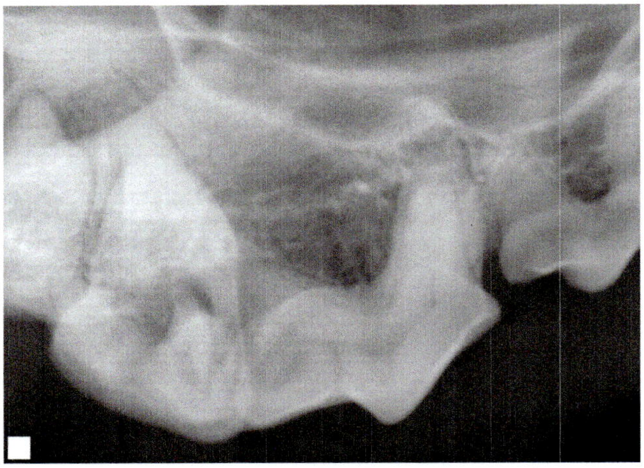

Figure 9.21 The same area as in Figure 9.20. Reduced exposure allow for appropriate evaluation of the furcation area in 108.

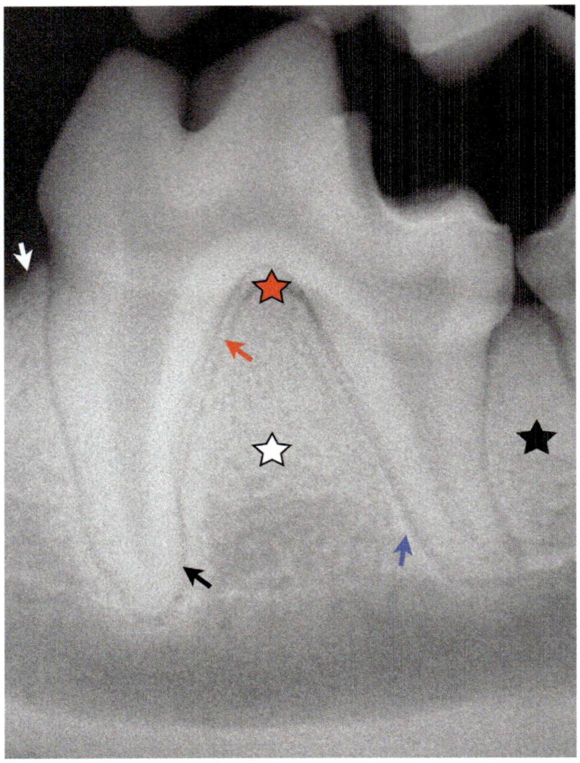

Figure 9.22 Radiograph of the left mandibular first molar (309). The following periodontal structures are evident: radiopaque alveolar bone with increased density of the lamina dura and an alveolar edge. The alveolar process is comprised of cancellous bone, which shapes the interalveolar septa and interradicular area. The alveolar wall margin as well as buccal and lingual (palatal) surfaces consists of compact bone. The radiolucent zone between cementum and lamina dura is the PDL space. In all feline teeth and most canine the PDL space is radiographically linear. In dogs, some of the roots (particularly mandibular molars) appear as a double radiolucent line. This is created by the presence of the developmental radicular grooves, which strenghten the resistance for twisting movements. White arrow-alveolar ridge, red arrow-radicular groove, blue arrow-lamina dura, white star-interradicular space, black star-interalveolar space, and red star-furcation area.

Radiographic appearance of normal periodontal anatomy

The radiographic appearance of periodontal structures and normal anatomic features refers to both the deciduous and permanent dentition. The radiopaque periodontal tissues are

1. The alveolar bone with increased density of the lamina dura.
2. The alveolar process, which is comprised of cancellous bone that shapes the interalveolar septa and interradicular area.
3. The alveolar wall and margin and buccal and lingual (palatal) surfaces consisting of compact bone.

The radiolucent zone between cementum and lamina dura is the periodontal ligament (PDL) space. In all feline and most canine teeth, the PDL space is radiographically linear. In some tooth roots of dogs (particularly the mandibular molars), this space appears as a double radiolucent line. This is created by the presence of developmental radicular grooves, which strengthen the resistance for twisting movements (Figure 9.22).[25]

The process of creation of the periodontal structures occurs during root development and subsequent eruption. This process is visible in the radiographs taken at the age of 10 and 16 weeks (Figures 9.23 and 9.24). After eruption is complete, the healthy periodontium keeps the same radiographic appearance (Figures 9.25 and 9.26). Age in and of itself does not seem to play a role in it, although in older patients the alveolar bone is less elastic and more prone to fracture. This is also true in cats (Figures 9.27 and 9.28).[1,12,15,27]

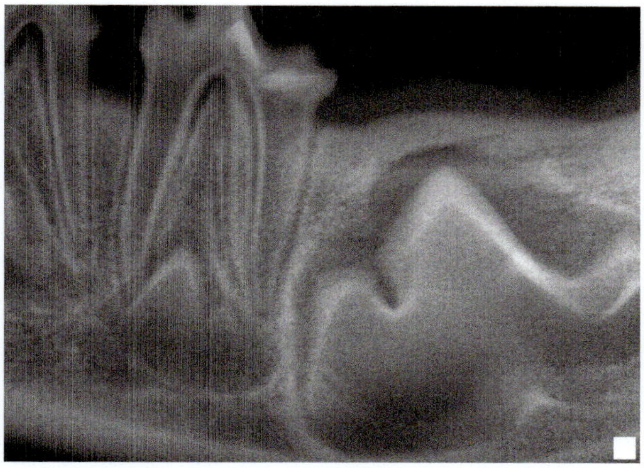

Figure 9.23 Radiograph of the left mandible in a 10-week-old puppy. Periodontal structures of deciduous dentition are perfectly developed. The roots in secondary dentition are at the beginning of development.

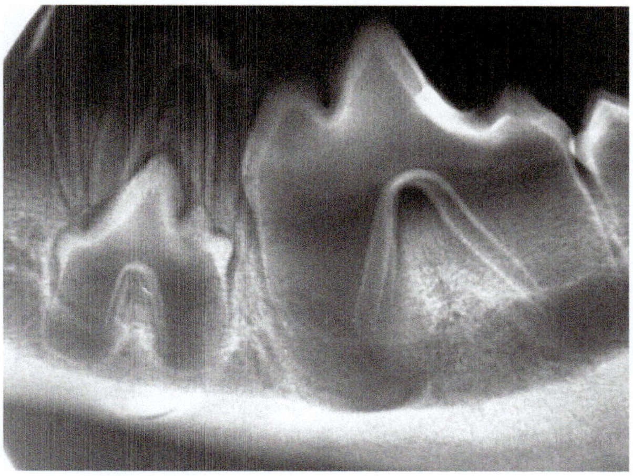

Figure 9.24 Radiograph of the left mandible in a puppy at the age of 16 weeks. The development of the roots is accompanied by development of the periodontal structures.

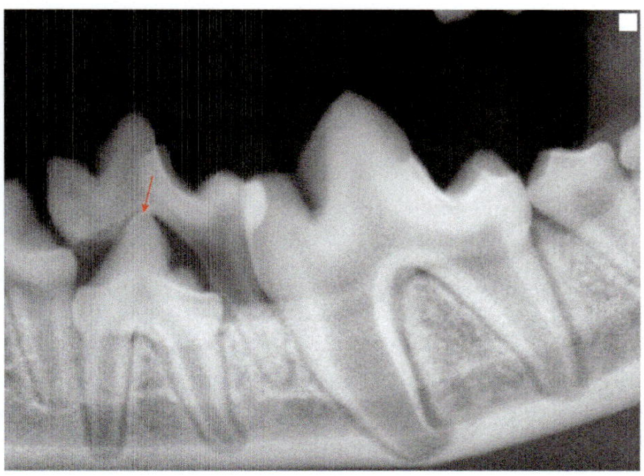

Figure 9.25 When the periodontal structures of the secondary dentition are created, the deciduous periodontium undergoes resorption. This puppy is 6 months old. A persistent deciduous 708 (red arrow) is present over the retained 308.

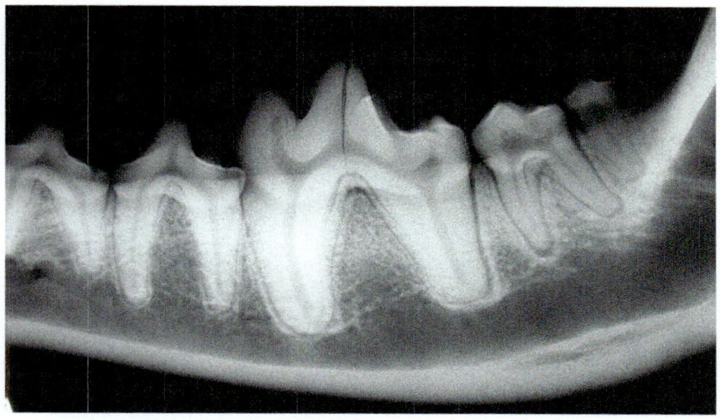

Figure 9.26 After eruption is completed, the healthy periodontium keeps the same radiographic appearance. Radiograph of left mandible of 6-year-old German Shepherd.

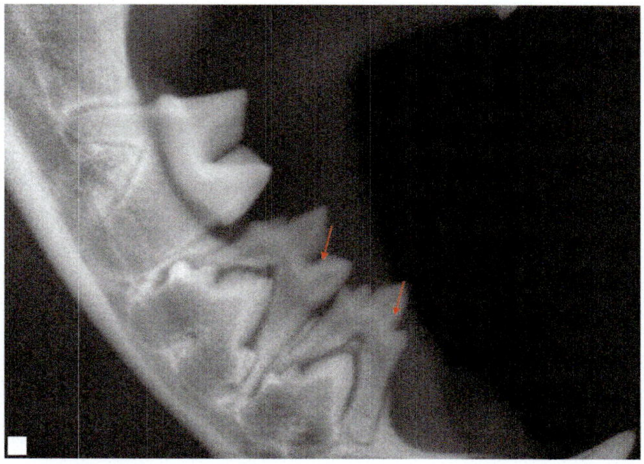

Figure 9.27 Radiograph of a 5-month-old kitten's right mandible. Root and periodontal structures of the secondary dentition (307, 308) are under process of development. Roots and periodontal structures of deciduous teeth (707, 708) (red arrows) undergo resorption.

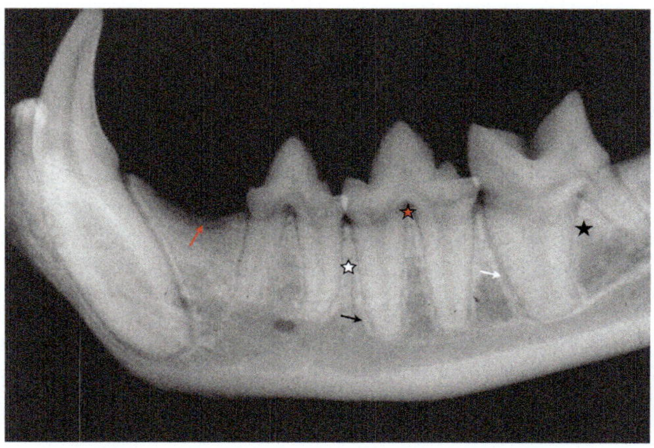

Figure 9.28 2-year-old feline's left mandible. Visible normal periodontal structures: lamina dura, periodontal space, alveolar ridge, interalveolar septum, interradicular septum, furcation area.

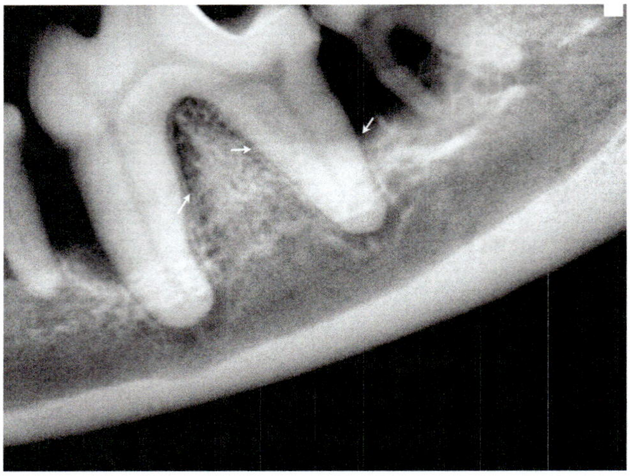

Figure 9.29 Radiograph of the left mandible (teeth 309 and 310). Loss of lamina dura (white arrows) is an indicator of periodontal disease.

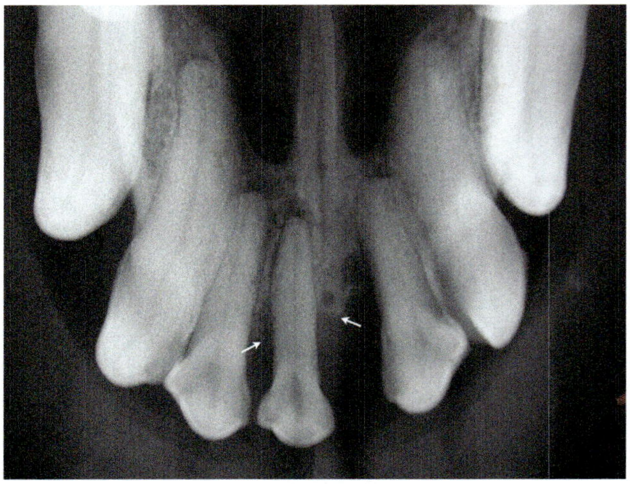

Figure 9.30 The loss of sharp edges of the interalveolar septa (white arrows) is a very important symptom in human periodontology.

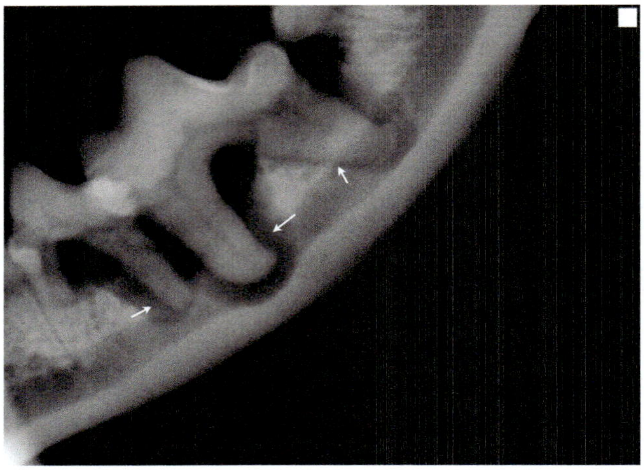

Figure 9.31 Periodontal ligament space in periodontal disease is widened and irregular (white arrows).

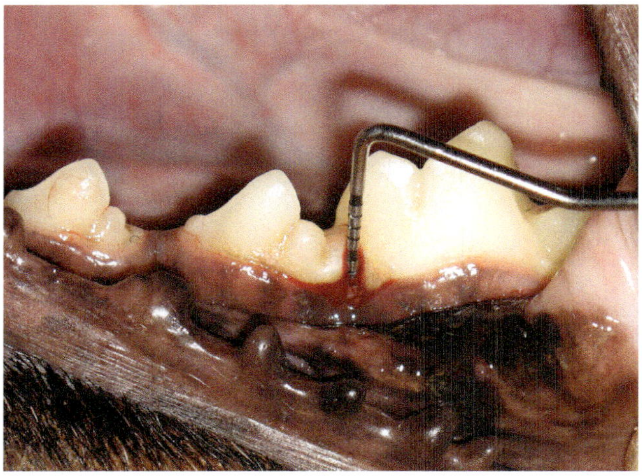

Figure 9.32 Periodontal pocket (7 mm) revealed in one location between 308 and 309.

Radiography in periodontal disease and other pathologic conditions

Numerous mechanical, metabolic, inflammatory, and microbiological factors influence the quality, density, and structure of periodontal tissues, resulting in radiographic changes. Listed below are various lesions and their respective images that characterize the process of the attachment destruction, bone loss, and other changes accompanying periodontal disease.

Note that most of the vertical bone loss images were taken of artificially created pathology in order to achieve educational-quality images (see Figures 9.34–9.39).

Clinically, all possible types of lesions can be (and often are) combined on one tooth, making it much less obvious.

1. Lamina dura normal appearance should be visible, continuous, linear, and even. In periodontal disease, the lamina dura loses its anatomic character (Figure 9.29).
2. The interalveolar septa edges lose their sharpness; this is a very important symptom of periodontal disease in humans (Figure 9.30).
3. The periodontal ligament space becomes widened and irregular in periodontal disease (Figure 9.31).
4. Vertical bone loss occurs when there is one area of recession with the surrounding tissue being higher and closer to the CEJ[27] (Figures 9.32 and 9.33).
   a. Early stage of bone loss: three-wall bony pocket; the defect is defined by the root as one wall and three surfaces of the alveolar bone (Figures 9.34 and 9.35).
   b. Further development of previous defect extends the lesion interdentally to communicate with a root of the adjacent tooth, creating

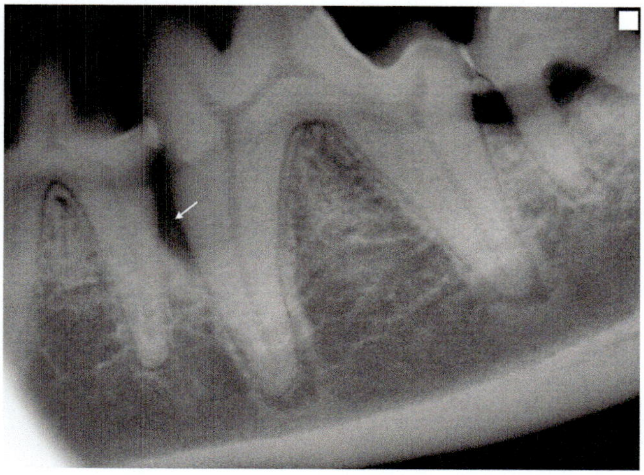

Figure 9.33 Radiograph of the same area as in Figure 9.32. Vertical bone loss (white arrows) occurs when there is one area of recession with the surrounding tissue being higher and closer to the CEJ.

a two-wall crater defect. Another type of two-wall defect refers to the situation where instead of a communication with the adjacent tooth, the lingual or facial wall of the three-wall pocket is destroyed, and the remaining two bony walls create a two-wall defect (Figures 9.36 and 9.37).

c. A one-wall defect is an extension of the two-wall defect that involves only one tooth. Destruction of both lingual and facial bony walls creates a one-wall defect (Figure 9.38).

d. A four-wall or circumferential defect occurs when the bone loss surrounds the entire tooth[28] (Figure 9.39).

(a)

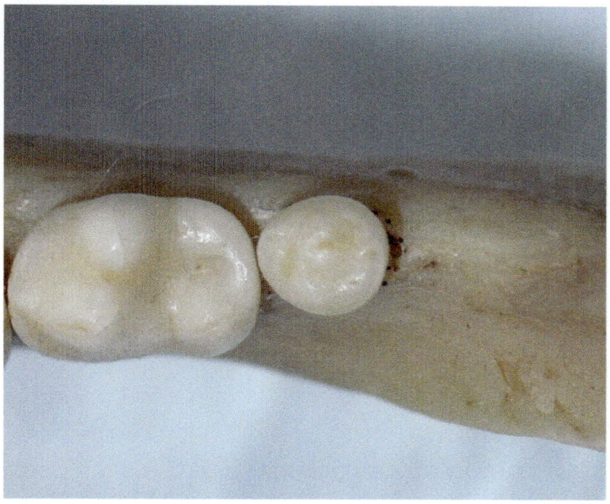

(b)

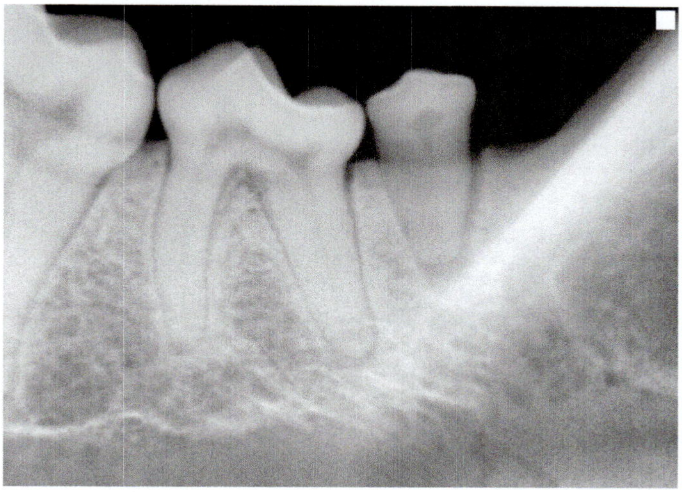

Figure 9.34 (a) Left mandibular third molar (311) with intact periodontium. (b) Radiograph of 311.

(a)

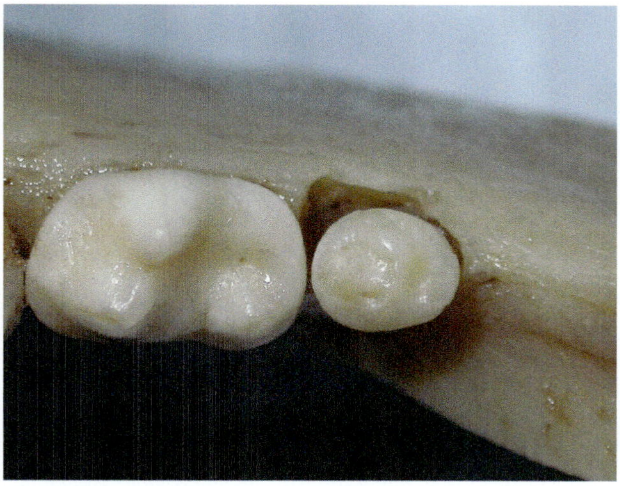

(b)

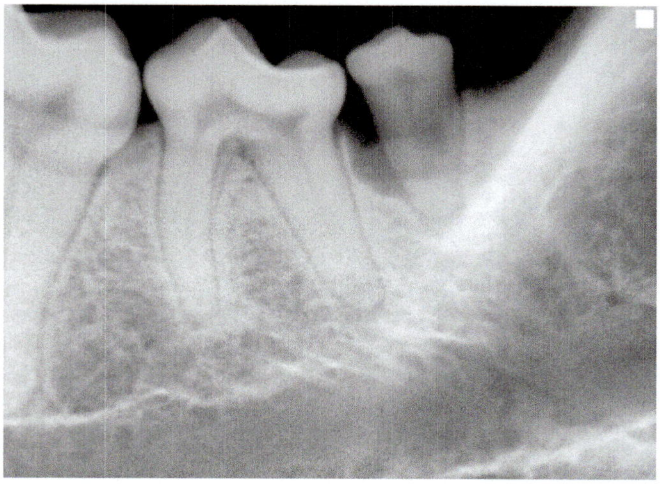

Figure 9.35 (a) Three-wall bony pocket defect created in the periodontal tissue of 311. (b) The corresponding dental radiograph from Figure 9.35a.

(a) (b)

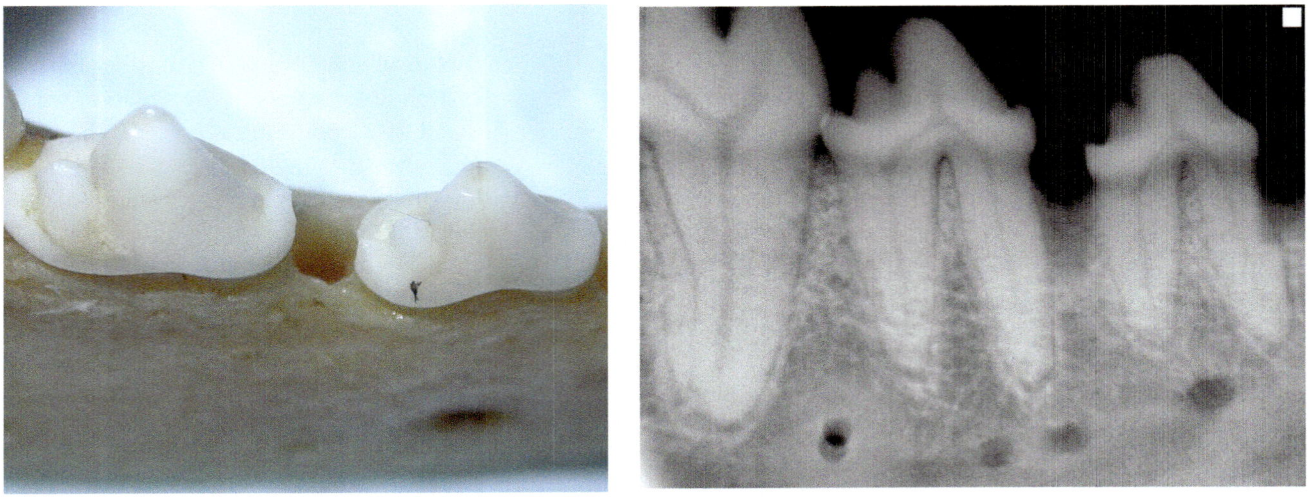

Figure 9.36 Further development of the three-wall defect extends the lesion interdentally; communication with the root of the adjacent tooth is what makes a two-wall crater defect. (a) Defect created between 407 and 408. (b) Corresponding radiograph from Figure 9.36a.

(a) (b)

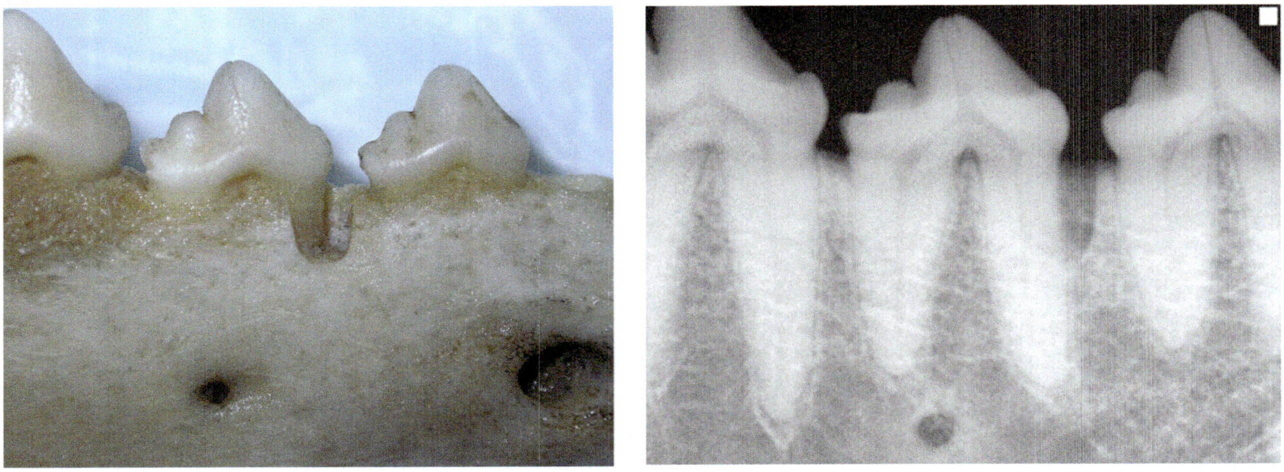

Figure 9.37 When the lingual or facial wall of the three-wall pocket is destroyed, the remaining two bony walls create a two-wall defect. (a) Defect created between 406 and 407. (b) Corresponding radiograph from Figure 9:37a.

(a) (b)

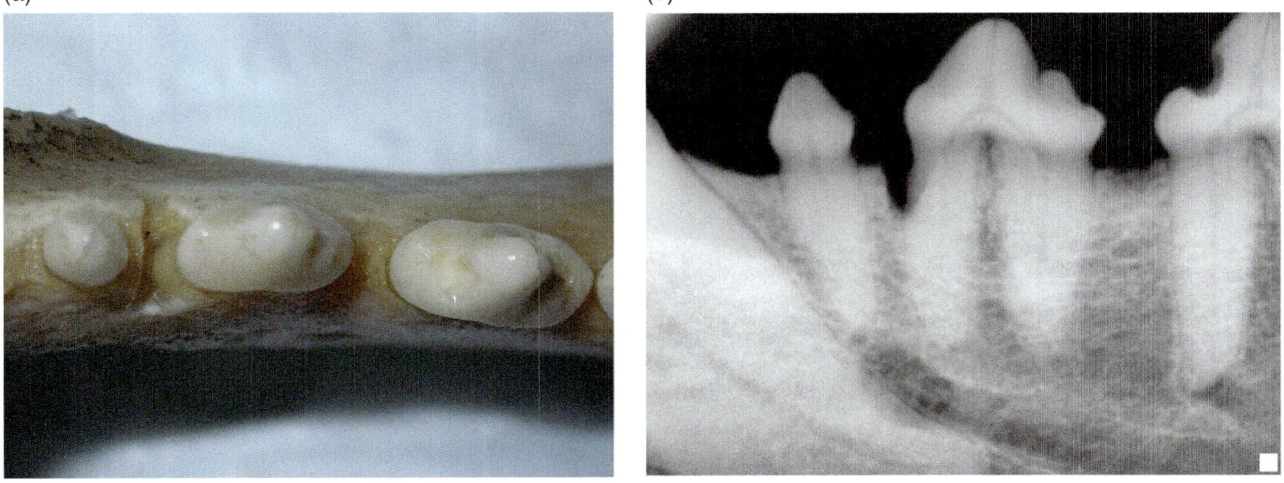

Figure 9.38 The one-wall defect is an extension of the two-wall defect that involves only one tooth. Destruction of both lingual and facial bony walls makes the defect one wall. (a) Defect created in mesial part of 306. (b) Corresponding radiograph from Figure 9.38a.

(a) (b)

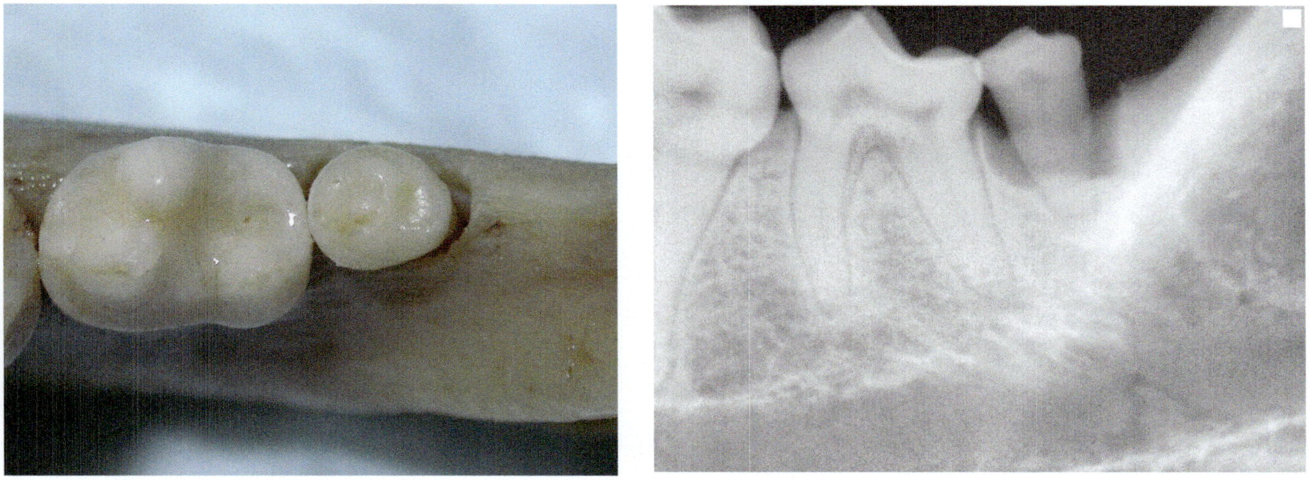

Figure 9.39 Four-wall defect or a circumferential one occurs when the bone loss surrounds the entire tooth. (a) Destruction created in 311. (b) Corresponding radiograph from Figure 9.39a.

(a) (b)

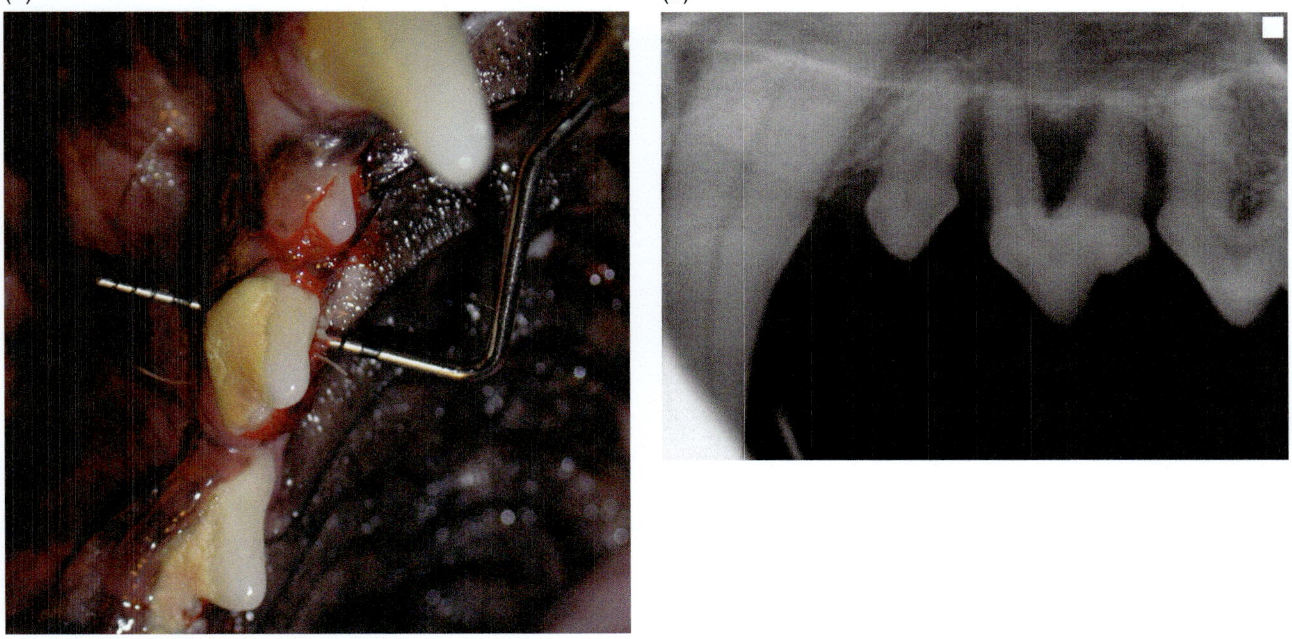

Figure 9.40 Furcation involvement appeares as a loss of density and lack of substance at the coronal aspect of the interradicular bone. Stage 3 of furcation involvement allows the periodontal probe to go through the furcation area from the buccal to lingual/palatal site of the examined tooth. (a) Stage 3 involvement of 206. (b) Radiographed 206 from Figure 9.40a.

5. Furcation involvement appears as a loss of density and lack of substance at the coronal aspect of the interradicular bone. Clinically, it has 3 grades (grade 0 has no furcation involvement) (see chapter 19):
   a. Grade 1—the periodontal probe may be inserted into the furcation area but the destruction is less than one-third of the horizontal width.
   b. Grade 2—the probe explores the furcation but does not pass through it.
   c. Grade 3—total involvement; the probe passes through the furcation from one side to another of the multirooted teeth (Figure 9.40).
6. Radiographic appearance of calculus: visible subgingival deposits and tartar bridges joining adjacent teeth (Figure 9.41). Because calculus is radiodense, in order to avoid interference of dental deposits

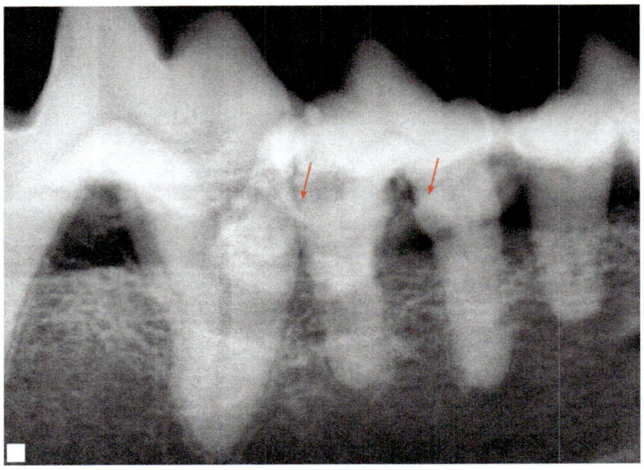

Figure 9.41 Radiographic appearance of tartar: visible subgingival deposits in 408 and 409 (white arrows) and tartar bridges joining adjacent teeth 407, 408, and 409.

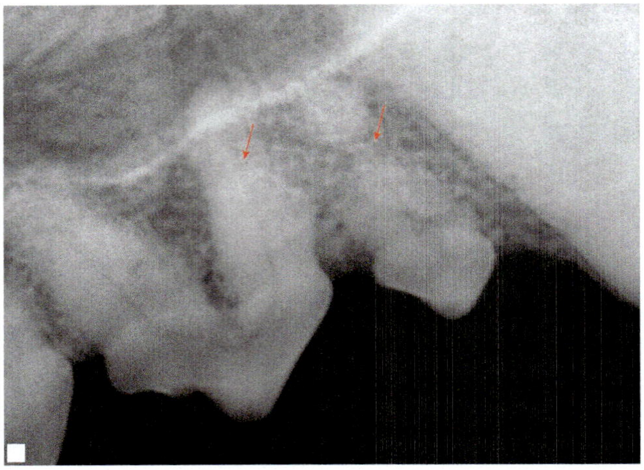

Figure 9.43 Ankylosis of the periodontal attachment appearing as the lack of PDL space (red arrows). Illustrated ankylosis in 105 and 106.

(a)

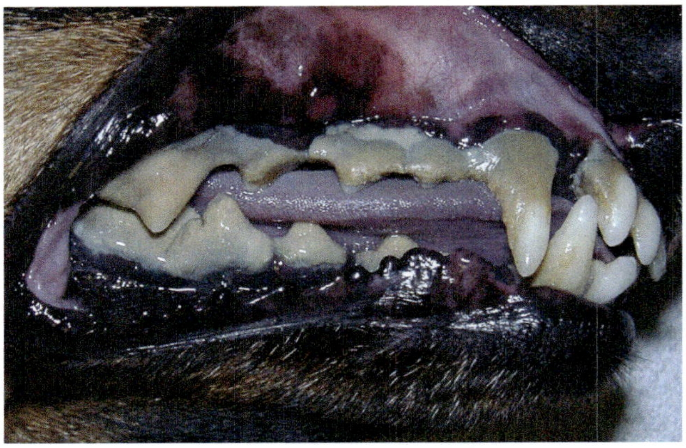

(b)

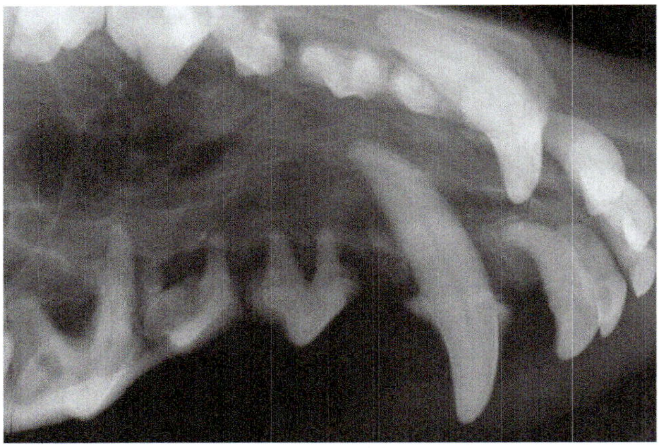

Figure 9.42 (a) Right maxillary premolars covered by tartar. (b) Radiographed right maxillary premolars of the dog from Figure 9.42a. Horizontal bone loss is defined as an osteolytic process leading to decreasing height of the alveolar ridge and root exposure.

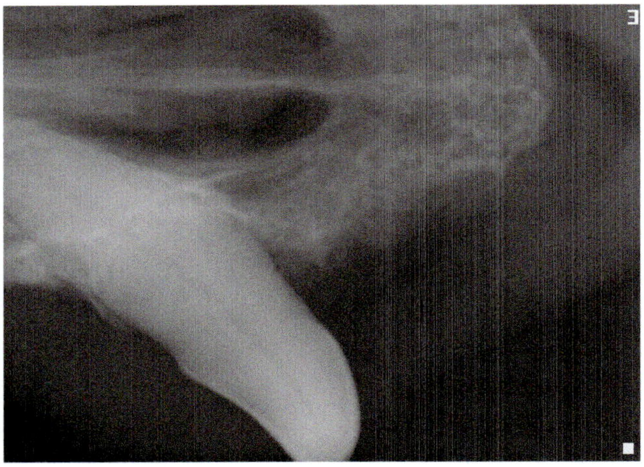

Figure 9.44 Cancellous bone had replaced pre-existing interalveolar septa in incisive part of maxilla 6 months after the extraction of the maxillary incisors.

on the final image, it is reasonable to radiograph cleaned and scaled dentition.

7. Horizontal bone loss (Figure 9.42) is defined as an osteolytic process leading to a decreased height of the alveolar ridge and root exposure.[27,29]
8. Ankylosis of the periodontal attachment appears as the lack of a PDL space. The alveolar bone and root substance have no significant border line. Resorption of cementum is often followed by bone replacement of resorbed tissue (Figure 9.43).[30]
9. Toothless periodontium 6 months after extraction. Cancellous bone has replaced pre-existing interalveolar septa in incisive part of maxilla (Figure 9.44). In humans, edentulous areas undergo atrophy.
10. Chronic periodontitis may cause osteomyelitis of the entire maxilla or mandible (Figures 9.45 and 9.46). This is a serious complication of periodontal

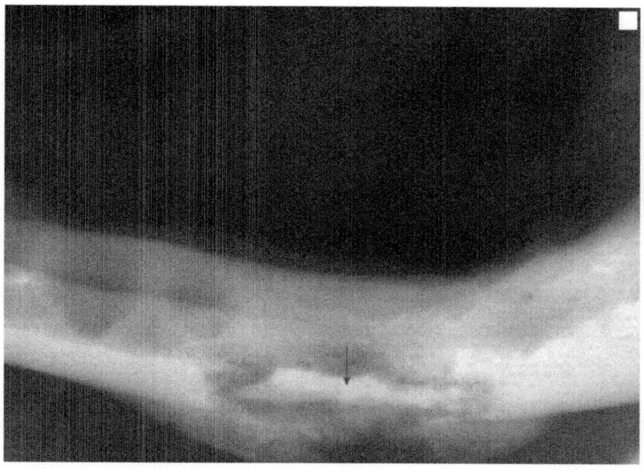

Figure 9.45 Chronic periodontitis in a 4-year-old dog caused complete loss of dentition, osteomyelitis, and bone sequestra in the mandible (red arrow).

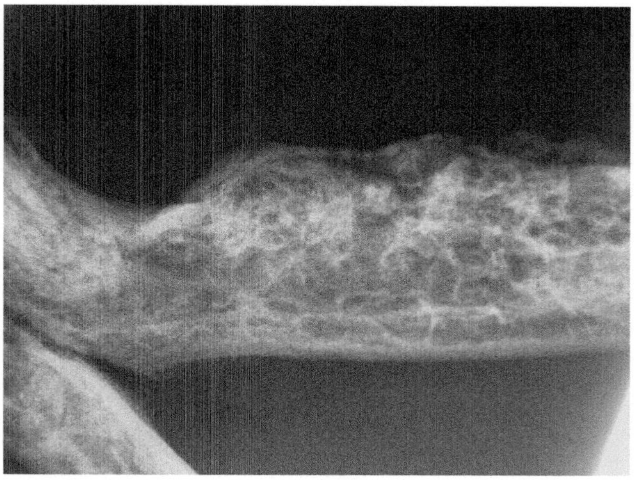

Figure 9.46 Chronic periodontitis and tooth resorption in a 16-year-old cat has resulted in osteomyelitis.

disease that influences the quality of life of the patient (with pain and malfunction of the jaws) and the potential for further complications such as distant infection, immune response, or pathologic fracture. The complementary and necessary diagnostic tool apart from radiography is histopathologic evaluation of the affected bone.

11. Tooth luxation due to periodontal disease. The tooth is pushed out from the alveolus (Figure 9.47). This is a long-term and atypical process. Usually the tooth becomes loose (mobile).
12. Perio-endo lesions (class II) have primarily periodontal character with secondary endodontic involvement (Figure 9.48).
13. Endo-perio lesions (class I) have primarily endodontic with subsequent periodontal involvement.

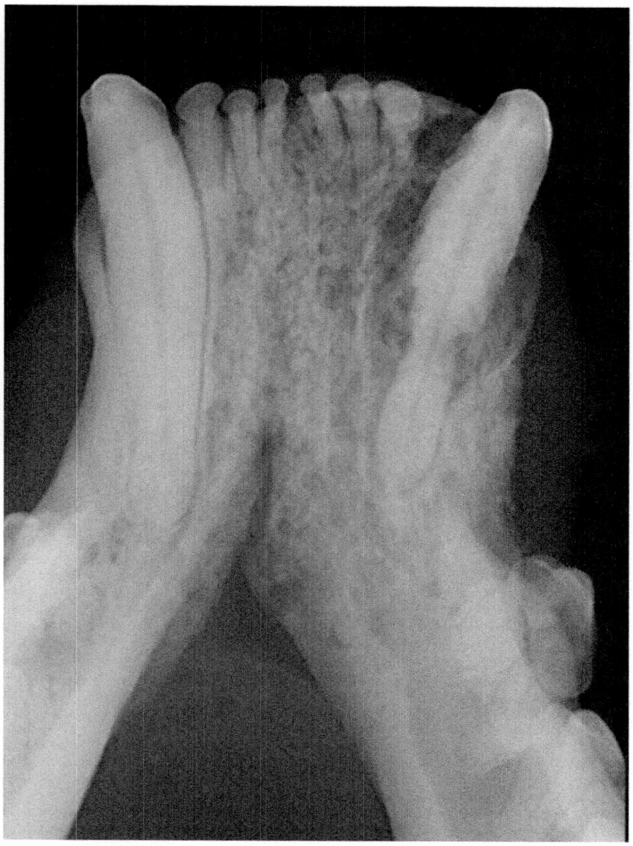

Figure 9.47 Tooth luxation due to periodontal disease. The left mandibular canine (204) is pushed out from the alveolus.

Quite often, class I lesions have fistulation. To distinguish the origin of the fistula, it helps to expose the radiograph after inserting a gutta percha point into the intaroral opening (Figure 9.49).

14. Radiograph of a "swimming tooth" with complete loss of periodontal attachment and level III mobility (Figure 9.50). High mobility of the tooth can be caused by loss of attachment as well as root fracture or neoplastic process. Radiographic assesment is necessary for diagnosis. Histopathology should be considered if there is any question as to the cause of the bone loss.

The appearance of the periodontium in specific conditions

The appearance of the periodontium in specific conditions is as follows:

1. Dentin hypoplasia—lack of roots, decreased mineralization of the hard dental tissues (generally associated with enamel hypocalcification) (Figure 9.51).

(a) (b)

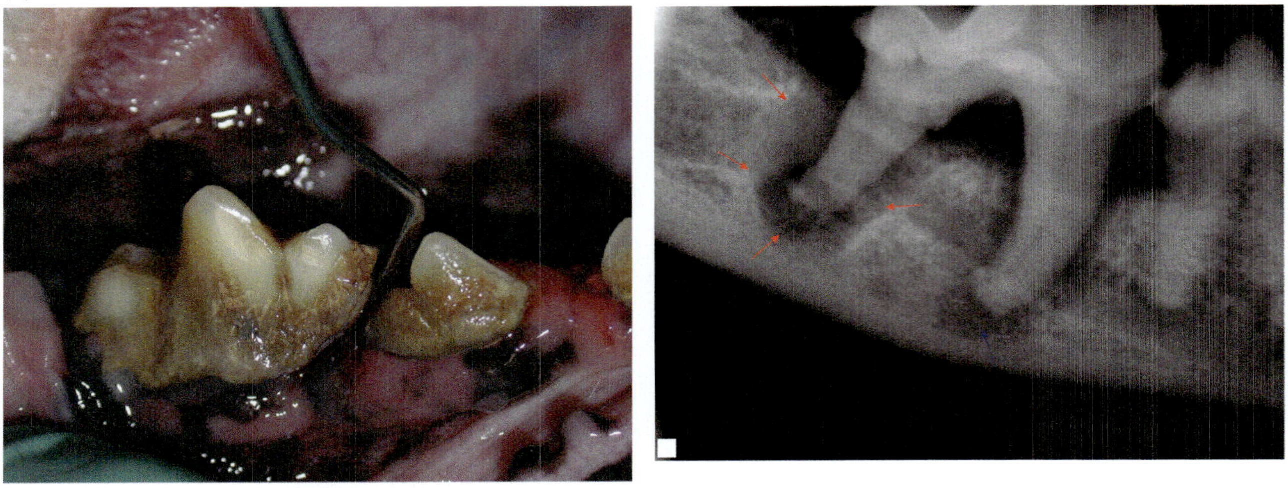

Figure 9.48 (a) Clinical examination revealed 15 mm periodontal pocket between 408 and 409 and grade 3 mobility of 309. There was no fracture of the examined tooth crown. (b) Radiographed 409 from Figure 9.48a. Perio-endo lesions (class II) have primarily periodontal character (red arrows) with secondary endodontic involvement (blue arrow).

(a) (b)

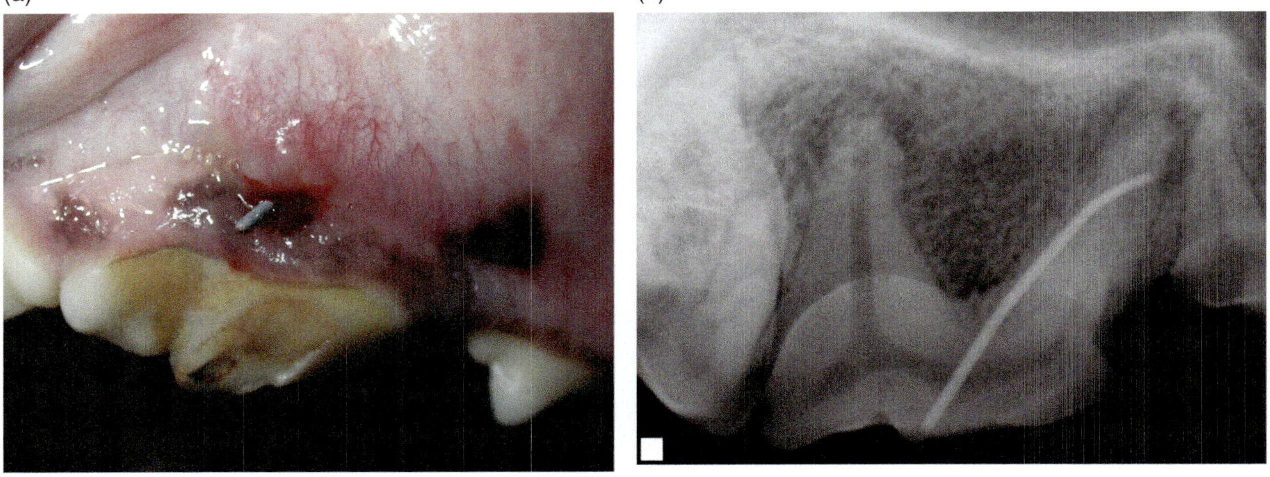

Figure 9.49 (a) Clinical examination of 108 in a dog revealed a complicated crown fracture and draining tract at the buccal aspect of oral mucoca 6 mm over furcation area of the fractured tooth. (b) Radiograph of 108 from Figure 9.49a with the use of a GP point inserted into the intaroral fistula. Endo-perio lesions (class I) have primarily endodontic with subsequent periodontal involvement.

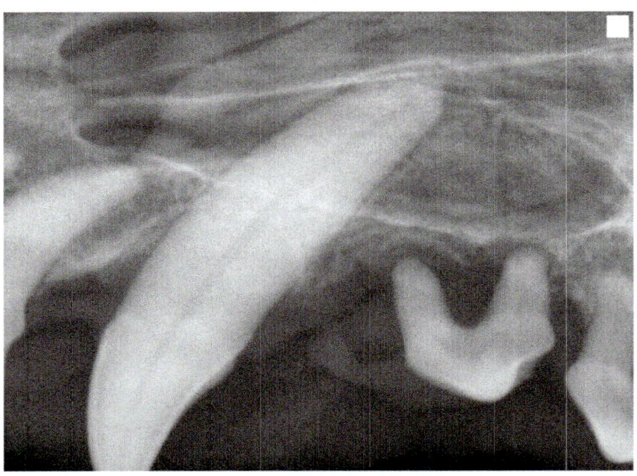

Figure 9.50 Radiograph of "swimming tooth" 206 with complete loss of periodontal attachment and level III mobility.

2. Craniomandibular osteopathy (Figure 9.52)—this disease affects the alveolar bone, which has an abnormal radiologic appearance.
3. Hyperparathyroidism associated with renal insufficiency (Figure 9.53)—decalcification of the bone in the jaws is particularly quick due to very high calcium turnover in alveolar bone metabolism. Clinically, teeth are mobile without causing pain and/or bleeding. Radiographs show the lack of bone structure: no lamina dura, interalveolar bone, or PDL space. This condition is also called "rubber jaw" syndrome.
4. Tooth resorption in cats—related to periodontal disease and type of resorption. A significantly

(a) (b)

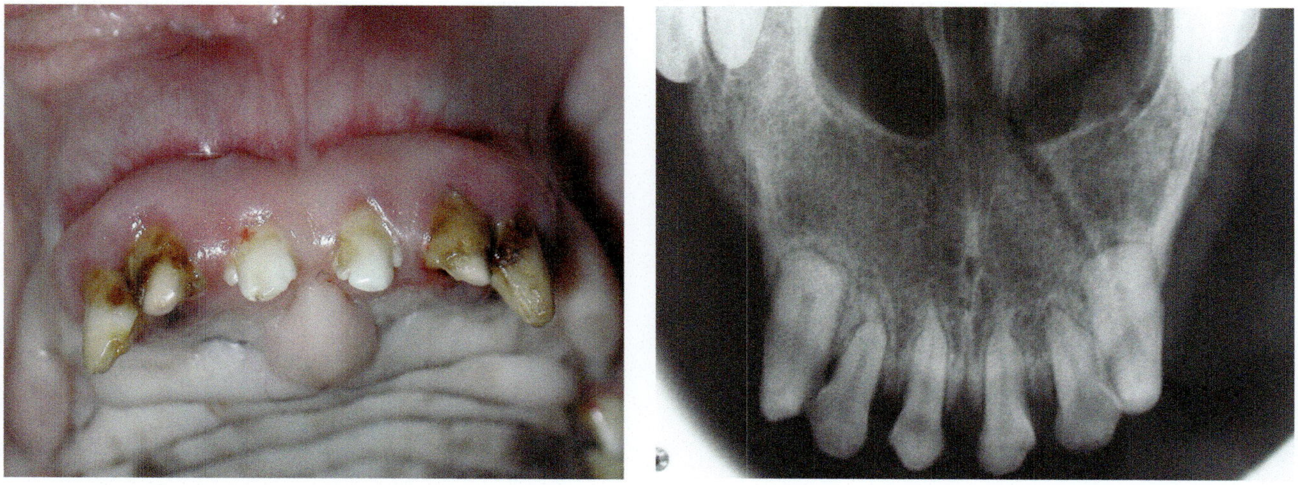

Figure 9.51 (a) Clinical examination of maxillary incisors of 8-month-old Dog de Bordeaux. All examined teeth are affected by enamel hypoplasia and hypocalcification. (b) Radiograph of maxillary incisors presented in Figure 9.51a. Dentinal hypoplasia—lack of roots and decreased mineralization of the hard dental tissues (generally associated with enamel hypocalcification).

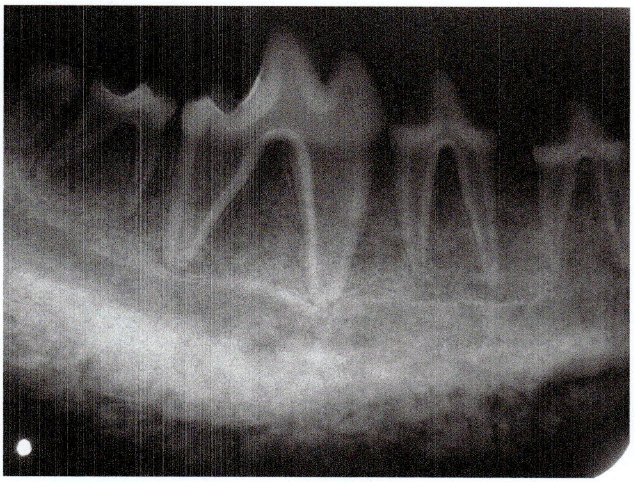

Figure 9.52 Radiograph of the right mandible. Craniomandibular osteopathy in 8-month-old female Doberman Pinscher. Alveolar bone is affected with remarkable loss of the trabecular structure.

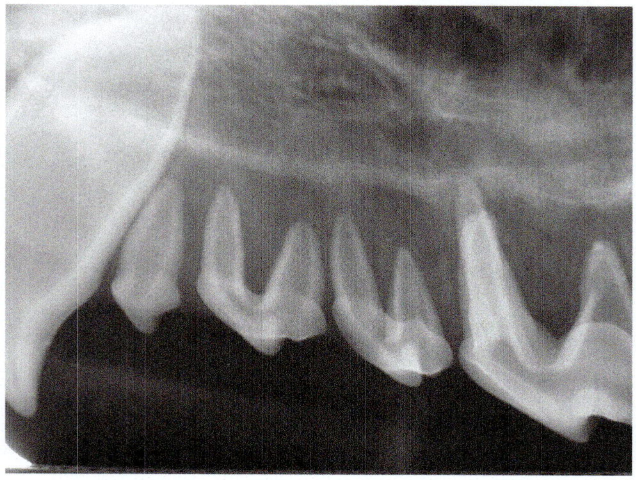

Figure 9.53 Radiograph of the left maxilla of a 6-month-old Bernese affected by hyperparathyroidism associated with renal insufficiency. Complete decalcification and loss of density of the alveolar bone.

lower occurrence of root replacement in cats' teeth with resorptive lesions and periodontitis (type 1) has been described in the literature[31,32] (Figure 9.54).

5. Tooth resorption in a dog (Figure 9.55).
6. Hypercementosis, which is often associated with tooth resorption (Figure 9.56).
7. Proliferative conditions—gingival hyperplasia or neoplastic diseases. Some of these conditions are radiodense, such as when calcification occurs or the process has an osseous character. Others appear as radiolucent areas with infiltrative lesions or circumferenced character. Destruction of periodontal space and ankylosis is not seen with benign lesions such as gingival hyperplasia (Figure 9.57), but is seen in more aggressive lesions such as squamous cell carcinoma (Figure 9.58). This can be crucial knowledge in treating oral growths (Figures 9.57 and 9.58).

Clinical applications of periodontal radiography

Clinical applications of periodontal radiography include the following:

1. Treatment plan before performing extractions (deciduous and/or permanent teeth).[33]
2. Postoperative radiographs in extraction cases to ensure complete removal of the roots.

(a)

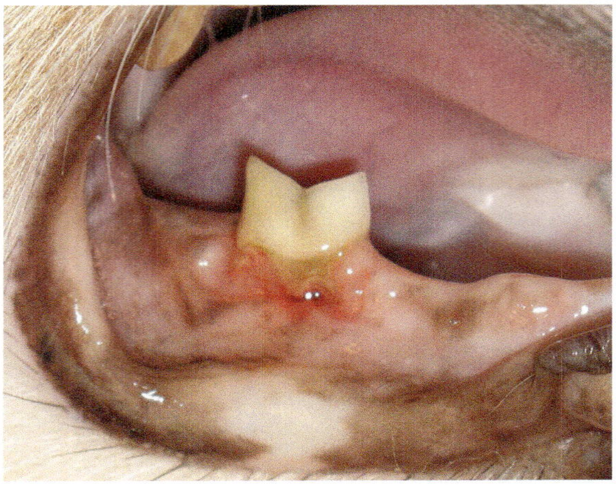

(b)

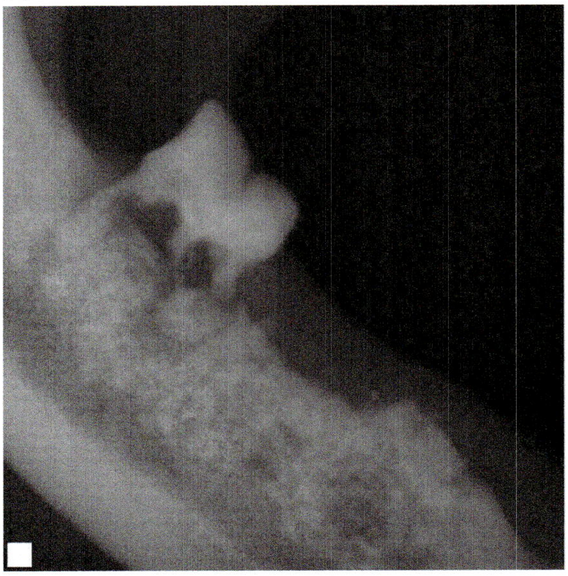

Figure 9.54 (a) Right mandibular first molar (409) in 10-year-old cat with periodontal pockets, grade 3 mobility, and furcation involvement. (b) Radiographed tooth from Figure 9.54a. Bone loss and tooth resorption affecting the same tooth.

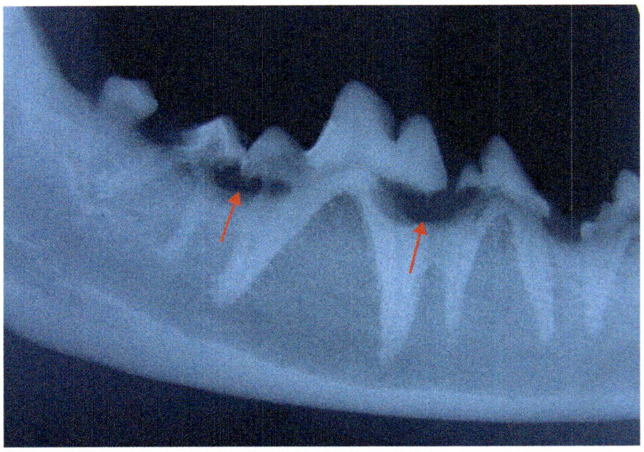

Figure 9.55 Tooth resorption in a dog (red arrows). Mandibular dentition in 9-year-old Dachshund.

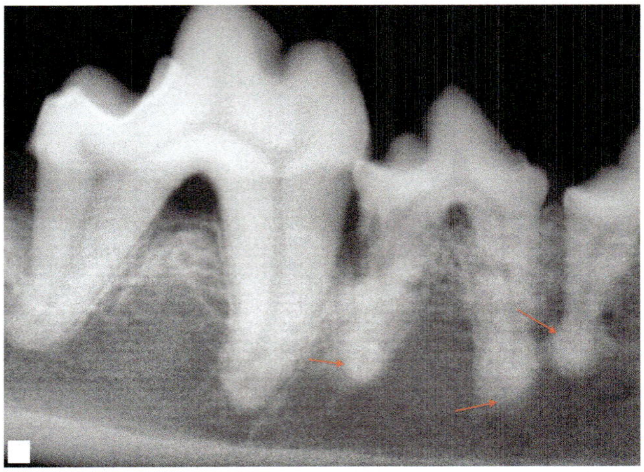

Figure 9.56 12-year-old Dachshund with teeth affected by resorption accompanied by hypercementosis.

(a)

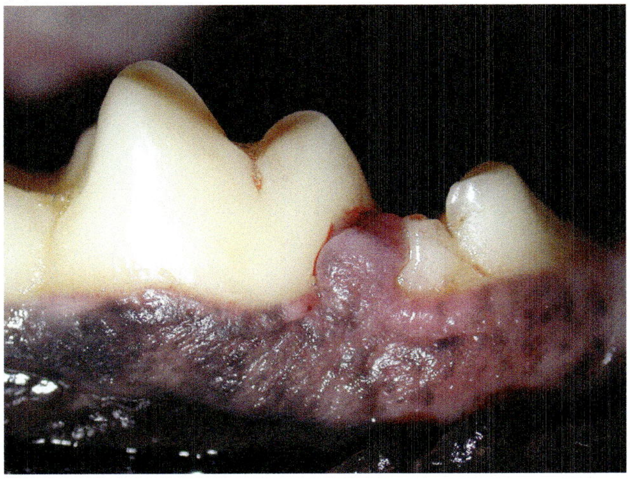

(b)

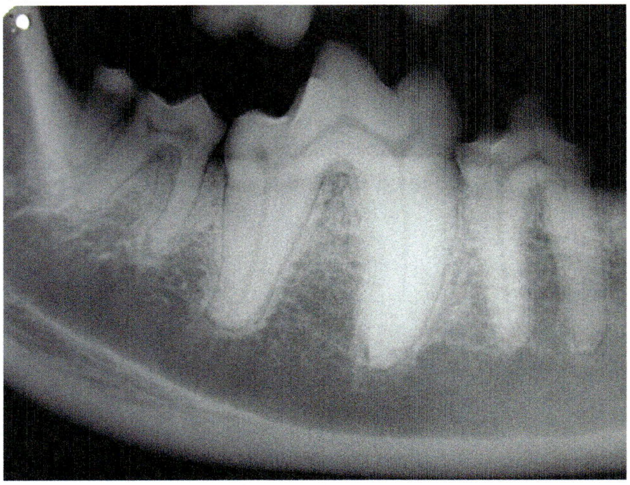

Figure 9.57 (a) Gingival hyperplasia between 408 and 409 (confirmed by histopathologic evaluation). Local pseudopocket present in affected area. (b) Radiograph of the area illustrated in Figure 9.57a. No evidence of periodontal pathology.

(a) (b)

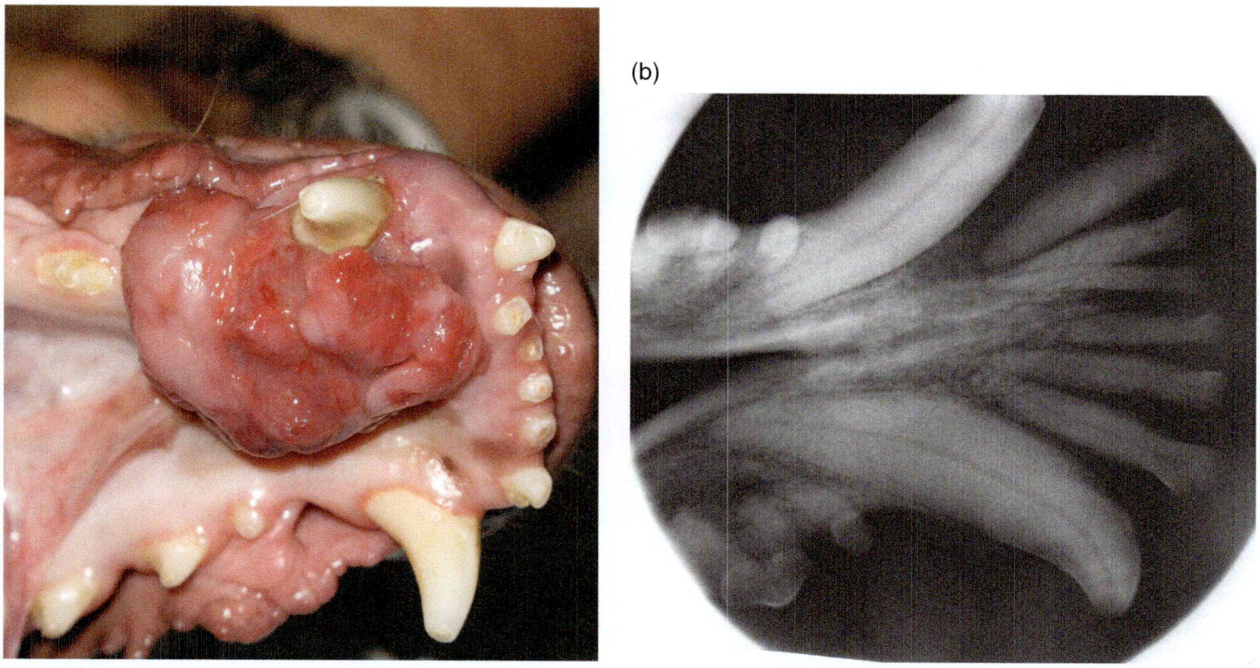

Figure 9.58 (a) Squamous cell carcinoma in a 1.5-year-old dog. Third stage of growth. (b) Radiograph of the affected mandible. Bone loss of the interalveolar space between 304 and 303.

(a) (b) (c)

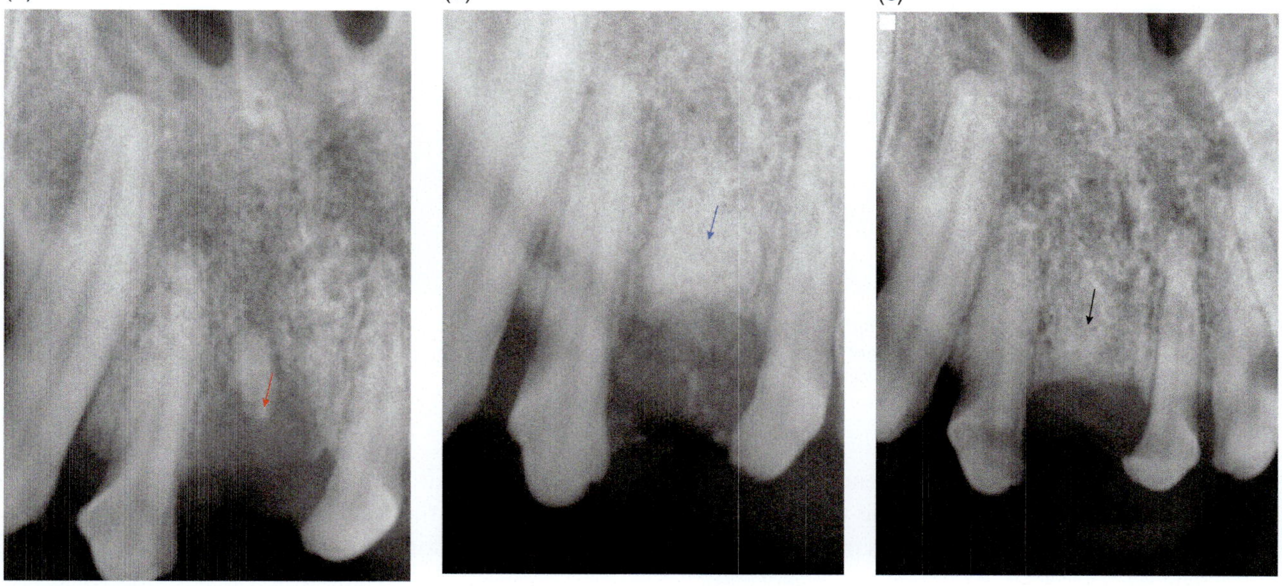

Figure 9.59 (a) Radiograph of the maxilla of a 5-year-old dog. 101 was lost due to injury. The root remnant causes inflammation in the alveolar socket (red arrow). (b) After debridement the socket was augmented with the use of bioglass material (blue arrow). (c) 6-month follow-up. The alveolar process is recovered and ready for the implant procedure (black arrow).

3. Treatment plan for periodontal surgery. Based on results of the clinical examination and radiographic appearance of periodontal lesions (i.e., the extent, size, and accompanying pathologies), a prognosis can be assigned. If the tooth is to be saved, the best treatment decision can be made; that is, closed or open root planing, pocket reduction, or guided tissue regeneration , or extraction.[34]
4. Results of treatment: alveolar socket augmentation, healing, GTR requires follow-ups and reliable evaluation of the healing process[34,35] (Figure 9.59). The material applied for the bone augmentation

(a) (b)

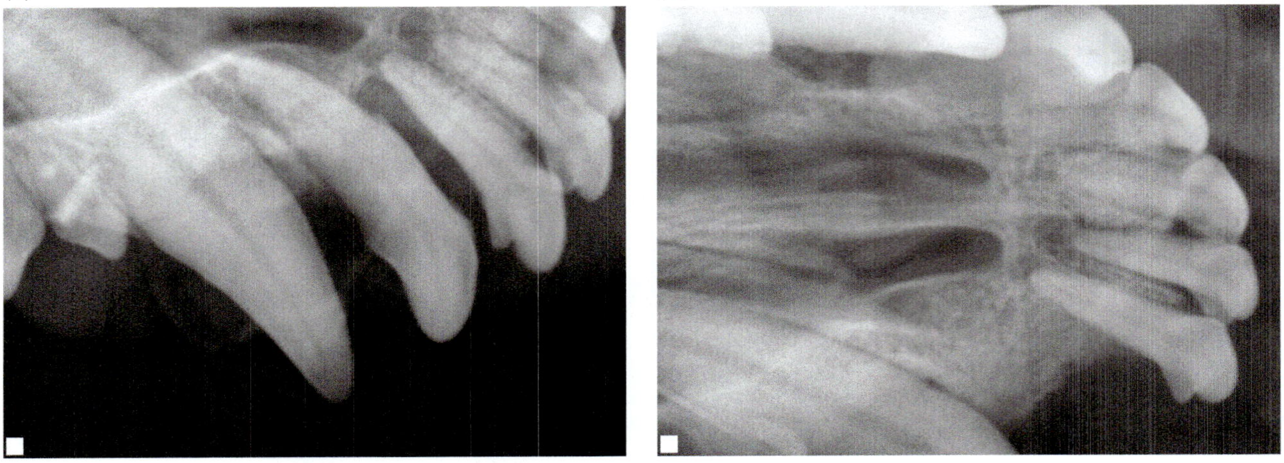

Figure 9.60 (a) Radiograph of 103 and 102 in dog. The 103, due to its mobility, was planned for extraction; the adjacent 102 was planned to be saved. (b) After extraction of 103 and meticulous debridement, the alvelolar socket was augmented with the use of bone graft material.

(a) (b)

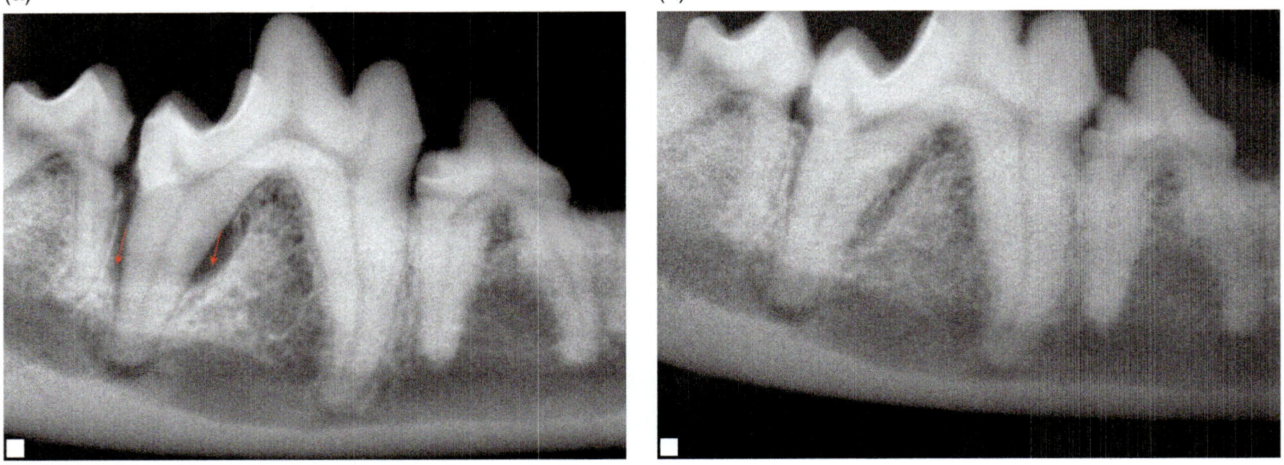

Figure 9.61 (a) Radiograph of the right mandible in 11-year-old Dachshund. Distal root is affected by periodontal disease and has an infrabony pocket (red arrows). Open root planing was performed as was local application of antibiotic. (b) 13 month follow-up revealing bony regrowth.

influences the quality of regenerated bone and may also play a role in planing the implant after traumatic loss of the tooth. It is important to evaluate whether after extraction and alveolar socket debridement the augmentation is packed properly (Figure 9.60).[36] Radiography is also proven to be the most reliable method for evaluation of the bone remodelling process (Figure 9.61).[37] The long-term radiographic follow-up after periodontal treatment shows the results of surgical efforts and the efficacy of homecare provided (Figure 9.62).

5. Endo-perio lesions (class I): A 6-month follow-up evaluation of the endodontic treatment is always required,[38] primarily because it is the only way to evaluate the result of treatment, and secondly to evaluate for any periodontal reactions that may be caused by certain root canal filling materials[39] (Figure 9.63).
6. Implantology requires proper radiographic evaluation of the remaining alveolar bone to determine if the healing process is sufficient (see Figure 9.59). In addition, therapeutic decisions such as the appropriate size of the implant and/or the depth/angle of placement can be directed via radiology (Figure 9.64).[40] Further evaluation of the alveolar bone surrounding the implant is also required (Figure 9.65).

(a)

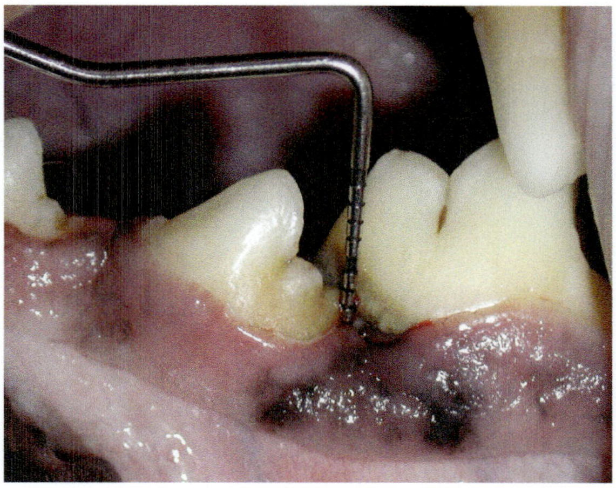

(b)

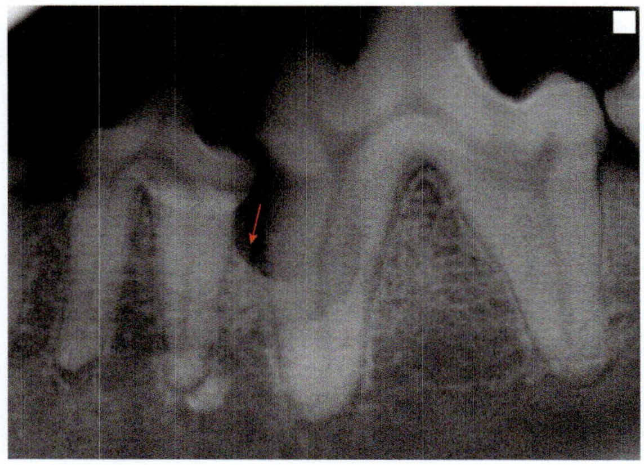

(c)

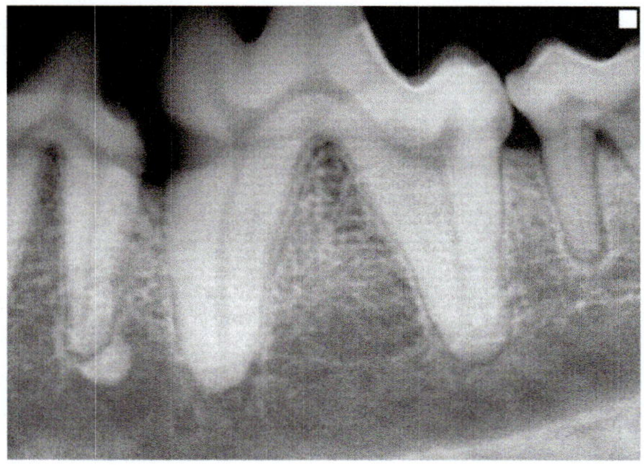

Figure 9.62 (a) 7 mm pocket of the mesial root of the left mandibular first molar (309); 7-year-old male Cocker Spaniel. (b) Radiograph of affected tooth from Figure 9.62a confirming bone loss (red arrow). (c) Radiograph of 6-month follow-up after GTR procedure in mesial root of 309 revealing regeneration of bone.

(a)

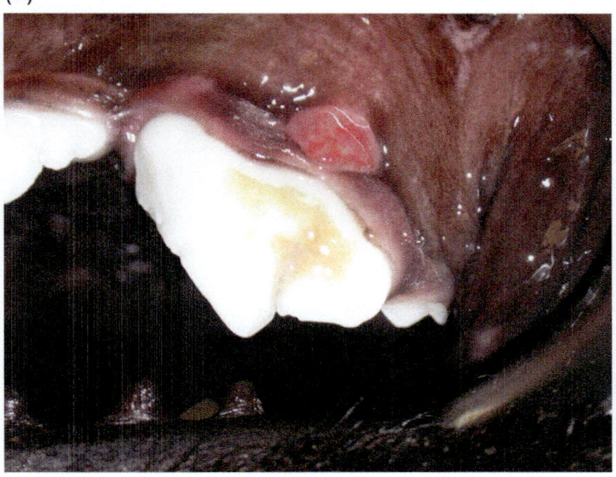

(b)

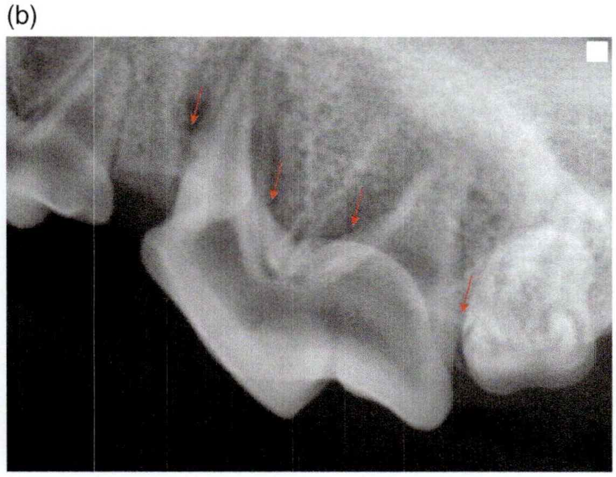

(c)

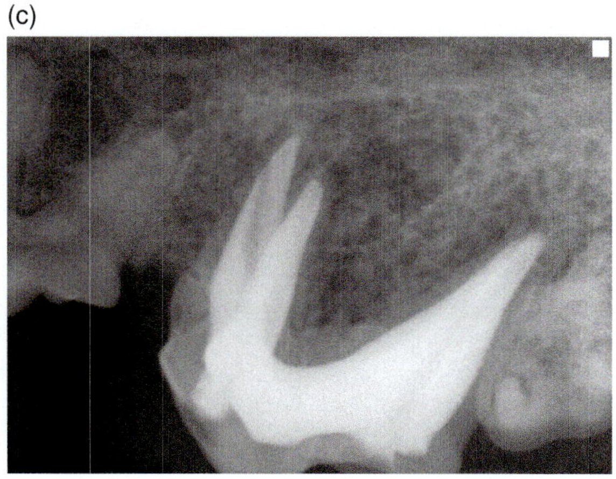

Figure 9.63 (a) Fistula at the area of the left maxillary fourth premolar (208). (b) Radiograph for the root canal treatment of 208 with class I endo-perio lesion showing excessive radiolucent periodontal lesions in all 3 roots (red arrows). (c) Radiograph at 5-year follow-up. The periodontium is healthy and radiodense.

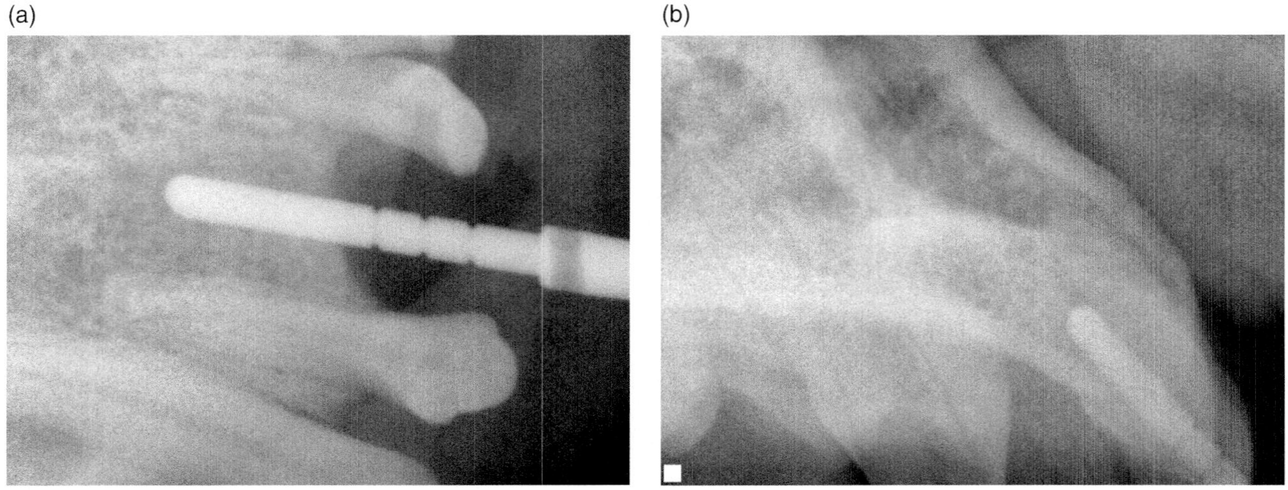

Figure 9.64 Radiograph of the implant probe inserted to drilled bone to measure the depth of the preparation, its angulation, and location. (a) Bite projection. (b) Lateral projection.

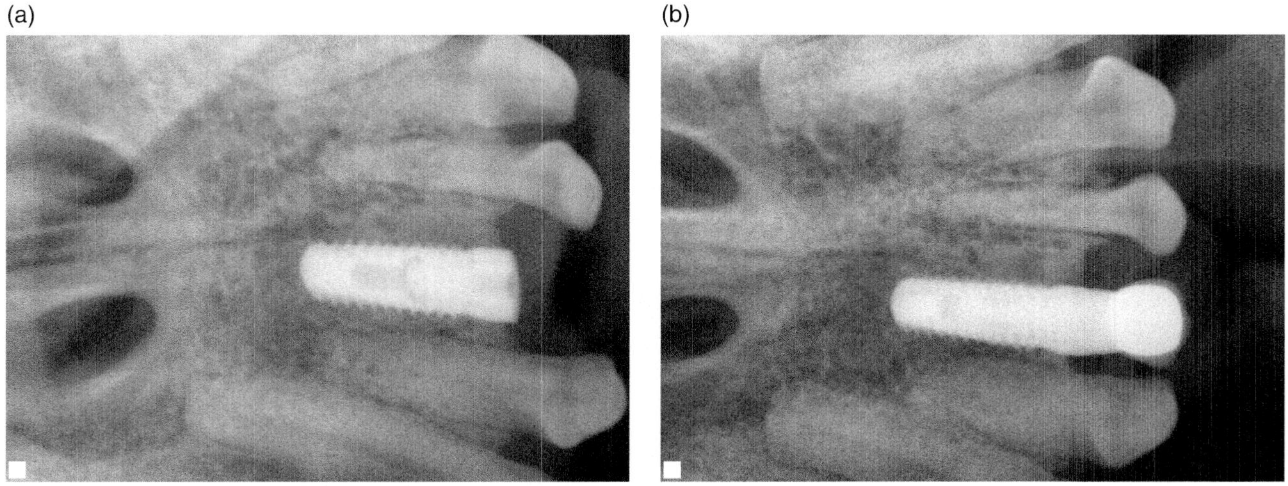

Figure 9.65 (a) Implant placed in location of 101. (b) 8-month follow-up.

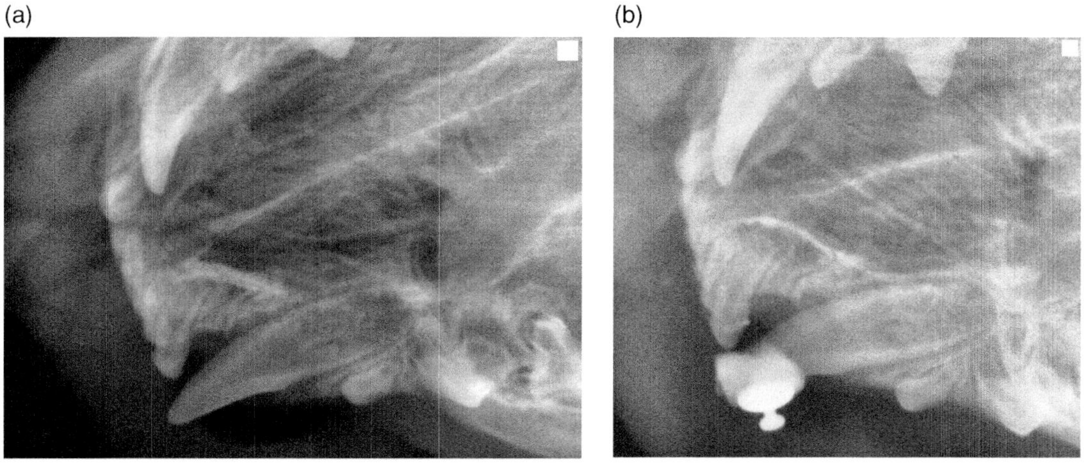

Figure 9.66 (a) Radiograph of mesioccluded left maxillary canine (204) in 7-month-old female Maine Coon cat. (b) Installation of the orthodontic bracket and beginning of orthodontic treatment.

(c)

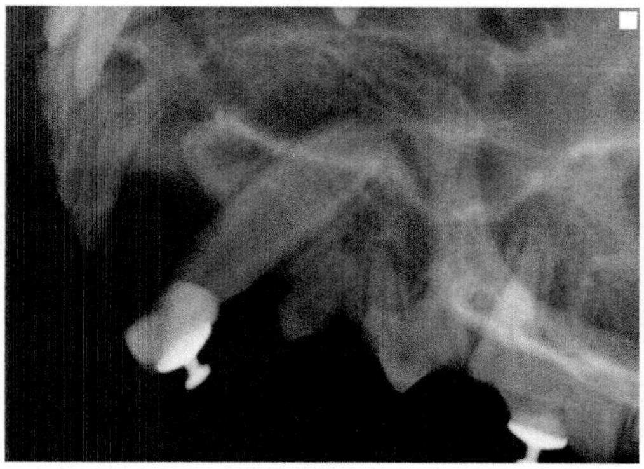

(d)

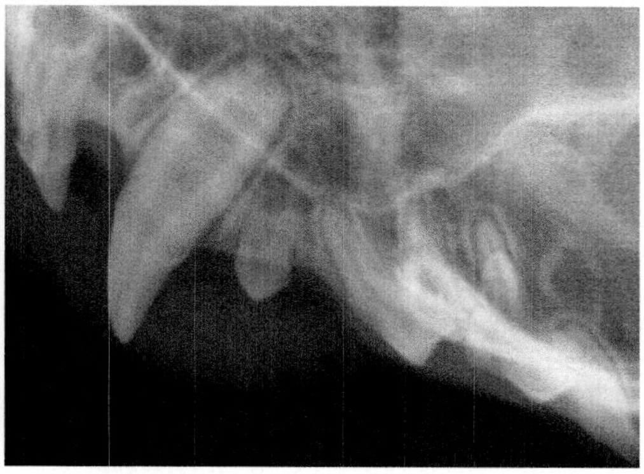

Figure 9.66 (cont'd) (c) Radiograph 8 weeks after initial treatment. (d) Radiograph 1 year after treatment, revealing normal periodontal tissues.

7. The periodontal appearance in orthodontic treatment: Evaluation of the periodontal tissues of orthodontically treated teeth is mandatory in each case. Attention is given to the PDL space and quality of the periapical area (Figure 9.66).[41]

Box 9.1 Key points

- Periodontal examination is not complete without radiography.
- Full mouth radiography is an obligatory part of the diagnostic plan in older animals or in those more prone to periodontal disease.
- Dental radiographs for periodontal assessment should be made slightly underexposed.
- Before any radiographs are taken it is useful to clean the teeth, as the dental calculus is radiodense and can obscure pathological lesions on a radiograph.
- Radiography is proven to be the most reliable method of evaluation of the results of treatment in periodontology, endodontics, implantology, and extractions.

References

1. Hoffman S. Diagnostic imaging in veterinary dental practice. Focal advanced periodontal disease. JAVMA 228(11):1683–1684, 2006.
2. Ivanusa T, Babic A, Petelin M. Diagnostic systems for assessing alveolar bone loss. Stud Health Technol Inform. 43 Pt B:478–481, 1997.
3. Colmery B. The gold standard of veterinary oral health care. Vet Clin Small Anim. 35:781–787, 2005.
4. Gorrel C. Radiographic evaluation. Vet Clin North Am Small Anim Pract. 28(5):1089–1110, 1998.
5. Verstraete FJ, Kass PH, Terpak CH. Diagnostic value of full-mouth radiography in dogs. Am J Vet Res. 59(6):686–691, 1998.
6. Verstraete FJ, Kass PH, Terpak CH. Diagnostic value of full-mouth radiography in cats. Am J Vet Res. 59(6):692–695, 1998.
7. Lang NP, Hill RW. Radiography. J Clin Periodontol. 4:16–28, 1977.
8. Gawor J, Reiter A, Jodkowska K, Kurski G, Wojtacki MP, Kurek A. Influence of diet on oral heath in cats and dogs. J Nutr. 136:7S, 2006.
9. Yun JH, Hwang SJ, Kim CS, Cho KS, Chai JK, Kim CK, Choi SH. The correlation between the bone probing, radiographic and histometric measurements of bone level after regenerative surgery. J Periodontal Res. 40(6):453–460, 2005.
10. Jeffcoat MK. Radiographic methods for the detection of progressive alveolar bone loss. J Periodontol. 63(4 Suppl):367–372, 1992.
11. Smith MM, Zontine WJ, Willits NH. A correlative study of the clinical and radiographic signs of periodontal disease in dogs. JAVMA 186(12):1286–1290, 1985.
12. Mulligan T, Williams C. Atlas of Canine and Feline Dental Radiography. Trenton, NJ: Veterinary Learning Systems, 1998, p. 126.
13. Verstreate FJ. Self Assessment Colour Review of Veterinary Dentistry. London: Manson, 1999, p. 194.
14. Tutt C. Radiographic differentiation between vertical and horizontal bone loss. Proceedings of the 16th ECVD, The Hague, 2007, p. 44.
15. DuPont G, DeBowes LJ. Atlas of Dental Radiography in Dogs and Cats. Philadelphia: Saunders, 2009, pp. 134–135.
16. Eriksen T, Koch R, Nautrup CP. Microradiography of the feline marginal periodontium with a microfocal high-resolution x-ray system. Scand J Dent Res. 102(5):284–289, 1994.
17. Gorrel C. Small Animal Dentistry. New York: Saunders-Elsevier, 2008, pp. 22–68.
18. DuPont G, DeBowes LJ. Atlas of Dental Radiography in Dogs and Cats. Philadelphia: Saunders, 2009, p. 232.
19. Niemiec BA, Gilbert T, Sabatino D. Equipment and basic geometry of dental radiography. J Vet Dent. 21(1):48–52, 2004.
20. Tetradis S, Carranza FA, Fazio RC, Takei HH. Radiographic aids in the diagnosis of periodontal disease. In: Carranza's Clinical Periodontology. New York: Elsevier-Saunders, 2006, p. 562.
21. Tsugawa AJ, Verstraete FJ, Kass PH, Gorrel C. Diagnostic value of the use of lateral and occlusal radiographic views in comparison with periodontal probing for the assessment of periodontal attachment of the canine teeth in dogs. Am J Vet Res. 64(3):255–261, 2003.
22. Wiggs B. Lobprise H. Oral anatomy and physiology. In: Veterinary Dentistry, Principles and Practice. Philadelphia: Lippincott-Raven, 1997, p. 78.
23. Tsugawa AJ, Verstraete FJ. How to obtain and interpret periodontal radiographs in dogs. Clin Tech Small Anim Pract. 15(4): 204–210, 2000.

24. Rózylo KT, Rózylo-Kalinowska I. Radiologia Stomatologiczna Wydawnictwo Lekarskie PZWL Warszawa, 2007, p. 175.
25. Tutt C. Radiography. In: Small Animal Dentistry. Ames, IA: Blackwell, 2006, pp. 120–121.
26. Wang LZ, Li DY. [Study on odontal & periodontal tissue of guinea pigs, dogs and monkeys.] Shanghai Kou Qiang Yi Xue. 13(2):122–125, 2004.
27. Niemiec BA. Dental radiographic interpretation. J Vet Dent. 22(1):53–59, 2005.
28. Wiggs RB, Lobprise H. Veterinary Dentistry, Principles and Practice. Philadelphia: Lippincott-Raven, 1997, pp. 203–204.
29. Morgan JP, Miyabayashi T, Anderson J, Klinge B. Periodontal bone loss in the aging beagle dog. A radiographic study. J Clin Periodontol. 17(9):630–635, 1990.
30. Arnbjerg J. Idiopathic dental root replacement resorption in old dogs. J Vet Dent. 13(3):97–99, 1996.
31. DuPont GA, DeBowes LJ. Comparison of periodontitis and root replacement in cat teeth with resorptive lesions. J Vet Dent. 19(2):71–75, 2002.
32. Girard N, Servet E, Biourge V, Hennet P. Periodontal health status in a colony of 109 cats. J Vet Dent. 26(3):147–155, 2009.
33. Niemiec BA. Case based dental radiology. Top Companion Anim Med. 24(1):4–19, 2009.
34. Beckman BW. Treatment of an infrabony pocket in an American Eskimo dog. J Vet Dent. 21(3):159–163, 2004.
35. Eickholz P, Hörr T, Klein F, Hassfeld S, Kim TS. Radiographic parameters for prognosis of periodontal healing of infrabony defects: Two different definitions of defect depth. J Periodontol. 75(3):399–407, 2004.
36. Urabe M, Hosokawa R, Chiba D, Sato Y, Akagawa Y. Morphogenetic behavior of periodontium on inorganic implant materials: an experimental study of canines. J Biomed Mater Res. 49(1):17–24, 2000.
37. Kim M, Kim JH, Lee JY, Cho K, Kang SS, Kim G, Lee MJ, Choi SH. Effect of bone mineral with or without collagen membrane in ridge dehiscence defects following premolar extraction. In Vivo. 22(2):231–236, 2008.
38. DeForge DH. Images in veterinary dental practice. Class II endodontic-periodontic lesion. JAVMA 224(4):515–516, 2004.
39. Kundzinia RS, Komnova ZD, Volozhin AI. [The periodontal reaction to root canal obturation with different filling materials.] Stomatologiia (Mosk). 72(1):4–7, 1993.
40. Hong AI, Qing-feng XU, Hong-fei LU, Zhi-hui MAI, Ai-qun AN, Guo-ping LUI. Rapid tooth movement through distraction osteogenesis of the periodontal ligament in dogs. Chin Med J (Engl). 121(5):455–462, 2008.
41. Nackaerts O, Jacobs R, Quirynen M, Rober M, Sun Y, Teughels W. Replacement therapy for periodontitis: Pilot radiographic evaluation in a dog model. J Clin Periodontol. 35(12):1048–1052, 2008.

10

The complete dental cleaning

Introduction

There are numerous therapeutic options available (classic and new) for periodontal disease; however, the basis of periodontal therapy remains plaque control. The cornerstone of plaque control and the first step for any periodontal therapy is a *thorough dental prophylaxis*. Newer names for this procedure include complete oral health assessment and treatment (COHAT) and oral assessment, treatment, and prevention (Oral ATP).[1] The new names are designed to convey the fact that a proper dental procedure in veterinary medicine is more than a cleaning and generally involves treatment rather than just prevention of disease.

General anesthesia should be multimodal and balanced (i.e., not inhalant only). In addition, the endotracheal tube must be properly inflated to avoid aspiration of procedural water, oral contaminants (plaque and calculus), or gastroesphageal regurgitation, which could lead to an aspiration pneumonia. This will also minimize the anesthesia gas contamination of the operatory. Finally, since these can be lengthy procedures, it is critical that the patient be provided heat support and be well monitored (EKG, blood pressure, temperature, pulse ox at a minimum).[7] (See chapter 21 for a detailed discussion of anesthesia/patient care.) Finally, the head should be angled downward or the neck supported to encourage fluid drainage.[4]

It is important to note that proper periodontal/dental/oral therapy takes time and patience. A minimum of 1 hour should be allotted for *all* dental cases and much more in many instances. Professional periodontal therapies must be performed with quality (not quantity) in mind.

> **Box 10.1** Key clinical point
>
> Regardless of the name, the goal of this procedure is not only clean and smooth teeth but also to evaluate the periodontal tissues as well as the entire oral cavity. Any professional periodontal therapy for veterinary patients *must* be performed under general anaesthesia, with a well–cuffed endotracheal tube.[2–5] Only when the patient is properly anesthetized can a safe and effective cleaning and oral evaluation be performed.[6] In addition, anesthesia provides a much more pleasant experience for the dentalpatient (see Box 10.2).

Procedure

A complete dental prophylaxis should include the following steps (as detailed below).[3,5,8,9] Note that there are almost as many recipes for a dental prophylaxis as there are veterinary dentists. The instructions below are this author's personal recommendations and may or may not correspond with those of other veterinary dentists. However, the basic procedure is essentially the same. The reader is encouraged to research the procedure in other texts and develop the protocol he or she is most comfortable with.

Step 1: Presurgical exam and consultation

This is a commonly neglected step of the professional dental prophylaxis.[3,6,8,10] The veterinarian should perform a complete physical and oral exam. The physical exam, in combination with preoperative testing, screens for general health issues that may exacerbate periodontal

Veterinary Periodontology, First Edition. Brook A. Niemiec.

Box 10.2 Non-anesthetic dentistry (NAD)

As this chapter demonstrates, a complete dental procedure or "prophylaxis" is a very involved process. It takes time as well as significant attention to detail to be effective. There are numerous steps required to create a positive medical benefit, including *supra* and *sub*gingival scaling, polishing, sulcal lavage, oral exam (including periodontal probing), and charting.

Of all these critical steps, only the first (supragingival scaling) can be performed without anesthesia. Furthermore, even this simple and mostly cosmetic step is generally poorly performed, especially on the lingual/palatal surfaces and in the back of the mouth (Figures 10.a and 10.b).

With NAD, the teeth are scaled by *non-professionals* in a conscious patient. The combination of unskilled operators and movement of the patient often leads to roughened tooth surfaces (Figure 10.c). These factors combined with the lack of polishing lead to much faster recurrence of disease. Furthermore, unskilled operators working without anesthesia can cause significant iatrogenic trauma such as gingival lacerations.

(a1) (a2)

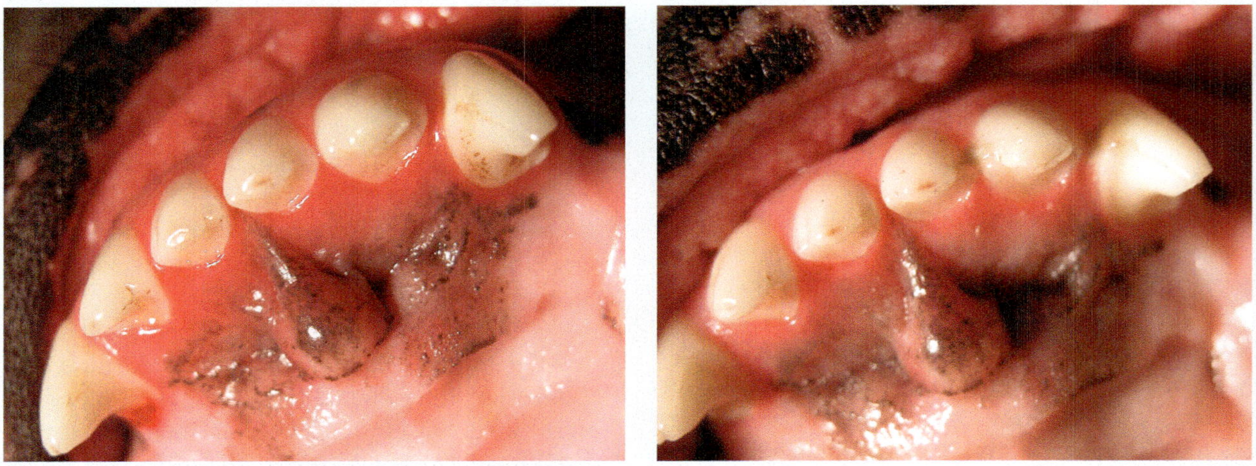

Figure 10.a Intraoral pictures of a patient who received NAD 1 week previous. (1) Presentation of the palatal surface of the maxillary incisors (note the significant amount of residual calculus). (2) The same area following a professional scaling under general anesthesia (note how clean the teeth are now).

(b1) (b2)

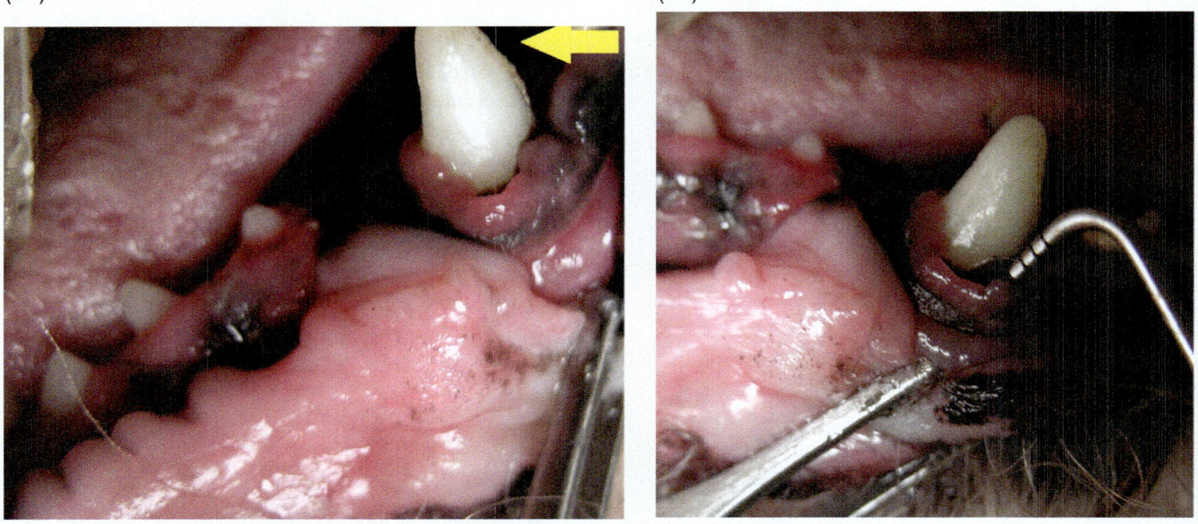

Figure 10.b These images are from a dog who had received NAD on a monthly basis (most recently 2 weeks previous) for 3 years. The patient was presented for persistent bad breath and was recommended by the NAD provider "to come every week for a while." (1) Evaluation under general anesthesia revealed the large amount of dental calculus on the lingual surface of the right mandibular canine (404) (yellow arrow), whereas the remainder of the teeth looked clean. (2) Periodontal probing revealed the deep periodontal pocket on the lingual and facial surfaces of the tooth.

(b3)

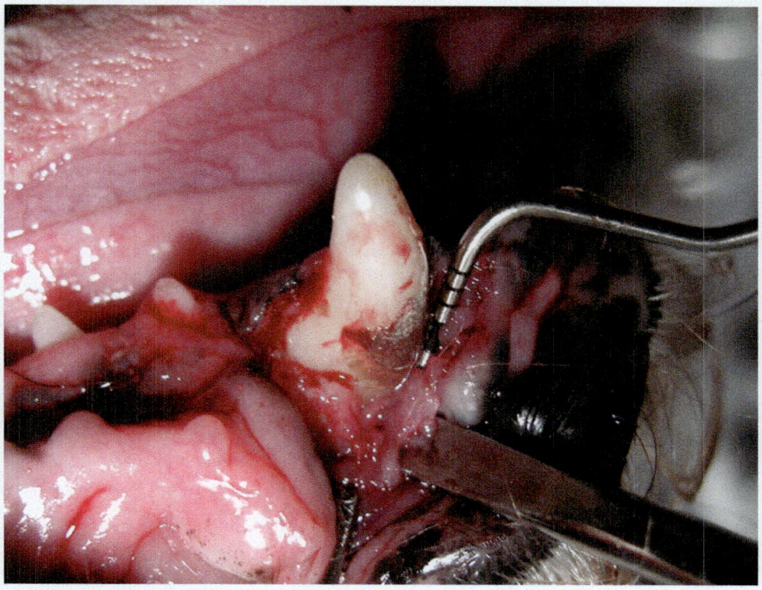

(b4)

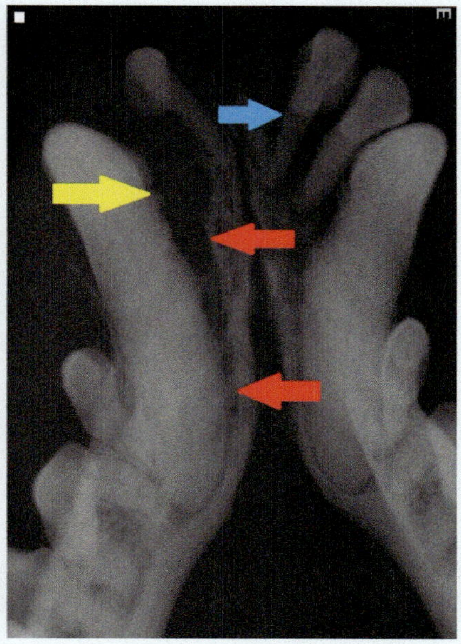

Figure 10.b (cont'd) (3) Following flap creation for surgical extraction, the subgingival dental calculus is evident. (4) Finally, the dental radiograph confirms the subgingival calculus (yellow arrow) and severe alveolar bone loss in the area (red arrows) predisposing the patient to a pathologic fracture (see chapter 6). In addition, note the severe alveolar bone loss to the left incisors (blue arrow).

Moreover, the single most important step of a prophylaxis (subgingival scaling) *cannot* be performed without general anesthesia. Simply said, what animal patient would allow you to place a sharp instrument under its gums? Patients are often seen following NAD with clean crowns but with significant areas of subgingival calculus (Figures 10.b and 10.d). This may be the most damaging issue with this service, as it gives the client a false sense that he or she is improving the dental health of the pet. This author has routinely dealt with clients who are very upset when dental disease is diagnosed despite "clean" crowns. These clients feel that they have "failed" their pet, allowing them to progress to disease despite well-intentioned efforts.

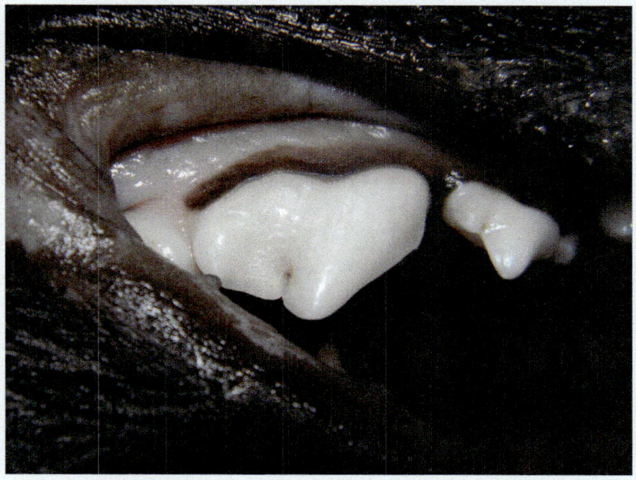

Figure 10.c Right maxillary fourth premolar (108) of a patient who recently received NAD. Note the significant damage to the enamel of the tooth. This will result in much faster plaque accumulation (see chapter 2).

An oral exam is a very important but mostly underappreciated step of a dental cleaning. As evidenced throughout this book, oral pathology can have very subtle clinical signs, yet with significant infection (Figures 10.e through 10.g). Without anesthesia, a complete oral exam is *impossible*. Furthermore, dental radiographs are necessary for proper diagnosis and treatment (Figure 10.g2). This valuable diagnostic tool cannot be performed without general anesthesia.

The lack of proper cleaning and evaluation is not the only reason that NAD is contraindicated as a means of treating oral disease. There is also a strong possibility of iatrogenic damage to the patient. Without chemical restraint, the sharp instruments necessary for a proper cleaning can easily lacerate the delicate gingival tissues if the patient moves. This has been repeatedly seen throughout the country. Furthermore, jaw fractures and neck injuries have been reported following restraint for "non-anesthesia dentals." Finally, the risk of aspiration pneumonia from the lack of intubation is significant.

These concerns are not just the opinion of this author. Based on the numerous limitations and dangers of NAD, the American Veterinary Dental College has drafted a position statement against this procedure (http://avdc.org/Dental_Scaling_Without_Anesthesia.pdf). In fact, some states (including California) have laws that make the practice illegal unless performed under the supervision of a veterinarian. Some providers of NAD are getting around these laws by providing the service within

(d1) (d2)

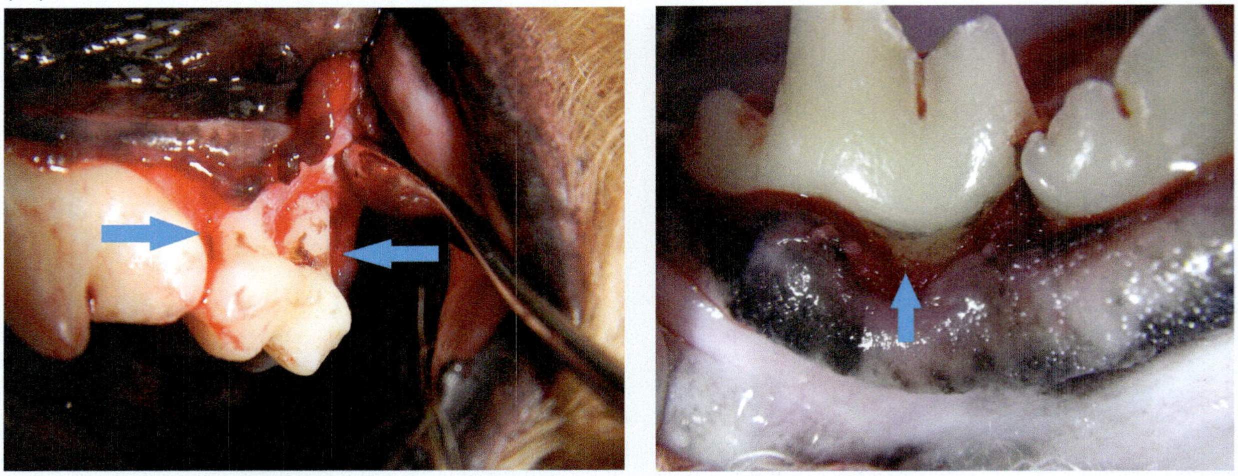

Figure 10.d Intraoral pictures of the left maxillary first molar (209) (1) and the right mandibular first molar (409) (2) in two patients who recently received NAD. Note that the crowns of the tooth are clean, but there is significant *sub*gingival calculus.

(e1) (e2) (e3)

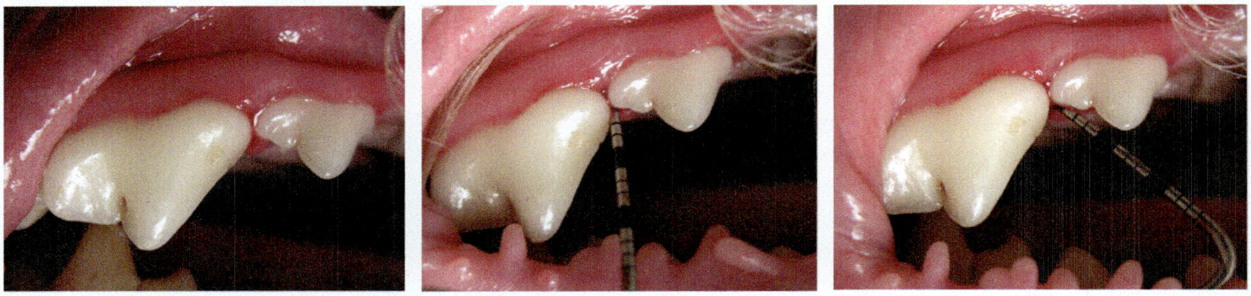

Figure 10.e Intraoral dental pictures of the maxillary right fourth premolar (108) of a patient who has been receiving NAD on a regular basis. Note that the teeth appear outwardly clean (1). However, there is a significant periodontal pocket (2) and furcation exposure level II (3) on this tooth. This would have been diagnosed and treated much earlier (or entirely avoided) with proper oral care.

(f1) (f2)

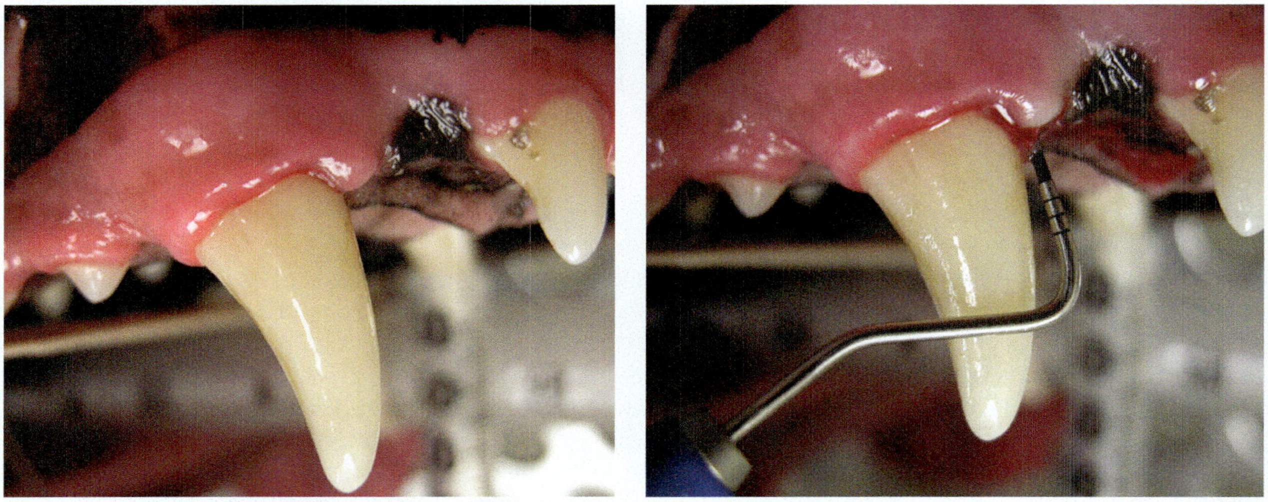

Figure 10.f Intraoral dental pictures of the right maxillary canine (104) of a dog who has been receiving NAD on a regular basis. (1) Note that the teeth appear outwardly clean. (2) However, there is a significant periodontal pocket on this tooth. This would have been diagnosed and treated much earlier (or entirely avoided) with proper oral care.

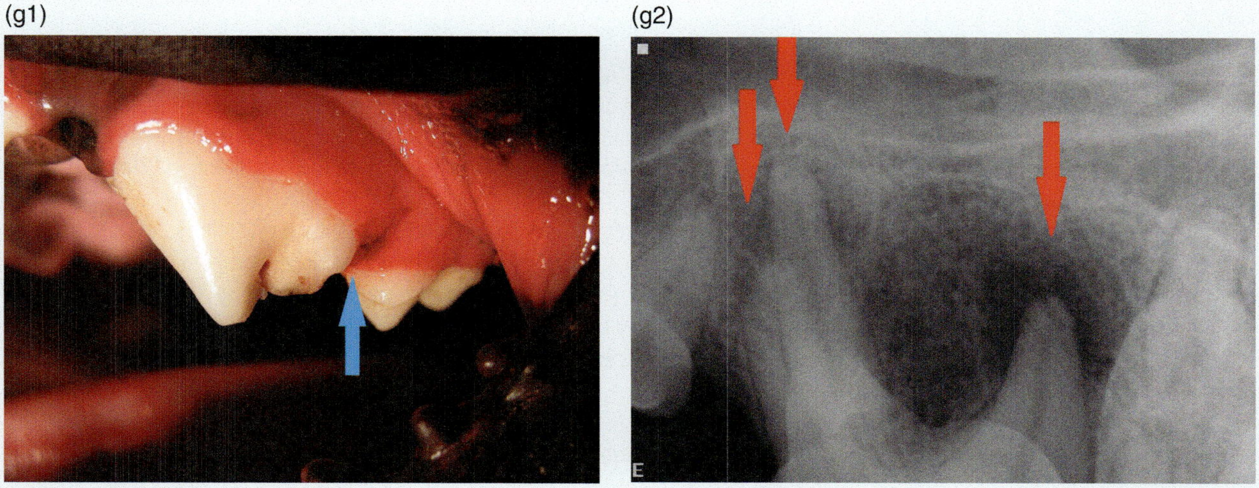

Figure 10.g (1) Intraoral picture of the left maxillary fourth premolar (208) of the canine patient in Figure 10.a that received NAD 1 week ago. The patient was presented for a carnassial abscess. Conscious oral exam by a trained professional revealed the small fracture to the distal aspect of the tooth (blue arrow). (2) Intraoral dental radiographs revealed periapical rarefaction (red arrows) confirming the source of the infection. Note that these infections are generally present for a long time prior to creating a clinical abscess and that bone destruction is also a fairly lengthy process. Therefore, this infection has been present but undiagnosed for a significant period of time. Proper oral care with a thorough oral exam and/or dental radiology would have allowed for much earlier treatment of this significant infection.

veterinary hospitals. While this is legal, it is considered below the standard of practice. No AVDC diplomate would be likely to support a veterinarian in a malpractice suit if this was the inciting cause. It should also be noted that in these cases, it is the prescribing (i.e., practice owner) veterinarian's license at risk, NOT the contracted service provider. Therefore, think carefully before allowing this procedure in your practice.

There is an also an emerging and concerning trend toward "sedation" dentistry within veterinary practices. While possibly more effective than NAD, it still shares many of its limitations and dangers. Of large concern, there is still no protection for the lungs and typically no catheter for emergency treatment. Pain control is absent or very limited and no procedures beyond a cleaning can be performed. Finally, sedation is no safer and in some cases is more dangerous than balanced and monitored anesthesia.

In conclusion, the best way to challenge this dangerous and non-beneficial practice is client education. In the minds of most clients (and some veterinarians), this service seems like an excellent alternative to general anesthesia. This is reinforced by the fact that the visible areas of the mouth are generally fairly clean. However, every veterinary dentist has scores of cases demonstrating its ineffectiveness as well as those showing its dangers.

disease (e.g., diabetes or uremia) or compromise anesthetic safety (cardiopulmonary disease, anemia, hepatopathy).[6,11] The conscious oral examination should identify most obvious oral pathologies (fractured, intrinsically stained, or mobile teeth; oral masses; and large tooth resorptive [TR] lesions) as well as allow for a preliminary assessment of periodontal status.

An additional exam room diagnostic tool is provided by a periodontal diagnostic strip.[A] This product measures the production of thiols, which are produced by periodontal pathogens. A quick swipe of the maxillary gingival margin will reveal visual evidence of the severity of periodontal infection, improving compliance with dental recommendations. While this product is certainly a valuable tool for any patient, there are several presentations in which it is particularly valuable. This includes patients with significant periodontal disease despite a lack of gingival inflammation or significant calculus and also those with dark pigmented gingiva. Finally, small and toy breed dogs quite often have severe disease involving the molar teeth while the rest of the mouth is fairly healthy. Moreover, these teeth are typically difficult or impossible to evaluate on conscious oral exam, but infection would be demonstrated on the test strip.[6,11,12]

Following the conscious oral examination, the veterinarian can then discuss with the owner the various disease processes found on the examination as well as the available treatment options. It is best to utilize visual educational materials during discussions with clients, to aid in their understanding. A list of resources for these

Box 10.3 Scheduling of dental procedures

It is impossible to fully evaluate the conscious veterinary patient. Therefore, it is quite common for dental procedures to take much longer than anticipated when unexpected pathology is discovered during the anesthetized exam. Furthermore, providing appropriate periodontal therapy (as presented in this text), including thorough subgingival scaling, charting, and radiology, is time-consuming. It is important to note, however, that only by performing appropriate periodontal assessment and cleaning are the financial investment and anesthetic risk justified.

These factors make scheduling dental procedures within a general practice challenging, which often leads to overscheduling. This results in either unhappy staff, inappropriate patient care, or both. A proper presurgical exam will minimize but not eliminate this issue. Provided below is a rough guide for the *minimum* amount of time that should be allotted for various dental procedures. Note that this will be affected by the quality of equipment as well as staff skills. Finally, remember to allow time to treat any non-periodontal pathology (such as fractured teeth, tooth resorption, or oral masses) that is noted on conscious exam.

Utilizing the AVDC periodontal disease classification below, assign a time slot to each prophylaxis procedure and limit the case to the available time. Note that the classifications and stage-related guidelines are an educated guess. To truly designate the level of disease, periodontal probing and dental radiographs are required, and these steps can only be performed *after* the patient is anesthetized.

Periodontal Disease Classification (AVDC Nomenclature Committee, www.avdc.org)

- Normal (PD0): Clinically normal; no gingival inflammation or periodontitis clinically evident.
- Stage 1 (PD1): Gingivitis only, without attachment loss. The height and architecture of the alveolar margin are normal.
- Stage 2 (PD2): Early periodontitis; less than 25% of attachment loss, or at most there is a stage 1 furcation involvement in multirooted teeth. There are early radiographic signs of periodontitis. The loss of periodontal attachment is less than 25% as measured either by probing of the clinical attachment level or radiographic determination of the distance of the alveolar margin from the cementoenamel junction relative to the length of the root.
- Stage 3 (PD3): Moderate periodontitis; 25–50% of attachment loss as measured either by probing of the clinical attachment level or radiographic determination of the distance of the alveolar margin from the cementoenamel junction relative to the length of the root, or there is a stage 2 furcation involvement in multirooted teeth.
- Stage 4 (PD4): Advanced periodontitis; more than 50% of attachment loss as measured either by probing of the clinical attachment level or radiographic determination of the distance of the alveolar margin from the cementoenamel junction relative to the length of the root, or there is a stage 3 furcation involvement in multirooted teeth.

Stage-Related Guidelines for *Minimum* Time Scheduling for Dental Procedures

Dog:

- Stage 1: 60–75 minutes
- Stage 2: 75–90 minutes
- Stage 3: 90–120 minutes
- Stage 4: 120–180 minutes

Cat

- Stage 1: 30 min
- Stage 2: 30–60 min
- Stage 3: 60–120 min
- Stage 4: 120–150 min

materials is included in appendix 4, and/or clinics can create their own "smile" book or computer slideshow of common cases for these conversations. This face-to-face discussion will improve client understanding of the disease processes and associated sequela and should therefore increase client understanding and acceptance of proposed therapy.

Based on the oral examination findings, the practitioner can create a more accurate estimate both of procedure time and financial costs to the client. The client should be made aware at this point that a complete oral examination is *not* possible on a conscious patient. Therefore, the preoperative estimate is only preliminary, and the client should be warned that it can (and often will) increase. In addition, the prudent practitioner will allot for a certain number of dental procedures per day based on the anticipated time involved for each case, as dental procedures vary widely in the required amount of

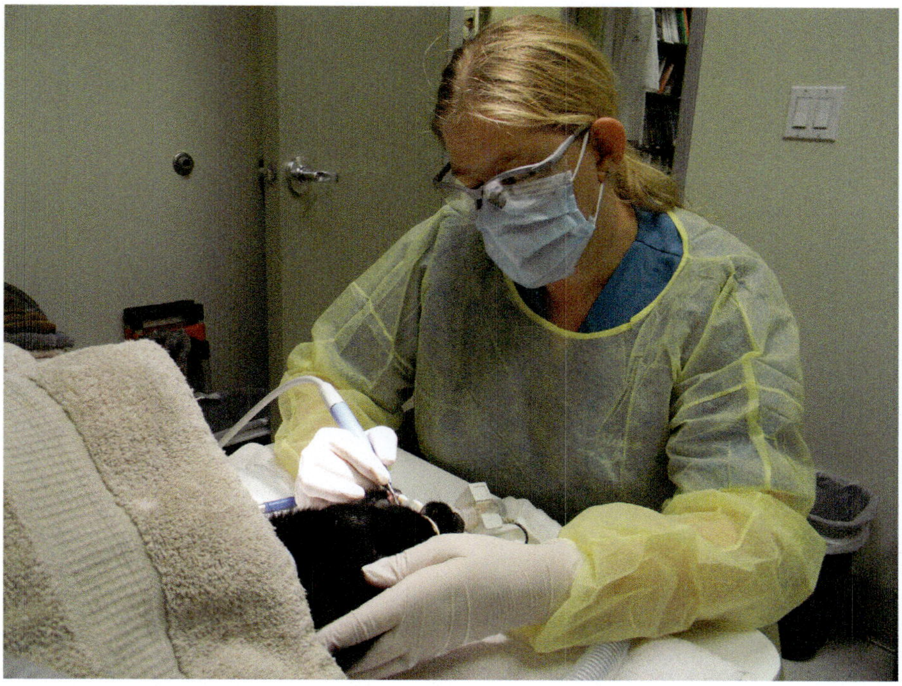

Figure 10.1 Properly attired dental technician performing a dental cleaning. Her eyes, lungs, and hands are well protected from the aerosolized bacteria. Furthermore, the gown protects her clothes from contamination, which decreases the spread throughout the hospital. Finally, note that this procedure is being performed in a dedicated dental surgery suite.

time. For example, two stage IV dental procedures can take longer than five stage I and II procedures (see Box 10.3). By scheduling patients as assigned by stage or severity of dental disease, the veterinarian and his or her support team will not be rushed, which improves patient care and staff morale (and possibly their health too).[12] This small investment of time prior to the procedure will improve the experience of everyone involved (veterinarian, technician, receptionist, client, and patient).

Staff and patient protection

Numerous studies have shown that ultrasonic and sonic scalers create significant pathogenic aerosols (see "Mechanical Scalers" below). These aerosols are highly contaminated and contain not only bacteria but also fungi and viruses.[13–15] The infectious organisms are not only supplied by the patient's mouth but there are also significant numbers of infectious organisms within the water lines of the mechanized hand-pieces (sonic and ultrasonic scalers, as well as high-speed hand-pieces).[16–18] Therefore, a bacterial water filter or chlorhexidine flushing of the system is recommended to decrease contamination.[19]

In addition, low levels of aerosolization occur during hand scaling as well as simple oral examination.[20] These pathogenic aerosols have been linked to numerous deleterious effects on the staff of human dental practices (see below). Staff members performing dental prophylactic (or *any* dental) procedures should be instructed to wear personal protective equipment (mask, goggles, and gloves) at all times to decrease contamination (Figure 10.1).[4,8,12,21,22] Dental procedures also must *not* be performed in "sterile" environments such as surgical suites. Furthermore, they should not be performed near any sick or compromised patients or near any clean procedures (including blood draws and catheterizations [intravenous or urinary]).[19] Dental procedures are best confined to their own designated room, ideally with filters (HEPA) on the ventilation ducts, as airborne aerosols have been shown to affect the entire office.[23–26] Finally, it is important to remember that aerosols will contaminate the clothing of the operator and can then be spread throughout the entire hospital.[20] Therefore, gowns are recommended to be worn in the dental operatory and to be discarded or washed following the procedure (see Figure 10.1).[12]

Step 2: Chlorhexidine lavage

The oral cavity is a contaminated area and thorough dental cleanings are mildly invasive. This means that dental cleanings often result in a transient bacteremia,[27] which is more severe in patients with periodontitis.[28,29] Dental cleanings cause bacterial aerosolization and contamination of the office environment when ultrasonic instruments are employed (as above). Finally, while the incidence of pneumonia is positively related to the duration of intubation, it can occur with even

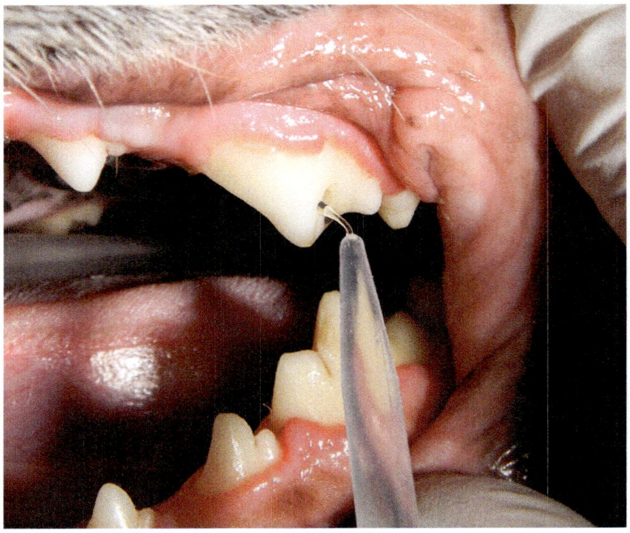

Figure 10.2 Chlorhexidine lavage.

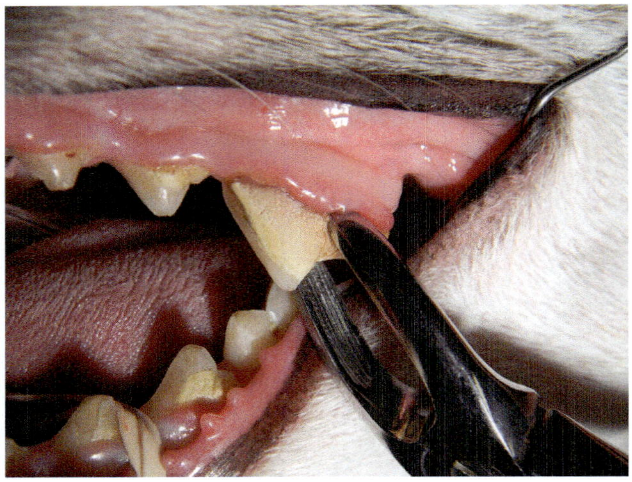

Figure 10.3 Careful removal of a large accumulation of dental calculus with an extraction forceps.

short surgical procedures, so it is ideal to minimize the number of oral pathogens whenever intubation is planned.[30] Rinsing the oral cavity with a 0.12% or 0.2% solution of chlorhexidine gluconate[B] (Figure 10.2) prior to commencing the prophylaxis has been shown to decrease the bacterial load.[3,8,31–34] Allowing 1 minute of contact time has been recommended as an effective minimum. This very short step has been shown to decrease the degree of bacteremia following extractions[35] and would be expected to be effective in cases of periodontal therapy as well. The effectiveness of this procedure can be surmised from a study that showed that open heart surgery patients had better survival rates if their mouths were rinsed with chlorhexidine gluconate prior to surgery.[36] Not only does the reduction of oral bacteria benefit the patient, it also lowers the number of aerosolized bacteria and thus reduces the degree of staff contamination.[32,37]

Step 3: Supragingival cleaning

Very large accumulations of calculus can be quickly removed with a calculus forceps (Figure 10.3).[8,38] However, this must be done very carefully to avoid tooth and gingival damage.[39] Because current mechanical scalers are very effective in removing large calculus deposits,[21] this author does not often use forceps.

Supragingival cleaning can be performed via mechanical or hand scaling but is best performed using a combination of the modalities.[21]

Mechanical scalers

Mechanical scalers include both sonic and ultrasonic types. The most common type of mechanical scaler in veterinary dentistry today is the ultrasonic model. There are two main types (magnetostrictive and piezoelectric).[40] Both of these ultrasonic scalers vibrate at approximately 25,000–45,000 Hz.[4,21,40] *Magnetostrictive* units have an elliptical pattern of vibration, so all sides of the instrument are useful.[4] *Piezoelectric* systems, however, are thought to have a linear pattern of vibration and ergo only the sides (not the front or back) of the instrument are effective at plaque removal.[4,32] A recent study has shown, however, that piezoelectrics also have an elliptical motion, concluding that they can actually be used on all surfaces.[41] An additional advantage of piezoelectrics is that they produce significantly less heat than magnetostrictives and are less damaging to the enamel, which means they may be the safer choice.[39]

Both types of ultrasonic scalers are very efficient and provide the additional benefit of creating an antibacterial effect in the coolant spray (cavitation).[4,32,42,43]

Sonic scalers run on compressed air and vibrate at only 2,000–6,500 Hz,[4,21,32,39] although speeds of up to 9,000 Hz have been reported.[4] Most reports indicate that this slower speed results in longer scaling time compared to ultrasonics;[44] however, some report equal time,[45] and at least one report indicated that sonic scalers are actually faster.[46] At slower speeds they generate minimal heat, and therefore may be a safer alternative to ultrasonics.[47] Sonic scalers also have an elliptical pattern of vibration, so all sides of the instrument are useful.[32] It was classically believed that they do not offer the antibacterial effects of the ultrasonics; however, this fundamental belief is being challenged.[48,49] Sonic scalers run on a higher amplitude (10 times or more as compared to ultrasonics), which may be more damaging to the root surface.[4,50] (See chapter 23 for a complete discussion of mechanical scalers.)

Mechanical scaling

When using any of the mechanical scalers, the first concern is the power setting of the instrument. Ultrasonic tips have a recommended vibrational velocity (Hz) range, and this should be determined and set prior to initiating scaling. The power should be set low and adjusted upward to the *minimum* required power.[21] Note that there may be a different setting for the same instrument/tip when it is utilized subgingivally. The area of maximum vibration for ultrasonic scalers is 1–3 mm from the tip.[39,51] Piezoelectric scalers only function in the last 3 mm from the tip; however, magnetostrictive scalers are useful (but not nearly as effective) over a much larger area, which is up to 12 mm for the ferrite rod type.[4] Do not use the very tip of the instrument as it is not effective for calculus removal and can potentially damage the tooth (Figure 10.4).[4,21]

Next, it is important to ensure that there is adequate coolant being delivered through the working end of the scaler. A fine but significant spray should be evident when the unit is activated (Figure 10.5).[21] If minimal or excessive coolant is released, adjust the water flow to an appropriate level. Utilizing a mechanical scaler without sufficient coolant can cause numerous deleterious effects including tooth death.[5,52] It is important to note that standard periodontal tips must *not* be introduced under the gingival margin.[32,40] The water coolant will not reach the working area of the instrument, which results in overheating and possible tooth damage, especially when using magnetostrictive scalers. Specific low-powered periodontal tips are available for subgingival use, and clinicians and staff should familiarize themselves with this equipment prior to their use. (See chapters 11 and 23 for detailed information on subgingival tips.)

The instrument should be *gently* grasped with the fingers of the dominant hand (Figure 10.6).[10,21] Avoid using a whole palm grip as this tends to reduce tactile sensitivity, increase operator fatigue, and result in both decreased operator ability to sense residual calculus and a tendency toward placing too much downward pressure on the tooth (see below).

Next, the *side* of the instrument is placed in contact with the tooth surface (Figure 10.7) with a very light (feather) touch.[5,21,38,51] Too much pressure on the instrument will *not* improve its efficiency. In fact, applying excessive pressure on the tooth surface will dampen the vibration, which may actually make the instrument *less*

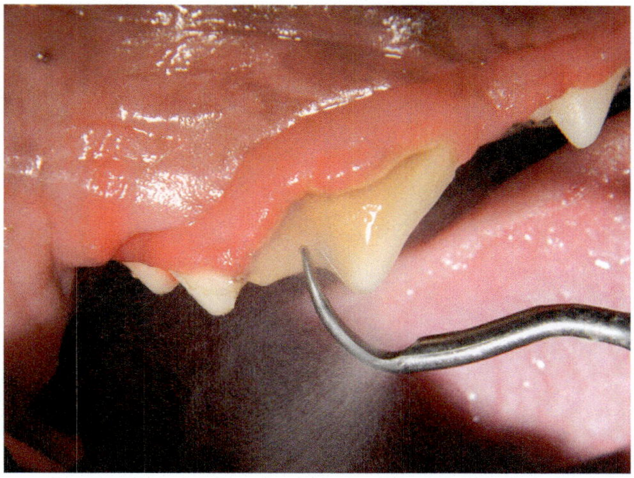

Figure 10.5 The fine spray of coolant fluid. This indicates proper operation of the unit.

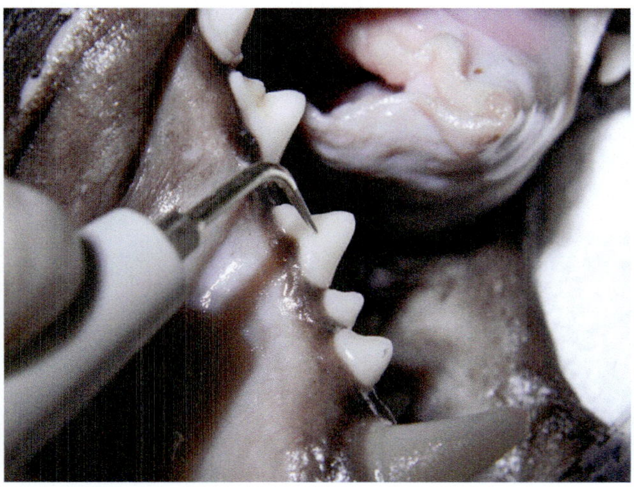

Figure 10.4 Inappropriate use of an ultrasonic scaler. The tip is ineffective for scaling and can damage the tooth.

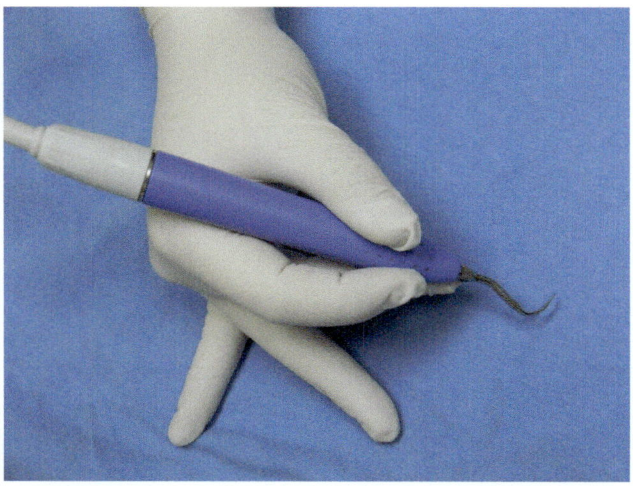

Figure 10.6 Proper grip for the use of a mechanical scaler. It is gently held with the tips of the fingers (like a pencil) while the other two fingers are resting on a surface.

effective[53] and can result in damage to both the instrument and the tooth.[5,54]

Use the side surface of the terminal portion of the instrument, keeping the tip parallel to the tooth, and then run across the *entire* tooth surface using numerous overlapping strokes in different directions.[21,39] Keep the instrument in motion at all times to avoid tooth damage.[21]

It has long been recommended to strictly limit the amount of time ultrasonic scalers linger on one tooth. Typically, it is recommended that they be kept in constant contact with tooth for no more than 15 seconds,[21,38,39] but some authors recommend only 5–7 seconds.[51] Interestingly, however, an exhaustive literature search can find no primary research that indicates a length of time that actually causes pulp damage *providing that the instrument has adequate water cooling.*[52,55] Although the classic recommendations may therefore be somewhat arbitrary, this author agrees that if the calculus is not removed from a tooth in 15 seconds, it may be best to move to another tooth and then return. This lengthy cleaning could also indicate that either the equipment is not working properly (inappropriate power setting or broken/worn tip/stack) or that the user's technique is faulty. In these cases, check the equipment thoroughly and then redirect the instrument so that the terminal 3 mm of the side of the instrument is in contact with the tooth.

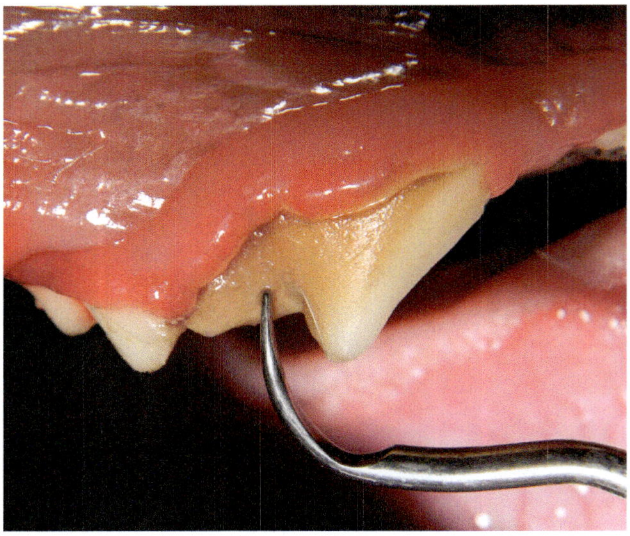

Figure 10.7 Proper position of the ultrasonic scaler on a tooth. The side of the instrument, very near the tip, is applied gently to the tooth surface.

Once the instrument loses contact with the tooth, the scaler can no longer be effective. The instrument should be kept in constant motion, running *slowly* over the tooth surface in overlapping, wide, sweeping motions to cover each mm^2 of every tooth surface.[21,39,56] Plaque and early calculus is difficult to visualize. Therefore, the operator should assume that the entire tooth is affected and clean each tooth completely.

It should be further noted that most mechanical scalers have a particular spot where they are most effective at calculus removal.[39] If calculus appears "tough," consider rotating the instrument slightly to ensure the proper orientation. This tiny adjustment may result in dramatic improvement in cleaning efficiency. If calculus is still not being removed relatively quickly, check the tip for wear and check the power settings, as these may be the culprit.[57] It has been shown that damage affecting the terminal 1 mm of the tip reduces efficiency of an ultrasonic scaler by 25%, and 2 mm by 50%[58] (Figure 10.8).

Mechanical scalers are very efficient in plaque and calculus removal. In addition, they tend to less operator fatigue (vs. hand scaling), which may decrease the

(a) (b)

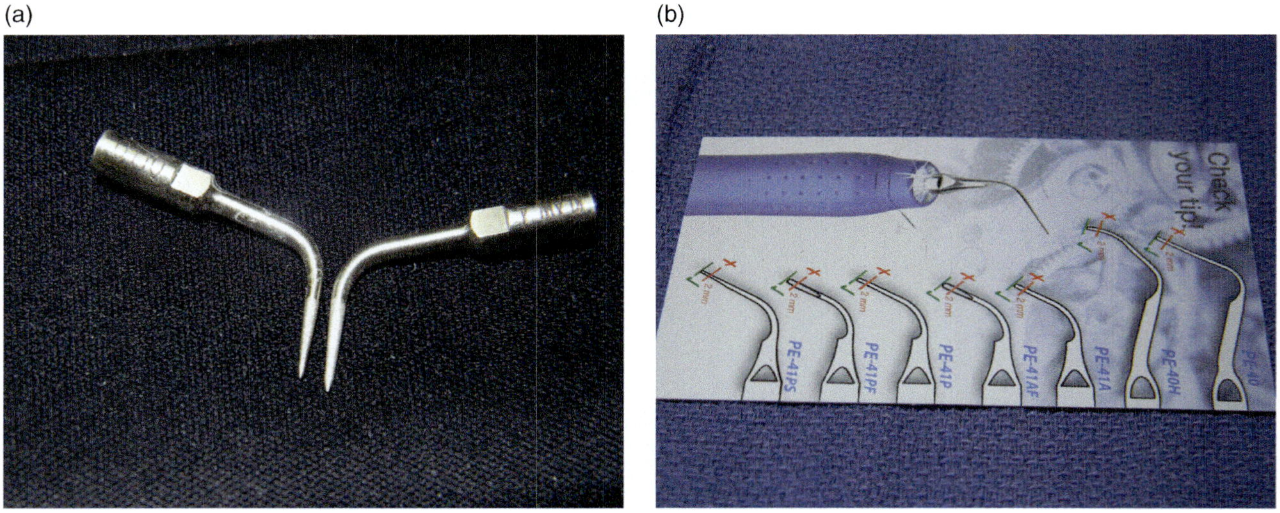

Figure 10.8 Measuring tip wear. (a) Image showing a new (right) and used (left) ultrasonic tip. Note that the used tip has lost approximately 2 mm of its tip. This decreases its efficiency by approximately 50%. (b) Commercial wear chart.

incidence of repetitive motion injuries (such as carpal tunnel).[32,59] They can, however, be more damaging to the tooth[56,60] and may leave some calculus behind. Therefore, it is recommended that a combination of hand scaling and ultrasonic scaling be performed to ensure the complete removal of calculus.[21,56]

Another concern with mechanical scalers is the production of a bacteria-laden aerosol, which affects the entire practice.[14,22,33,61–63] Therefore, the use of these instruments must be coupled with good infection control (see "Staff and Patient Protection" above).

Finally, it should be noted that rotosonic scaling, while popular in the past, is no longer a recommended form of scaling.[4] This is due to the fact that these instruments produce a significantly rougher surface compared to hand and ultrasonic/sonic power scalers.[54] In addition, they are *by far* the most damaging mechanical scaling instrument.[39,40]

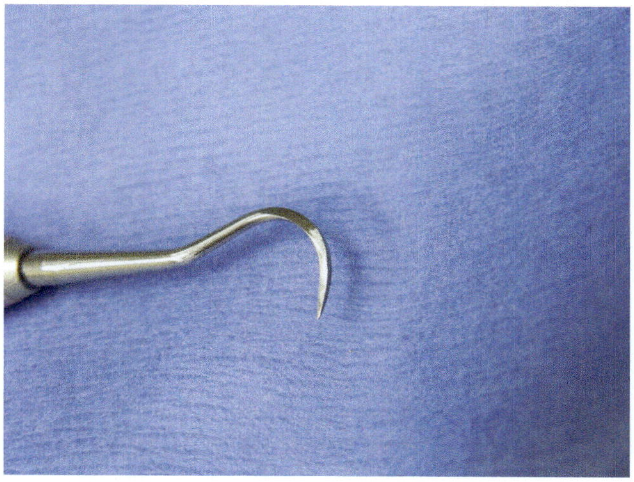

Figure 10.9 Hand scalers: This sickle instrument is triangular in shape with sharp edges and tip. Use for *supra*gingival scaling only.

Hand scaling

Equipment

Supragingival hand scaling is best performed with a scaler. This is a triangular instrument with two sharp cutting edges and a sharp tip (Figure 10.9).[4,21,40,56] Typically, the blade is positioned at a 90-degree angle to the shaft, and this is called a universal scaler.[21] However, area-specific scalers with different terminal angles are also available, and these may improve cleaning ability in some areas (especially distal).[21,39] Scalers are designed for *supra*gingival use only, as the shape of the instrument as well as the sharp back and tip can easily damage the gingiva.[21,40,56] This sharp tip is very useful in reaching tight interproximal spaces.[4] (See chapter 22 for a detailed description of periodontal hand instrumentation.)

Note: Periodontal hand instruments are only effective when sharp. This means they need to be sharpened on a regular basis (at least weekly if used regularly). If a curette or scaler has not been sharpened in over a few months, it will likely need to be professionally sharpened or replaced. For sharpening instructions please see appendix 3.

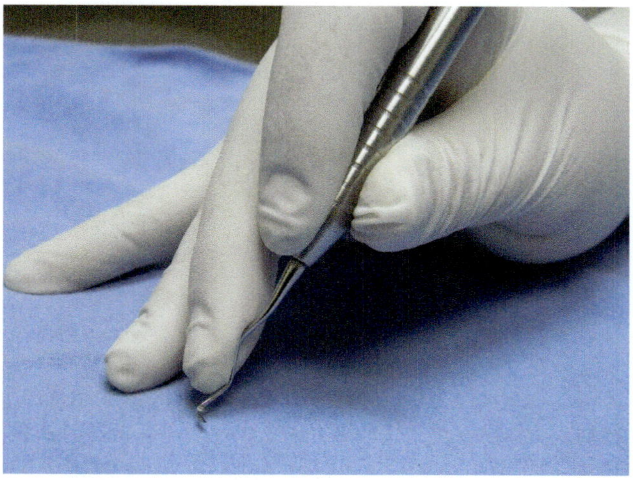

Figure 10.10 Modified pencil grasp.

Technique

Scalers (as well as curettes) are typically held with a modified pencil grasp (Figure 10.10),[5,21,56] but other grips such as the extended or open grasp or long reach can be necessary in certain situations (particularly distal in the mouth).[39] The instrument is gently held at the textured or rubberized end, between the *tips* of the thumb and index finger. The middle finger is placed near the terminal end of the shaft and is used to feel for vibrations that signal residual calculus or diseased/rough tooth/root surfaces. Finally, the ring and pinkie fingers are rested on a stable surface, generally the target tooth or nearby teeth (Figure 10.11). Other stabilization points for the fingers or "finger rests" include the cross arch, opposite arch, and finger on finger rests.[5,21] This grasp and described method of cleaning allow for maximum control during the scaling procedure.[21]

Hand instruments must also be used with a gentle touch.[21,56] The instrument is held with the terminal shank parallel to the tooth surface (if using a universal scaler, the handle is also parallel) and the blade placed at the gingival margin (Figure 10.12). Hand scalers are used in a pull stroke fashion (Figure 10.13), which helps avoid inadvertent laceration of the gingiva by pulling away from the soft tissue.[39,56] The scaler's cutting surface should be run drawn against the tooth numerous times in overlapping strokes until the tooth feels smooth.[21]

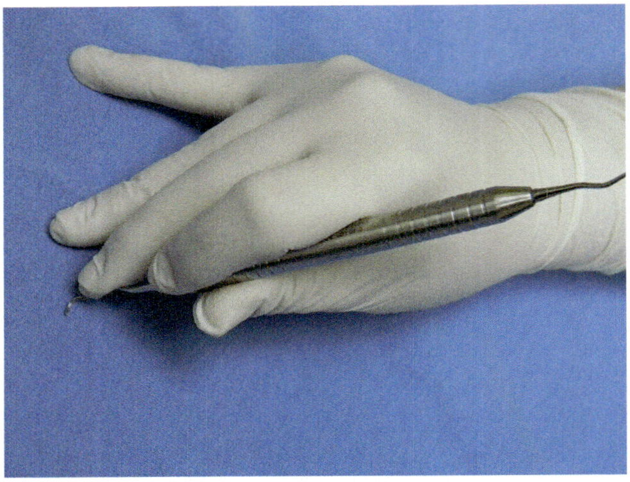

Figure 10.11 Ring and pinkie finger rest for the modified pencil grip.

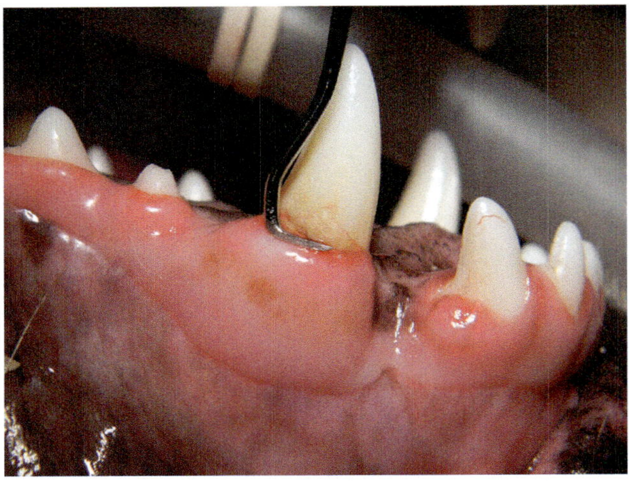

Figure 10.12 Hand scaler correctly placed against the tooth. The shank is placed parallel to the tooth and the blade starts at the gingival margin.

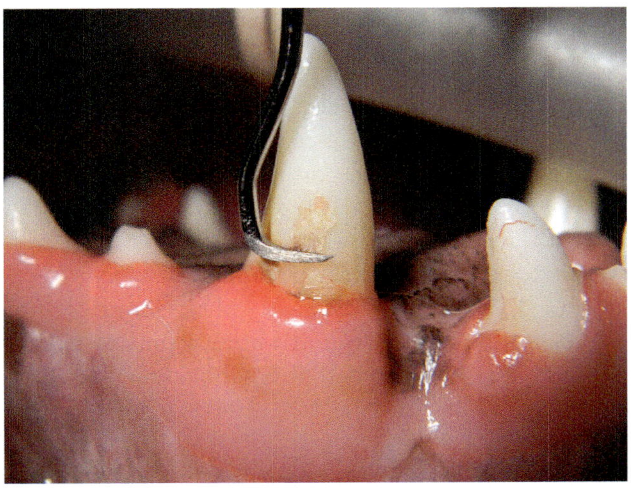

Figure 10.13 Pressure is placed against the tooth and the scaler moved coronally in a firm, controlled movement. This removes the calculus from the surface.

Step 4: Subgingival plaque and calculus scaling

This is *the most important* step of the dental cleaning, as *supra*gingival plaque control is insufficient to treat periodontal disease.[39,56,64] Unfortunately, for several reasons, this step is also the most difficult.[21] First, *sub*gingival calculus is harder than *supra*gingival and tends to be locked into tooth surface irregularities.[65,66] Second, visualization of the subgingival crown and root surfaces is difficult and may be further limited by bleeding from the inflamed tissues (requiring good tactile sense). Finally, the gingival sulcus or periodontal pocket limits the movement of the instrument.[21] Because of these limitations, the incidence of residual calculus increases with increasing pocket depth.[67]

Subgingival scaling has classically been performed by hand with a curette, but advances in sonic and ultrasonic tips now allow their use under the gingival margin.[21,40] Numerous studies have shown that sonic and ultrasonic scaling is equal in effectiveness to traditional hand scaling.[68–72] One study actually found them to be superior to hand scaling for cleaning class II and III furcations.[73] It is therefore currently recommended to use a combination of ultrasonic (or sonic) and hand scaling for best results.[21]

Hand scaling

A curette has two cutting edges with a blunted toe and bottom (Figure 10.14).[21,40,56] The blunted bottom will not cut through the delicate periodontal attachment, as long as excess force is not applied.[21] There are two types of standard curette, universal and *Gracey*. Universal curettes usually have a 90-degree angle and are designed to be used throughout the mouth providing that the instrument is adapted to the tooth correctly. *Gracey* curettes are area specific and are designed with different angles to provide superior adaptation to specific areas of the dentition. The proper curette should be selected based on its angulation. Curettes are labelled by numbers that correlate as the lower the number (i.e., 1–2) the smaller the terminal angle of the shank, and the further rostral in the mouth the instrument is used.[21,56] (See chapter 22 for a complete discussion of hand instruments.)

Manual subgingival scaling is a very technically demanding procedure, and although it will be described here, the practitioner is directed to continuing education programs to hone his or her skills.[47] (See appendix 4 for a list of hands-on training labs.) Subgingival scaling is performed as follows.[10,21,38,56] First, place the blade of the instrument on the tooth surface just coronal to the free gingival margin, with the lower shank parallel

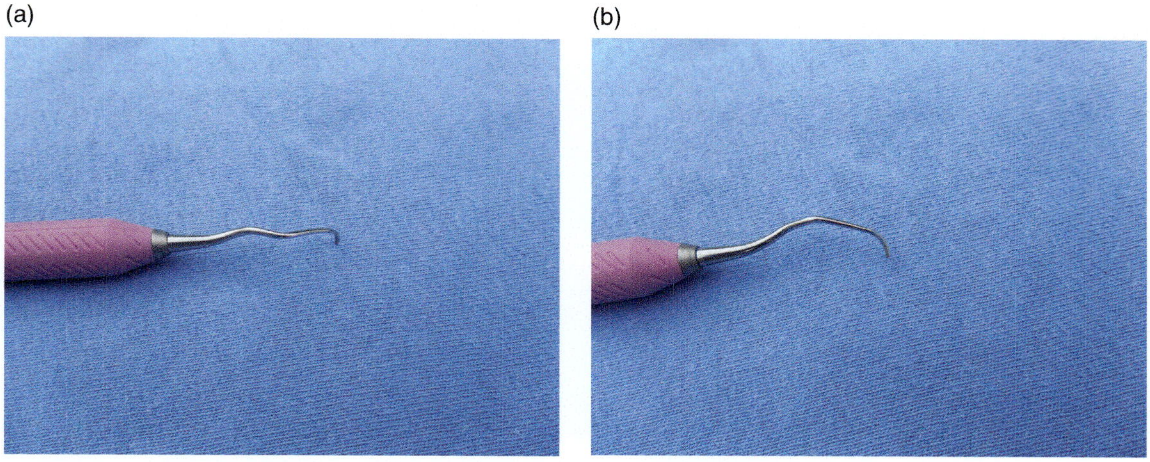

Figure 10.14 (a and b) A dental curette: Note that the back and tip of the instrument are blunted.

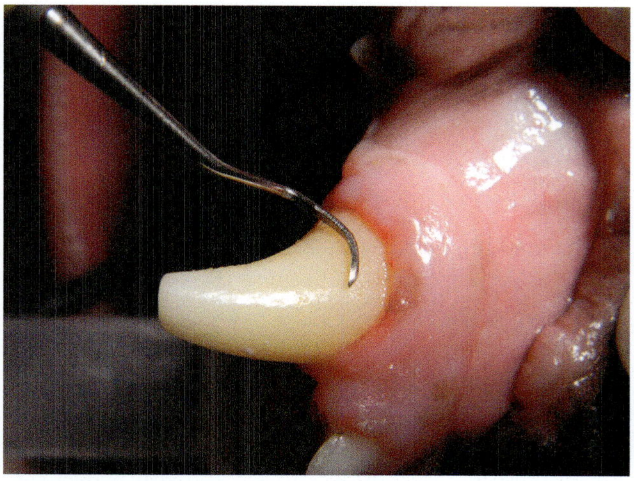

Figure 10.15 Starting position for subgingival scaling. The blade is placed against the tooth surface just coronal to the free gingival margin, with the lower shank parallel to the tooth.

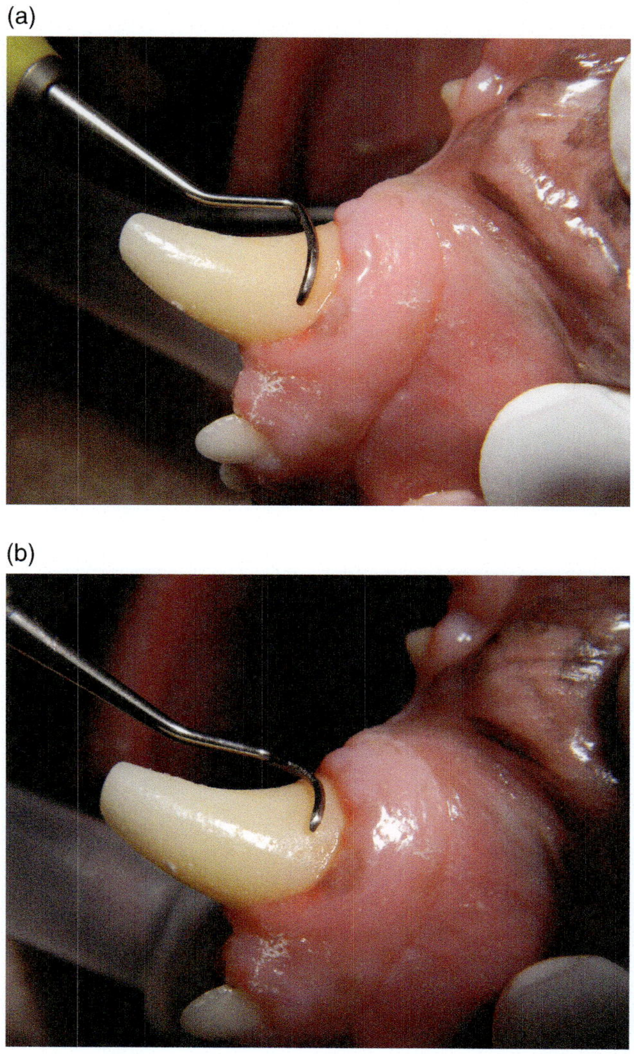

Figure 10.16 (a and b) The curette is rotated so that the flat "face" of the blade is against the tooth surface.

to the tooth surface (Figure 10.15). Next, the curette is rotated so that the flat "face" of the blade is against the tooth surface (Figure 10.16). This is done to minimize the width of the instrument during insertion and to allow the blade to slide under the calculus and engage it. Next, insert the instrument *gently* to the base of the sulcus or pocket (Figure 10.17). Once the bottom of the pocket is reached, the instrument is rotated to create a 90-degree working angulation (Figure 10.18). **When the terminal portion (or shank) is parallel to the tooth, a 90-degree angle is created.** This positioning places the sharp/working edge of the instrument perpendicular to the tooth surface, which is the correct orientation for cleaning. Once properly positioned, *slight* pressure is applied down onto the tooth surface. Finally, the instrument is removed in the coronal direction from within the pocket with a firm/short stroke (Figure 10.19). This

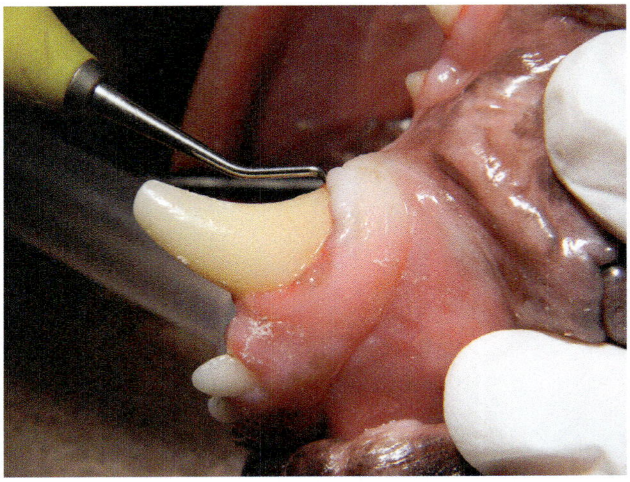

Figure 10.17 The instrument is inserted *gently* to the base of the pocket.

(a)

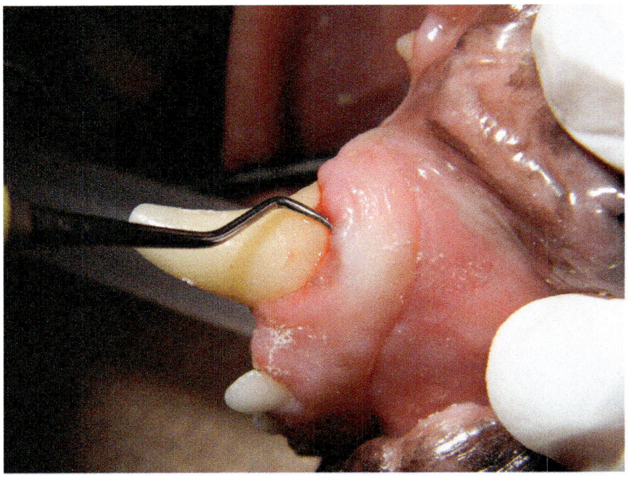

(b)

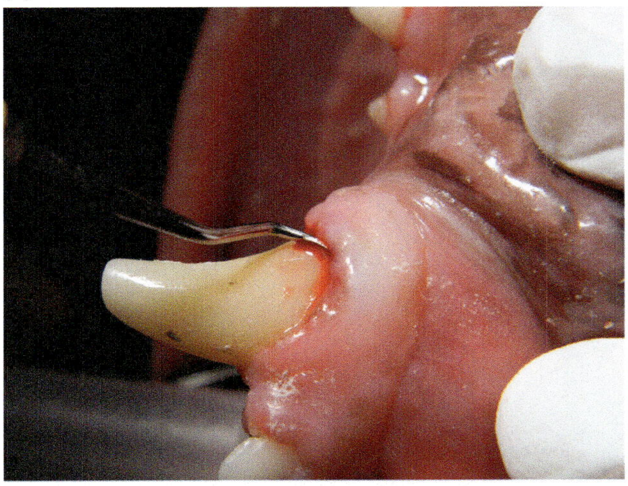

Figure 10.18 (a and b) Once the bottom of the pocket is reached, the instrument is rotated to create a 90-degree working angulation.

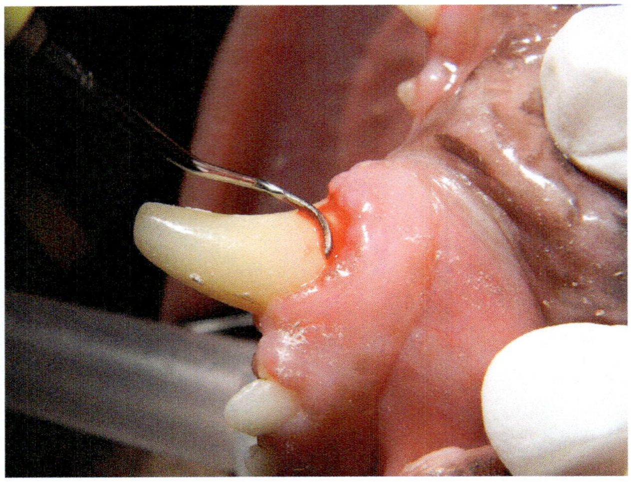

Figure 10.19 The instrument is removed from within the pocket with a firm, short stroke.

technique is repeated with numerous overlapping strokes in different apical to coronal directions until the tooth/root feels smooth.[56]

Mechanical scaling

Traditional ultrasonic scalers (especially magnetostrictive) should not be used subgingivally to avoid damage to the gingiva, periodontal tissues, and pulp.[32] This damage occurs due to excessive power settings as well as too big of a tip for the tight subgingival area. However, the most common damage is thermal, because the water coolant cannot reach the tip of the instrument. Recently, sonic and ultrasonic scalers with specialized periodontal tips have been developed for subgingival use (Figure 10.20).[21] These instruments are much easier to use and thus may provide a superior cleaning in the hands of novices; however, this has not been confirmed by clinical studies.[74,75] In addition, ultrasonic scaling may result in decreased levels of bacteria and endotoxins on the root surface.[76] This owes to the fact that ultrasonic waves produce cavitational activity, acoustic turbulence, and acoustic microstreaming within the coolant spray, resulting in bacterial disruption.[8,32,43,77] These activities may improve plaque reduction and cleanliness of the root surface.[77,78]

To accomplish subgingival scaling, these instruments are used in a similar fashion as supragingival scaling described above, but more care should be taken not to damage the root surface. Again, this technique is performed with a *gentle* touch using numerous overlapping strokes until the root feels smooth (Figure 10.21).[21]

For detailed information on subgingival cleaning (hand and mechanical), please see chapter 11.

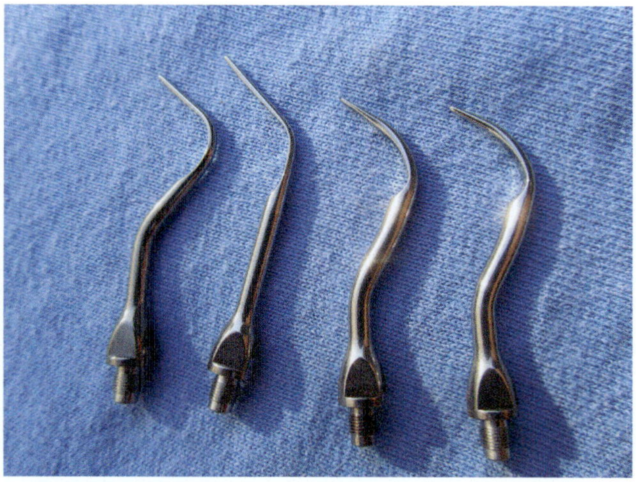

Figure 10.20 Selection of piezoelectric scaler tips. The thinner subgingival tips are pictured on the left, with the thicker supragingival tips on the right.

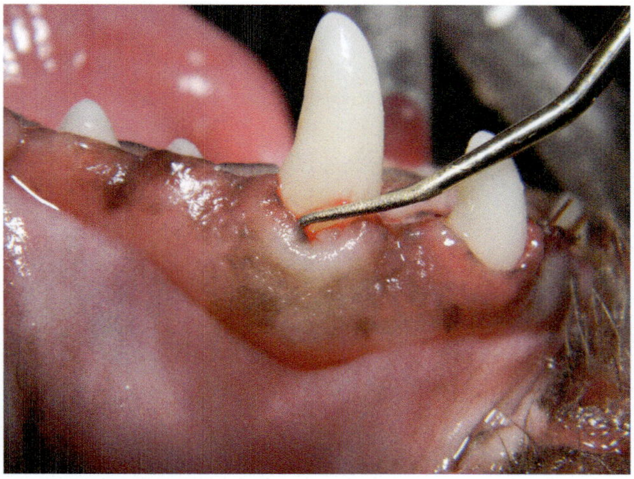

Figure 10.21 Correct use of a fine *subgingival* piezoelectric scaler under the gingival margin.

Step 5: Residual plaque and calculus identification

After scaling, it is recommended to check the teeth with an explorer (Figure 10.22), feeling for any rough areas that indicate small areas of dental pathology (such as diseased cementum or enamel) or residual calculus.[5,21] Residual plaque and calculus may also be identified by utilizing a plaque-disclosing solution[C] (Figure 10.23) or by drying the tooth surfaces with air (residual calculus will appear chalky [Figure 10.24]).[5,8,79]

Step 6: Polishing

Dental scaling (both mechanical and hand) will result in microabrasion and roughening of the tooth surface,[8,38] which will result in increased plaque adherence.[39,80,81]

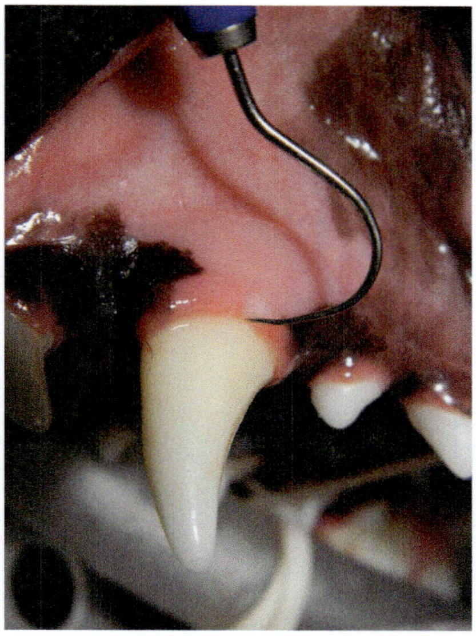

Figure 10.22 Using a dental explorer along the gingival margin to feel for residual calculus.

(a)

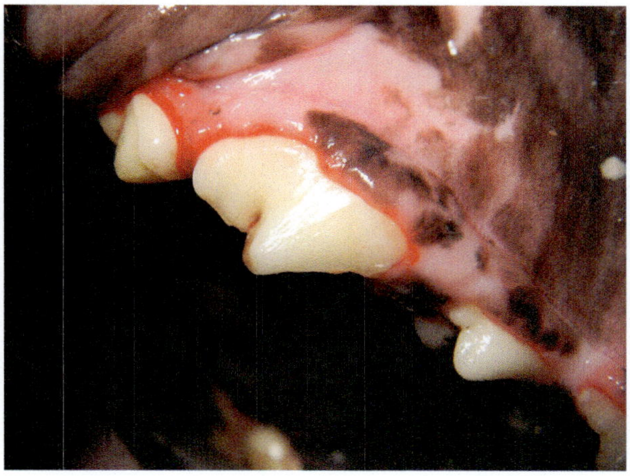

(b)

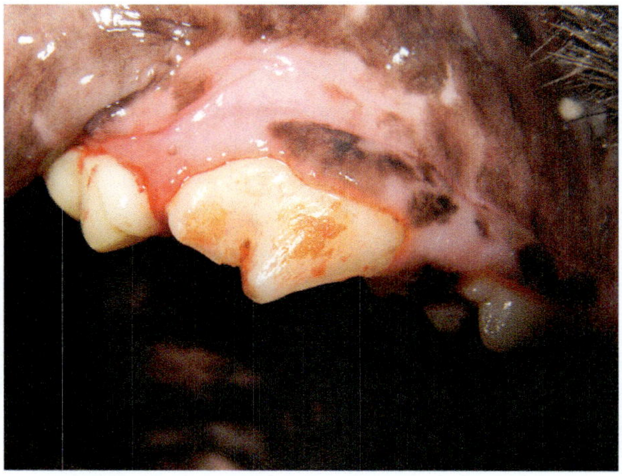

Figure 10.23 Plaque-disclosing solution: (a) Picture of postoperative cleaning that appears to be complete. (b) After the disclosing solution is applied, the significant amount of residual calculus is apparent.

(a) (b)

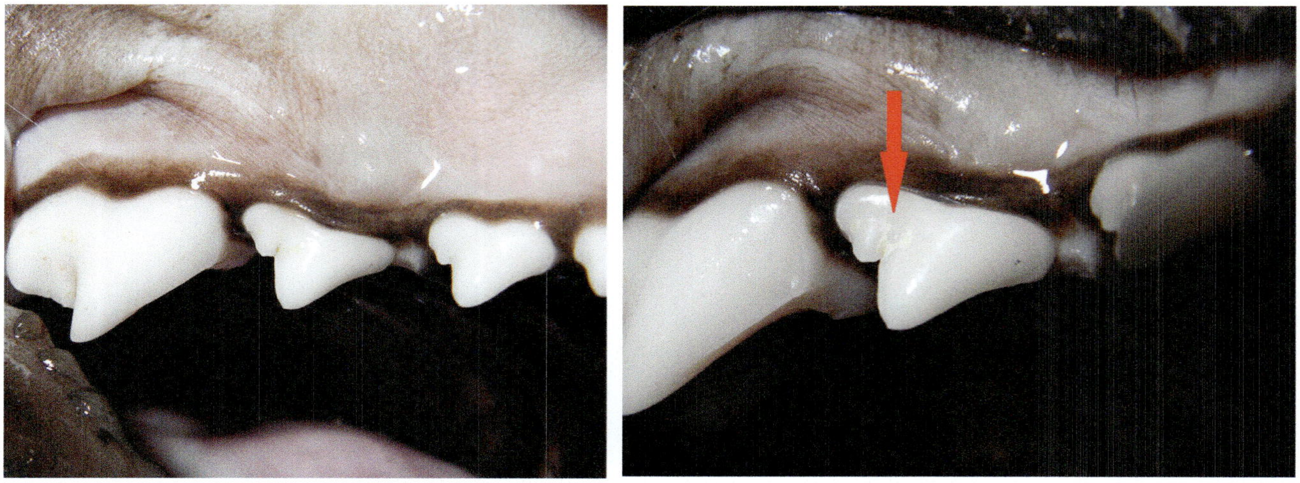

Figure 10.24 Effect of drying: (a) Picture of postoperative cleaning that appears to be complete. (b) However, when the tooth is dried, the residual calculus is evident (red arrow).

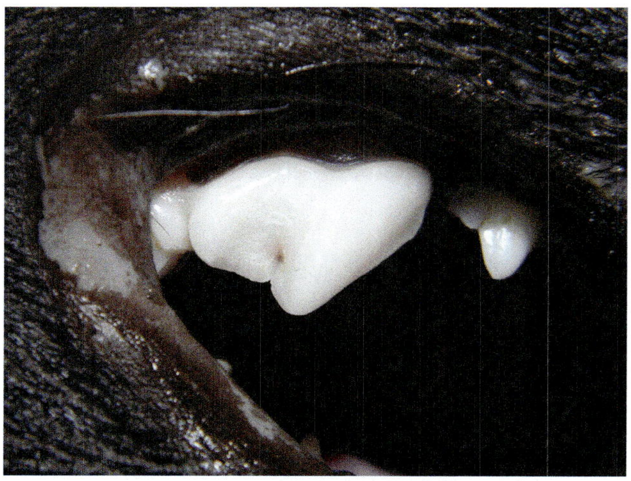

Figure 10.25 Postscaling picture of a maxillary fourth premolar. Notice the significant gouging of the surface. This will lead to a fast recurrence of plaque and calculus. (See chapter 2.)

Polishing smoothes the surface of the teeth, thus retarding plaque attachment.[8] In human dentistry, the polishing step is controversial due to the cumulative loss of enamel throughout the lifetime of the patient and the fact that proper scaling with either hand or ultrasonic instruments has been shown to leave a very smooth surface.[21] However, veterinary dental cleanings are often performed by less experienced operators who may leave the tooth surface (especially the root) rough, leading to increased plaque attachment (Figure 10.25). For this reason, polishing continues to be recommended in veterinary patients.[3,38,51,60]

Practices can choose to use a commercially available polish, or make their own. This author recommends a slurry of flour of pumice and chlorhexidine solution. These can be mixed in a dappen dish for each patient (Figure 10.26a). This not only is less messy than standard prophy paste, it contains an antimicrobial and does not contain other products (e.g., propylene glycol) that may interfere with restorative procedures (if indicated).

The polishing procedure is typically performed with a rubber prophy cup on a slow-speed hand-piece with a 90-degree angle (prophy angle).[21,60,82] The hand-piece should be run at a slow speed, no greater than 3,000 RPM.[38,56] Faster rotation will not improve the speed or quality of the procedure and may result in overheating the tooth. In addition, it is important to use an adequate amount of polish at all times. Running the prophy cup without paste is not only inefficient; it may also overheat the tooth.[21] Therefore we recommend coating the teeth with the polishing substance prior to polishing (Figure 10.26b) and then supplementing the prophy cup as needed. This will also save time, as the technician will not need to return to the polishing supply as often.

As with scaling, every mm^2 of tooth surface should be polished. *Slight* pressure must be placed down onto the tooth to flare the edges of the prophy cup so as to polish the subgingival areas (Figure 10.27). One tooth may be polished for a maximum of 5 seconds at a time, to avoid overheating.[1,38,39] The tooth can be further polished after a short break (during which other teeth are polished).

Step 7: Sulcal lavage

During the cleaning and polishing steps, debris such as calculus and prophy paste (some of which is bacteria laden) accumulates in the gingival sulcus (or periodontal pockets).[38,56] In some cases there are visible deposits, but in *all* cases there is microscopic debris. The presence of these substances allows for continued infection and inflammation, and therefore a gentle lavage of the sulcus

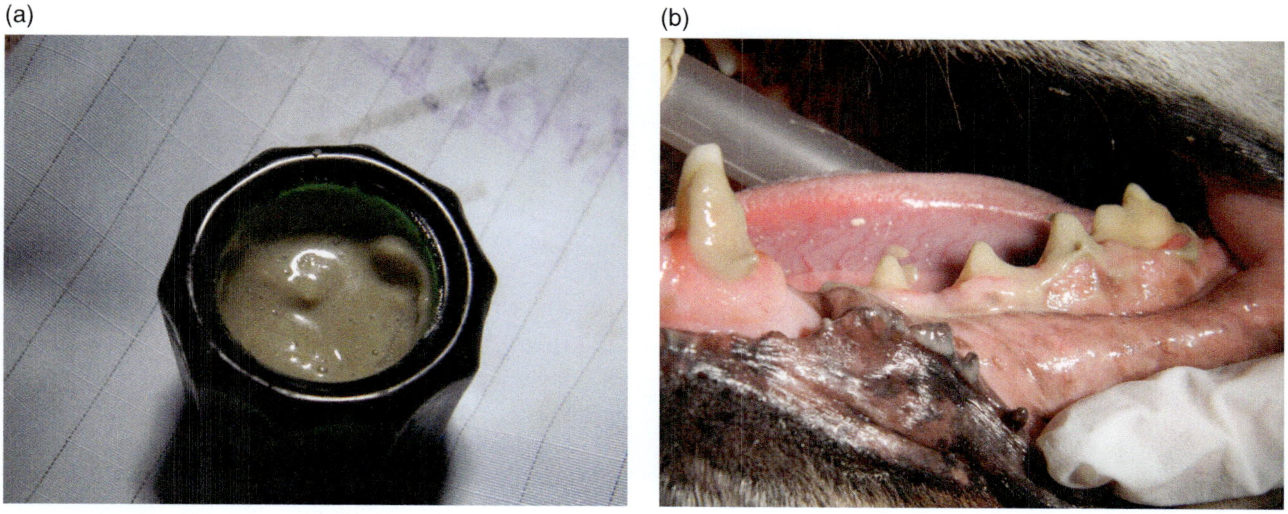

Figure 10.26 Prophy paste: (a) Properly mixed polishing paste. (b) Pumice applied to the teeth prior to polishing. This will decrease the polishing time and lessen the chances of overheating the tooth.

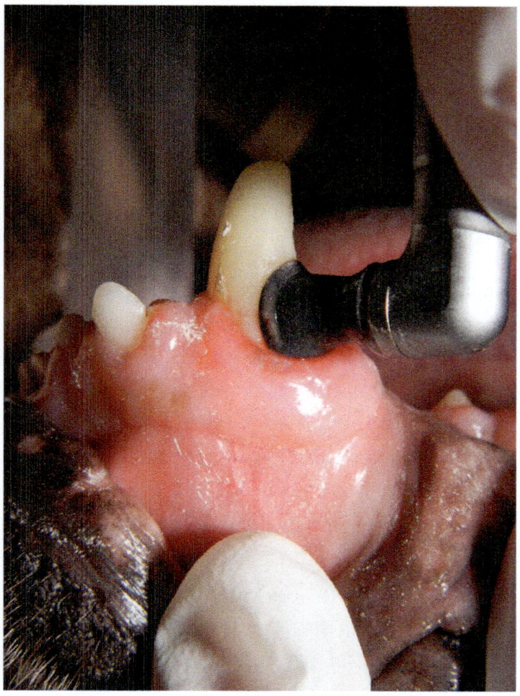

Figure 10.27 Prophy cup applied to the tooth. Pressure is applied against the tooth to flare out the cup and get it under the gingival margin.

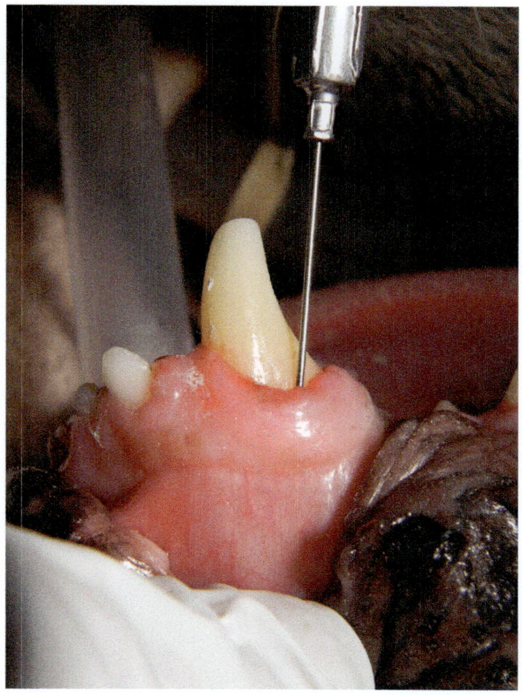

Figure 10.28 Sulcal lavage. The sulcus is gently rinsed utilizing a 22-gauge blunt-ended cannula.

is strongly recommended to improve healing.[5,38,56] Sulcal lavage is performed with a small (22–25) gauge blunt-ended cannula. The cannula is placed gently into the sulcus and the solution injected while slowly moving along the arcades (Figure 10.28).

Sterile saline can be used as a lavage solution, but most dentists favor a 0.12% chlorhexidine solution.[8,38,83,D] The use of chlorhexidine was refuted by some veterinary dentists due to the cytotoxic effects on periodontal ligament cells in vitro.[84] However, recent studies have proven that chlorhexidine does not delay wound healing and may even speed recovery and decrease pain.[83,85,86] Finally, there is evidence that postoperative chlorhexidine may actually improve healing and alveolar bone height.[87]

Step 8: Fluoride therapy (Optional)

This is a controversial step, with some dentists recommending that it be performed in all cases, and some dentists recommending that it never be done.[5,8] The positive

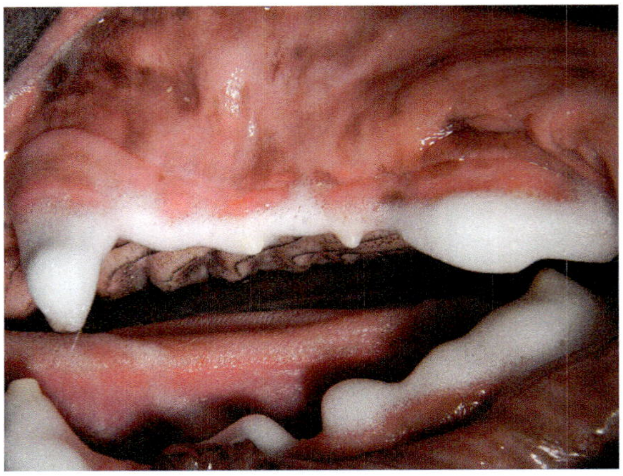

Figure 10.29 Fluoride application.

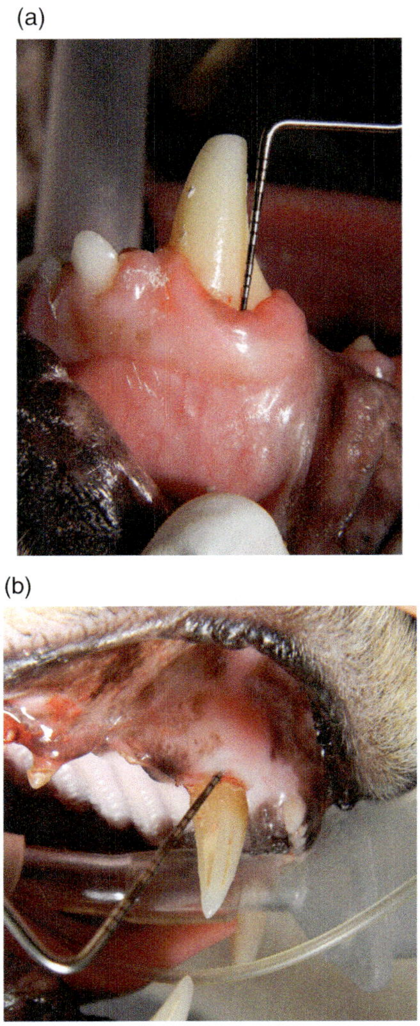

Figure 10.30 Periodontal probing (a) in a dog and (b) in a cat.

aspects of fluoride include antiplaque and antibacterial activities, hardening tooth structure, and decreasing tooth sensitivity.[1,5,8,38,88] Minimizing tooth sensitivity is most important in patients with gingival recession and secondary root exposure. When root planing is performed, cementum is removed, which may expose underlying dentin.[89] This leads to sensitivity of the teeth, which is worst in the cervical area.[89,90] Human literature reports that approximately 50% of patients experience sensitivity following subgingival scaling and root planing.[91] The application of fluoride should help decrease this sensitivity.[8,89]

Fluoride preparations are placed on the teeth and allowed to sit for the manufacturer's recommended contact time (3 minutes for foam and 10 minutes for gel) (Figure 10.29). After the appropriate contact time, the fluoride should be removed either by wiping or blowing it off with compressed air.[8] Fluoride should not be rinsed away with water, as rinsing will decrease its efficacy.[8,89]

Additional methods of managing tooth sensitivity include dentin bonding agents or the use of lasers.[89,92] Discussion of these techniques is beyond the scope of this book and should only be practiced after advanced training.

Step 9: Periodontal probing, oral evaluation, and dental charting

This is a *critically* important step of a complete dental prophylaxis but is unfortunately often poorly performed or completely omitted.[5,8] The *entire* oral cavity must be systematically evaluated using both visual and tactile senses. Careful visual examination should be performed along with the periodontal evaluation. Salient findings include (but are not limited to) fractured, mobile, or intrinsically stained teeth; foreign bodies; tooth defects such are caries or tooth resorption; and oral masses. This author recommends that the patient be placed in dorsal recumbency for this step, as it will improve visualization.[6]

The periodontal evaluation should begin with determining the plaque, calculus, and gingivitis indices (see chapter 4 and appendix 5 for a description of these indices). These key pieces of information are frequently noted prior to the dental cleaning. Following this, the periodontal status is measured. The only accurate method for detecting and measuring periodontal pockets is with a periodontal probe, as pockets are not always diagnosed by radiographs.[82,93,94]

The periodontal evaluation should be initiated at the first incisor of one of the quadrants. The measurements are then continued distally one tooth at a time. Starting at midline and moving systematically distal in this fashion will decrease the chance of a tooth being skipped. Periodontal probing is performed by gently inserting the probe into the pocket until it stops and then slowly "walking" the instrument around the tooth (Figure 10.30).[8,56,93] Depth measurements should be taken at six spots around *every* tooth.[4,5,56,93] The normal sulcal depth in dogs is 0–3 mm, and in cats is 0–0.5 mm.[8,51,79,82] This author considers normal sulcal depth in toy breed dogs to be less than or equal to 2 mm (see Box 10.4).

All abnormal findings (visual as well as periodontal probing depths) must be recorded on the dental chart. Dental charting is easier and more efficient if performed four-handed.[6,19] This means that one person evaluates the mouth and calls out the findings of pathology to the assistant, who records it on the chart. Using the modified Triadan system will also greatly increase efficiency of this step.

The modified Triadan system uses numbers to identify the teeth.[6,56,95] First, each quadrant is numbered starting with the maxillary right quadrant as the 100 series. This progresses clockwise so that the maxillary left is 200, mandibular left is 300, and the mandibular right is the 400 series. Next, starting at the rostral midline, the teeth are counted distally starting with the first incisor, which is tooth 01. The canines are always number 04 and the first molars are 09. For example, the left maxillary fourth premolar is tooth 208. This has been extrapolated from the fact that the complete dentition of the ancestral carnivore has been determined by anatomists to consist of each quadrant containing 3 incisors, 1 canine tooth, 4 premolars, and 3 molars. (See appendix 2.)

Box 10.4 Probing

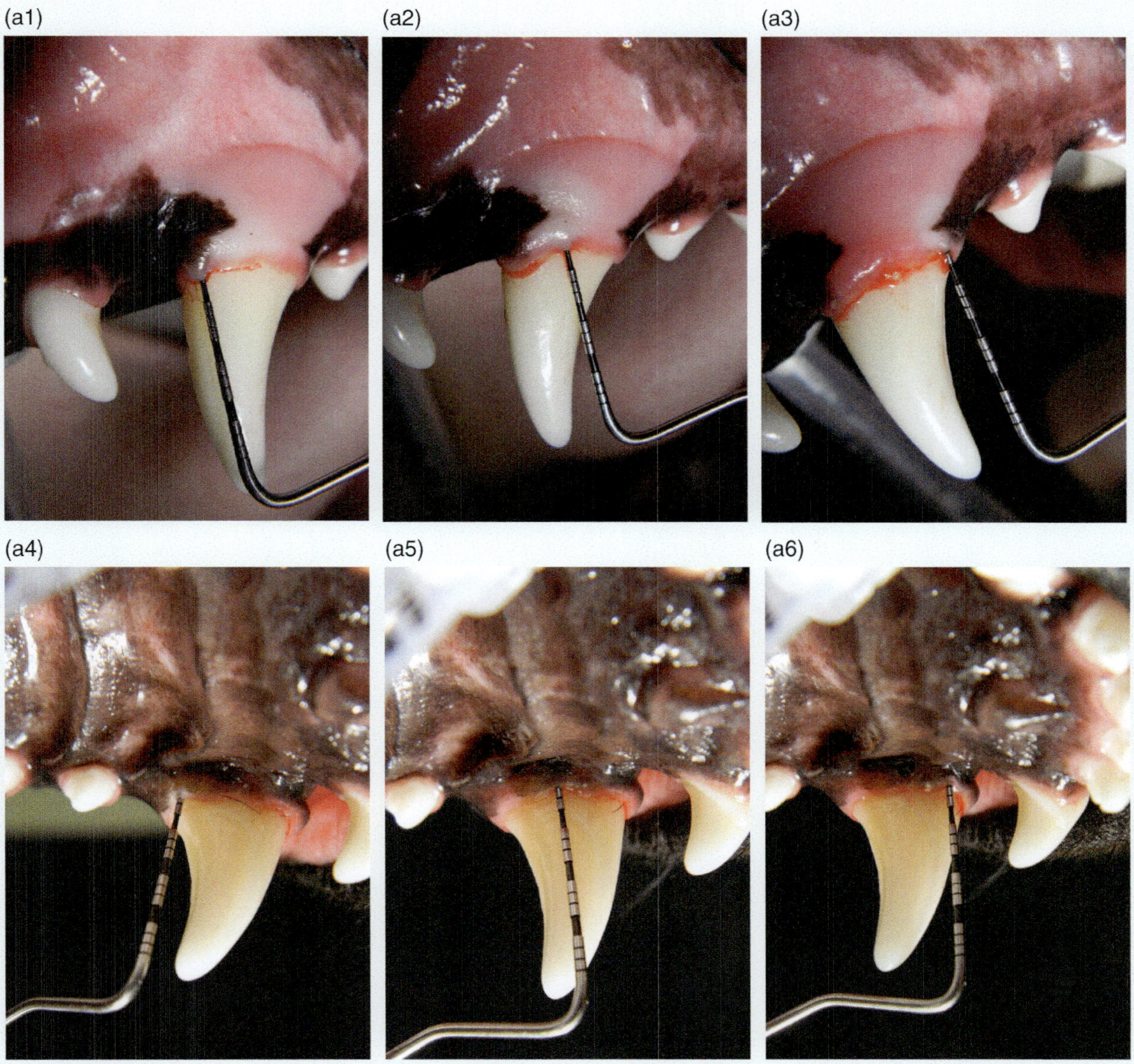

Figure 10.a Periodontal probing at six locations on the left maxillary canine of a dog—(1) mesio-buccal, (2) buccal, (3) disto-buccal, (4) disto-palatal, (5) palatal, and (6) mesio-palatal.

(b1) (b2)

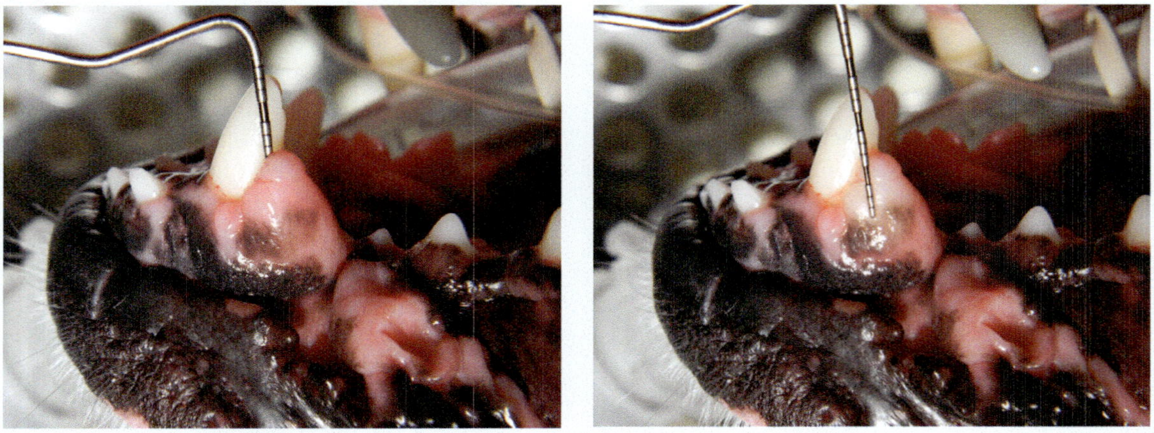

Figure 10.b Probing a patient with gingival enlargement. The attachment loss is the probing depth *minus* the gingival enlargement. The periodontal probe measures a 6–7 mm pocket on the buccal aspect of the left mandibular canine (304). Although this is a significant depth, when measured from the normal gingival margin, the area of enlargement is also 6–7 mm. This means that there is actually no attachment loss.

(c1) (c2)

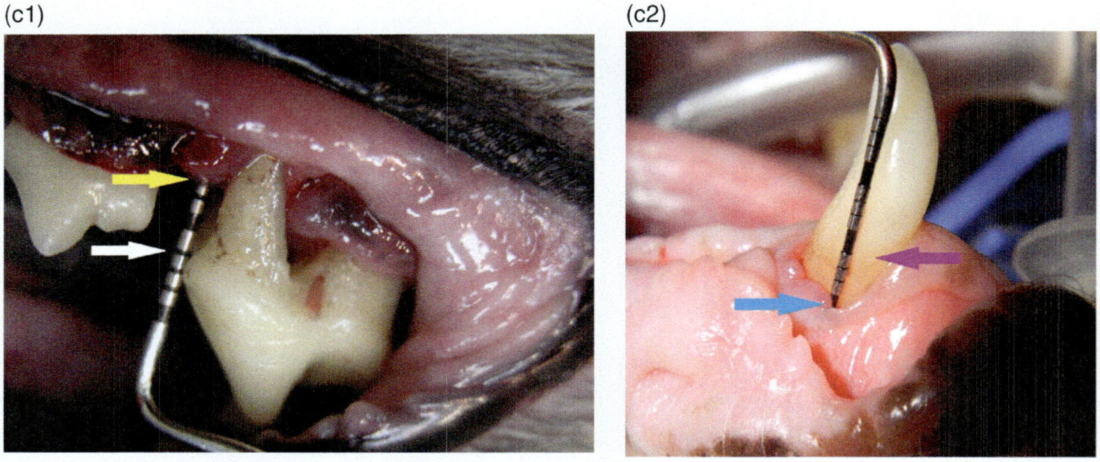

Figure 10.c Probing a patient with gingival recession. The attachment loss is the probing depth *plus* the gingival recession. (1) The periodontal probe measures a 6 mm pocket on the mesial aspect of the left maxillary fourth premolar (208) (yellow arrow). Although this is just a moderate depth, when measured from the cementoenamel junction (white arrow), the attachment loss is 11 mm, which is very significant. (2) Similarly, there is a mild 5.5 mm periodontal pocket on the buccal aspect of the right mandibular canine (404) (blue arrow), but with 3.5 mm of gingival recession from the CEJ (purple arrow), this means 9 mm of attachment loss, which is very significant.

(d1) (d2) (d3)

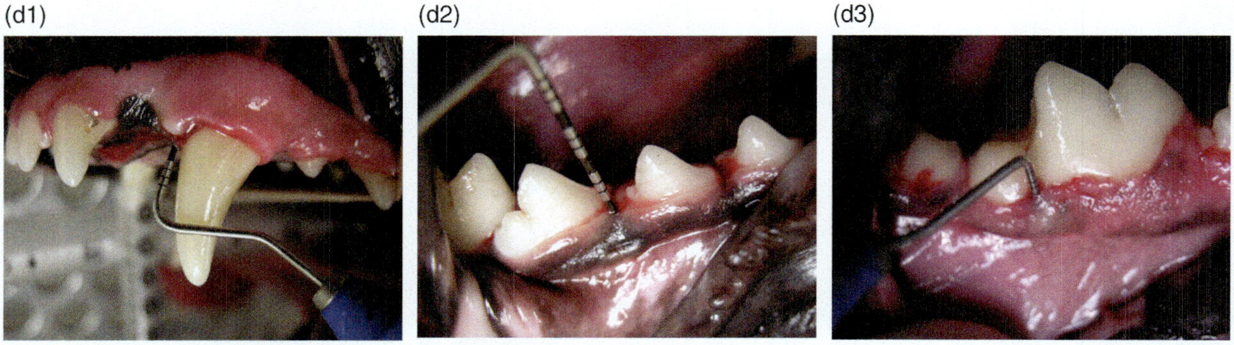

Figure 10.d The outward appearance of the gingiva is not reliable to determine if disease is present. All teeth must be probed regardless of outward appearance. Following are some examples of cases with significant attachment loss with no outward signs of disease (i.e., no to minimal gingivitis). (1) Left maxillary canine (204) in a dog with a 9 mm pocket. (2) Right mandibular third and fourth premolar in a dog with a 4 mm pocket. (3) Right mandibular first molar in a dog with a 13 mm periodontal pocket and normal appearing gingiva.

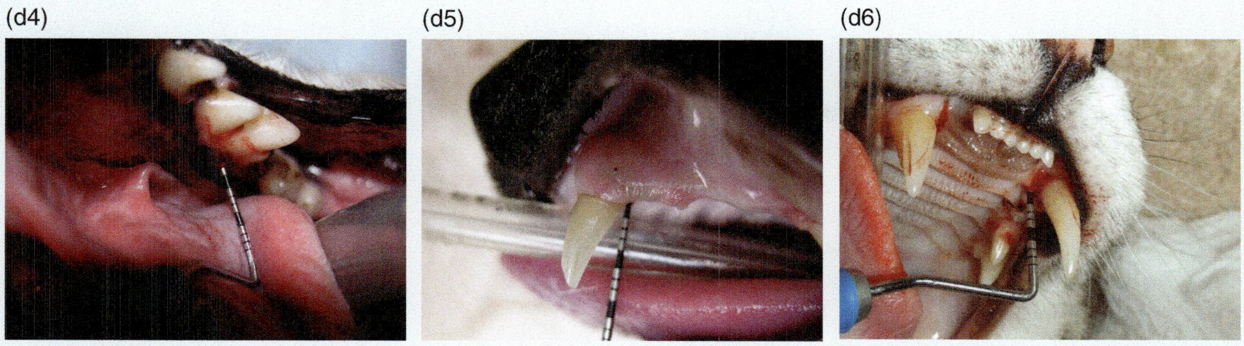

Figure 10.d (cont'd) (4) Lingual surface of the right mandibular first molar (409) in a dog with a class II furcation. (5) Distal surface of the left maxillary canine (204) of a cat with a 4 mm pocket. (6) Palatal surface of the left maxillary canine (204) of a cat with a 4 mm pocket.

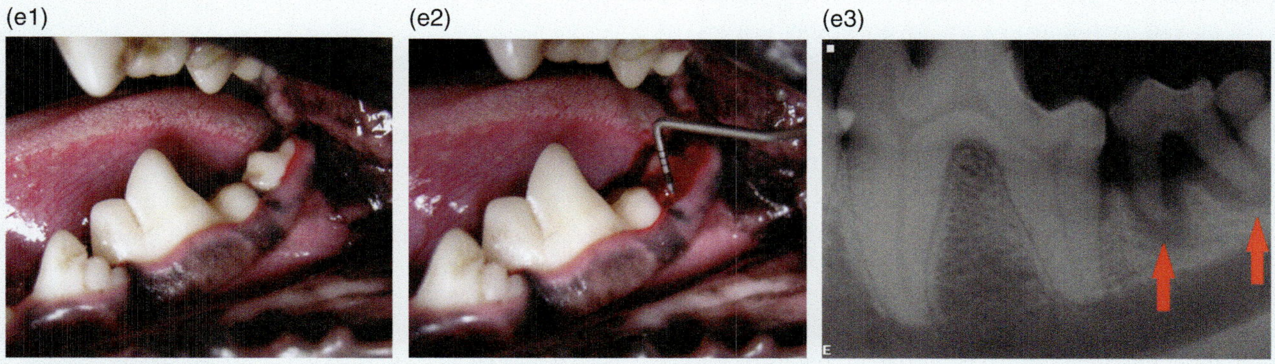

Figure 10.e Example of a patient with a severely infected left mandibular second molar (310). This patient had recently been treated for halitosis via a "dental" at a general practice. There was no dental charting performed. (1) The patient outwardly had clean teeth and minimal evidence of disease. (2) However, when probed, there was a deep and significantly infected pocket between the first and second molars. (3) Dental radiographs revealed the severe bone loss as well as the periapical rarefaction around 310 (red arrows), confirming the locus of infection. In this case, periodontal probing would have elucidated the infection and allowed for proper therapy much earlier.

It is important that dental charts be of sufficient size to allow for accurate placement of pathology. This is especially true when practitioners are performing quality periodontal evaluations. There must be incisal as well as lateral views of the teeth for accurate recording of pathology. Furthermore, the incisal view must have enough space to accommodate the six measurements. The minimum size for an acceptable dental chart is half of a page; however, most veterinary dentists utilize full-page charts (See appendix 2.) Sample charts are available for free download at www.vetdentalrad.com.

Step 10: Dental radiographs

Dental radiographs should be taken at a minimum of every area of pathology noted on dental exam. This includes any periodontal pocket that is larger than normal, fractured or chipped teeth, masses, swellings, or missing teeth. In addition, numerous studies support full mouth radiographs on all dental patients to further eliminate missed pathology.[96–98]

Dental radiographs are a critical aid in the evaluation of dental pathology; however, they are NOT a substitute for the clinical exam, for several reasons.[94,99] First, a change in the radiographic exposure (especially vertical angulation) can greatly affect the apparent level of bone.[82,94] Next, it is well known that the earliest stages of bone loss will not be seen radiographically.[100–102] Finally, periodontal bone loss does not become radiographically evident until 30–50% of the mineralization is lost.[99,103] Therefore, radiographic findings will always *underestimate* bone loss.[82,104] This can be somewhat (but not completely) ameliorated by taking occlusal as well as standard lateral views.[105] Help with radiographic interpretation is available for any questionable cases via telemedicine review at www.vetdentalrad.com. (See chapter 9 for a complete discussion of periodontal dental radiology.)

Step 11: Treatment planning

In this step, the practitioner uses all available information (visual, tactile, and radiographic findings) to determine appropriate therapy. It is important to consider overall patient health, *the owner's interest and willingness to perform homecare,* and all necessary follow-up.[56] After forming an appropriate dental treatment plan for the patient, the estimate should be revised and the client contacted for consent. There are numerous therapeutic possibilities (including referral) depending on the type of pathology. The reader is directed to the following chapters for more advanced periodontal therapies. In addition, the pursuit of advanced training in other areas of veterinary dentistry (endodontic, exodontic, and restorative) is strongly recommended. This type of training can be found in texts or preferably learned in hands-on labs.

It is very important to note that if a patient requires extensive treatment that would entail a lengthy anesthesia, or if the practitioner would be unduly rushed, rescheduling the remainder of the dental work is definitely an acceptable alternative. The two parameters that directly affect long-term morbidity and mortality in anesthetized patients are hypothermia and hypotension,[106,107] which become more pronounced with extended anesthesia time. Hypothermia is especially a concern in smaller patients.[108] In fact, anesthetic length has been shown to increase the complication rate in both humans and animals.[107,109] However, if the patient is stable and all parameters (especially blood pressure and temperature) are within normal physiologic parameters, there is no universally recommended predetermined cutoff for anesthesia. (See chapter 21 for a thorough discussion of anesthesia.)

Step 12 (Optional): Application of a barrier sealant

The barrier sealant[E] is a waxy substance that is clinically proven to decrease plaque and calculus.[110] This author has seen positive effects in clinical practice; however, some veterinary dentists dispute the efficacy of the product.[111] Although it has yet not been proven to decrease gingivitis and subsequent periodontal disease, due to its placement at and below the gingival margin, it should theoretically work. Following a prophylaxis, the teeth are dried and the product is then applied according to the manufacturer's directions (Figure 10.31). Continued applications are performed by the client at home on a weekly basis.

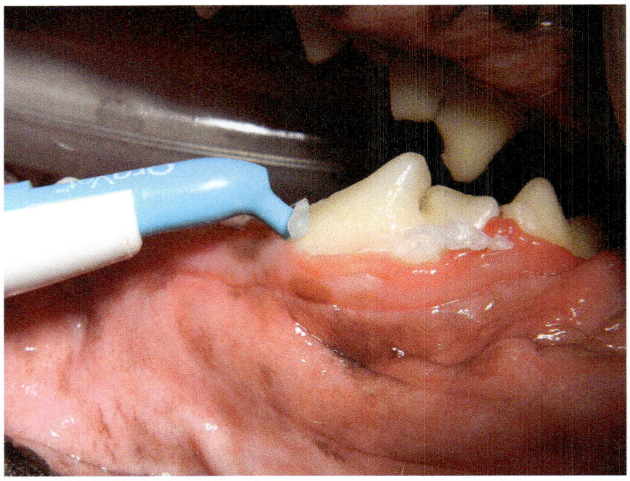

Figure 10.31 Application of the barrier sealant.

Step 13: Client education

The postsurgical discharge appointment is an important step in periodontal therapy.[8,10] It provides an opportunity to review radiographs (and clinical photographs if available) with the client. This meeting with the client should also be used to reinforce clinical findings, discuss the performed treatments, and finally to discuss periodontal disease in general. It is important to cover both immediate postoperative instructions and long-term periodontal care, including homecare to be provided by the client. It is important to note that long-term success of periodontal treatment frequently hinges on the client's commitment to providing homecare. In fact, professional therapy has been shown to be of little value without homecare.[112]

Box 10.5 Key points

- A complete dental prophylaxis is an involved procedure with numerous steps.
- All dental prophylactic procedures must be performed under general anesthesia.
- Each step must be properly performed to achieve a positive outcome.
- Sufficient time must be allotted for the procedure to have significant clinical benefit.
- *Sub*gingival scaling is the most important step of a prophylaxis.
- A complete oral exam and charting is a critical part of the procedure.
- Hands-on laboratories will improve the efficiency and quality of cleanings.

Notes

A. OraStrip, PDx BioTech.
B. CET Oral Hygiene Rinse, Virbac Animal Health.
C. Reveal, Butler Schein.
D. CET Oral Hygiene Rinse, Virbac Animal Health.
E. Oravet, Merial Limited.

Suggested reading

Huffman LJ. Oral examination. In: Small Animal Dental, Oral and Maxillofacial Disease, a Color Handbook (Niemiec BA ed.). London: Manson, 2010, pp. 39–61.

Holmstrom SE, Frost P, Eisner ER. Dental prophylaxis. In: Veterinary Dental Techniques for the Small Animal Practitioner. 2nd ed. Philadelphia: Saunders, 1998, pp. 133–166.

References

1. Bellows J. Treatment of periodontal disease. In: Feline Dentistry: Oral Assessment, Treatment, and Preventative Care. Ames, IA: Wiley-Blackwell, 2010, pp. 181–195.
2. Colmery B. The gold standard of veterinary oral health care. Vet Clin North Am. 35(4):781–787, 2005.
3. Niemiec BA. Professional teeth cleaning. J Vet Dent. 20(3): 175–180, 2003.
4. Bellows J. Equipping the dental practice. In: Small Animal Dental Equipment, Materials, and Techniques, a Primer. Ames, IA: Blackwell, 2004, pp. 13–55.
5. Holmstrom SE, Frost P, Eisner ER. Dental prophylaxis and periodontal disease stages. In: Veterinary Dental Techniques, for the Small Animal Practitioner. 3rd ed. Philadelphia: Saunders, 2004, pp. 175–232.
6. Huffman LJ. Oral examination. In: Small Animal Dental, Oral and Maxillofacial Disease, a Color Handbook (Niemiec BA ed.). London: Manson, 2010, pp. 39–61.
7. Colmery B. The gold standard of veterinary oral health care. Vet Clin North Am Small Anim Pract. 35(4):781–787, 2005.
8. Bellows J. Periodontal equipment, materials, and techniques. In: Small Animal Dental Equipment, Materials, and Techniques, a Primer. Ames, IA: Blackwell, 2004, pp. 115–173.
9. Wiggs RB, Lobprise HB. Periodontology. In: Veterinary Dentistry, Principles and Practice. Philadelphia: Lippincott-Raven, 1997, pp. 186–231.
10. Holmstrom SE, Frost P, Eisner ER. Periodontal therapy and surgery. In: Veterinary Dental Techniques for the Small Animal Practitioner. 2nd ed. Philadelphia: Saunders, 1998, pp. 167–213.
11. Joubert KE. Pre-anesthetic screening of geriatric dogs. J S Afr Vet Assoc. 78(1):31–35, 2007.
12. Holmstrom SE, Frost P, Eisner ER. Ergonomics and general health safety in the dental workplace. In: Veterinary Dental Techniques for the Small Animal Practitioner. 2nd ed. Philadelphia: Saunders, 1998, pp. 497–506.
13. Szymanska J. Dental bioaerosol as an occupational hazard in a dentist's workplace. Ann Agric Environ Med. 14(2):203–207, 2007.
14. Harrel SK. Airborne spread of disease—the implications for dentistry. J Calif Dent Assoc. 32(11):901–906, 2004.
15. Pederson ED, Stone ME, Ragain JC Jr, Simecek JW. Waterline biofilm and the dental treatment facility: A review. Gen Dent. 50(2):190–195, 2002.
16. Shearer BJ. Biofilm and the dental office. J Am Dent Assoc. 127:181–189, 1996.
17. Meiller TF, Depaola LG, Kelley JI, Baqui AA, Turng BF, Falkler WA. Dental unit waterlines: Biofilms, disinfection and recurrence. J Am Dent Assoc. 130(1):65–72, 1999.
18. Wirthlin MR, Marshall GW Jr, Rowland RW. Formation and decontamination of biofilms in dental unit waterlines. J Periodontol. 74(11):1595–1609, 2003.
19. Bellows J. The dental operatory. In: Small Animal Dental Equipment, Materials, and Techniques, a Primer. Ames, IA: Blackwell, 2004, pp. 3–12.
20. Huntley DE, Campbell J. Bacterial contamination of scrub jackets during dental hygiene procedures. J Dent Hyg. 72(3):19–23, 1998.
21. Pattison AM, Pattison GL. Scaling and root planing. In: Carranza's Clinical Periodontology. St. Louis: Saunders, 2006, pp. 749–797.
22. Harrel SK, Barnes JB, Rivera-Hildalgo F. Aerosol and splatter contamination from the operative site during ultrasonic scaling. J Am Dent Assoc. 129:1241, 1998.
23. Legnani P, Checchi L, Pelliccioni GA, D'Achille C. Atmospheric contamination during dental procedures. Quintessence Int. 25(6):435–439, 1994.
24. Osorio R, Toledano M, Liébana J, Rosales JI, Lozano JA. Environmental microbial contamination. Pilot study in a dental surgery. Int Dent J. 45(6):352–357, 1995.
25. Leggat PA, Kedjarune U. Bacterial aerosols in the dental clinic: A review. Int Dent J. 51(1):39–44, 2001.
26. Al Maghlouth A, Al Yousef Y, Al-Bagieh NH. Qualitative and quantitative analysis of microbial aerosols in selected areas within the College of Dentistry, King Saud University. Quintessence Int. 38(5):e222–228, 2007.
27. Lafaurie GI, Mayorga-Fayad I, Torres MF, Castillo DM, Aya MR, Barón A, Hurtado PA. Periodontopathic microorganisms in peripheric blood after scaling and root planing. J Clin Periodontol. 34(10):873–879, 2007.
28. Forner L, Larsen T, Kilian M, Holmstrup P. Incidence of bacteremia after chewing, tooth brushing and scaling in individuals with periodontal inflammation. J Clin Periodontol. 33(6):401–407, 2006.
29. Daly CG, Mitchell DH, Highfield JE, Grossberg DE, Stewart D. Bacteremia due to periodontal probing: A clinical and microbiological investigation. J Periodontol. 72(2):210–214, 2001.
30. Okuda M, Kaneko Y, Ichinohe T, Ishihara K, Okuda K. Reduction of potential respiratory pathogens by oral hygienic treatment in patients undergoing endotracheal anesthesia. J Anesth. 17(2): 84–91, 2003.
31. Fine DH, Yip J, Furgang D, Barnett ML, Olshan AM, Vincent J. Reducing bacteria in dental aerosols: Pre-procedural use of an antiseptic mouthrinse. J Am Dent Assoc. 124(5):56–58, 1993.
32. Jahn CA. Sonic and ultrasonic instrumentation. In: Carranza's Clinical Periodontology. St. Louis: Saunders, 2006, pp. 828–835.
33. Harrel SK, Molinari J. Aerosols and splatter in dentistry: A brief review of the literature and infection control implications. J Am Dent Assoc. 135(4):429–437, 2004.
34. Day CJ, Sandy JR, Ireland AJ. Aerosols and splatter in dentistry—a neglected menace? Dent Update 33(10):601–602, 604–606, 2006.
35. Tomas I, Alvarez M, Limeres J, Tomas M, Medina J, Otero JL, Diz P. Effect of chlorhexidine mouthwash on the risk of post-extraction bacteremia. Infect Control Hosp Epidemiol. 28(5):577–582, 2007.
36. Limeback H. Implications of oral infections on systemic diseases in the institutionalized elderly with a special focus on pneumonia. Ann Periodontol. 3(1):262–275, 1998.
37. Fine DH, Mendieta C, Barnett ML, Furgang D, Meyers R, Olshan A, Vincent J. Efficacy of preprocedural rinsing with an antiseptic in reducing viable bacteria in dental aerosols. J Periodontol. 63(10):821–824, 1992.
38. Wiggs RB, Lobprise HB. Periodontology. In: Veterinary Dentistry, Principles and Practice. Philadelphia: Lippincott-Raven, 1997, pp. 186–231.
39. Holmstrom SE, Frost P, Eisner ER. Dental prophylaxis. In: Veterinary Dental Techniques for the Small Animal Practitioner. 2nd ed. Philadelphia: Saunders, 1998, pp. 133–166.
40. Wiggs RB, Lobprise HB. Dental equipment. Wiggs RB, Lobprise HB. Periodontology. In: Veterinary Dentistry, Principles and Practice. Philadelphia: Lippincott-Raven, 1997, pp. 1–28.

41. Lea SC, Felver B, Landini G, Walmsley AD. Three-dimensional analyses of ultrasonic scaler oscillations. J Clin Periodontol. 36(1):44–50, 2009.
42. Felver B, King DC, Lea SC, Price GJ, Damien Walmsley A. Cavitation occurrence around ultrasonic dental scalers. Ultrason Sonochem. 16(5):692–697, 2009.
43. Arabaci T, Ciçek Y, Canakçi CF. Sonic and ultrasonic scalers in periodontal treatment: A review. Intl J Dent Hyg. 5(1):2–12, 2007.
44. Loose B, Kiger R. An evaluation of basic periodontal therapy using sonic and ultrasonic scalers. J Clin Periodontol Res. 14:29–33, 1987.
45. Lie T, Leknes KN. Evaluation of the effect on root surfaces of air turbine scalers and ultrasonic instrumentation. J Periodontol. 56(9):522–531, 1985.
46. Clinical Research Associates. Sonic and ultrasonic scalers. Provo, UT. 6:1, 1982.
47. Holmstrom SE, Frost P, Eisner ER. Dental equipment and care. In: Veterinary Dental Techniques for the Small Animal Practitioner. 3rd ed. Philadelphia: Saunders, 2004, pp. 31–106.
48. Hermann JS, Rieder C, Rateitschak KH, Hefti AF. Sonic and ultrasonic scalers in a clinical comparison. A study in non-instructed patients with gingivitis or slight adult periodontitis. Schweiz Monatsschr Zahnmed. 105(2):165–170, 1995.
49. Derdilopoulou FV, Nonhoff J, Neumann K, Kielbassa AM. Microbiological findings after periodontal therapy using curettes, Er:YAG laser, sonic, and ultrasonic scalers. J Clin Periodontol. 34(7):588–598, 2007.
50. Jacobson L, Blomlö J, Lindskog S. Root surface texture after different scaling modalities. Scand J Dent Res. 102(3):156–160, 1994.
51. Debowes LJ. Problems with the gingiva. In: Small Animal Dental, Oral and Maxillofacial Disease, a Color Handbook (Niemiec BA ed.). London: Manson, 2010, pp. 159–181.
52. Nicoll BK, Peters RJ. Heat generation during ultrasonic instrumentation of dentin as affected by different irrigation methods. J Periodontol. 69(8):884–888, 1998.
53. Trenter SC, Landini G, Walmsley AD. Effect of loading on the vibration characteristics of thin magnetostrictive ultrasonic scaler inserts. J Periodontol. 74(9):1308–1315, 2003.
54. Brine EJ, Marretta SM, Pijanowski GJ, Siegel AM. Comparison of the effects of four different power scalers on enamel tooth surface in the dog. J Vet Dent. 17(1):17–21, 2000.
55. Vérez-Fraguela JL, Vives Vallés MA, Ezquerra Calvo LJ. Effects of ultrasonic dental scaling on pulp vitality in dogs: An experimental study. J Vet Dent. 17(2):75–79, 2000.
56. Niemiec BA. Periodontal therapy. Top Companion Anim Med. 23(2):81–90, 2008.
57. Lea SC, Landini G, Walmsley AD. The effect of wear on ultrasonic scaler tip displacement amplitude. J Clin Periodontol. 33(1): 37–41, 2006.
58. Bellows J. Small Animal Dental Equipment, Materials, and Techniques, a Primer. Ames, IA: Blackwell, 2004.
59. Holmstrom SE, Frost P, Eisner ER. General health, safety, and ergonomics in the veterinary dental workplace. In: Veterinary Dental Techniques for the Small Animal Practitioner. 3rd ed. Philadelphia: Saunders, 2004, pp. 637–664.
60. Fichtel T, Chra M, Langerova E, Biberaur G, Vlain M. Observations on the effects of scaling and polishing methods on enamel. J Vet Dent. 25(4):231–235, 2008.
61. Huntley DE, Campbell J. Bacterial contamination of scrub jackets during dental hygiene procedures. J Dent Hyg. 72(3):19–23, 1998.
62. Miller RL, Micik RE, Abel C, et al. Studies on dental aerobiology. II. Microbial splatter discharged from the oral cavity of dental patients. J Dent Res. 50:621, 1971.
63. Legnani P, Checchi L, Pelliccioni GA, D'Achille C. Atmospheric contamination during dental procedures. Quintessence Int. 25(6):435–439, 1994.
64. Westfelt E, Rylander H, Dahlen G, Lindhe J. The effect of supragingival plaque control on the progression of advanced periodontal disease. J Clin Periodontol. 25(7):536–541, 1998.
65. Canis MF, Kramer GM, Pameijer CM. Calculus attachment: Review of the literature and findings. J Periodontol. 50:406, 1979.
66. Zander HA. The attachement of calculus to root surfaces. J Periodontol. 24:16, 1953.
67. Caffesse RG, Sweeney PL, Smith BA. Scaling and root planing with and without periodontal flap surgery. J Clin Periodontol. 13(3):205–210, 1986.
68. Copulos TA, Low SB, Walker CB, Trebilcock YY, Hefti AF. Comparative analysis between a modified ultrasonic tip and hand instruments on clinical parameters of periodontal disease. J Periodontol. 64(8):694–700, 1993.
69. Odeid PR, D'Hoore W, Bercy P. Comparative clinical responses related to the use of periodontal instrumentation. J Clin Periodontol. 31(3):193–199, 2004.
70. Beuchat M, Busslinger A, Schmidlin PR, Michel B, Lehmann B, Lutz F. Clinical comparison of the effectiveness of novel sonic instruments and curettes for periodontal debridement after 2 months. J Clin Periodontol. 29(7):1145–1150, 2001.
71. Obeid PR, D'Hoore W, Bercy P. Comparative clinical responses related to the use of various periodontal instrumentation. J Clin Periodontol. 31(3):193–199, 2004.
72. Thornton S, Garnick J. Comparison of ultrasonic to hand instruments in the removal of subgingival plaque. J Periodontol. 53(1):35–37, 1982.
73. Leon LE, Vogel RI. A comparison of the effectiveness of hand scaling and ultrasonic debridement in furcations evaluated by differential dark field microscopy. J Periodontol. 58(2):86–94, 1987.
74. Kocher T, Rühling A, Momsen H, Plagmann HC. Effectiveness of subgingival instrumentation with power-driven instruments in the hands of experienced and inexperienced operators. A study on manikins. J Clin Periodontol. 24(7):498–504, 1997.
75. Kocher T, Riedel D, Plagmann HC. Debridement by operators with varying degrees of experience: A comparative study on manikins. Quintessence Int. 28(3):191–196, 1997.
76. Drisko CH. Root instrumentation. Power-driven versus manual scalers, which one? Dent Clin North Am. 42(2):229–244, 1998.
77. Walsley AD, Laird WR, Williams AR. Dental plaque removal by cavitational activity during ultrasonic scaling. J Clin Periodontol. 15:539, 1988.
78. Khambay BS, Walmsley AD. Acoustic microstreaming: Detection and measurement around ultrasonic scalers. J Periodontol. 70:626, 1999.
79. Wiggs RB, Lobprise HB. Oral exam and diagnosis. In: Veterinary Dentistry, Principles and Practice. Philadelphia: Lippincott-Raven, 1997, pp. 87–103.
80. Silness J. Fixed prosthodontics and periodontal health. Dent Clin North Am. 24(2):317–329, 1980.
81. Berglundh T, Gotfredsen K, Zitzmann NU, Lang NP, Lindhe J. Spontaneous progression of ligature induced peri-implantitis at implants with different surface roughness: An experimental study in dogs. Clin Oral Implants Res. 18(5):655–661, 2007.
82. Niemiec BA. Veterinary dental radiology. In: Small Animal Dental, Oral and Maxillofacial Disease, a Color Handbook (Niemiec BA ed.). London: Manson, 2010, pp. 63–87.
83. Jahn CA. Supragingival and subgingival irricgation. In: Carranza's Clinical Periodontology. St. Louis: Saunders, 2006, pp. 836–844.

84. Chang YC, Huang FM, Tai KW, Chou MY. The effect of sodium hypochlorite and chlorhexidine on cultured human periodontal ligament cells. Oral Surg Oral Med Oral Pathol Oral Radiol Endod. 92(4):446–450, 2001.
85. Tatnall FM, Leigh IM, Gibson JR. Comparative study of antiseptic toxicity on basal keratinocytes, transformed human keratinocytes and fibroblasts. Skin Pharmacol. 3:157–163, 1990.
86. Quirynen M, Mongardini C, de Soete M, et al. The role of chlorhexidine in the one-stage full-mouth disinfection treatment of patients with advanced adult periodontitis. Long-term clinical and microbiological observations. J Clin Periodontol. 27(8): 578–589, 2000.
87. Brägger U, Schild U, Lang NP. Effect of chlorhexidine (0.12%) rinses on periodontal tissue healing after tooth extraction. (II). Radiographic parameters. J Clin Periodontol. 21(6):422–430, 1994.
88. Spackman SS, Bauer JG. Periodontal treatment for older adults. In: Carranza's Clinical Periodontology. St. Louis: Saunders, 2006, pp. 675–692.
89. Klokkevold PR, Takei HH, Carranza FA. General principals of periodontal surgery. In: Carranza's Clinical Periodontology. St. Louis: Saunders, 2006, pp. 887–901.
90. Fischer C, Wennberg A, Fischer ZRG, Attstrom R. Clinical evaluation of pulp and dentine sensitivity after supragingival and subgingival scaling. Endod Dent Traumatol. 7(6):259–265, 1991.
91. Von Troil B, Needleman I, Sanz M. A systemic review of the prevalence of root sensitivity following periodontal therapy. J Clin Periodontol. 29(Suppl 3):173–177, 2002.
92. Lan WH, Liu HC, Lin CP. The combined occluding effect of sodium fluoride varnish and Nd:YAG laser irradiation on human dental tubules. J Endodont. 25(6):424–426, 1999.
93. Carranza FA, Takei HH. Clinical diagnosis. In: Carranza's Clinical Periodontology. St. Louis: Saunders, 2006, pp. 540–560.
94. Tetradis S, Carranza FA, Fazio RC, Takei HH. Radiographic aids in the diagnosis of periodontal disease. In: Carranza's Clinical Periodontology. St. Louis: Saunders, 2006, pp. 561–578.
95. Floyd MR. The modified Triadan system: Nomenclature for veterinary dentistry. J Vet Dent. 8(4):18–19, 1991.
96. Tsugawa AJ, Verstraete FJ. How to obtain and interpret periodontal radiographs in dogs. Clin Tech Small Anim Pract. 15(4):204–210, 2000.
97. Verstraete FJ, Kass PH, Terpak CH. Diagnostic value of full-mouth radiography in cats. Am J Vet Res. 59(6):692–695, 1998.
98. Verstraete FJ, Kass PH, Terpak CH. Diagnostic value of full-mouth radiography in dogs. Am J Vet Res. 59(6):686–691, 1998.
99. Niemiec, BA. Case based dental tadiology. Top Companion Anim Med. 24(1):4–19, 2009.
100. Ramadan AB, Mitchell DF. A roentgenographic study of experimental bone destruction. Oral Surg Oral Med Oral Pathol. 15:934–943, 1962.
101. Bender IB, Seltzer S. Roentgenographic and direct observation of experimental lesions in bone: I. 1961. J Endod. 29(11):702–706, 2003.
102. Bender IB, Seltzer S. Roentgenographic and direct observation of experimental lesions in bone: II. 1961. J Endod. 29(11):707–712, 2003.
103. Mulligan TM, Aller MS, Williams CE. Interpretation of periodontal disease. In: Atlas of Canine and Feline Dental Radiography. Trenton, NJ: Veterinary Learning Systems, 1998, pp. 104–123.
104. Rees TD, Biggs NL, Collings CK. Radiographic interpretation of periodontal osseous lesions. Oral Surg Oral Med Oral Pathol. 32(1):141–153, 1971.
105. Tsugawa AJ, Verstraete FJ, Kass PH, Görrel C. Diagnostic value of the use of lateral and occlusal radiographic views in comparison with periodontal probing for the assessment of periodontal attachment of the canine teeth in dogs. Am J Vet Res. 64(3): 255–261, 2003.
106. Torossian A. Thermal management during anaesthesia and thermoregulation standards for the prevention of inadvertent perioperative hypothermia. Best Pract Res Clin Anaesthesiol. 22(4):659–668, 2008.
107. Broadbelt DC, Pfeiffer DU, Young LE, Wood JLN. Results of the confidential enquiry into perioperative small animal fatalities regarding risk factors for anesthetic-related death in dogs. JAVMA 233(7):1096–1103, 2008.
108. Hall LW, Clarke KW, Trim CM. Veterinary Anesthesia. 10th ed. London: Saunders, 2001.
109. Tiret L, Desmonts JM, Hatton F, Vourc'h G. Complications associated with anaesthesia—a prospective survey in France. Can Anaesth Soc J. 33:336–344, 1986.
110. Gengler WR, Kunkle BN, Romano D, Larsen D. Evaluation of a barrier sealant in dogs. J Vet Dent. 22(3):157–159.
111. Roudebush P, Logan E, Hale, FA. Evidence-based veterinary dentistry: A systematic review of homecare for prevention of periodontal disease in dogs and cats. J Vet Dent. 22(1):6–15, 2005.
112. Needleman I, Suvan J, Moles DR, Pimlott J. A systematic review of professional mechanical plaque removal for prevention of periodontal diseases. J Clin Periodontol. 32 Suppl 6:229–282, 2005.

11

Advanced non-surgical therapy

Introduction

Periodontal pockets are present in many small animal patients, especially older small and toy breed dogs. Any pockets deeper than normal for the species (i.e., 3 mm in a dog and 1 mm in a cat) are pathologic and in need of therapy.[1,2] A thorough oral exam including dental radiographs performed under general anesthesia will reveal these pockets and allow for proper therapy.

Non-surgical periodontal therapy involves removing the infection (i.e., plaque, calculus, and granulation tissue) from the root surface and then smoothing the diseased/roughened root surface (if necessary).[1,3] This therapy markedly decreases the numbers of subgingival bacteria and also changes the bacterial composition. More specifically, the bacterial flora returns to a predominantly gram-positive aerobic population that is compatible with gingival health.[4,5] This significant reduction in periodontal pathogens reduces or even eliminates periodontal inflammation.[6,7] Decreasing the infection and inflammation in turn allows for gingival reattachment, leading to a decrease in pocket depth.[8]

In dogs, pockets between 3 mm and 5 mm (and possibly up to 6 mm) that are not associated with tooth mobility or other pathology (furcation, root caries) are best treated with scaling and closed root planing.[1–3,9] Pockets deeper than 5 mm (Figure 11.1) and/or those associated with other pathology (especially furcation level II and III exposure) (Figure 11.2) will *not* be effectively cleaned without direct root visualization.[1,10–13] Root visualization is best afforded by periodontal flap surgery.[1,8,13] In other words, a periodontal flap procedure is necessary in these cases or the infection will continue.[14] (See section 4 for a thorough description of surgical periodontal therapy.)

Scaling is defined as the removal of plaque and calculus from the tooth surface (both *supragingival* and *subgingival*) *without* the intentional removal of tooth substance. *Root planing* is the procedure of removing embedded calculus along with cementum to leave a smooth and clean root surface.[1,3] These are not actually separate procedures, but they differ notably in the amount of applied pressure (or force) against the tooth surface.[3]

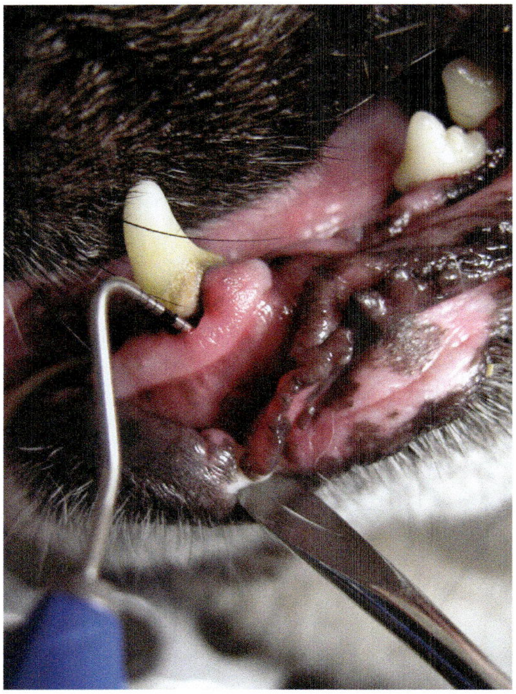

Figure 11.1 Intraoral dental picture of the left mandibular canine (304) in a dog with a 9 mm periodontal pocket. This is too deep for closed root planing; periodontal flap surgery or extraction is indicated.

Veterinary Periodontology, First Edition. Brook A. Niemiec.

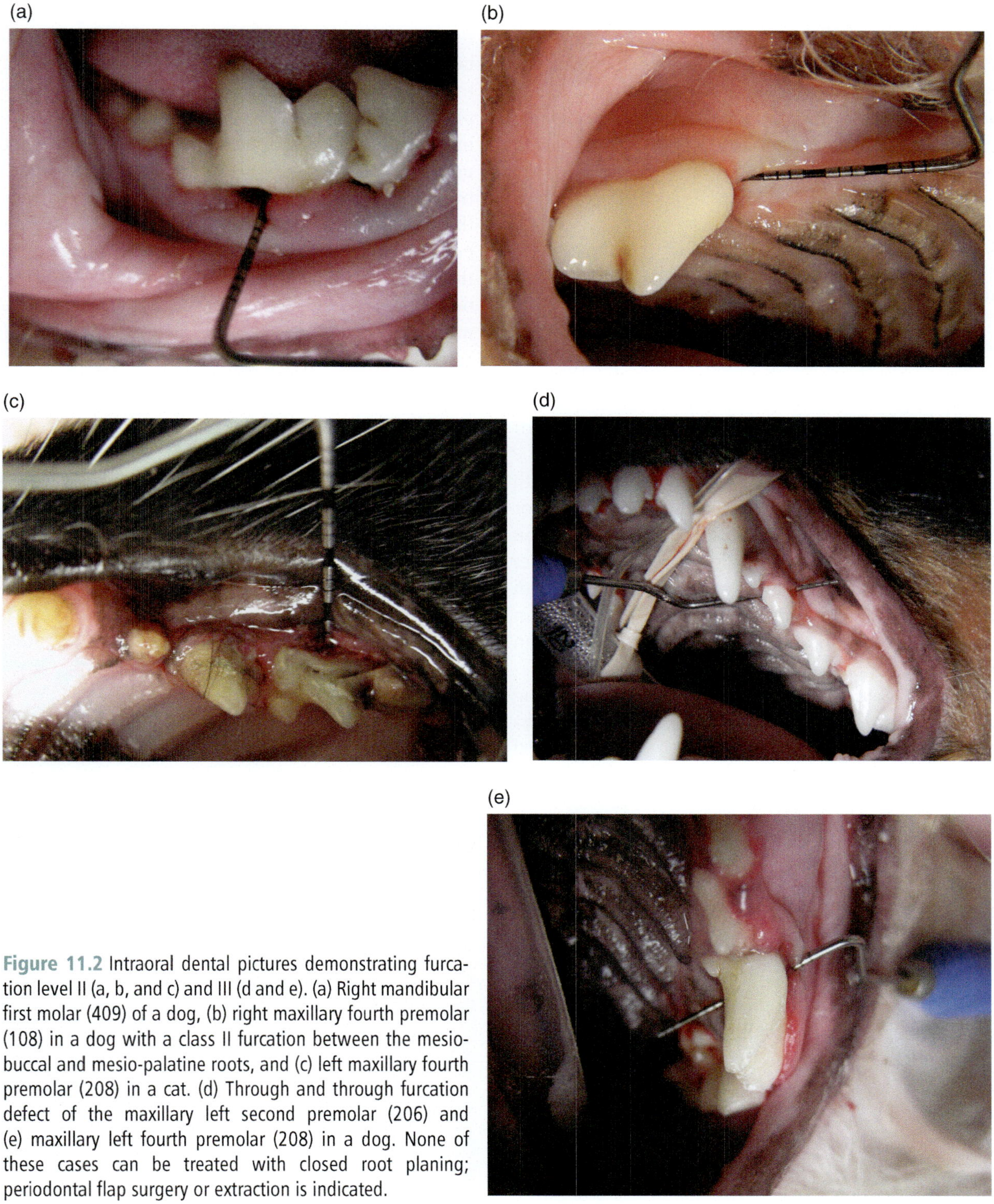

Figure 11.2 Intraoral dental pictures demonstrating furcation level II (a, b, and c) and III (d and e). (a) Right mandibular first molar (409) of a dog, (b) right maxillary fourth premolar (108) in a dog with a class II furcation between the mesiobuccal and mesio-palatine roots, and (c) left maxillary fourth premolar (208) in a cat. (d) Through and through furcation defect of the maxillary left second premolar (206) and (e) maxillary left fourth premolar (208) in a dog. None of these cases can be treated with closed root planing; periodontal flap surgery or extraction is indicated.

Root planing is performed with more tooth-ward force than simple scaling. The increased force necessary for root planing may result in damage to the root surface, ergo more precision is required.[3] More surgical time should therefore be allotted for root planing.

Healthy enamel is smooth, and thus plaque and calculus deposits on its surface are loosely attached and easily removed with simple scaling. However, the *root* surface is coated with cementum which is very irregular. Numerous studies have shown that calculus deposits on the root surface are commonly embedded in these irregularities.[15–17] Furthermore, if dentin is directly exposed, its tubules may become infected.[15] Finally, exposure of the root surface allows contamination with numerous toxic substances (particularly endotoxins).[18,19] Consequently, removing a small amount of root surface is required to render the root surface free of infection.[3] This is typically cementum, but unfortunately in some cases, the removal of a small amount of dentin is necessary.[3] It is important to note that this infection/contamination does not penetrate deep into the root,[20–22] which means that excessive tooth substance removal is unnecessary and should be avoided.[3,23]

Options for therapy

There are two major techniques currently used for treating minor periodontal pockets. These include hand and mechanical (typically ultrasonic) scaling methods.[2,13] Both of these methods are effective but have distinct advantages and disadvantages. This author recommends using a combination of these methods for best results.

The classic form of therapy is performed by hand with a curette.[8] It is known as scaling/root planing (SRP) or closed root planing. This is an exceedingly common procedure performed routinely in human dental offices and should be performed in veterinary hospitals with similar frequency. It is proven to be highly effective in cleaning the root surface and thereby establishing an environment for healing to occur.

Over the last few decades, however, ultrasonic scaling has become more and more accepted as a method of subgingival plaque and calculus removal. There are several reasons for its increasing popularity. Ultrasonic scaling is less technically demanding, requires less surgical time, and has the ability to sterilize the root surface.[3,13,24–28] In fact, when properly performed, mechanical scaling is equally effective as hand instrumentation for plaque control, root smoothness, and clinical results.[29–40]

Hand scaling/root planing

SRP by hand has been the standard of care for decades. It is highly effective in plaque and calculus removal, as well as removing the granulation tissue from the periodontal pocket (subgingival curettage), which in turn reduces pocket depth and controls infection.

The major advantage of hand scaling (when performed correctly) is the ability to achieve complete removal of subgingival plaque and calculus (to a depth of 5 mm). Furthermore, it can reliably smooth the root surface and therefore improve reattachment.

The major disadvantage of this form of therapy is that it is very technically demanding,[3,24] which is true for several reasons.[3] First, subgingival calculus is harder than supragingival calculus and it tends to be locked in root surface irregularities. Second, the overlying tissues restrict subgingival instrumentation. Finally, bleeding (or hemorrhage) as well as overlying inflammatory tissues can restrict visualization (Figure 11.3). Therefore, tactile sensitivity is critical to quality non-surgical therapy. If SRP is not meticulously performed, bacterial plaque will remain on the tooth, resulting in continued infection.[13] This is of special concern in general veterinary practices where assistants with minimal to no training commonly perform this important method of therapy. Practitioners are strongly recommended to become proficient in this skill in order to better teach their staff these techniques. Hands-on wet-labs should be a must for every practice, and ideally for every staff member entrusted to perform this therapy.[41] (See appendix 4 for a listing of hands-on laboratories.) Additionally, this method of plaque removal is more

(a)

(b)

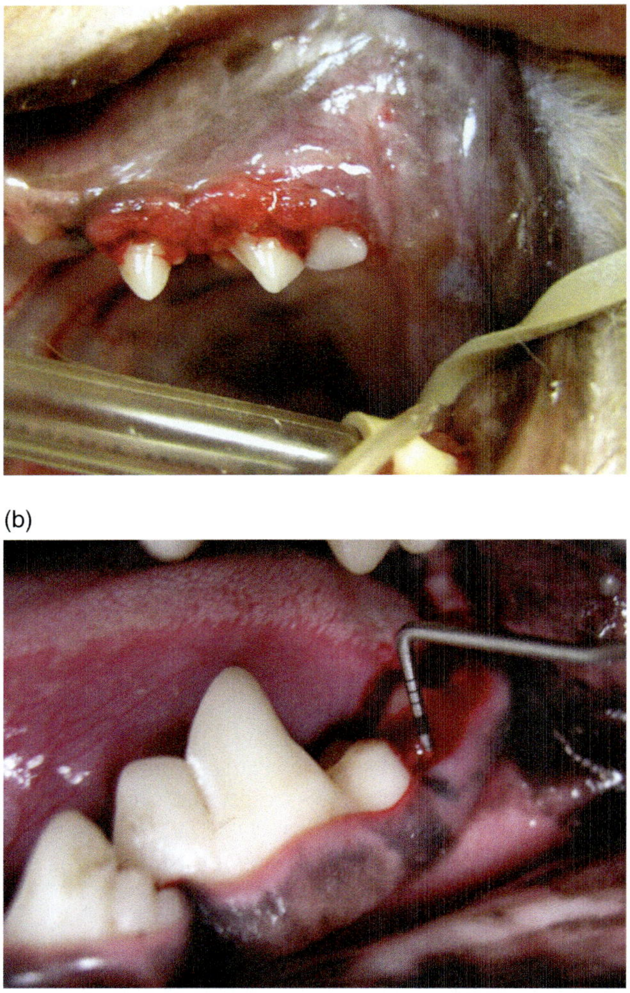

Figure 11.3 Situations where closed root planing is more challenging due to local conditions. These situations will hamper visualization. (a) Intraoral picture of the maxillary left of a cat with significant inflammatory gingival enlargement. (b) Intraoral picture of the mandibular left of a dog. The periodontal probing has elicited significant hemorrhage from the inflamed tissues.

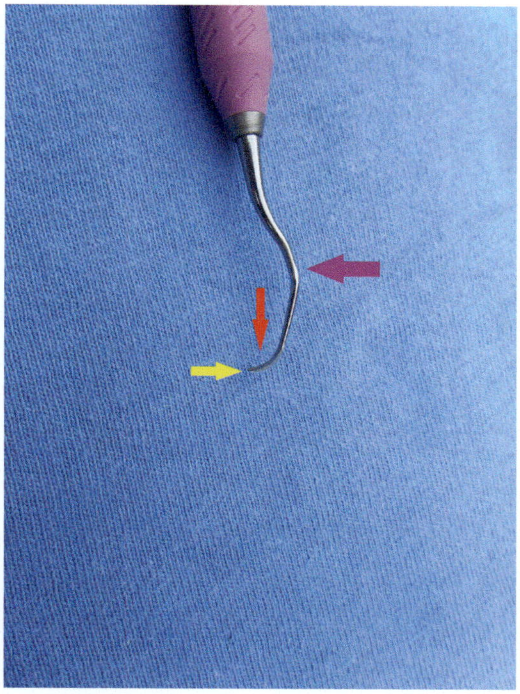

Figure 11.4 Side view of a 7-8 Gracey curette. Note the curved face (red arrow), blunt toe (yellow arrow), and extra bend at the shank (purple arrow).

time-consuming and can result in longer procedures.[13,27,28] Provided that the patient is stable, the increased anesthesia time is worth the benefits afforded by proper dental care. *In fact, a dental cleaning procedure is of little to no value if periodontal pockets are not effectively treated.* It is also noteworthy to mention that repetitive motion injuries are common in human hygienists if ergonomics are not followed. Again, proper training should reduce the chances of this occurring.

Equipment needs for hand SRP

This procedure requires only a supply of *sharp* dental curettes (Figure 11.4) (although a fine dental explorer and probe are necessary for diagnostics). Large hand instruments such as hoes, sickles, and files are too big for proper adaptation to the root surface, and therefore the quality of cleaning suffers.[41] In addition, these large instruments are more likely to inflict damage to the delicate gingival tissues. There are fine varieties of these instruments available that are effective subgingivally and may be considered for advanced practitioners.[3] Several curettes are needed to access the various areas of the mouth. The different types of curettes and the appropriate use of each are discussed in chapter 22. Having at least one of each angulation/size of curette is ideal, but this may be excessive for the needs of many practices. This author recommends that each practice have the following hand equipment at minimum: a dental mirror, periodontal probe, explorer (preferably pigtail), a two-ended scaler (jacquette and sickle), and finally a 1/2, 7/8, and 12/13 Gracey curette. This minimum list of equipment has been packaged and is currently commercially available.[A,B] Additional curettes may improve the cleanliness of the root as well as the experience of the operator and are recommended for practices providing advanced periodontal care. Other basic needs should include sharpening equipment[14,41] and a sterilization cassette.[42] It is absolutely critical that curettes and *all* periodontal surgery equipment be kept sharp, as proper and effective therapy depends on sharp instruments.[42,43]

See appendix 3 for a sharpening guide.

Preparation for SRP

Following a complete dental prophylaxis, evaluation, and intraoral dental radiographs, the pockets are ready for therapy. Appropriate antibiotic and pain management protocols should also be in place prior to initiating therapy. (See chapters 14 and 21 respectively for information on these steps.)

Begin by selecting the proper instrument for the area/teeth to be cleaned. In general, this should be an area-specific *Gracey* curette. A more detailed guide is presented in chapter 22, but typically the lower the number of the instrument, the more rostral in the mouth it is utilized. However, the practitioner should adjust this based on clinical presentation and individual preference.

Once the correct instrument is chosen, the next step involves proper handling of the curette. Moreover, the instrument should be gripped properly. For the vast majority of procedures, this will be the modified pencil grip described in chapter 10. In some instances, however, alternate grips are necessary.[3] These situations generally involve difficult areas to access such as the distal teeth in small breed dogs.[44] When slightly more reach is necessary, an open or extended grasp may be used, which separates the middle and ring fingers. If even more distance is needed, a long reach grip can be employed, which grips the instrument further back on the handle. This allows for work in tight spaces but sacrifices strength and control.[44]

Detection skills

The first step in ensuring complete subgingival plaque and calculus removal is detection.[3] Many human periodontologists feel that detection skills are as important as properly performed scaling and closed root planing. Detection of subgingival calculus requires a combination of visual and tactile senses.[3] Visual detection can be aided by the use of disclosing solutions[C] (Figure 11.5), proper lighting, and magnification.[42,44,D] In addition, residual calculus can be detected by drying the root

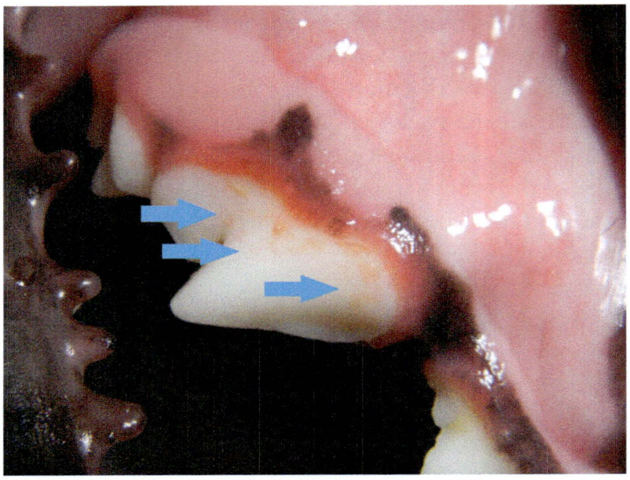

Figure 11.5 Intraoral picture of a patient showing plaque revealed (blue arrows) with the use of a disclosing solution.

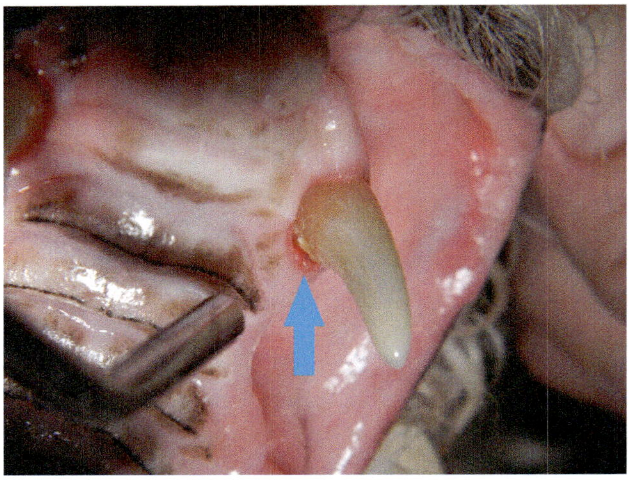

Figure 11.6 Intraoral picture of the left maxillary canine (204) in a dog. The tooth was already "cleaned"; however, when compressed air is used to dry the tooth and open the gingival sulcus, the residual calculus (blue arrow) is revealed for further cleaning.

surface with a gentle stream of compressed air, which reveals the calculus as appearing chalky white (Figure 11.6).[44,45] Using the compressed air directed into the gingiva also opens up the gingival space for easier viewing. Tactile exploration of the pocket should be performed with a fine explorer or probe. The explorer is held in a soft modified pencil grasp and used with great care. The instrument is inserted *gently* within the sulcus to the nadir (bottom) of the pocket (Figure 11.7). Once the bottom of the pocket is determined, the instrument is run over the tooth surface in light strokes. The instrument should be rotated in the operator's hands/fingers, in order to move around the tooth surface while maintaining the tip in contact with the tooth surface. When calculus or diseased tooth structure is

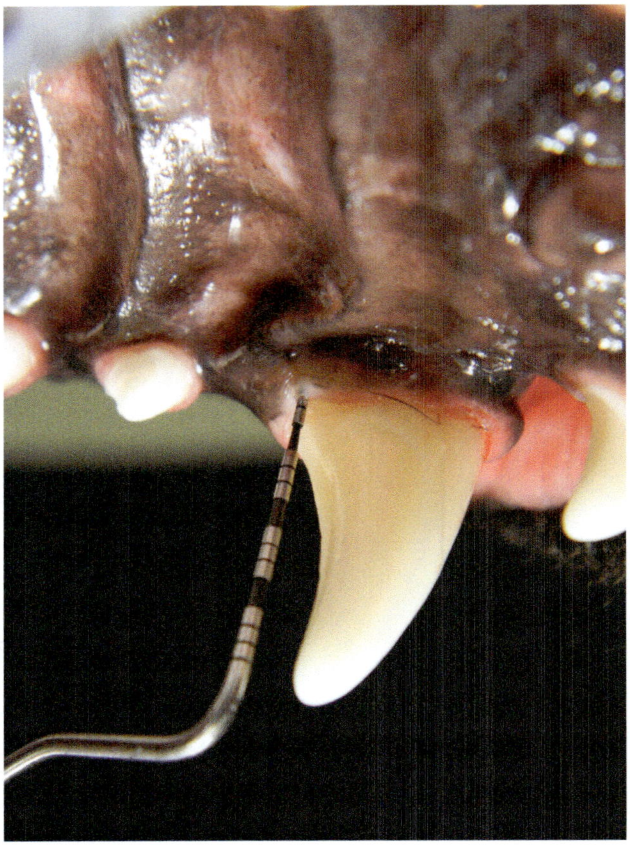

Figure 11.7 "Mapping" the periodontal pocket on the palatal surface of the left maxillary canine (204) of a dog prior to treatment.

encountered, the instrument should be carefully run over the deposit to "map" it. The operator must then use this mental map to thoroughly clean the root surfaces. Finally, an intraoral dental radiograph should be exposed to determine the level of alveolar bone as well as any root disease (such as resorption or endodontic disease), which may complicate therapy. After determining the level of disease, the proper instrument choice, and the indicated grip, the practitioner is ready to begin pocket cleansing.

Scaling/root planing

First, place the blade of the instrument on the tooth surface just coronal to the gingival margin with the lower shank parallel to the tooth surface (Figure 11.8).[1,3,13] Next, the curette is rotated so that the flat "face" of the blade is against the tooth surface (Figure 11.9). This is done to minimize the width of the instrument during insertion and to allow the blade to slide over the calculus and engage it apically. The blade is then inserted *gently* to the base of the pocket (Figure 11.10). The expected pocket depth can be estimated by reviewing the probing depths. Excessive force can damage the delicate gingival attachment. Once

(a)

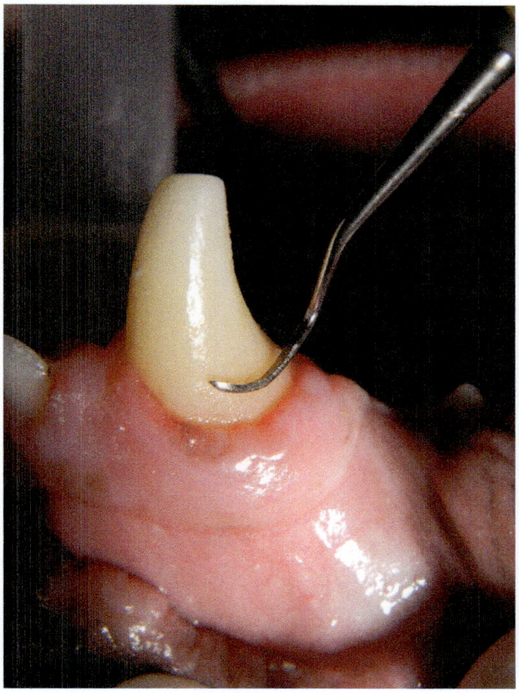

(b)

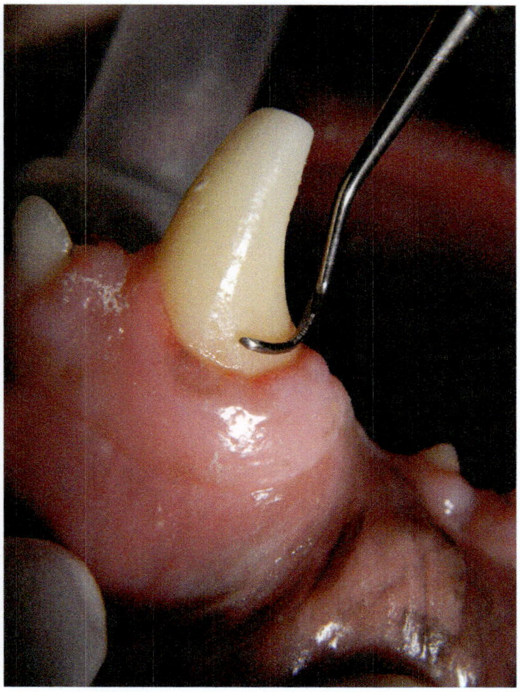

Figure 11.8 (a and b) The curette is placed against the tooth surface just above the gingival margin. It is best to begin with the shank parallel to the tooth in the "working position." This will familiarize the operator with the correct angulation when scaling.

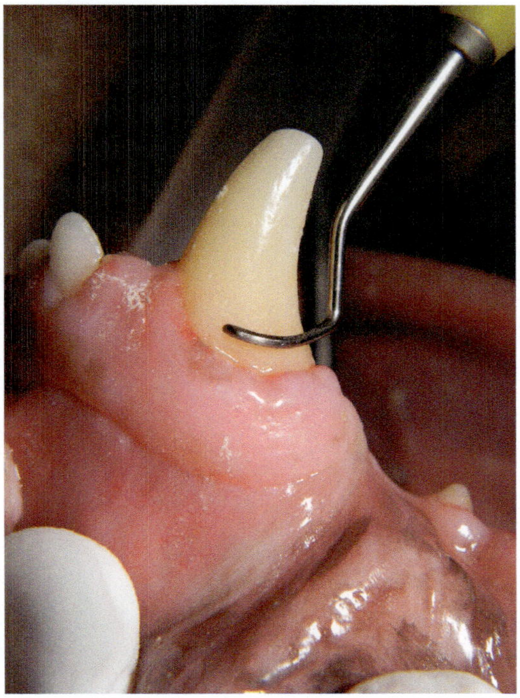

Figure 11.9 The instrument is then rotated toward the tooth surface to flatten the "face" of the instrument against the tooth. This minimizes the profile of the instrument, which allows for easier insertion into the pocket as well as the ability to slide over the calculus.

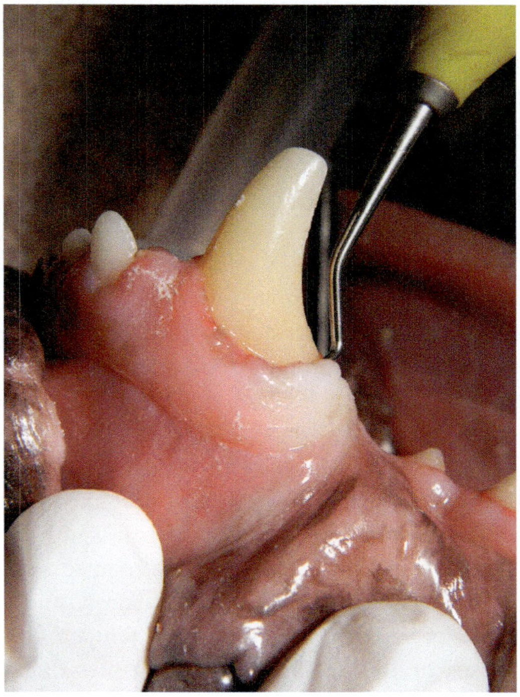

Figure 11.10 The curette is then *gently* inserted to the nadir of the pocket. Practitioners should be cognizant of the depth to be attained based upon the preoperative exam (probing). If the bottom of the pocket is not reached, calculus will be left behind and the treatment will fail. Be careful, however, not to pass through the delicate gingival sulcus.

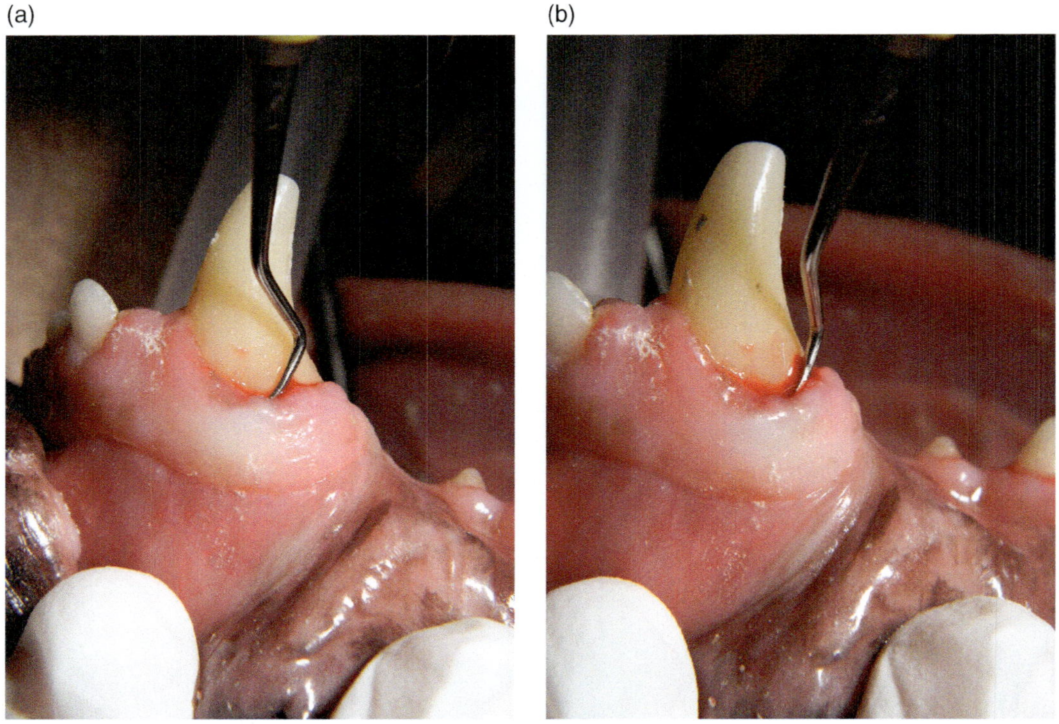

Figure 11.11 (a and b) The instrument is then rotated to bring the shank parallel to the root surface. Note that the angle of the root and tooth may be different, and therefore the angle of the shank needs to be adjusted (see Box 11.1). This situation is one of the many reasons that a firm knowledge of anatomy is necessary for proper treatment.

the bottom of the pocket is reached, the instrument is rotated to create a 70- to 90-degree working angulation (closer to 90 is ideal). **When the terminal portion (or shank) is parallel to the tooth, a 90-degree angle is created** (Figure 11.11). This positioning will place the sharp/working edge of the instrument perpendicular to the tooth surface, which is the correct orientation for cleaning. Once positioned, slight pressure is applied down onto the root surface.[46] Finally, the instrument is removed from the pocket in a firm/short stroke (Figure 11.12).

This procedure is repeated in numerous overlapping strokes in slightly different directions. It is important to remember that teeth are not flat but rather generally curved to circular in shape. Therefore, the instrument must be rotated through the hand during the cleaning to keep the proper surface (or "sweet-spot") in contact with the contours of the tooth surface. Also, it is important to note that different areas of the mouth require a different approach to maintain proper angulation and form. Therefore, practitioners should not be reluctant to move themselves or the patient numerous times during the cleaning in order to stay in proper position. In general, proper operator positioning is opposite the gingiva of the quadrant being instrumented.

In addition, it is critical to pay particular attention to the interproximal areas of teeth with tight interproximal contacts (incisors and molars) (Figure 11.13). These "con-

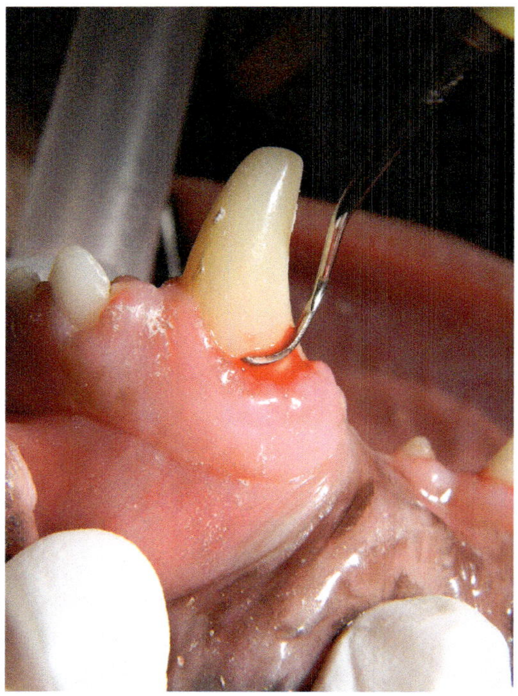

Figure 11.12 Pressure is placed against the tooth and the instrument removed from the pocket in a firm, short, and *controlled* pull. The instrument should not move more than a few mm above the gingival margin when finished. If it does move more than a few mms, then too much effort is being used, which can damage the delicate gingiva.

tacts" are prone to development of calculus due to the fact that they are protected from the natural cleaning ability of an animal's mouths as well as homecare attempts. It is these areas in humans that makes flossing of paramount importance. Not only are these areas likely to develop calculus, they are very hard to clean, and it is very difficult to effectively instrument these areas. This is especially true in small and toy breed dogs with very small mouths.

Box 11.1 Key clinical point

Note, the proper 90 degree cleaning angle is created to the root, which is not necessarily the same as the crown. For instance, the buccal and palatal aspects of the canine teeth are fairly straight and therefore the angle is the same for root and crown (Figure 11.a). However, other teeth have a significant angle between the roots and the crown, which will affect the cleaning angle. For example, the maxillary fourth premolar has an approximately 25-degree angle (Figure 11.b) and the facial surface of the incisors and mesial and distal of the canines gradually curve distally to an approximate 40-degree angle.[47–50] (Figure 11.c). A firm grasp of anatomy is necessary for proper instrumentation.

(a1) (a2)

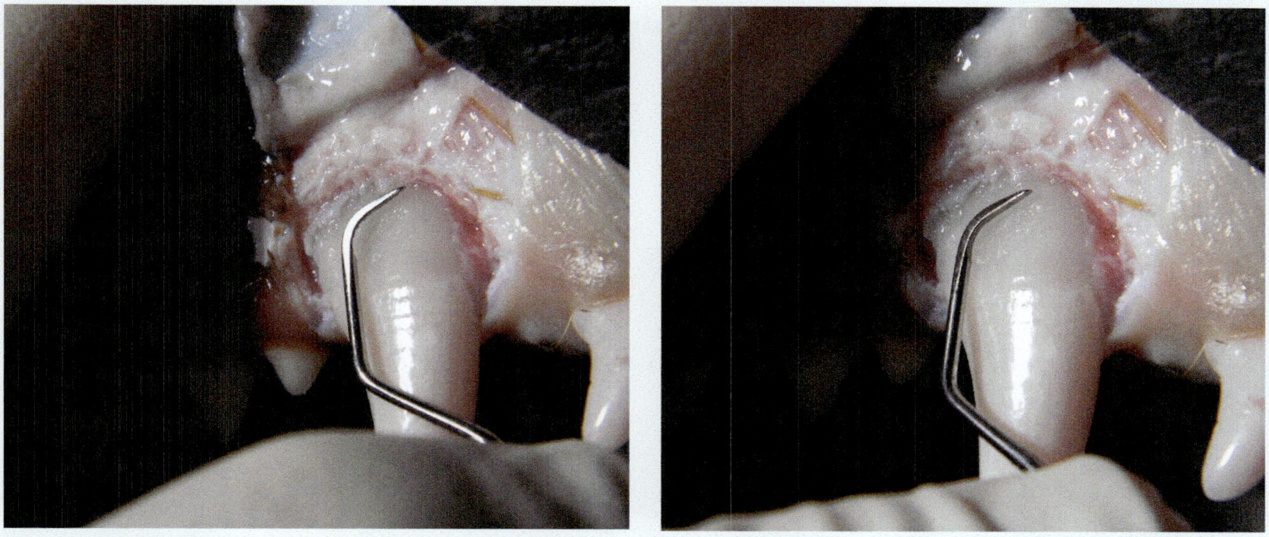

Figure11.a (1 and 2) Intraoral cadaver pictures of scaling the buccal surface of the maxillary canine in a dog. Note, the root and crown are parallel, which means that the shank should be parallel to the crown for proper scaling position.

(b1) (b2)

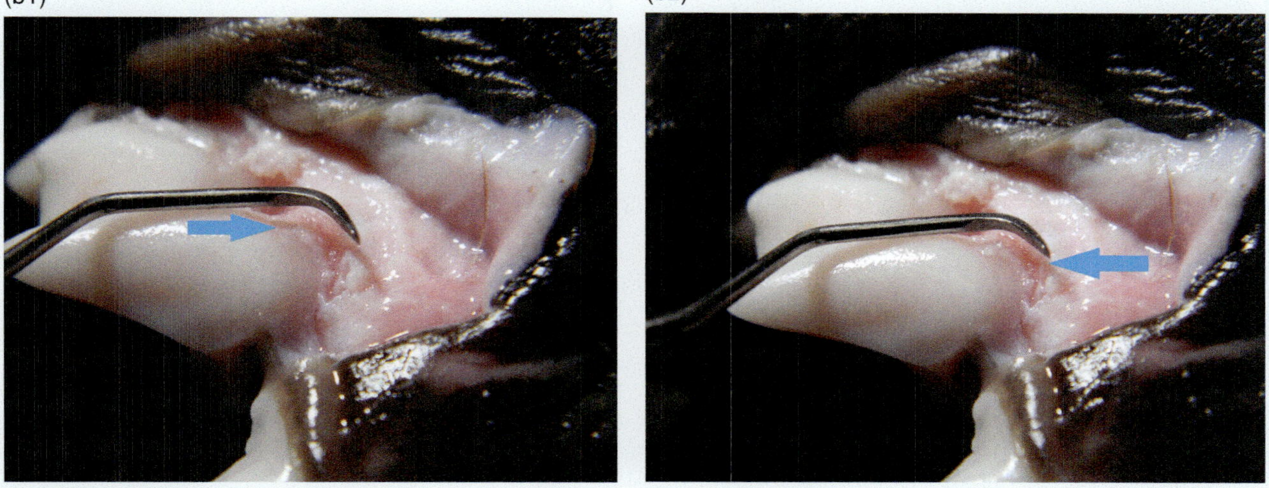

Figure 11.b Intraoral cadaver picture of scaling the buccal surface of the maxillary fourth premolar in a dog. Note the root and crown are *not* parallel. Thus, if the shank is parallel to the crown it is not in proper contact with the root (1 and 2). For the blade to achieve proper scaling position, the shank must be angled off the crown approximately 25 degrees (3 and 4) (red arrows).

(b3)

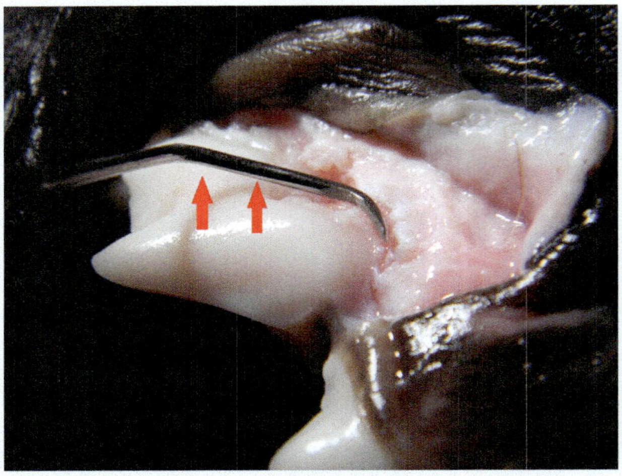

(b4)

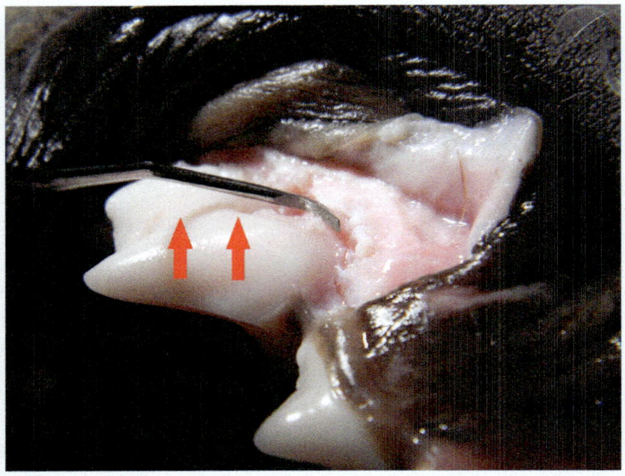

Figure 11.b (cont'd)

(c1)

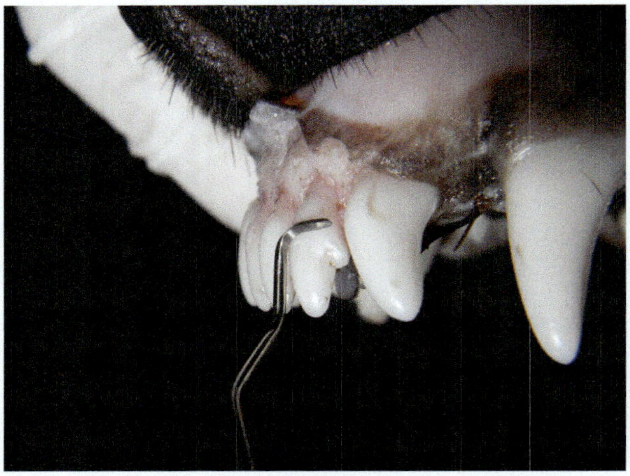

(c2)

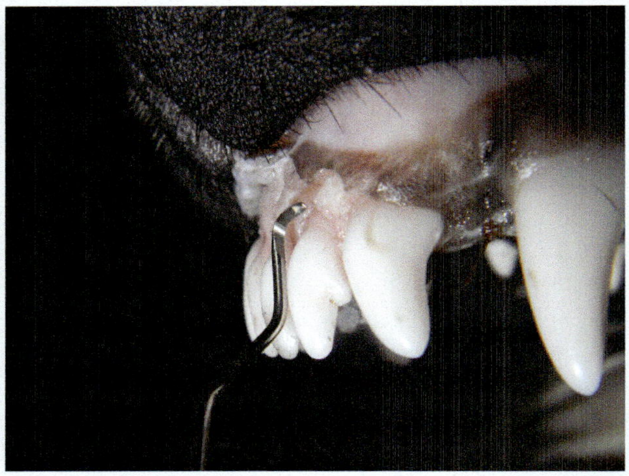

(c3)

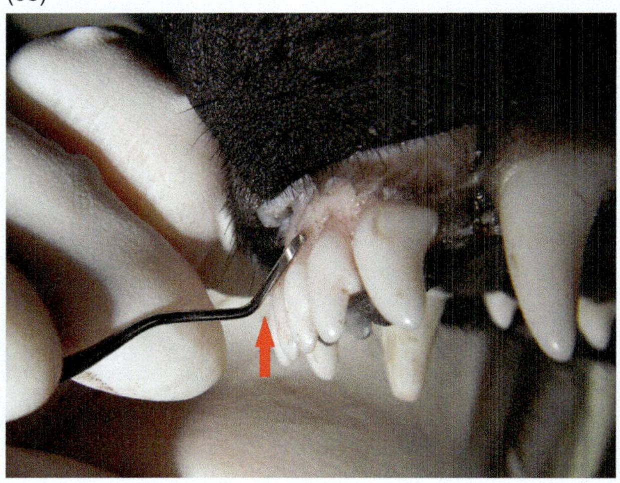

Figure 11.c Intraoral cadaver picture of scaling the facial surface of the maxillary incisors in a dog. Note the root and crown are *not* parallel. Thus, if the shank is parallel to the crown (1) it is not in proper contact with the root (2). For the blade to achieve proper scaling position, the shank must be angled off the crown approximately 40 degrees (3) (red arrow).

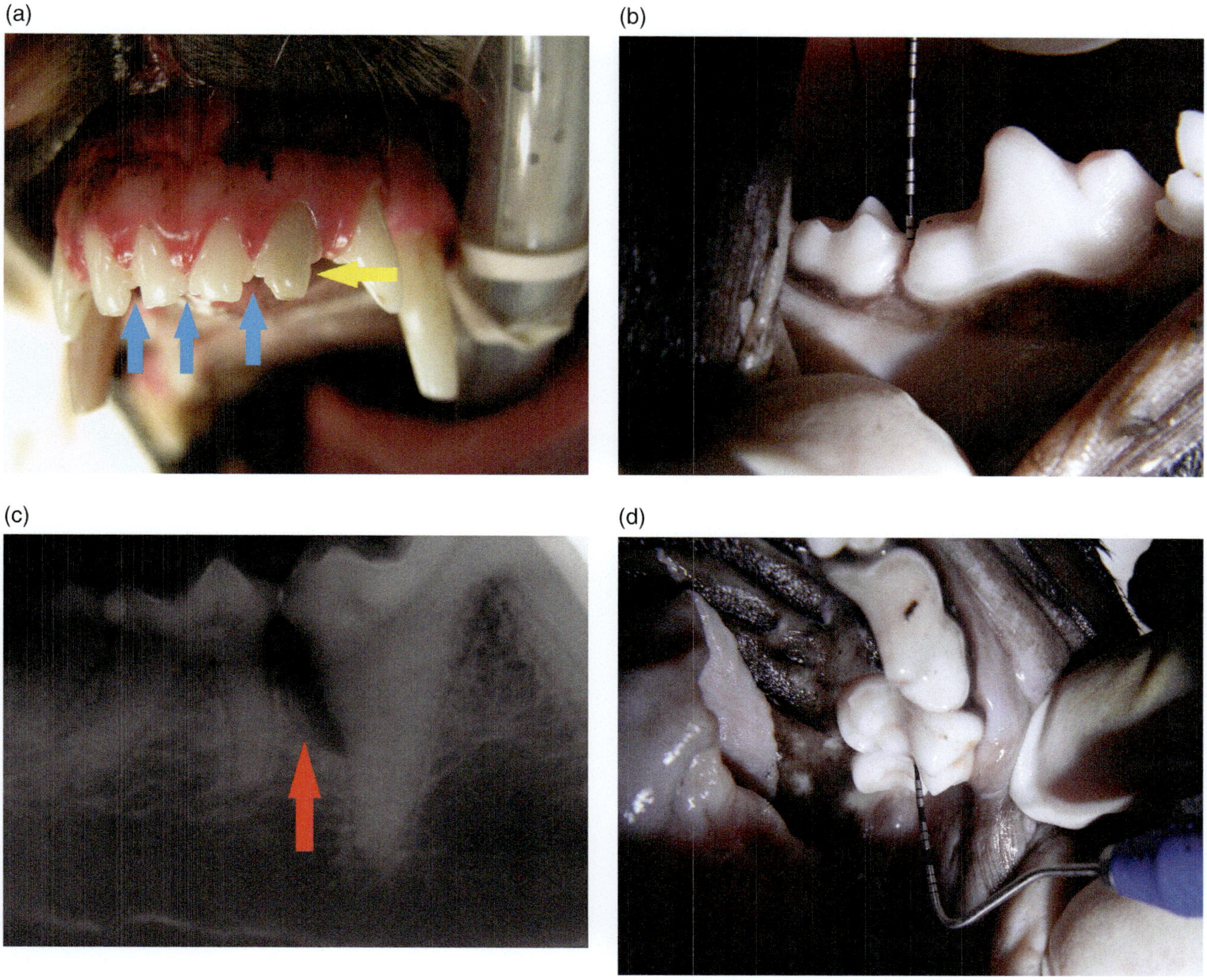

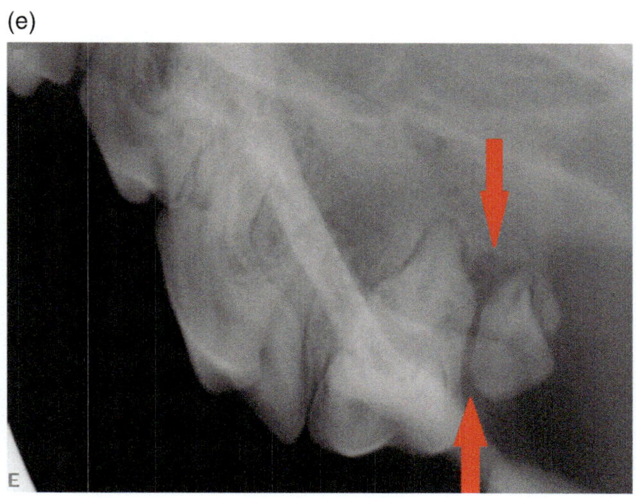

Figure 11.13 Areas of tight contact where probing and cleaning are very challenging. This can lead to ineffective cleaning if great care is not taken. (a) Maxillary incisors. Note the very tight contacts between the teeth (blue arrows). Incidentally, the left second incisor is non-vital (yellow arrow). (b) Intraoral picture of the right mandibular first and second molar (409–410) in a dog. Note that the probe cannot pass between the teeth. However, the dental radiograph (c) reveals severe alveolar bone loss (red arrow). This case reinforces the importance of a proper oral exam and thorough scaling. (d) Intraoral picture of the left maxillary first and second molar (209–210) in a dog. Note that the probe cannot pass between the teeth. However, the dental radiograph (e) reveals severe alveolar bone loss (red arrows). This case further reinforces the importance of a proper oral exam and thorough scaling.

Proper cleaning of these areas typically requires special, small, highly angled instruments as well as extended or cross-arch rests. Remember that the lower shank must be parallel to the tooth surface (or at least very close) to provide effective cleaning. When instrumenting these areas, make sure to extend the stroke at least midway across the proximal surface to ensure complete cleaning, and clean effectively from *both* sides (Figure 11.14).

It is important to note that it is much easier to remove successive small areas of calculus from large deposits,

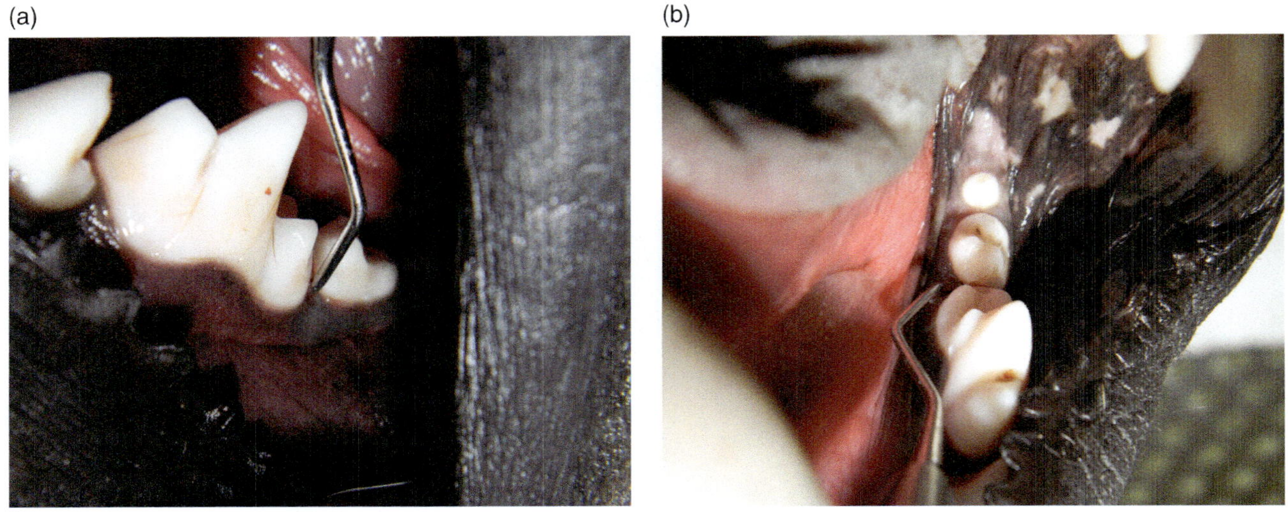

Figure 11.14 Intraoral picture of the left mandibular first molar (309) in a dog undergoing closed root planing. The tooth is thoroughly scaled from the buccal (a) as well as the lingual (b) surfaces for a complete cleaning.

rather than trying to remove it all in one stroke. In the latter effort, the force is spread out over the whole instrument rather than just a small part (decreased PSI). Removal of large calculus deposits should be performed by engaging an edge of the calculus with the terminal one-third of the curette and breaking off small pieces with each stroke as one advances along the tooth. This will not only decrease operator strain; it will also decrease the chance of trauma from a vigorous stroke.

After the initial few strokes, the resistance lessens until only a slight roughness remains. As this occurs, the strokes should become longer and with less force applied to the tooth in order to smooth the surface. This is an important point, since excessive strokes with firm pressure damage the root surface unnecessarily. Root planing should continue until the entire root surface is clean and feels smooth. This is a good indication of complete cleaning. Finally, a fine explorer should be carefully run along the root surface (see "Detection Skills" above) to check for irregularities that may indicate residual calculus or root pathology (Figure 11.15).

SRP is continued across all affected teeth. Once all pockets have been treated, they should be thoroughly lavaged to remove any debris. This may be followed by the instillation of a product for local antibacterial effects (see chapter 12).

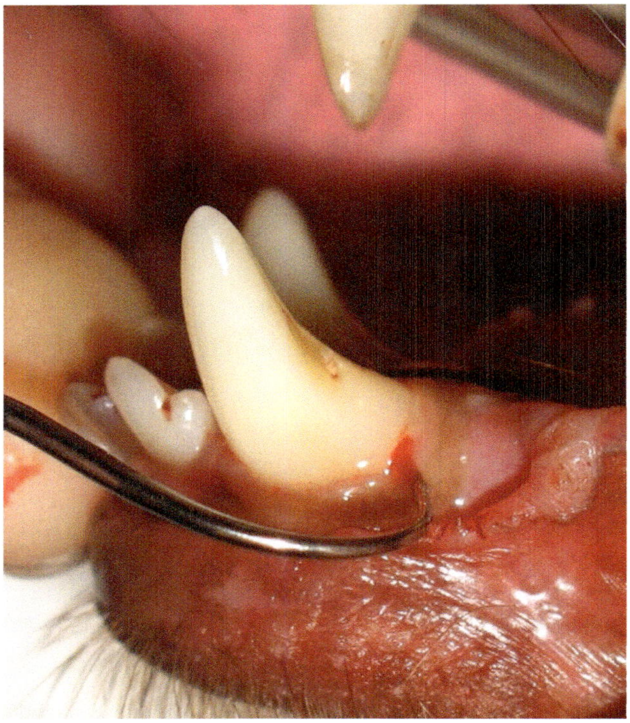

Figure 11.15 Utilizing a dental explorer to feel for residual calculus.

Mechanical (ultrasonic) therapy

Recent advances in ultrasonic scalers[1,3,13] have resulted in the creation of special tips that can be used subgingivally.[30] The major design changes include thinner tips with the coolant spray directed near the tip of the instrument.[24,42,51] In addition to proper tip selection, power is an important consideration. Most *sub*gingival tips are designed for use at lower power settings than standard *supra*gingival tips.[3,24] Practitioners should refer to the owner's manual for specific settings for individual equipment.

Although there are studies to the contrary,[52,53] it has been shown that the new, thinner ultrasonic periodontal tips produce root surfaces that are as smooth, if not smoother, than standard curettes.[30,54–56] Most studies report that they are more effective than standard curettes at cleaning furcational disease,[57,58] but other studies report that curettes are more effective in these areas.[59] One study did find improved healing following ultrasonic as compared to hand debridement.[60] Moreover, numerous reports have shown that when properly performed, hand and ultrasonic scaling are equally effective in cleaning teeth, removing bacteria, decreasing inflammation, and increasing attachment.[29,32–37,61,62]

There are several major advantages to the use of ultrasonic scalers in periodontal pockets. First, these instruments are much less technically demanding to use in comparison to hand curettes.[24] This means that a higher degree of cleaning may be achieved by less experienced operators. While this is certainly not ideal, it is the reality in the vast majority of veterinary practices. It should be noted, however, that proper therapy still requires significant training and experience and that improper use of these instruments can have significant deleterious effects. Consequently, proper training is still critical. In fact, some studies show that inexperienced operators do not perform any better with mechanical instruments verses hand instruments.[28,63] The incongruity of the ultrasonic method appearing more effective in the veterinary field is likely due to the degree of cleanliness achieved by experienced human dental hygienists compared to the average veterinary technician/assistant, where any improvement is vast.

Another advantage of mechanical scaling is decreased time under anesthesia. Ultrasonic scalers remove calculus much faster than hand scaling,[27,28,30,33,42,64] especially if the deposits are large (which is common in veterinary patients).[3] In addition, ultrasonic scalers require less movement and are more ergonomical,[13,24] decreasing chances of repetitive motion injuries.[26] When properly performed, ultrasonic debridement may be less traumatic than hand scaling, resulting in less patient discomfort; however, this was not seen in a human study.[60]

Furthermore, the small periodontal tips used with ultrasonic scalers may be superior to curettes in deep periodontal pockets (greater than 7 mm).[31] This is likely due to the fact that deep pockets are more restrictive to hand instruments.

Finally, and perhaps most importantly, ultrasonic scaling may result in decreased levels of bacteria and endotoxins on the root surface.[36] This owes to the fact that ultrasonic waves produce cavitational activity, acoustic turbulence, and acoustic microstreaming within the coolant spray, resulting in bacterial disruption.[2,24,65,66] These activities may improve plaque reduction and cleanliness of the root surface.[65,67] However, recent studies dispute the fact that the cavitational effect of the ultrasonics directly kills bacteria,[68] suggesting instead that it is the lavage that results in lower bacterial numbers.

Many texts as well as equipment manuals recommend the addition of dilute chlorhexidine to the coolant solution. This was recently shown to be of no additional value over standard ultrasonic cavitation.[69,70] However, these studies are based on perfectly performed scaling, which may not be the typical case in veterinary practice. Therefore inclusion of chlorhexidine to the coolant in the veterinary setting may still be indicated.

There are two major disadvantages of ultrasonic scaling. First, with improper use of the ultrasonic instrument, damage may occur to the root, pulp, and/or gingiva.[30] Tissue damage may be caused by inappropriate tip or power selection, excessive pressure on the tooth, long exposure of the tip to the root, insufficient water coolant, or a damaged instrument tip.[71] Any of these errors can have significant deleterious effects including tooth death. The other concern with ultrasonic scaling is the potential to create significant aerosolization of pathogenic bacteria. It is therefore very important to institute a protocol for infection control. (See chapter 10 for a thorough discussion of bacterial aerosols.)

Equipment needed for mechanical scaling

Mechanical debridement requires only an ultrasonic scaler and proper periodontal tips. A variety of tips are available depending on the location and size of the pocket, and therefore a good supply is recommended (Figure 11.16). The various types of mechanical scalers and tips are covered in detail in chapter 23. It is recommended for the practitioner to be very familiar with his or her equipment prior to using it.

Mechanical subgingival scaling procedure

The handle and ultrasonic insert should ideally be sterilized prior to use. To begin the procedure,[3,13] the tip should be inspected to ensure that it is not damaged and then carefully placed in the handle. Power settings should be checked to ensure appropriate levels for subgingival use. They should be at the minimum level required to remove calculus, as excessive power can damage root surfaces. The scaling unit is then started and the tip inspected for proper function. The water coolant should be adjusted to create a fine mist at the working tip (Figure 11.17).

After the unit is prepared, the instrument is held with a *light* modified pencil grasp and the hand (or a finger) rested on a surface to ensure maximum tactile sensitivity. The tip should be *carefully* introduced into the gingival sulcus/pocket and the unit activated. The tip is then directed against the tooth surface with a *minimum* amount of force (just touching).[1,3,44,46] Heavy forces

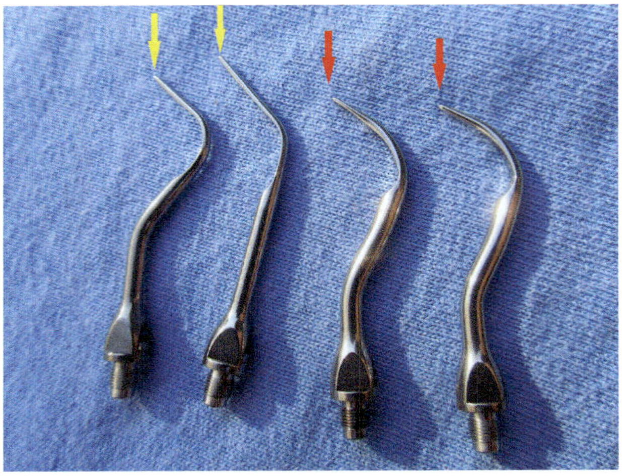

Figure 11.16 A selection of ultrasonic tips for a piezoelectric ultrasonic scaler. On the right are two shorter/thicker scalers for *supra*gingival scaling (red arrows). On the left are longer, thinner instruments for careful *sub*gingival scaling (yellow arrows).

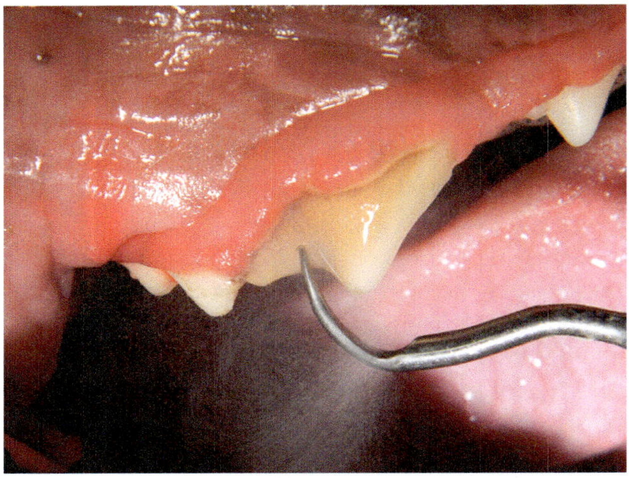

Figure 11.17 The fine but adequate cooling spray from a well-tuned ultrasonic scaler. (Note that this is a supragingival tip.)

should be avoided as they dampen the motion of the instrument, thus *decreasing* its effectiveness.[72] In addition, excessive downward force can damage the tooth surface and the instrument.[44,73] Using the side surface of the terminal portion of the instrument, while keeping the tip parallel to the tooth (Figure 11.18), the instrument is run over the *entire* affected root surface using numerous overlapping strokes in different directions.[3,74] It is important to keep the instrument in motion at all times to avoid root damage.[3] Typically, it is recommended that they be kept in constant contact with tooth for no more than 12–15 seconds,[1,3,74] but some authors recommend only 5–7 seconds.[46] Interestingly, however, an exhaustive literature search finds no primary research that indicates a length of time that causes pulp damage,

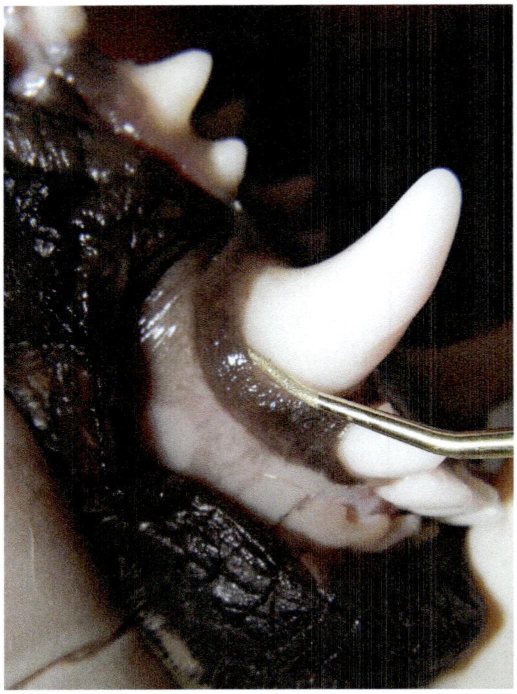

Figure 11.18 Intraoral picture of a small/fine ultrasonic scaler tip cleaning a periodontal pocket on the buccal surface of the right mandibular canine (404) of a dog.

providing that the instrument has adequate water cooling.[75,76] Therefore, these recommendations may be somewhat arbitrary. Regardless, the procedure should be interrupted on a regular basis to allow for fluid suction and tooth/root inspection.

This step should be continued until the root feels smooth. Further confirmation of the level of cleanliness should be evaluated visually by directing air into the sulcus or manually detecting with a fine explorer.[3] Residual calculus can be removed with a sharp curette. It is important to follow the scaling with subgingival lavage (as described in chapter 10), especially if an antiseptic was not used in the coolant supply.

Combined therapy using both hand and mechanical methods

Due to the unique properties of both hand and mechanical scaling methods, this author recommends they be combined to achieve the best results in the shortest time. The combined method is also favored by the majority of human periodontists.[3] By performing careful ultrasonic debridement, the vast majority of infectious material is removed in a very efficient manner. At the same time, the root surface receives an antibacterial treatment. Following the ultrasonic debridement, hand scaling should be performed to remove any residual calculus deposits and to further smooth the root surface.[3,8] This synergism results in the ideal healing environment in the most time-efficient fashion.

Box 11.2 Key points

- Meticulous cleaning and smoothing of the root surface is necessary for the removal of infection and the healing of pockets.
- Hand scaling is very effective at cleaning but is technically demanding and relatively slow.
- Ultrasonic debridement is very efficient and has an antibacterial effect on the tooth surface but may leave residual calculus.
- Careful ultrasonic debridement followed by meticulous hand scaling efficiently provides the best environment for healing.
- Hands-on CE labs will greatly improve operator speed and quality of patient care.

Notes

A. Weldin Periodontal Kit, Miltex.
B. Dentalaire Periodontal Pack, Dentalaire.
C. Reveal, Butler Schein.
D. Perioptix.

References

1. Wiggs RB, Lobprise HB. Periodontology. In: Veterinary Dentistry, Principles and Practice. Philadelphia: Lippincott-Raven, 1997, pp. 186–231.
2. Bellows J. Periodontal equipment, materials, and techniques. In: Small Animal Dental Equipment, Materials, and Techniques, a Primer. Ames, IA: Blackwell, 2004, pp. 115–173.
3. Pattison AM, Pattison GL. Scaling and root planning. In: Carranza's Clinical Periodontology. St. Louis: Saunders, 2006, pp. 749–797.
4. Mousques T, Listgarten MA, Phillips RW. Effect of scaling and root planing on the composition of human subgingival microbial flora. J Periodontal Res. 7:199, 1980.
5. Renvert S, Wikstrom M, Dahlen G, et al. Effect of root debridement on the elimination of Actinobacillus actinomycetemcomitans and Bacteroides gingivalis from periodontal pockets. J Clin Periodontol. 17:345, 1990.
6. Hughes TP, Caffesse RG. Gingival changes following scaling, root planing and oral hygiene, a biometric evaluation. J Periodontol. 49:245, 1978.
7. Lowenguth RA, Greenstein G. Clinical and microbiological response to non-surgical mechanical periodontal therapy. Periodontol 2000 9:14, 1995.
8. Niemiec BA. Periodontal therapy. Top Companion Anim Med. 23(2):81–90, 2008.
9. Cobb CM. Non-surgical pocket therapy: Mechanical. Ann Periodontol. 1(1):443–490, 1996.
10. Carranza FA, Takei HH. Phase II periodontal therapy. In: Carranza's Clinical Periodontology. St. Louis: Saunders, 2006, pp. 881–886.
11. Perry DA, Schmid MO, Takei HH. Phase I periodontal therapy. In: Carranza's Clinical Periodontology. St. Louis: Saunders, 2006, pp. 722–727, 2006.
12. Caffesse RG, Sweeney PL, Smith BA. Scaling and root planing with and without periodontal flap surgery. J Clin Periodontol. 13(3):205–210, 1986.
13. Holmstrom SE, Frost PF, Eisner ER. Periodontal therapy and surgery. In: Veterinary Dental Techniques. 2nd ed. Philadelphia: Saunders, 1998, pp. 167–213.
14. Bellows J. Equipping the dental practice. In: Small Animal Dental Equipment, Materials, and Techniques, a Primer. Ames, IA: Blackwell, 2004, pp. 13–55.
15. Adriaens P, Edwards C, DeBoever J, et al. Ultrastructural observations on bacterial invasion in cementum and radicular dentin of periodontally diseased human teeth. J Periodontol. 59: 493, 1988.
16. Zander HA. The attachment of calculus to root surfaces. J Periodontol. 24:16, 1953.
17. Moscow BS. Calculus attachment in cemental separations. J Periodontol. 40:125, 1969.
18. Aleo J, DeRenzis F, Farber P, et al. The presence and biological activity of cementum-bound endotoxins. J Periodontol. 45:672, 1974.
19. Hatfield CG, Baumhammers A. Cytotoxic effects of periodontally involved surfaces of human teeth. Arch Oral Biol. 16:465, 1971.
20. Hughes FJ, Auger DW, Smales FC. Investigation of the distribution of cementum associated lipopolysaccharides in periodontal disease with scanning electron microscope immunohistochemistry. J Periodontal Res. 23:10, 1998.
21. Smart JG, Wilson M, Davis EH, et al. The assessment of ultrasonic root surface debridement by determination of residual endotoxin levels. J Clin Periodontol. 17:174, 1990.
22. Moore J, Wilson M, Keiser JB. The distribution of bacterial lipopolysaccharide (endotoxins) in relation to periodontally diseased root surfaces. J Clin Periodotol. 13:748, 1986.
23. Garret JS. Effects of non-surgical periodontal therapy on periodontitis in humans: A review. J Clin Periodontol. 10:5151, 1983.
24. Jahn CA. Sonic and ultrasonic instrumentation. In: Carranza's Clinical Periodontology. St. Louis: Saunders, 2006, pp. 828–835.
25. Fichtel T, Chra M, Langerova E, Biberaur G, Vlain M. Observations on the effects of scaling and polishing methods on enamel. J Vet Dent. 25(4):231–235, 2008.
26. Holmstrom SE, Frost P, Eisner ER. General health safety and ergonomics in the veterinary dental workplace. In: Veterinary Dental Techniques for the Small Animal Practitioner. 3rd ed. Philadelphia: Saunders, 2004, pp. 637–664.
27. Tunkel J, Heinecke A, Flemmig TF. A systematic review of efficacy of machine-driven and manual subgingival debridement in the treatment of chronic periodontitis. J Clin Periodontol. 29 Suppl 3:72–81, 2002.
28. Kocher T, Rühling A, Momsen H, Plagmann HC. Effectiveness of subgingival instrumentation with power-driven instruments in the hands of experienced and inexperienced operators. A study on manikins. J Clin Periodontol. 24(7):498–504, 1997.
29. Oosterwall PJ, Matee MI, Mikx FHM, et al. The effect of subgingival debridement with hand and ultrasonic instruments on subgingival microflora. J Clin Periodontol. 14:528, 1987.
30. Dragoo MR. A clinical evaluation of hand and ultrasonic instruments on subgingival debridement. 1. With unmodified and modified ultrasonic inserts. Int J Periodont Restor Dent. 12(4):310–323, 1992.
31. Gagnot G, Mora F, Poblete MG, et al. Comparative study of manual and ultrasonic instrumentation of cementum surfaces:

Influence of lateral pressure. Int J Periodont Restor Dent. 24:137, 2004.

32. Santos FA, Pochapski MT, Leal PC, Gimenes-Sakima PP, Marcantonio E Jr. Comparative study on the effect of ultrasonic instruments on the root surface in vivo. Clin Oral Investig. 12(2):143–150, 2008.
33. Copulos TA, Low SB, Walker CB, et al. Comparative analysis between a modified ultrasonic tip and hand instruments on clinical parameters of periodontal disease. J Periodontol. 64:694,1993.
34. Stende GW, Schaffer EM. A comparison of ultrasonic and hand scaling. J Periodontol. 32:312, 1961.
35. Torfason T, Kiger R, Selvig KA, et al. Clinical improvement of gingival conditions following ultrasonic verses hand instrumentation of periodontal pockets. J Clin Periodontol. 6:165, 1979.
36. Drisko CH. Root instrumentation. Power-driven versus manual scalers, which one? Dent Clin North Am. 42(2):229–244, 1998.
37. Breininger DR, O'Leary TJ, Blumenshine RV. Comparative effectiveness of ultrasonic and hand scaling for the removal of subgingival calculus. J Periodontol. 58:9, 1987.
38. Derdilopoulou FV, Nonhoff J, Neumann K, Kielbassa AM. Microbiological findings after periodontal therapy using curettes, Er:YAG laser, sonic, and ultrasonic scalers. J Clin Periodontol. 34(7):588–598, 2007.
39. Obeid PR, D'Hoore W, Bercy P. Comparative clinical responses related to the use of various periodontal instrumentation. J Clin Periodontol. 31(3):193–199, 2004.
40. Thornton S, Garnick J. Comparison of ultrasonic to hand instruments in the removal of subgingival plaque. J Periodontol. 53(1):35–37, 1982.
41. Holmstrom SE, Frost P, Eisner ER. Dental equipment and care. In: Veterinary Dental Techniques for the Small Animal Practitioner. 3rd ed. Philadelphia: Saunders, 2004, pp. 31–106.
42. Bellows J. The dental operatory. In: Small Animal Dental Equipment, Materials, and Techniques, a Primer. Ames, IA: Blackwell, 2004, pp. 3–12.
43. Klokkevold PR, Takei HH, Carranza FA. General principles of periodontal surgery. In: Carranza's Clinical Periodontology. St. Louis: Saunders, 2006, pp. 887–901.
44. Holmstrom SE, Frost P, Eisner ER. Dental prophylaxis and periodontal disease stages. In: Veterinary Dental Techniques for the Small Animal Practitioner. 3rd ed. Philadelphia: Saunders, 2004, pp. 175–232.
45. Wiggs RB, Lobprise HB. Oral exam and diagnosis. In: Veterinary Dentistry, Principles and Practice. Philadelphia: Lippincott-Raven, 1997, pp. 87–103.
46. Debowes LJ. Problems with the gingiva. In: Small Animal Dental, Oral and Maxillofacial Disease, a Color Handbook (Niemiec BA ed.). London: Manson, 2010, pp. 159–181.
47. Niemiec BA, Furman R. Feline dental radiology. J Vet Dent. 21(4):252–257, 2004.
48. Niemiec BA, Furman R. Canine dental radiology. J Vet Dent. 21(3):186–1990, 2004.
49. Gracis M, Harvey CE. Radiographic study of the maxillary canine tooth in mesaticephalic dogs. J Vet Dent. 15(2):73–78, 1998.
50. Gracis M. Radiographic study of the maxillary canine tooth of four mesaticephalic cats. J Vet Dent. 16 (3):115–128, 1999.
51. Wiggs RB, Lobprise HB. Dental equipment. In: Veterinary Dentistry, Principles and Practice. Philadelphia: Lippincott-Raven, 1997, pp. 1–28.
52. Schlageter L, Rateitschak-Plüss EM, Schwarz JP. Root surface smoothness or roughness following open debridement. An in vivo study. J Clin Periodontol. 23(5):460–464, 1996.
53. Hunter RK, O'Leary TJ, Kafrawy AH. The effectiveness of hand versus ultrasonic instrumentation in open flap root planing. J Periodontol. 55(12):697–703, 1984.
54. Drisko CH. Scaling and root planing without over instrumentation: Hand vs. power driven scalers. Curr Opin Periodontol. 3:78, 1993.
55. Garnik JJ, Dent J. A scanning electron micrographical study of root surfaces and subgingival bacteria after hand scaling and ultrasonic instrumentation. J Periodontol 60:144, 1989.
56. Kawashima H, Sato S, Kishida M, Ito K. A comparison of root surface instrumentation using two piezoelectric ultrasonic scalers and a hand scaler in vivo. J Periodontal Res. 42(1):90–95, 2007.
57. Leon LE, Vogel RI. A comparison of hand scaling and ultrasonic debridement in furcations as evaluated by differential dark field microscopy. J Periodontol. 58:86, 1987.
58. Sugaya T, Kawanami M, Kato H. Effects of debridement with an ultrasonic furcation tip in degree II furcation involvement of mandibular molars. J Int Acad Periodontol. 4:132, 2002.
59. Ortero-Cagide FJ, Long BA. Comparative in vitro effectiveness of closed root debridement with fine instruments on specific areas of mandibular first molar furcations. I. Furcation area. J Periodontol 68:1098, 1997.
60. Walsh TF, Waite IM. A comparison of postsurgical healing following debridement by ultrasonic or hand instruments. J Periodontol. 49(4):201–205, 1978.
61. Beuchat M, Busslinger A, Schmidlin PR, Michel B, Lehmann B, Lutz F. Clinical comparison of the effectiveness of novel sonic instruments and curettes for periodontal debridement after 2 months. J Clin Periodontol. 28(12):1145–1150, 2001.
62. Garnick JJ, Dent J. A scanning electron micrographical study of root surfaces and subgingival bacteria after hand and ultrasonic instrumentation. J Periodontol. 60(8):441–447, 1989.
63. Kocher T, Riedel D, Plagmann HC. Debridement by operators with varying degrees of experience: A comparative study on manikins. Quintessence Int. 28(3):191–196, 1997.
64. Yukna RA, Scott JB, Aichelmann-Reidy ME, LeBlanc DM, Mayer ET. Clinical evaluation of the speed and effectiveness of subgingival calculus removal on single-rooted teeth with diamond-coated ultrasonic tips. J Periodontol. 68(5):436–442, 1997.
65. Walsley AD, Laird WR, Williams AR. Dental plaque removal by cavitational activity during ultrasonic scaling. J Clin Periodontol. 15:539, 1988.
66. Arabaci T, Ciçek Y, Canakçi CF. Int J Dent Hyg. 5(1):2–12, 2007.
67. Khambay BS, Walmsley AD. Acoustic microstreaming: Detection and measurement around ultrasonic scalers. J Periodontol. 70:626, 1999.
68. Schenk GY, Flemmig T, Lob S, Ruckdeschel G, Hickel R. Lack of antimicrobial effect on periodontopathic bacteria by ultrasonic and sonic scalers in vitro. J Clin Periodontol. 27:116–119, 2000.
69. Taggart JA, Plamer RM, Wilson RF. A clinical and microbiological comparison of the effects of water and 0.02% chlorhexidine as coolants during ultrasonic scaling and root planing. J Clin Periodontol. 17:32, 1990.
70. Grossi SG, Skrepcinski FB, DeCaro T, et al. Treatment of periodontal disease in diabetics reduces glycated hemoglobin. J Periodontol. 68:713, 1997.
71. Lea SC, Landini G, Walmsley AD. The effect of wear on ultrasonic scaler tip displacement amplitude. J Clin Periodontol. 33(1): 37–41, 2006.
72. Trenter SC, Landini G, Walmsley AD. Effect of loading on the vibration characteristics of thin magnetostrictive ultrasonic scaler inserts. J Periodontol. 74(9):1308–1315, 2003.

73. Brine EJ, Marretta SM, Pijanowski GJ, Siegel AM. Comparison of the effects of four different power scalers on enamel tooth surface in the dog. J Vet Dent. 17(1):17–21, 2000.
74. Holmstrom SE, Frost P, Eisner ER. Dental prophylaxis. In: Veterinary Dental Techniques. 2nd ed. Philadelphia: Saunders, 1998b, pp. 133–166.
75. Nicoll BK, Peters RJ. Heat generation during ultrasonic instrumentation of dentin as affected by different irrigation methods. J Periodontol. 69(8):884–888, 1998.
76. Vérez-Fraguela JL, Vives Vallés MA, Ezquerra Calvo LJ. Effects of ultrasonic dental scaling on pulp vitality in dogs: An experimental study. J Vet Dent. 17(2):75–79, 2000.

12

Local antibiotic usage

One of the current methods being used to promote gingival reattachment is local treatment with antimicrobials. There are several human products available,[A-E] as well as veterinary-labelled doxycycline and clindamycin gels.[F,G] These products are designed to create a long-term/high-dose antimicrobial effect directly within the periodontal space, with minimal systemic absorption.[1-3] Studies have shown that they develop local antimicrobial concentrations exceeding 1,300 ug/ml,[4] in contrast to the 4–8 ug/ml seen with systemic administration.[5]

Local antimicrobial administration has been shown to decrease bacterial counts further than SRP alone.[6,7] They are effective in decreasing periodontal inflammation and increasing attachment gains (reduced pocket depth)[8-25] and are safe for routine use.[23,26] Finally, the use of these products without SRP was shown to be as effective in pocket depth reduction as SRP alone.[24,27,28]

Tetracycline derivatives also offer several additional (i.e., non-antimicrobial) benefits that include:

1. *An anti-inflammatory effect* (specifically anticollagenase).[29-39] This is important since it has been shown that host modulation is an important factor in controlling periodontal disease. Moreover, it has been shown that these products have a direct effect on cytokines and chemokines.[40]
2. *Improved wound healing.*[41] This also holds true in periodontal healing,[42] and therefore the addition of a tetracycline product to any periodontal or oral surgery should be beneficial.
3. *Direct reduction of osteoclast function.* One study reported that chemically modified tetracyclines (CMT-3 and CMT-8 of doxycycline and minocycline, respectively) are potent inhibitors of osteoclastogenesis and directly induce osteoclast apoptosis.[43] This may have a direct effect on reducing bone loss.

It is important to note, however, that only the clindamycin product is licensed for use in cats. There have been occasional anecdotal adverse reactions reported with the doxycycline product in this species. Therefore, practitioners should use caution and inform clients of the risks of off-label use before treating a feline patient with one of these products.

Once a suitable periodontal pocket is discovered (Figure 12.1), it should first be treated with closed root planing. Local antibiotic therapy is an aid to standard SRP, *not a substitute for it*.[48] After the tooth is scaled and root cleanliness is confirmed, the pocket/sulcus is lavaged. The pocket is then ready for the application of the medication. (See chapter 11 for details on closed root planning.)

The technique for preparation and application of the veterinary-labelled doxycycline product is described below.[48-50] (For instructions on the human-labelled and clindamycin products, refer to the package insert.)

The product is thoroughly mixed (according to package directions) to ensure a homogeneous mixture (Figure 12.2). The product is then concentrated in syringe A, and syringe B is separated and discarded. Next, the 22-gauge blunt-ended cannula (supplied) is

Box 12.1 Key clinical point

Local antibiotics are best suited for use in periodontal pockets between 3 mm (or maximum normal depth for the species) and 5 mm. Pockets greater than 5 mm are too deep to effectively clean with closed root planing alone and therefore require surgical therapy.[44-48] Practitioners can choose to use the antimicrobial products in these pockets after the surgical procedure.

Veterinary Periodontology, First Edition. Brook A. Niemiec.

(a) (b)

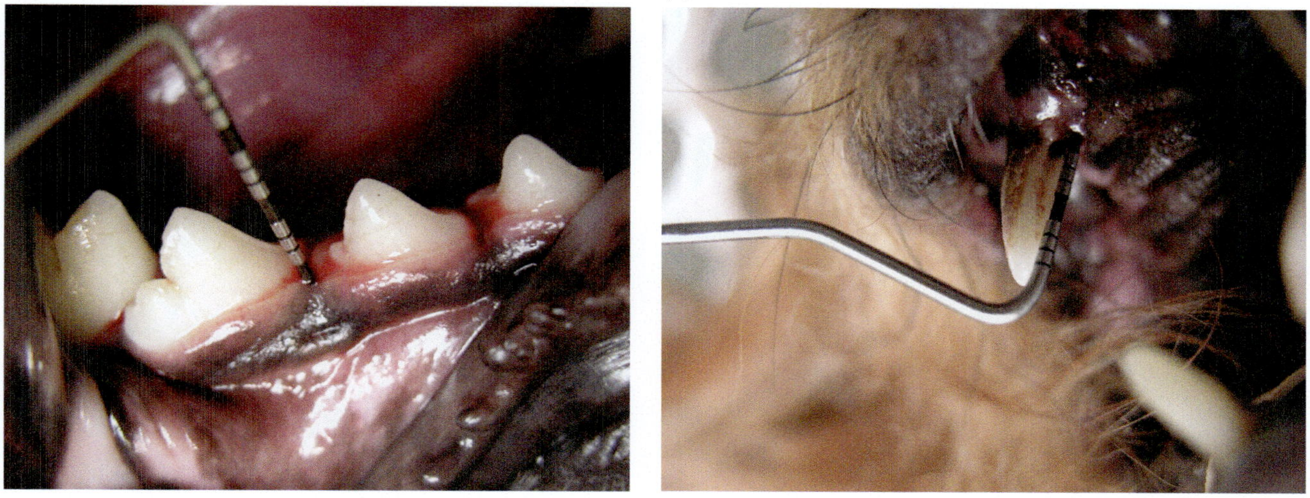

Figure 12.1 Appropriate sites for application of perioceutic. (a) 4 mm pocket between the mandibular third and fourth premolars. (b) 5 mm periodontal pocket on the palatal aspect of the right maxillary canine (104).

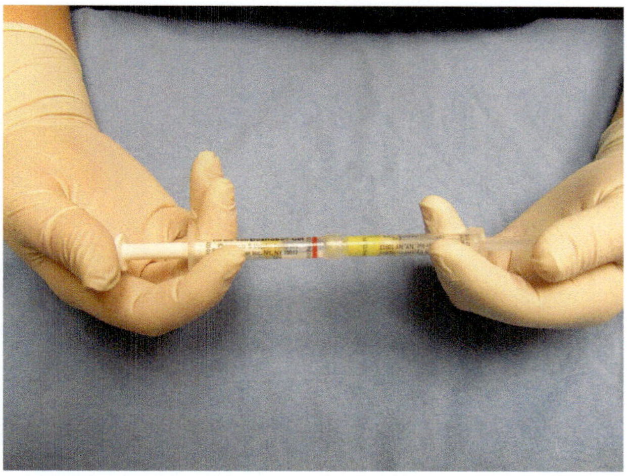

Figure 12.2 Mixing the perioceutic.

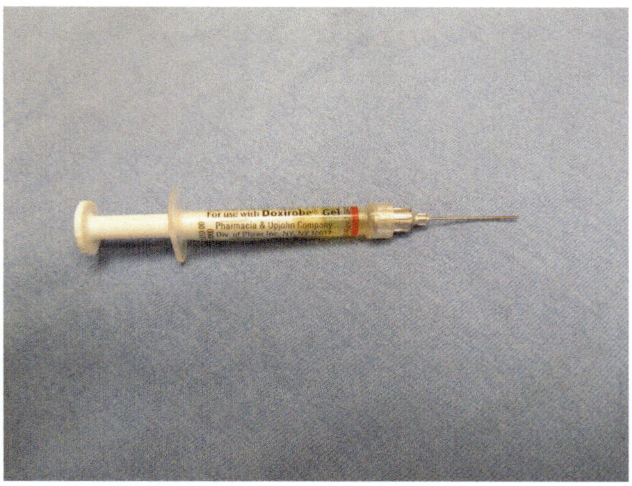

Figure 12.3 Mixed product with the cannula attached, ready for placement into the pocket.

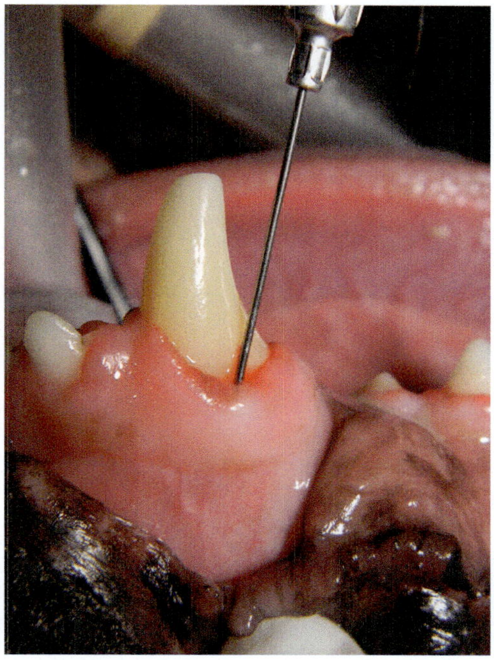

Figure 12.4 The cannula is placed *gently* to the base of the pocket.

attached to the syringe and the air is removed (Figure 12.3).

After being properly prepared, the cannula is inserted *gently* to the base of the pocket (Figure 12.4). Once it has been determined that the bottom of the pocket is reached, the product is slowly injected. Injection is continued until the applied product is just barely overflowing the pocket (Figure 12.5). Overfilling the pocket will not improve clinical gains and will make the procedure of

(a)

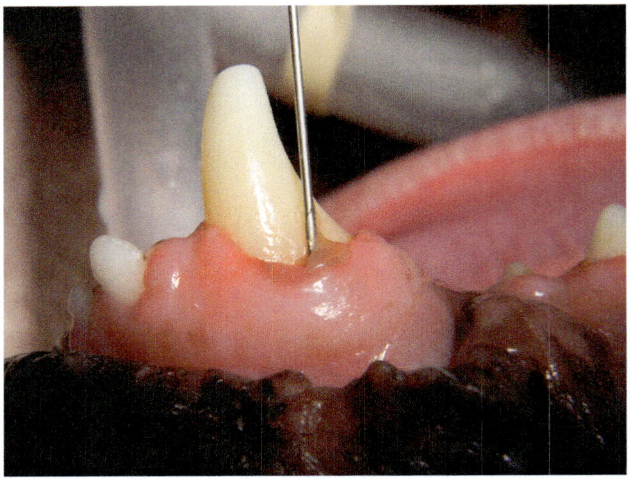

(b)

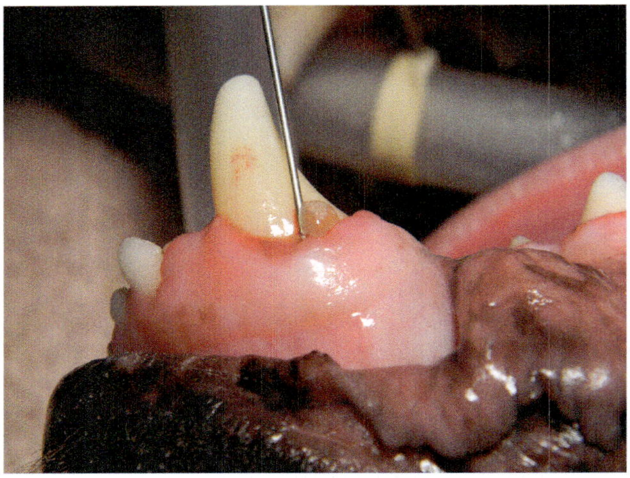

Figure 12.5 (a) The product is slowly inserted until it is *just* overflowing. (b) Excessive application does not add efficiency, it actually makes the placement into the pocket much more difficult, and should be avoided.

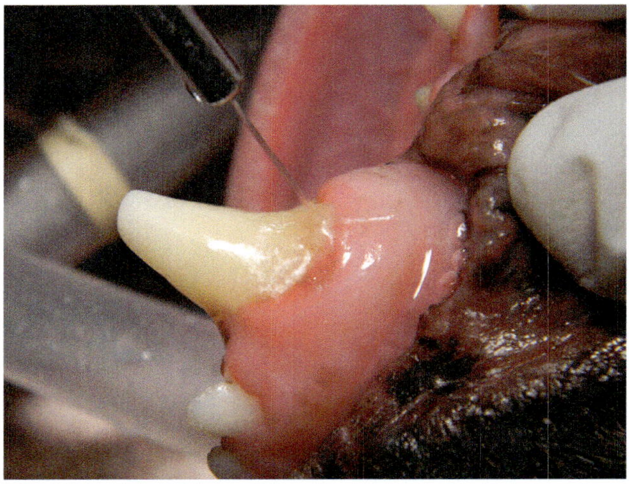

Figure 12.6 Wetting the product gently with water from an air-water syringe.

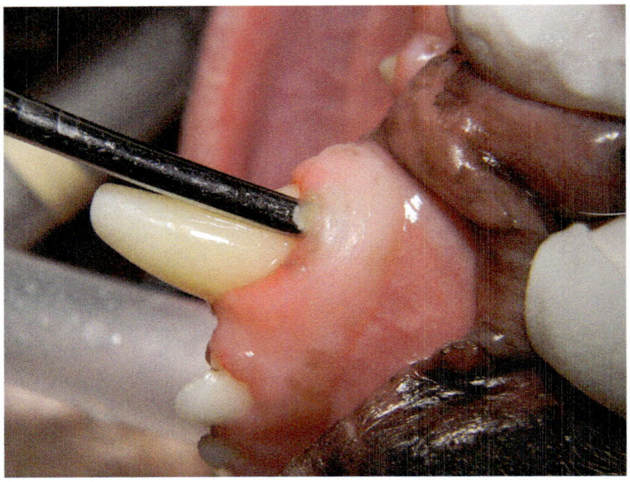

Figure 12.7 Gently pushing the product apically into the pocket.

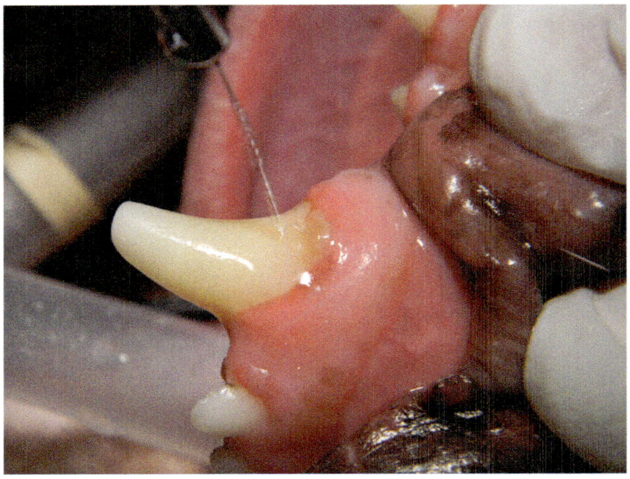

Figure 12.8 Rewetting the extruded product gently with water from an air-water syringe.

filling the pocket much more difficult. Next, the exposed gel is gently but completely wetted with water or saline (Figure 12.6). (Do not use the air from the air-water syringe.) The water hardens (or plasticizes) the gel instantly. Following this step, the product is gently tapped into the sulcus (Figure 12.7). An instrument with sufficient surface area (i.e., a 3 mm elevator as opposed to a periodontal probe) is used to decrease the chances of inadvertent piercing of the product, which can result in its removal from the pocket. It is common for some of the subgingival product (which did not get wet) to extrude from the pocket. This gel will likely become stuck to the placing instrument and result in removal of the product. To avoid this scenario, as soon as any leakage is perceived, the filling instrument is removed and the exposed gel is rewetted (Figure 12.8) and compaction is reinitiated (Figure 12.9). These steps should be

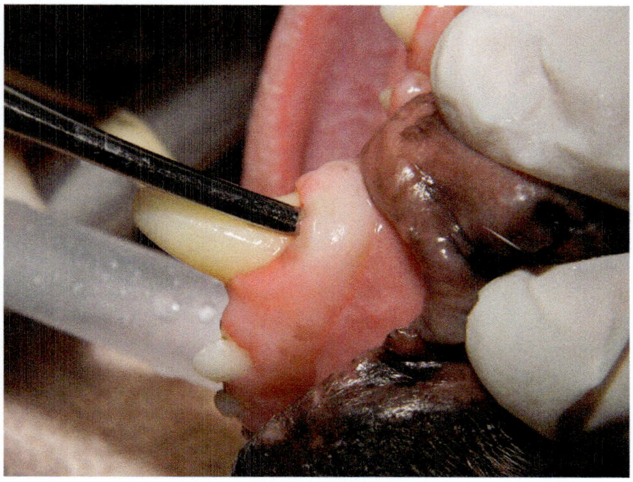

Figure 12.9 The tamping and wetting steps are repeated until the product is below the gingival margin.

Box 12.2 Key points

- Local antibiotics are an effective adjunct therapy to meticulous SRP.
- These products are best used in pockets between 3 and 5 mm (as pockets deeper than 5 mm require surgical therapy).
- Topical tetracycline products provide a high level of antimicrobial and anti-inflammatory effects directly where they are needed, without the systemic side effects.
- Doxycycline products are not licensed for use in felines.
- A helpful tip in the application of the veterinary labeled doxycycline product is to wet the gel early and often for more successful placement.
- The veterinary labelled clindamycin product is best applied to a dry tooth.

repeated until no product is visible above the gingival margin, which decreases the chances of the patient dislodging the product before natural dissolution.

To further avoid premature dislodgement of the product, the client should be advised to avoid brushing the areas where the product was placed for 4 weeks. The remainder of the mouth can be brushed normally. During this time, alternate forms of plaque control (chlorhexidine rinses or barrier sealants) should be utilized.

The patient should be rechecked 4–6 weeks after placement of the subgingival antibiotics, primarily to ensure that the surgical site is healing well with no inflammation. Additionally, it allows for a preliminary assessment of homecare and another opportunity for the practitioner to discuss continued care with the client.

Notes

A. Actisite, ALZA Corporation.
B. Arestin, OraPharma, Inc.
C. Atridox, TOLMAR, Inc.
D. PerioChip, Dexcel Pharma Technologies.
E. Periofilm, Molteni Farmaceutici.
F. Doxirobe, Pfizer Animal Health.
G. Clindorol, TriLogic Pharma.

References

1. Rapley JW, Cobb CM, Killoy WJ, Williams DR. Serum levels of tetracycline during treatment with tetracycline-containing fibers. J Periodontol. 63:817–820, 1992.
2. Ranadive KS, Bhat KM. Local antimicrobial delivery in periodontal therapy. Indian J Dent Res. 9(4):124–130, 1998.
3. Tonetti M, Cugini MA, Goodson JM. Zero-order delivery with periodontal placement of tetracycline-loaded ethylene vinyl acetate fibers. J Periodontal Res. 25(4):243–249, 1990.
4. Walker CB, Gordon JM, McQuilkin SJ, Niebloom TA, Socransky SS. Tetracycline: Levels achievable in gingival crevice fluid and in vitro effect on subgingival organisms. Part II. Susceptibilities of periodontal bacteria. J Periodontol. 52(10):613–616, 1981.
5. Gordon JM, Walker CB, Murphy JC, Goodson JM, Socransky SS. Tetracycline: Levels achievable in gingival crevice fluid and in vitro effect on subgingival organisms. Part I. Concentrations in crevicular fluid after repeated doses. J Periodontol. 52(10):609–612, 1981.
6. Goodson JM. Antimicrobial efficacy of Arestin in periodontitis therapy. Presented at the 35th Annual Meeting of the American Association for Dental Research, Orland, FL, March 8–11, 2006.
7. Walker CB, Gordon JM, McQuilkin SJ, Niebloom TA, Socransky SS. Tetracycline: Levels achievable in gingival crevice fluid and in vitro effect on subgingival organisms. Part II. Susceptibilities of periodontal bacteria. J Periodontol. 52(10):613–616, 1981.
8. Salvi GE, Mombelli A, Mayfield L, Rutar A, Suvan J, Garrett S, Lang NP. Local antimicrobial therapy after initial periodontal treatment. J Clin Periodontol. 29(6):540–550, 2002.
9. Skaleric U, Schara R, Medvescek M, Hanlon A, Doherty F, Lessem J. Periodontal treatment by Arestin and its effects on glycemic control in type 1 diabetes patients. J Int Acad Periodontol. 6 (4 Suppl):160–165, 2004.
10. Hellström MK, McClain PK, Schallhorn RG, Bellis L, Hanlon AL, Ramberg P. Local minocycline as an adjunct to surgical therapy in moderate to severe, chronic periodontitis. J Clin Periodontol. 35(6):525–531, 2008.
11. Ciancio SG, Cobb CM, Leung M. Tissue concentration and localization of tetracycline folowing site-specific tetracycline fiber therapy. J Periodontol. 63:849–853, 1992.
12. Goodson JM, Tanner A. Antibiotic resistance of the subgingival microbiota following local tetracycline therapy. Oral Microbiol Immunol. 7(2):113–117, 1992.
13. Pappalardo S, Baglio OA, Cappello C, Guarrera S, DeBenedittis M, Petruzzi M, Grassi RF. Local delivery of antimicrobial drugs in the treatment of chronic adult periodontitis. Minerva Stomatol. 55(11–12):655–661, 2006.
14. Preshaw PM, Ryan ME, Giannobile WV. Host modulation agents. In: Carranza's Clinical Periodontology. St. Louis: Saunders, 2006, pp. 813–827.
15. Dean JW, Branch-Mays GL, Hart TC, et al. Topically applied minocycline microspheres: Why it works. Compendium 24: 247–257, 2003.

16. Williams RC, Paquette DW, Offenbacher S, et al. Treatment of periodontitis by local administration of minocycline microspheres: A controlled trial. J Periodontol. 72:1535–1544, 2001.
17. Fleischer HC, Mellonig JT, Brayer WK, Gray JL, Barnett JD. Scaling and root planing efficacy in multirooted teeth. J Periodontol. 60(7):402–409, 1989.
18. Paquette DW, Hanlon A, Lessem J, Williams RC. Clinical relevance of adjunctive minocycline microspheres in patients with chronic periodontitis: Secondary analysis of a phase 3 trial. J Periodontol. 75:531–536, 2004.
19. Garrett S, Johnson L, Drisko CH, et al. Two multi-center studies evaluating locally delivered doxycycline hyclate, placebo control, oral hygiene, and scaling and root planing in the treatment of periodontitis. J Periodontol. 70:490–503, 1999.
20. Wennstrom JL, Newman HN, MacNeill SR, et al. Utilisation of locally delivered doxycyline in non-surgical treatment of chronic periodontitis. A comparative multi-center trial of 2 treatment approaches. J Clin Periodontol. 28:753–761, 2001.
21. Polson AP, et al. Periodontal pocket treatment in beagle dogs using subgingival doxycycline from a biodegradable system. J Periodontol. 67:1176–1184, 1996.
22. Zetner K, Rothmueller G. Treatment of periodontal pockets with doxycycline in beagles. Vet Ther. 3(4):441–452, 2002.
23. Jeffcoat MK, Bray KS, Ciancio SG, et al. Adjunctive use of a subgingival controlled-release chlorhexidine chip reduces probing depth and improves attachment level compared with scaling and root planing alone. J Periodontol. 69(9):989–997, 1998.
24. Hanes PJ, Purvis JP. Local anti-infective therapy: Pharmacological agents. A systematic review. Ann Periodontol. 8(1):79–98, 2003.
25. Martorelli de Lima AF, Cury CC, Palioto DB, Duro AM, da Silva RC, Wolff LF. Therapy with adjunctive doxycycline local delivery in patients with type 1 diabetes mellitus and periodontitis. J Clin Periodontol. 31:648–653, 2004.
26. ARESTIN (minocycline hydrochloride) 1 mg Microspheres [Prescribing Information]. Warminster, PA: OraPharma, Inc., 2005.
27. Garrett S, Johnson L, Drisko CH, et al. Two multi-center studies evaluating locally delivered doxycycline hyclate, placebo control, oral hygiene, and scaling and root planing in the treatment of periodontitis. J Periodontol. 70(5):490–503, 1999.
28. Drisko CH. The use of locally delivered doxycycline in the treatment of periodontitis. Clinical results. J Clin Periodontol. 25(11 Pt 2):947–952, 1998.
29. Garcia-Alvarez L, Oteo JA. Nonantimicrobial effects of tetracyclines. Rev Esp Quimioter. 23(1):4–11, 2010.
30. Greenwald RA, Simonson BG, Moak SA, Rush SW, Ramamurthy NS, Laskin RS, Golub LM. Inhibition of epiphyseal cartilage collagenase by tetracyclines in low phosphate rickets in rats. J Orthop Res. 6(5):695–703, 1988.
31. Golub LM, Goodson JM, Lee HM, Vidal AM, McNamara TF, Ramamurthy NS. Tetracyclines inhibit tissue collagenases. Effects of ingested low-dose and local delivery systems. J Periodontol. 56 (11 Suppl):93–97, 1985.
32. Golub LM, Wolff M, Lee HM, McNamara TF, Ramamurthy NS, Zambon J, Ciancio S. Further evidence that tetracyclines inhibit collagenase activity in human crevicular fluid and from other mammalian sources. J Periodontal Res. 20(1):12–23, 1985.
33. Sorsa T, Ingman T, Suomalainen K, Halinen S, Saari H, Konttinen YT, Uitto VJ, Golub LM. Cellular source and tetracycline-inhibition of gingival crevicular fluid collagenase of patients with labile diabetes mellitus. J Clin Periodontol. 19(2):146–149, 1992.
34. Sorsa T, Ding Y, Salo T, Lauhio A, Teronen O, Ingman T, Ohtani H, Andoh N, Takeha S, Konttinen YT. Effects of tetracyclines on neutrophil, gingival, and salivary collagenases. A functional and western-blot assessment with special reference to their cellular sources in periodontal diseases. Ann NY Acad Sci. 732:112–131, 1994.
35. Webster G, Del Rosso JQ. Anti-inflammatory activity of tetracyclines. Dermatol Clin. 25(2):133–135, 2007.
36. Golub LM, Lee HM, Ryan ME, Giannobile WV, Payne J, Sorsa T. Tetracyclines inhibit connective tissue breakdown by multiple non-antimicrobial mechanisms. Adv Dent Res. 12:12–26, 1998.
37. Guerin C, Laterra J, Masnyk T, Golub LM, Brem H, et al. Selective endothelial growth inhibition by tetracyclines that inhibit collagenase. Biochem Biophys Res Commun. 188:740–745, 1992.
38. Boyle JR, McDermott E, Crowther M, Wills AD, Bell PR, Thompson MM. Doxycycline inhibits elastin degradation and reduces metalloproteinase activity in a model of aneurismal disease. J Vasc Surg. 27:354–361, 1998.
39. Solomon A, Rosenblatt M, Li DQ, et al. Doxycycline inhibition of interleukin-1 in the corneal epithelium. Invest Ophth Vis Sci. 41:2544–2557, 2000.
40. Krakauer T, Buckley M. Doxycycline is anti-inflammatory and inhibits Staphylococcal exotoxin-indued cytokines and chemokines. Anitimicrob Agents Chemother. 47:3630–3633, 2003.
41. Pirila E, Parikka M, Ramamurthy NS, et al. Chemically modified tetracycline (CMT-8) and oestrogen promote wound healing in ovariectomised rats, effects on matrix metalloproteinase-2 membrane type1 matrixmetalloproteinase, and laminin-5 gamma2-chain. Wound Repair Regen. 10:38–51, 2002.
42. Gapski R, Barr JL, Sarment DP, Layher MG, Socransky SS, Giannobile WV. Effect of systemic matrix metalloproteinase inhibition on periodontal wound repair, a proof of concept trial. J Periodontol. 75:493–494, 2004.
43. Holmes SG, Still K, Buttle DJ, Bishop NJ, Grabowski PS. Chemically modified tetracyclines act through multiple mechanisms directly on osteoclast precursors. Bone 35: 471–478, 2004.
44. Caffesse RG, Sweeney PL, Smith BA. Scaling and root planing with and without periodontal flap surgery. J Clin Periodontol. 13(3):205–210, 1986.
45. Perry DA, Schmid MO, Takei HH. Phase I periodontal therapy. In: Carranza's Clinical Periodontology. St. Louis: Saunders, 2006, pp. 722–727.
46. Zetner K, Rothmueller G. Treatment of periodontal pockets with doxycycline in beagles. Vet Ther. 3(4):441–452, 2002.
47. Carranza FA, Takei HH. Phase II periodontal therapy. In: Carranza's Clinical Periodontology. St. Louis: Saunders, 2006, pp. 881–886.
48. Bellows J. Periodontal equipment, materials, and techniques. In: Small Animal Dental Equipment, Materials, and Techniques, a Primer. Ames, IA: Blackwell, 2004, pp. 115–173.
49. Doxirobe, Pfizer Animal Health, Exton, PA, package insert.
50. Niemiec BA. Periodontal disease. Top Companion Anim Med. 23(2):72–80, 2008.

13

Home plaque control

Introduction

Homecare is a *critical* aspect of periodontal therapy. The initial phase of plaque accumulation is pellicle formation on the surface of the teeth, which starts within *nansoeconds* of a prophylaxis.[1] In addition, true bacterial plaque colonizes clean tooth surfaces within 24 hours of cleaning.[2,3] Finally, without homecare, gingival infection and inflammation quickly recurs.[4–8] In fact, one author emphatically states, "Forty years of experimental research, clinical trials, and demonstration projects in different geographical and social settings have confirmed that effective removal of dental plaque is essential to dental and periodontal health throughout life".[9] Furthermore, it was found in a human review that professional cleanings were of little value without homecare.[10]

With regards to established disease, a recent study found that periodontal pockets become reinfected within 2 weeks of a prophylaxis if homecare is not performed.[6] This same study showed that pocket depth returns to pretreatment depths within 6 weeks of therapy. Therefore, the performance of advanced periodontal procedures for clients who can/will not perform homecare on their pets is of dubious value.

Homecare discussion/instructions

The benefits of routine homecare must be conveyed to each client on a regular basis. Dental care (including homecare) should be discussed with clients on their *first visit* to the practice, which is often the well puppy/kitten or vaccination visit.[2] This client education is of much greater benefit if it comes from the entire staff.[2] The early institution of homecare not only leads to the greatest benefit, it also makes the introduction to the pet and training easier. The importance of homecare should be discussed again following each dental cleaning with detailed instructions provided. Finally, the client's intention and ability to perform consistent homecare should be confirmed prior to performing advanced periodontal procedures. With consistency, home plaque control will slow the progression of periodontal disease and greatly improve periodontal health. However, it will not eliminate the need for professional cleanings.[11]

Goals of home plaque control

The primary goal of home plaque control is to limit or reduce the amount of plaque on the teeth.[12] This in turn should decrease the level of gingival inflammation and ultimately periodontal disease.

Keep this in mind when reviewing various homecare options and when discussing them with clients. Information on the suitability of different methods for marginal and subgingival plaque control is covered along with their descriptions below.

Brushing is *by far* the most effective means to mechanically remove plaque.[11] Chew-based products can be effective if properly formulated (see below). However, oral sprays, rinses, and water additives are

Box 13.1 Key clinical point

It is important to note that *supra*gingival plaque and calculus has little to no effect on periodontal disease. It is the plaque at the gingival margin and in the *sub*gingival area that creates inflammation and initiates periodontal disease.[13–15] Therefore, controlling the plaque at and below the gingival margin is the key to maintaining periodontal health.

Veterinary Periodontology, First Edition. Brook A. Niemiec.

generally an insufficient means of plaque control, due to the tenacity with which plaque adheres to the teeth, and the increased resistance of the plaque biofilm to antiseptics (which is reported to be up to 500,000 times that of singular bacteria[16]).[1]

Types of homecare

The two major types of home plaque control are active and passive. Both types can be effective if performed correctly and consistently, but active homecare is currently the gold standard. Active homecare involves the participation of the pet's owner, such as brushing or rinsing. Passive methods are typically based on chewing behaviors via treats or specially formulated diets. It has been shown that active homecare is most effective on the rostral teeth (incisors and canines).[17] In contrast, passive homecare (chew-based) is more effective on the distal teeth (premolars and molars).[17,18] This difference is intuitive because the front teeth are easier for clients to access, while passive homecare is more effective on the distal teeth, where chewing occurs. In addition, water and food additives are also currently available.

Active homecare

Active homecare is defined as the client actively participating in the removal of plaque from the tooth surface. This can be achieved either by brushing or rinsing/applying antiseptic/antiplaque solutions.

Tooth brushing

When properly performed, tooth brushing has been proven to be the most effective means of plaque control.[11] Therefore, it should be the goal of all veterinarians to promote tooth brushing for all of their patients by educating their clients.

Materials and methods for tooth brushing

Brushes (Figure 13.1)

The only critical piece of equipment necessary is a tooth brush. There are numerous veterinary brushes available,[A] and a proper brush should be selected based on patient size. Double- and triple-sided[B,C] as well as circular feline brushes[D] are effective products and should be considered along with the standard veterinary brushes depending on patient size and temperament. This author does not recommend the "finger brushes" as they do not effectively address the subgingival areas of the teeth, which are the most important areas to clean, and they increase the chances of the owner being bitten. Gauze and washcloths are not recommended for the same reasons.[19]

In addition to the veterinary products, human tooth brushes may be substituted. A soft-bristled tooth brush is always recommended. A child's tooth brush is often the correct size for small patients and may be more effective than the larger veterinary version. An infant brush may work best for toy breed dogs, cats, or juvenile patients.

An important point to consider is the degree of contamination that accumulates on the bristles of a tooth brush. This infection (viral and bacterial) multiplies on the brush and is then reintroduced into the mouth.[20–22] This is NOT to suggest that brushing should be abandoned, rather that brushes should not be shared between pets and should be changed regularly.

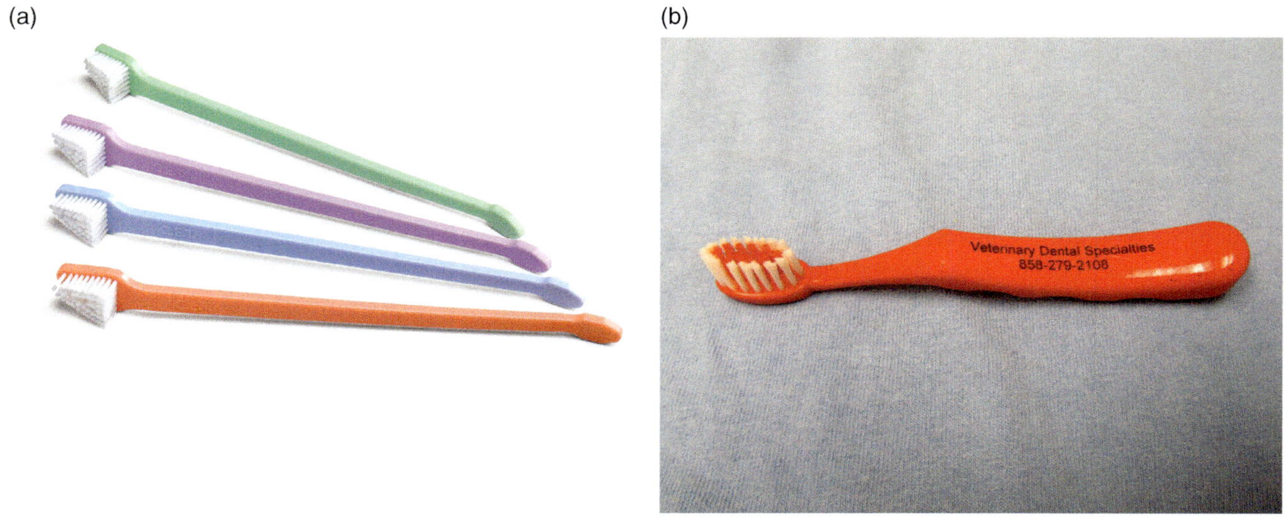

Figure 13.1 Various standard tooth brushes: (a) Double-ended canine tooth brush[A], (b) small, soft tooth brush that is personalized with the clinic information.

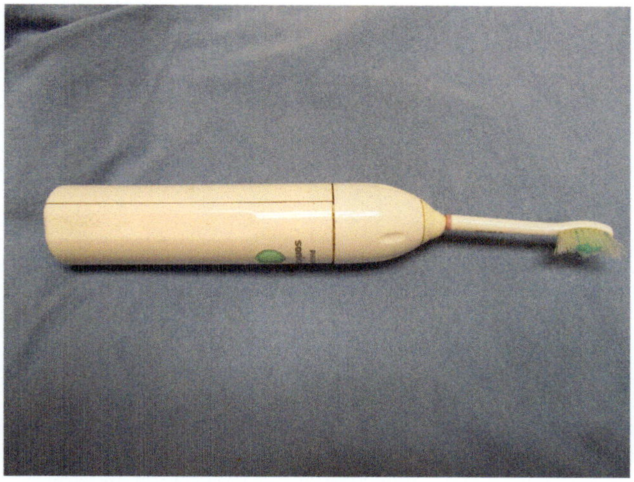

Figure 13.2 Human sonic tooth brush.

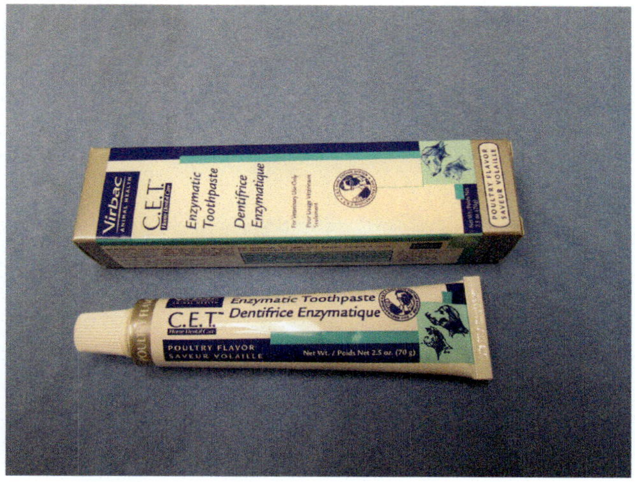

Figure 13.3 Veterinary toothpaste.

Mechanized (sonic[E] and rotary[F]) brushes (Figure 13.2) have been shown to be superior to standard brushes in human studies.[23,24] In addition to the numerous human product options, there is currently a mechanized veterinary brush available.[G] These products are likely superior for use in veterinary patients as well and should make the process more time efficient, which is important in animal patients for acceptance reasons. The only negative aspect to these brushes is that the movement/vibration of these instruments can feel awkward and/or may scare the patients.[19] Therefore, mechanized brushes should only be used on patients with accepting temperament. This author recommends initiating brushing very slowly with a standard tooth brush, and then potentially progressing to a mechanical type after acceptance of the standard brush is achieved.

Pastes (Figure 13.3)

There are a number of veterinary toothpastes available,[H] which greatly increase the acceptance of the tooth brush by the pet. Toothpastes typically contain a calcium chelator[I] that has been shown to decrease the level of calculus deposits on the teeth.[25-27] It is important to note, however, that calculus itself is largely non-pathogenic.[2] As such, the paste is not a significant player in the reduction of plaque and gingivitis. The mechanical removal of plaque by the movement of the brush/instrument is the key to control.[11] Consequently, palatability can be increased by using alternate flavorings.[2,28] Tuna juice (especially for cats), garlic powder, and beef broth are all excellent means of increasing palatability, as is dipping the brush in the patient's favorite canned food. This author recommends these options be used initially, and the additional benefits of the pastes be added once acceptance of brushing is achieved.

Antimicrobial preparations[J] (see "Antiseptic Rinses" below) are also available. These products will improve plaque and gingivitis control beyond that of pastes when used with brushing, and therefore should be considered instead of toothpaste in high-risk patients and in cases of established periodontal disease.[29-34] Human toothpastes and products such as baking soda (sodium bicarbonate) are *not* recommended as they contain detergents or fluoride that may cause gastric upset or fluorosis if swallowed.[2,28]

Brushing technique

The ideal technique to safely and effectively initiate tooth brushing in veterinary patients is described in the following text.[2,19] Keep in mind, however, that the ideal technique may only be possible in the most agreeable patients. Clients should be encouraged to work toward this level of care but to accept any degree of homecare success as valuable. Forcing homecare on a patient is counterproductive and may decrease the client-animal bond.[19] Similarly, coercing clients too harshly may drive them away from your practice.[19] Therefore, as with everything, balance is critical.

The keys to compliance with brushing can be stated as follows. First, start early, because young patients are more amenable to training.[19] Second, go slow; start with just holding the mouth and then progress to a finger and finally start brushing slowly. Next, be consistent; make this a learned behavior. And finally, make it positive; using food, treats, or playtime as a reward will greatly increase the likelihood of acceptance. While brushing prior to eating is counterintuitive, it is actually perfectly acceptable. In humans we are brushing mainly for cavity control, while in animals it is primarily for periodontal disease control. It is an important point to ensure that

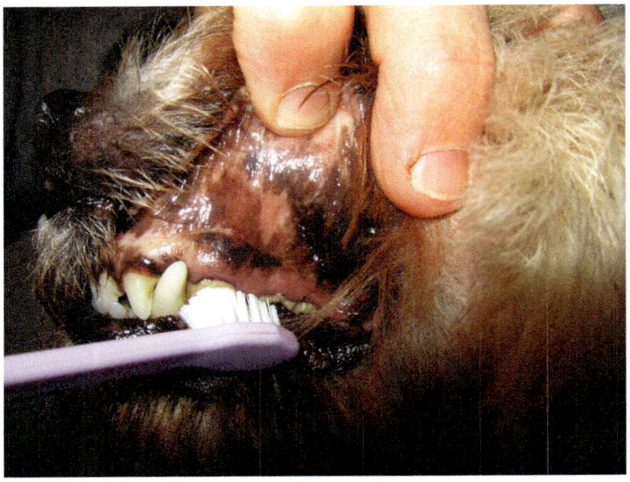

Figure 13.4 Proper position of the brush against the tooth.

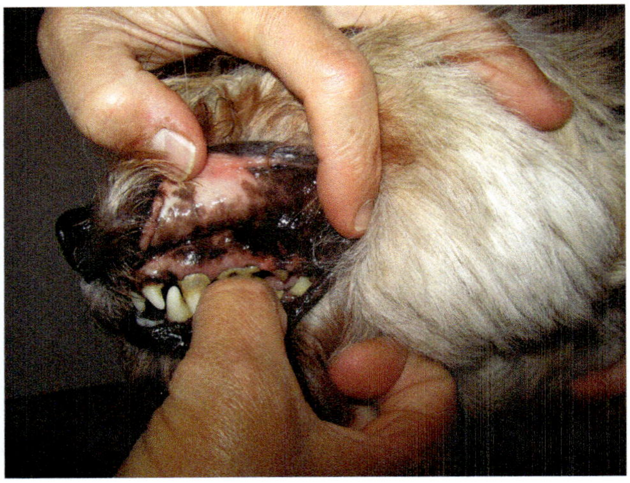

Figure 13.6 Placing a finger behind the canines to allow access to the mandibular cheek teeth.

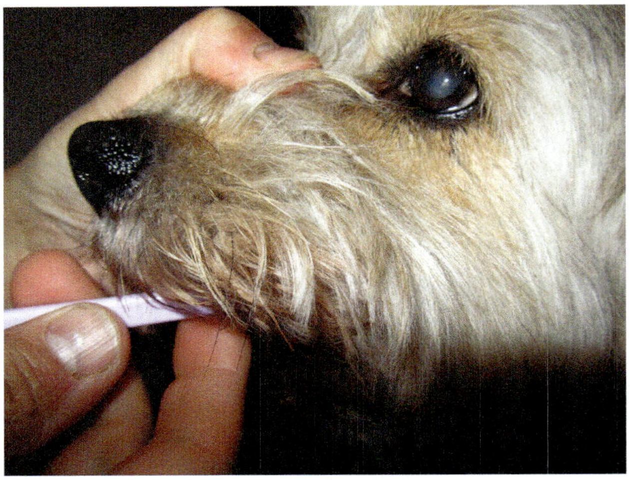

Figure 13.5 Brushing the buccal surface of the distal teeth.

the patient's temperament is acceptable for this process. Advise your clients that getting bitten is not worth it.[19]

Proper tooth brushing technique begins with the brush held at a 45-degree angle to the long axis of the tooth (Figure 13.4). The brush is then placed at the gingival margin and moved along the arcades utilizing a rotary motion. The buccal surfaces of the teeth are the most accessible and fortunately are the most important, as these are the surfaces that generally have higher levels of calculus deposition. Make sure to counsel owners not to attempt to open the pet's mouth on initiation of this procedure. Most veterinary patients greatly dislike their mouth being forced open, and this approach may result in increased resistance. Instead, clients should be instructed to begin by effectively brushing the buccal surfaces with the mouth closed (Figure 13.5). The distal teeth can be accessed by gently inserting the brush inside the cheek to reach these teeth, relying on tactile feel and experience to ensure proper positioning.

If the patient is amenable and tractable, the client should progress to caring for the palatal/lingual surfaces of the teeth. These surfaces *must* be treated if periodontal surgery has been performed on them. This is most common in cases of deep vertical/angular pockets on the palatal surfaces of the maxillary canine teeth (especially in chondrodystrophic breeds). To open the mouth, begin by placing the thumb of the non-dominant hand behind the mandibular canines (Figure 13.6). This allows for some leverage and is also the safest place in the mouth.

The 2-week postsurgical recheck is an excellent time to provide homecare instructions to your clients. This will make it more effective but also reinforce that you believe it is important. Having a technician demonstrate proper brushing procedures is an ideal technique. More detailed homecare instructions are available at www.dogbeachdentistry.com.

Regarding the frequency of brushing, once a day is ideal, as this level of care is required to stay ahead of plaque formation.[2,28] Furthermore, every other day brushing was not found to be effective at gingivitis control.[35] Three days a week is considered the *minimum* frequency for patients *in good oral health*.[36] Brushing once a week is not considered sufficient to maintain good oral health. For patients with established periodontal disease (even gingivitis), daily brushing is required to maintain oral health, and twice daily may be recommended.[2,28,35,37–39] Finally, it should be noted that consistency with homecare is critical. If brushing is suspended for as little as a month, the level of gingival inflammation will return to the same level as patients with no therapy.[40]

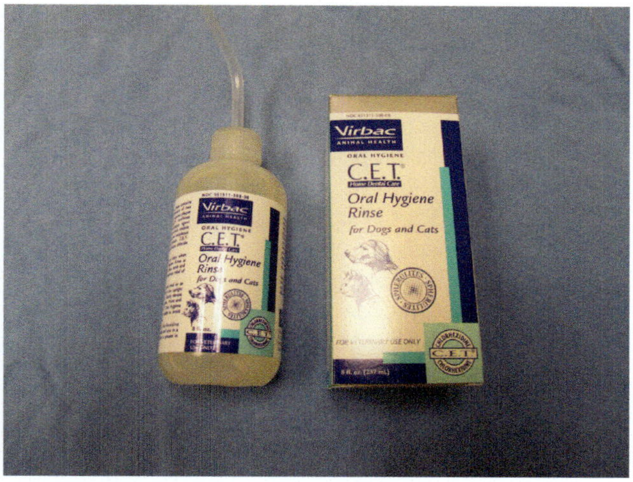

Figure 13.7 Veterinary-labelled chlorhexidine solution.

Antiseptic rinses

The other option for active homecare is the application of antiseptic/antiplaque solutions. There are numerous products available and it is recommended that veterinary professionals review the literature to determine for themselves whether or not to recommend a particular product.[41] It is best to evaluate the research behind product claims and not simply read the marketing hype. An invaluable tool for the busy practitioner is the Veterinary Oral Health Council (VOHC). This group of veterinary dentists have evaluated the research and given a seal of approval to worthy products. A list of these can be found on the website www.vohc.org. Remember, however, that the seal may be given for plaque and/or calculus control, which may or may not correlate with decreased periodontal disease. Below is a description of several products that this author recommends based on his review of the literature. This discussion is not comprehensive and new information/products are continually available.

The traditional antiseptic of choice is chlorhexidine (Figure 13.7).[K,L] The method of action for this product is that it disrupts the bacterial cell walls and penetrates the cells, creating a precipitation of the cytoplasm.[42] There is no known method of bacterial resistance to this product, and it is very safe.[41,43] Chlorhexidine has been shown in numerous studies to decrease gingivitis if applied consistently over time.[29–32,34,44–49] Chlorhexidine reportedly has a quick onset and minimal systemic uptake, making it an excellent choice for oral disinfection.[50] An additional benefit of this product is that it maintains antiseptic effects for up to 7 hours after application.[51–53] Furthermore, it appears that the 0.2% strength products may be superior to the 0.12% solutions and should be considered in cases of established periodontal disease.[54]

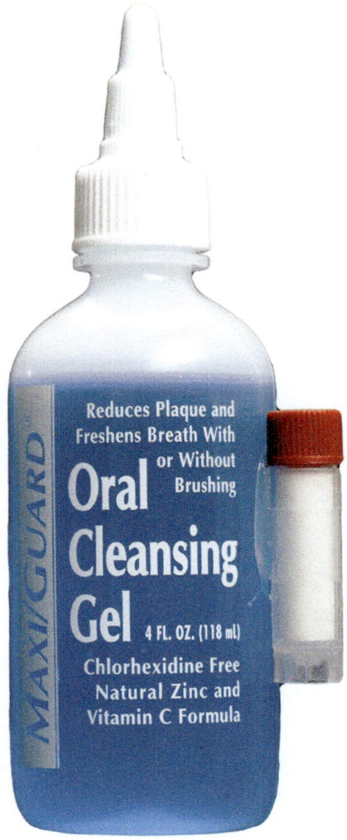

Figure 13.8 Commercial zinc ascorbate gel.

This author has seen good clinical results when clients are able to consistently apply these products. One concern with the use of these products is the lack of palatability, which may hinder homecare efforts.[19] Finally, chronic use of chlorhexidine has been shown to cause dental staining.[19,55] The staining is reversible and can be polished off, and this author has not actually seen it in an animal patient.

Proper application of these products requires only a small amount of the solution be used. Ideally, the rinse should be directly applied to the surface of the teeth and gingiva. In most cases, however, getting the solution between the cheek and teeth is the best the client can achieve. Although this is not ideal, it is better than no therapy.

An additional option for home oral care is the use of soluble zinc salts (Figure 13.8). In vitro studies showed that these products can be effective in decreasing viable plaque biomass.[56] One veterinary-labelled oral zinc ascorbate gel[M] has been proven to decrease plaque and gingivitis,[57] and it provides the additional advantage of being tasteless (which should improve acceptance, especially in cats). Furthermore, this product also contains ascorbic acid, shown to support/induce collagen synthesis,[19,58–60] which may improve healing following dental scaling and/or oral surgery.

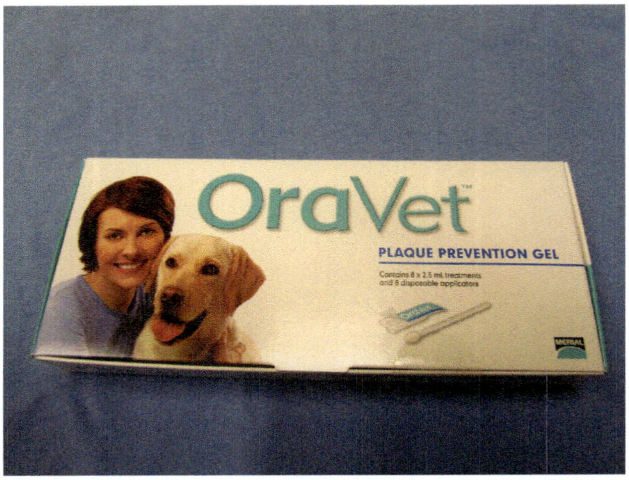

Figure 13.9 Barrier sealant.

> **Box 13.2** The validity of pet food claims
>
> In regards to marketing claims, it is critical to note that AAFCO (Association of American Feed Control Officials) regulations do *not* allow prevention or treatment claims for dental disease. However, manufacturers can claim that the mechanical actions of food products "cleanse, freshen, or whiten teeth" *without* any evidence of efficacy![64] Furthermore, the U.S. Food and Drug Administration Center for Veterinary Medicine has decided that if a product claims to be effective in "plaque or tartar reduction or prevention, or control of breath odor . . . only with respect to the product's abrasive action, enforcement would be a low priority."[64] Therefore, current regulations under AAFCO are inadequate for determining the effectiveness of a dental product.[65]

Barrier sealants

A final option for active homecare is the application of a commercially available barrier sealant[N] (Figure 13.9). This product works by changing the electrostatic charge of the teeth and creates a hydrophobic surface that is designed to prevent plaque attachment.[61] This has been shown to decrease the accumulation of plaque and calculus.[62] There are currently no published studies that prove effectiveness of these barrier sealants against gingivitis or periodontal disease. However, this author has anecdotally seen some positive effects, likely due to its placement at the gingival margin. It should be noted, however, that not all veterinary dentists support its use.[63] The review of this product using evidence-based means supports the use of the professional application but not the homecare version.[41] Therefore, it appears that barrier sealants may be most promising as a treatment in the postoperative phase, until the mouth is healed, inflammation resolves, and a more established means of homecare (such as brushing) can be instituted.

Passive homecare

Passive homecare is an alternative for minimizing periodontal disease and is achieved with special diets, chews, and treats and potentially water additives. Some of these methods are effective, but many are not. Some of the effective products are detailed below; however, there is not enough room here for a complete discussion of all products. Practitioners should perform their own research and utilize the VOHC to form proper client recommendations, rather than simply reading the marketing hype.

Since passive homecare requires no work by the owner, compliance is more likely. Compliance is especially important since long-term consistency is the key factor in the efficacy of home dental care.[66] It has been shown that the compliance rate with tooth brushing with *highly motivated* pet owners is only around 50% after 6 months.[67] In fact, one study showed that passive homecare may be superior to active homecare simply due to the fact that it is actually performed.[68] This should *not* be misconstrued to mean that it is more effective, just that the average client is poorly compliant.

The downfall of all chew-based passive homecare products involves the fact that pets typically do not chew with the entire mouth and therefore areas will be missed. Passive homecare is most effective on the carnassial and surrounding teeth, and in contrast, active homecare is superior for the incisor and canine teeth.[17] Therefore, a combination of active and passive homecare is best.

Tartar control diets

It has long been thought that traditional dry dog food is good for oral health, and one study appeared to support these claims.[69] However, an additional study showed that dry food was *not* superior to moist foods in regards to improving oral health.[70] There are, however, several prescription diets available that do decrease tartar and plaque buildup.[71] These products employ abrasives to scrape the teeth free of plaque. Additionally, the individual kibbles of these therapeutic diets tend to be larger than standard pet food[25,68] (Figure 13.10). This increases the amount of chewing performed and the efficacy of the abrasive aspects.[65] Many of the products also contain a calcium chelator[O] to further reduce dental calculus.[25–27,72,73] Finally, one product has added green tea polyphenols[P] (which are purported to be antibacterial) for an additional layer of defense.[74,75] These studies may support a larger role for nutraceuticals in the near future (see chapter 20). However, some studies have reported that it is the kibble size and not any antimicrobials that improve oral health,[76] and therefore further studies are needed. Numerous

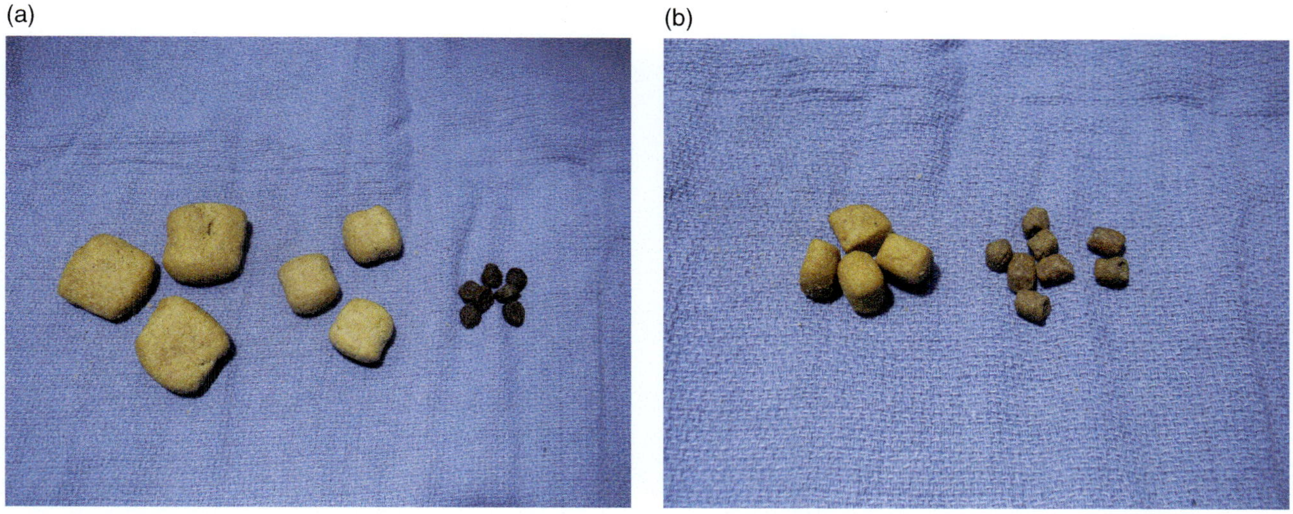

Figure 13.10 Commercially available dental diet, demonstrating size difference between a "dental diet" (Hill's Science Diet t/d) and a standard kibble. (a) From left: Canine t/d, Canine t/d "small bites," standard kibble. (b) Left: Feline t/d; right: standard kibble.

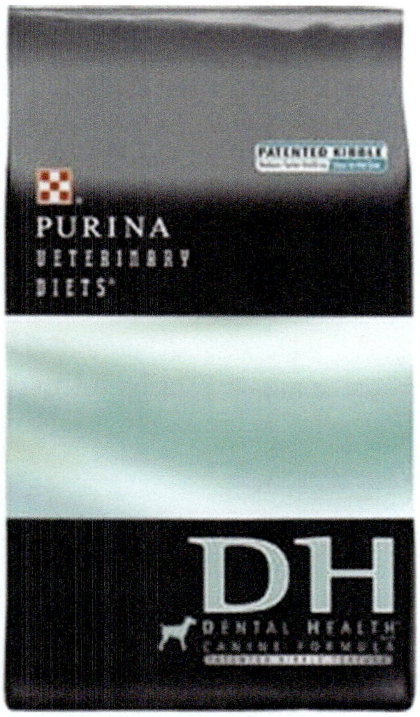

Figure 13.11 Canine "dental diet."

products have received the VOHC seal as effective in tartar (and in some cases plaque) reduction.[77,Q–U] One important point is that even though these products may decrease plaque and calculus, they are typically most effective on the areas around the cusp tips and not at the gingival margin.[72] Remember, supragingival plaque and calculus is generally non-pathogenic, and therefore minimal control of gingivitis is gained by calculus control.[41] Of the available diets, only one[v] has been clinically proven to decrease gingivitis (Figure 13.11).[78–80] The main reason for this product's effectiveness lies in the fiber arrangement within the kibble. This arrangement requires the tooth to fully enter the kibble prior to it breaking apart, allowing the entire tooth (including the marginal area) to be cleaned. The addition of antioxidants in this diet may also be beneficial.

Raw diets

It is widely believed that "raw" diets are effective at maintaining oral health. However, there are no current studies that document this benefit.[65] In fact, one study reported similar incidence of periodontal disease between African wild dogs when compared with domestic canines.[81] Furthermore, similar studies on feral cats whose diet consisted mostly of birds reported a similar level of periodontal disease as domestic felines on commercial pet food.[82,83] Therefore, until controlled, peer-reviewed studies are available, these diets should not be prescribed for improving dental health.

Tartar control treats

There are numerous treats available for passive homecare, the original and most common being the biscuit-style treats. Plain biscuits have not been shown to aid in the reduction of periodontal disease.[41] A better choice appears to be biscuits coated with HMP, although there are studies that support and detract from their efficacy as well.[84,85]

Over the last few years several new edible treats with varying efficacy have been brought to market. Many of the studies are unpublished; however, there are several products with VOHC approval in this class (Figure 13.12).[W,X,Y]

The most prevalent and proven effective products in this class are the rask type and rawhide chews (Figure 13.13).[73,86] These products work similarly to

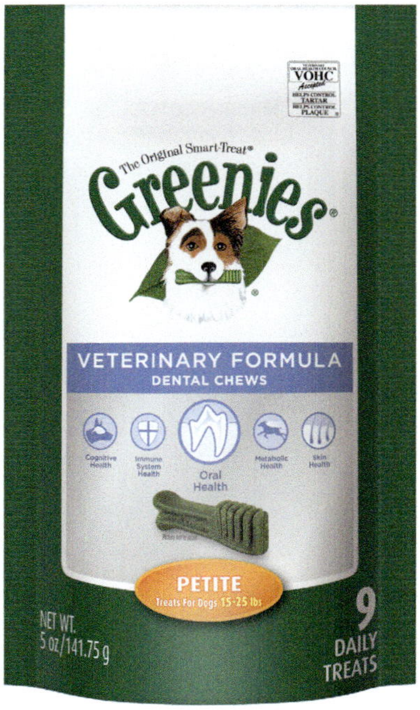

Figure 13.12 Commercial dental health treat.

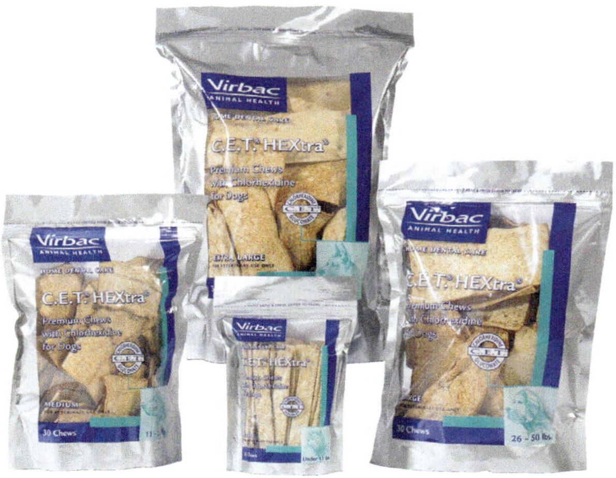

Figure 13.13 Commercial rawhide chews with added chlorhexidine.

tartar control diets, with the abrasives cleaning the tooth surface, but additionally may include calcium chelators (such as sodium hexametaphosphate) or other substances to further increase their antiplaque efficacy.[87] However, the addition of chlorhexidine was not found to further increase the efficacy of rawhide chews.[76] As with the diets discussed above, however, most of the beneficial effect is supragingival and on the cheek teeth. Of the available products, only a handful[Z,AA,BB] have been clinically proven to decrease gingivitis.[76,87–90] VOHC approval has been awarded to several of these products as well.[CC,DD]

Box 13.3 Key points

- Daily homecare is recommended since plaque accumulates in 24 hours.
- Without homecare, the efficacy of professional periodontal therapy is severely limited.
- Tooth brushing is the gold standard and is most effective on rostral teeth.
- Passive homecare methods may or may not be effective, and any provided benefit will be mainly on the distal teeth.
- A combination of active and passive methods is likely the best choice.
- Look for the VOHC seal on dental homecare products.

One important point to remember is that many chew treats that claim to help control dental disease are very hard in texture. The chewing of these products may (and often does) result in tooth fracture. A good rule of thumb is that if you cannot make an indentation into the product with your fingernail, it is too hard. Also, just because a product is effective for dental disease does not necessarily mean it is safe. Owners must be aware of the choking/obstructive possibilities of many treats. For this reason the VOHC has recently modified its requirements to include evidence of safety as well.

Water additives

This is a relatively new area of home dental care, and there are several products available in this category.[EE] While there are some studies on the human side that found that the active ingredients have some efficacy,[44,91] there is currently minimal to no peer-reviewed evidence that supports their use in controlling periodontal disease in veterinary patients. One product with xylitol[FF] was shown to decrease plaque and calculus in one study,[92] but the potential negative systemic effects of the product (possible hypoglycemia and liver derangement)[93–95] must be weighed against the possible oral benefit. There is one product,[GG] however, that does have unpublished data[96] supporting plaque control and has been accepted by the VOHC despite the lack of publication.

Conclusions

Homecare is a critical aspect of periodontal therapy, but it is often ignored. Early and consistent client education is the key to compliance. There are numerous options available, but tooth brushing remains the gold standard. Of the numerous products available for passive homecare, only a few are truly effective, and the reader is urged to critically review the clinical studies when deciding which products to endorse.

Notes

A. CET Dual-Ended Toothbrush, Virbac Animal Health.
B. Triple-Pet EZ Dog Toothbrush.
C. Quadbrush Cat Toothbrush.
D. CET Cat Toothbrush, Virbac Animal Health.
E. Sonicare toothbrush, Phillips.
F. Oral B Vitality toothbrush, Braun.
G. Sonic Canine Premium Pet toothbrush.
H. CET Enzymatic Toothpaste, Virbac Animal Health.
I. Sodium hexametaphosphate.
J. CET Oral Hygiene Rinse, Virbac Animal Health.
K. Nolvadent, Fort Dodge Animal Health.
L. CET Oral Hygiene Rinse, Virbac Animal Health.
M. Maxiguard oral hygiene gel, Addison Biological Laboratory.
N. Oravet, Merial Limited.
O. Sodium hexametaphosphate.
P. Royal Canin DD.
Q. Oral Care canine and feline, Hill's Pet Nutrition.
R. Chunk Dental Defense Diet for Dogs, Iams.
S. Eukanuba Adult Maintenance Diet for Dogs, Iams.
T. Purina Veterinary Diets DH Dental Health brand Canine and Feline Formulas, Purina Nestle Purina Petcare Company.
U. Friskies Feline Dental Diet, Purina Nestle Purina Petcare Company.
V. Prescription Diet Canine and Feline t/d, Hill's Pet Nutrition.
W. BlueChews, Vetradent Inc.
X. Canine Greenies, all sizes and formulations (lite, senior).
Y. Bright Bites and Checkups Chews for Dogs, Diamond Foods, Inc.
Z. CET hexachews, Virbac Animal Health.
AA. Pedigree Rask/Dentabone, Mars.
BB. Tartar Shield Soft Rawhide Chews for Dogs, Therametric Technologies, Inc.
CC. Purina Veterinary Diets Dental Chews brand Canine Treats, Purina Nestle Purina Petcare Company.
DD. Friskies Cheweez Beefhide Treats, Friskies Co., Purina Nestle Purina Petcare Company.
EE. Oxyfresh, Oxyfresh Worldwide.
FF. Aquadent, Virbac Animal Health.
GG. Healthymouth.

References

1. Quirynen M, Teughels W, Kinder Haake S, Newman MG. Microbiology of periodontal diseases. In: Carranza's Clinical Periodontology. St. Louis: Saunders, 2006, pp. 134–169.
2. Wiggs RB, Lobprise HB. Periodontology. In: Veterinary Dentistry, Principles and Practice. Philadelphia: Lippincott-Raven, 1997, pp. 186–231.
3. Boyce EN, Ching RJ. Logan EI. Hunt JH. Maseman DC. Gaeddert KL. King CT. Reid EE. Hefferren JJ. Occurrence of gram-negative black-pigmented anaerobes in subgingival plaque during the development of canine periodontal disease. Clin Infect Dis. 20 Suppl 2:S317–9, 1995.
4. Debowes LJ. Problems with the gingiva. In: Small Animal Dental, Oral and Maxillofacial Disease, a Color Handbook (Niemiec BA ed.). London: Manson, 2010, pp. 159–181.
5. Fiorellini JP, Ishikawa SO, Kim DM. Clinical features of gingivitis. In: Carranza's Clinical Periodontology. St. Louis: Saunders, 2006, pp. 362–372.
6. Rober M. Effect of scaling and root planing without dental homecare on the subgingival microbiota. Proceedings of the 16th European Congress of Veterinary Dentistry, 2007, pp. 28–30.
7. Corba NH, Jansen J, Pilot T. Artificial periodontal defects and frequency of tooth brushing in beagle dogs (II). Clinical findings after a period of healing. J Clin Periodontol. 13(3):186–189, 1986.
8. Payne WA, Page RC, Olgolvie AL, et al. Histopathologic features of the initial and early stages of experimental gingivitis in man. J Periodontal Res. 10:51, 1975.
9. Proceedings of the European Workshop on Mechanical Plaque Control, Chicago, 1998.
10. Needleman I, Suvan J, Moles DR, Pimlott J. A systematic review of professional mechanical plaque removal for prevention of periodontal diseases. J Clin Periodontol. 32 Suppl 6:229–282, 2005.
11. Hale FA. Home care for the veterinary dental patient. J Vet Dent. 20(1):52–54, 2003.
12. Perry DA. Plaque control for the periodontal patient. In: Carranza's Clinical Periodontology. St. Louis: Saunders, 2006, pp. 728–748.
13. Westfelt E, Rylander H, Dahlen G, Lindhe J. The effect of supragingival plaque control on the progression of advanced periodontal disease. J Clin Periodontol. 25(7):536–541, 1998.
14. Niemiec BA. Periodontal therapy. Top Companion Anim Med. 23(2):81–90, 2008.
15. Harvey CE, Emily PP. Periodontal disease. In: Small Animal Dentistry. St. Louis: Mosby, 1993, pp. 89–144.
16. Williams JE. Microbial contamination of dental lines. In: Current and Future Trends in Veterinary Dentistry: Proceedings of the Upjohn Worldwide Companion Animal Veterinary Dental Forum, 1995, pp. 8–11.
17. Capik I. Periodontal health vs. different preventative means in toy breeds—clinical study. Proceedings of the 16th European Congress of Veterinary Dentistry, 2007, pp. 31–34.
18. Bjone S, Brown W, Harris A, Genity PM. Influence of chewing on dental health in dogs. Proceedings of the 16th European Congress of Veterinary Dentistry, 2007, pp. 45–46.
19. Holmstrom SE, Frost P, Eisner ER. Dental prophylaxis. In: Veterinary Dental Techniques. 2nd ed. Philadelphia: Saunders, 1998, pp.133–166.
20. Bunetel L, Tricot-Doleux S, Agnani G, Bonnaure-Mallet M. In vitro evaluation of the retention of three species of pathogenic microorganisms by three different types of toothbrush. Oral Microbiol Immunol. 15(5):313–316, 2000.
21. Wetzel WE, Schaumburg C, Ansari F, Kroeger T, Sziegoleit A. Microbial contamination of toothbrushes with different principles of filament anchoring. J Am Dent Assoc. 136(6):758–765, 2005.
22. Glass RT, Martin ME, Peter LJ. Transmission of disease in dogs by toothbrushing. Quintessence Int. 20(11):819–824, 1989.
23. Moritis K, Jenkins W, Hefti A, Schmitt P, McGrady M. A randomized, parallel design study to evaluate the effects of a Sonicare and a manual toothbrush on plaque and gingivitis. J Clin Dent. 19(2):64–68, 2008.
24. Deery C, Heanue M, Deacon S, Robinson PG, Walmsley AD, Worthington H, Shaw W, Glenny AM. The effectiveness of manual versus powered toothbrushes for dental health: A systematic review. J Dent. 2004 Mar;32(3):197–211.
25. Hennet P, Servet E, Soulard Y, Biourge V. Effect of pellet food size and polyphosphates in preventing calculus accumulation in dogs. J Vet Dent. 24(4):236–239, 2007.
26. Liu H, Segreto VA, Baker RA, Vastola KA, Ramsey LL, Gerlach RW. Anticalculus efficacy and safety of a novel whitening dentifrice containing sodium hexametaphosphate: A controlled six-month clinical trial. J Clin Dent. 13(1):25–28, 2002.
27. White DJ, Cox ER, Suszcynskymeister EM, Baig AA. In vitro studies of the anticalculus efficacy of a sodium hexametaphosphate whitening dentifrice. J Clin Dent. 13(1):33–37, 2002.

28. Niemiec BA. Periodontal disease. Top Companion Anim Med. 23(2):72–80, 2008.
29. Maruniak J, Clark WB, Walker CB, Magnusson I, Marks RG, Taylor M, Clouser B. The effect of 3 mouthrinses on plaque and gingivitis development. J Clin Periodontol. 19(1):19–23, 1992.
30. Overholser CD, Meiller TF, DePaola LG, Minah GE, Niehaus C. Comparative effects of 2 chemotherapeutic mouthrinses on the development of supragingival dental plaque and gingivitis. J Clin Periodontol. 17(8):575–579, 1990.
31. Stratul SI, Rusu D, Didilescu A, Mesaros-Anghel M, Lala C, Tion L, Sculean A, Jentsch H. Prospective clinical study evaluating the long-time adjunctive use of chlorhexidine after one-stage full-mouth SRP. Int J Dent Hyg. 8(1):35–40, 2010.
32. Hase JC, Attstrom R, Edwardsson S, Kelty E, Kisch J. 6-month use of 0.2% delmopinol hydrochloride in comparison to 0.2% chlorhexidine digluconate and placebo, effect on plaque formation and gingivitis. J Clin Periodontol. 25(9):746–753, 1998.
33. Eaton KA, Rimini FM, Zak E, et al. The effects of a 0.12% chlorhexidine-digluconate containing mouthrinse versus a placebo on plaque and gingival inflammation over a 3-month period. A multicentre study carried out in general dental practices. J Clin Periodontol. 24(3):189–197, 1997.
34. Hennet P. Effectiveness of a dental gel to reduce plaque in beagle dogs. J Vet Dent. 19(1):11–14, 2002.
35. Gorrel C, Rawlings JM. The role of tooth-brushing and diet in the maintenance of periodontal health in dogs. J Vet Dent. 13(4): 139–143, 1996.
36. Tromp JA, Jansen J, Pilot T. Gingival health and frequency of tooth brushing in the beagle dog model. Clinical findings. J Clin Periodontol. 13(2):164–168, 1986.
37. Corba NH, Jansen J, Pilot T. Artificial periodontal defects and frequency of tooth brushing in beagle dogs (II). Clinical findings after a period of healing. J Clin Periodontol. 13(3): 186–189, 1986.
38. Corba NH, Jansen J, Pilot T. Artificial periodontal defects and frequency of tooth brushing in beagle dogs (I). Clinical findings after a period of healing. J Clin Periodontol. 13(3):158–163, 1986.
39. Tromp JA, van Rijn LJ, Jansen J. Experimental gingivitis and frequency of tooth brushing in the beagle dog model. Clinical findings. J Clin Periodontol. 13(3):190–194, 1986.
40. Ingham KE, Gorrel C. Effect of long-term intermittent periodontal care on canine periodontal disease. J Small Anim Pract. 42(2): 67–70, 2001.
41. Roudebush P, Logan EI, Hale FA. Evidence-based veterinary dentistry: A systematic review of homecare for prevention of periodontal disease in dogs and cats. J Vet Dent. 21(1):6–15, 2005.
42. Jenkins S, Addey M, Wade W. The mechanism of action of chlorhexidine. A study of plaque growth on enamel inserts in vivo. J Clin Periodontol. 15:415–424, 1988.
43. Robinson JG. Chlorhexidine gluconate—the solution to dental problems. J Vet Dent. 12(1):29–31, 1995.
44. Hamp SE, Emilson CG. Some effects of chlorhexidine on the plaque flora of the beagle dog. J Periodontol Res. 12:28–35, 1973.
45. Hull PS, Davies RM. The effect of a chlorhexidine gel on tooth deposits in beagle dogs. J Small Animal Pract. 13:207–212, 1972.
46. Hamp SE, Lindhe J, Loe H. Long term effects of chlorhexidine on developing gingivitis in the beagle dog. J Periodontol Res. 8:63–70, 1973.
47. Eaton KA, Rimini FM, Zak E, et al. The effects of a 0.12% chlorhexidine-digluconate containing mouthrinse versus a placebo on plaque and gingival inflammation over a 3-month period. A multicentre study carried out in general dental practices. J Clin Periodontol. 24(3):189–197, 1997.
48. Kantmann CL, Warrick JM, Stookey GK, Newman J, Ewing TH. The evaluation of the rate of gingivitis and plaque formation in cats treated with different antimicrobial solutions. Proceedings of the 19th Annual American Veterinary Dental Forum, Orlando, 2005.
49. Tepe JH, Leonard GJ, Singer R, et al. The long term effect of of chlorhexidine on plaque, gingivitis, sulcus depth, gingival recession, and loss of attachment in beagle dogs. J Periodontal Res. 18:452–458, 1983.
50. Salas Campos L, Gómez Ferrero O, Villar Miranda H, Martin Rivera B. Antiseptic agents: Chlorhexidine. Rev Enferm. 23(9):637–640, 2000.
51. Cousido MC, Tomás Carmona I, Garcia-Caballero L, Limeres J, Alvarez M, Diz P. In vivo substantivity of 0.12% and 0.2% chlorhexidine mouthrinses on salivary bacteria. Clin Oral Investig., Aug. 8, 2009.
52. Tomás I, Garcia-Caballero L, Cousido MC, Limeres J, Alvarez M, Diz P. Evaluation of chlorhexidine substantivity on salivary flora by epifluorescence microscopy. Oral Dis. 15(6):428–433, 2009.
53. Bonesvoll P. Oral pharmacology of chlorhexidine. J Clin Periodontol. 4:49–65, 1977.
54. Tomás I, Cousido MC, Tomás M, Limeres J, Garcia-Caballero L, Diz P. In vivo bactericidal effect of 0.2% chlorhexidine but not 0.12% on salivary obligate anaerobes. Arch Oral Biol. 53(12):1186–1191, 2008.
55. Olympio KP, Bardal PA, de M Bastos JR, Buzalaf MA. Effectiveness of a chlorhexidine dentifrice in orthodontic patients: A randomized-controlled trial. J Clin Periodontol. 33(6):421–426, 2006.
56. Wolinsky LE, Cuomo J, Quesada K, et al. A comparative pilot study of the effects of a dentifrice containing green tea bioflavonids, sanguinarine, or triclosan on oral bacterial biofilm formation. J Clin Dent. 11:535–559, 2000.
57. Clarke DE. Clinical and microbiological effects of oral zinc ascorbate gel in cats. J Vet Dent. 18(4):177–183, 2001.
58. Pinnel SR, Murad S, Darr D. Induction of collagen synthesis by ascorbic acid. A possible mechanism. Arch Dermatol. 123(12):1684–1686, 1987.
59. Murad S, Grove D, Lindberg KA, Reynolds G, Sivarajah A, Pinnell SR. Regulation of collagen synthesis by ascorbic acid. Proc Natl Acad Sci USA 78(5):2879–2882, 1981.
60. Booth BA, Uitto J. Collagen biosynthesis by human skin fibroblasts. III. The effects of ascorbic acid on procollagen production and prolyl hydroxylase activity. Biochim Biophys Acta. 675(1):117–122, 1981.
61. Homola AM, Dunton RK. Methods, compositions, and dental delivery systems for the protection of the surfaces of teeth. U.S. Patent No. 5,665,333 issued Sept. 9, 1997, and U.S. Patent No. 5,961,958 issued Oct. 5, 1999.
62. Gengler WR, Kunkle BN, Romano D, Larsen D. Evaluation of a barrier sealant in dogs. J Vet Dent. 22(3):157–159, 2005.
63. Personal communication with other diplomates of the AVDC.
64. Association of American Feed Control Officials, Inc. Official publication of the Association of American Feed Control Officials, Oxford, IN, 2010.
65. Larsen J. Oral products and dental disease. Compend Cont Educ Vet., Sept 2010, pp. E1–3.
66. Ingham KE, Gorrel C. Effect of long-term intermittent periodontal care on canine periodontal disease. J Small Anim Pract. 42(2): 67–70, 2001.
67. Miller BR, Harvey CE. Compliance with oral hygiene recommendations following periodontal treatment in client-owned dogs. J Vet Dent. 11(1):18–19, 1994.

68. Vrieling HE, Theyse LF, van Winkelhoff AJ, Dijkshoorn NA, Logan EI, Picavet P. Effectiveness of feeding large kibbles with mechanical cleaning properties in cats with gingivitis. Tijdschr Diergeneeskd. 130(5):136–140, 2005.
69. Gawor JP, Reiter AM, Jodkowska K, Kurski G, Wojtacki MP, Kurek A. Influence of diet on oral health in cats and dogs. J Nutr. 136:2021–2023 S, 2006.
70. Harvey CE, Shofer FS, Laster L. Correlation of diet, other chewing activities, and periodontal disease in North American client-owned dogs. J Vet Dent. 13:101–105, 1996.
71. Jensen L, Logan E, Finney O, Lowry S, Smith M, Hefferren J, Simone A, Richardson D. Reduction in accumulation of plaque, stain, and calculus in dogs by dietary means. J Vet Dent. 2(4): 161–163, 1995.
72. Stookey GK, Warrick JM. Calculus prevention in dogs provided diets coated with HMP. Proceedings of the 19th Annual American Veterinary Dental Forum, Orlando, 2005, pp. 417–421.
73. Lage A, Lausen N, Tracy R, Allred E. Effect of chewing rawhide and cereal biscuit on removal of dental calculus in dogs. JAVMA 197(2):213–219, 1990.
74. Hattori M, Kusumoto IT, Namba T, Ishigami T, Hara Y. Effect of tea polyphenols on glucan synthesis by glucosyltransferase from Streptococcus mutans. Chem Pharm Bull (Tokyo) 38(3):717–720, 1990.
75. Hirasawa M, Takada K, Makimura M, Otake S. Improvement of periodontal status by green tea catechin using a local delivery system: A clinical pilot study. J Periodontal Res. 37(6):433–438, 2002.
76. Brown WY, McGenity P. Effective periodontal disease control using dental hygiene chews. J Vet Dent. 22(1):16–19, 2005.
77. www.VOHC.org.
78. Logan EI, Finney O, Hefferren JJ. Effects of a dental food on plaque accumulation and gingival health in dogs. J Vet Dent. 19(1):15–18, 2002.
79. Logan EI, Proctor V, Berg ML, Coffman L, Hefferren JJ. Dietary effect on tooth surface debris and gingival health in cats. Proceedings of the 15th Annual American Veterinary Dental Forum, San Antonio, 2001, p. 377.
80. Logan EI, Berg ML, Coffman L, et al. Dietary control of feline gingivitis: Results of a six month study. Proceedings of the 13th Veterinary Dental Forum, 1999, p. 54.
81. Steenkamp G, Gorrel C. Oral and dental conditions in adult African wild dog skulls: A preliminary report. J Vet Dent. 16: 65–68, 1999.
82. Verstraete FJ, van Aarde RJ, Nieuwoudt BA, et al. The dental pathology of feral cats on Marion Island, part II: Periodontitis, external odontoclastic resorption lesions and mandibular thicking. J Comp Pathol. 115(3):283–297, 1996.
83. Clarke DE, Cameron A. Relationship between diet, dental calculus, and periodontal disease in domestic and feral cats in Australia. Aust Vet J. 76(10):690–693, 1998.
84. Stookey GK, Warrick JM, Miller LL, et al. Hexametphosphate-coated snack biscuits significantly reduce calculus formation in dogs. J Vet Dent. 13(1):27039, 1996.
85. Logan EI, Wiggs RB, Zetner K, et al. Dental disease. In: Small Animal Clinical Nutrition (Hand MS, Thacher CD, Remillard RL, Roudebush P eds.). 4th ed. Topeka, KS: Mark Morris Institute, 2000, pp. 475–492.
86. Hennet P, Servet E, Venet C. Effectiveness of an oral hygiene chew to reduce dental deposits in small breed dogs. J Vet Dent. 23(1): 6–12, 2006.
87. Warrick JM, Stookey GK, Inskeep GA, Inskeep TK. Reducing calculus accumulation in dogs using an innovative rawhide treat system coated with hexametaphosphate. Proceedings of the 15th Annual American Veterinary Dental Forum, San Antonio, 2001, pp. 379–382.
88. Gorrel C, Bierer TL. Long-term effects of a dental hygiene chew on the periodontal health of dogs. J Vet Dent. 16(3):109–113, 1999.
89. Stookey GK. Soft rawhide reduces calculus formation in dogs. J Vet Dent. 26(2):82–85, 2009.
90. Mariani C, Douhain J, Servet E, Hennet P, Biourge V. Effect of toothbrushing and chew distribution on halitosis in dogs. Proceedings of the 18th Congress of Veterinary Dentistry, Zurich, 2009, pp. 13–15.
91. Chapek CW, Reed OK, Ratcliff PA. Reduction of bleeding on probing with oral-care products. Compend Contin Educ Dent. 16(2):188, 190, 192, 1995.
92. Clarke DE. Drinking water additive decreases plaque and calculus accumulation in cats. J Vet Dent. 23:79–82, 2006.
93. Dunayer EK. New findings on the effects of xylitol ingestion in dogs. Vet Med. 101(12):791–797, 2006.
94. Dunayer EK. Hypoglycemia following canine ingestion of xylitol-containing gum. Vet Human Tox. 46(2):87–88, 2004.
95. Xia Z, He Y, Yu J. Experimental acute toxicity of xylitol in dogs. J Vet Pharma Thera. 32(5):465–469, 2009.
96. Dodds JW. Healthymouth Clinical Trials. Data on file at Healthymouth.

14

Antibiotics in periodontal disease

R. Michael Peak

Introduction

In the 1960s, microscopic examination and bacterial isolation of healthy and diseased peridontium found that specific plaque bacteria were responsible for periodontal disease.[1] In the early 1970s, Lindhe et al. found that plaque bacteria were indeed required for periodontal disease to develop in Beagle dogs.[2] Since the late 1920s, antibiotics have been known to kill bacteria or stop their growth, and have been used to prevent or treat oral infections.[3] As time has evolved, our knowledge of the specific types of bacteria involved with periodontal disease has changed, and certain antibiotics have proved more useful than others in treating this disease. Various modes of delivery for antibiotics have been advocated, from oral mouth rinses containing penicillin, to systemically administered antibiotics, and ultimately locally placed and delivered antibiotics to treat specific areas around teeth. We now know periodontal disease is a multifactorial disease affected by inherent risks that increase the likelihood for disease development, including the host response to bacteria in the oral cavity or lack thereof, the different types of bacteria, and environmental influences.

Antibiotics used for periodontal disease (Box 14.1)

In some instances, combinations of the aforementioned antibiotics may be most appropriate based on suspected periodontopathogens. Antibiotic combinations usually include metronidazole due to its ability to kill anaerobic bacteria. Common combinations include amoxicillin + metronidazole and amoxicillin-clavulinate + metronidazole. Ciprofloxacin + metronidazole has been suggested in human literature since metronidazole targets the obligate anaerobes and ciprofloxacin the facultative anaerobes.[4]

Box 14.1 Key clinical point

None of these antibiotics can be recommended as a monotherapy for periodontal disease. They are recommended as an adjunctive measure along with scaling, closed root planing and subgingival curettage, and/or periodontal surgery as indicated by the oral exam.

Table 14.1 Common Antibiotics Used in Periodontal Disease.

Drug	Dosage	Route of Administration	Frequency of Administration
Amoxicillin-clavulinate	11–22 mg/kg	PO	q 12 h
Clindamycin	5.5–33 mg/Kg	PO	q 12 h
Doxycycline	3–5 mg/kg	PO	q 12 h
Metronidazole	25–50 mg/kg	PO	q 12 h
Tetracycline	22 mg/kg	PO	q 8 h

Appropriate antibiotic selection

For most bacterial infections, the selection of the correct antibiotic relies on the appropriate drug (based on culture and sensitivity), the appropriate dose (based on minimum inhibitory concentrations and the target location of the infection), and the appropriate duration. The antibiotic of choice for periodontal infections ideally would be specific for periodontal pathogens, allogenic, non-toxic, substantive, not in general use for other

Veterinary Periodontology, First Edition. Brook A. Niemiec.

infections, easy to administer, and inexpensive.[4] Unfortunately, to date this drug does not exist.

For determination of the appropriate drug, plaque sampling along with culture and sensitivity would be ideal. Although subgingival antimicrobial sampling is available for human dental professionals, there are no commercially available tests for dogs/cats. Anaerobic sampling can be difficult and contamination of samples is a concern due to the normal flora of the oral cavity. In most cases, antibiotics are chosen empirically, based on previous studies and the likelihood of those bacteria playing a role in the periodontal disease process.[5] As a very general statement, in health, most of the oral flora along the gingival sulcus and margin is gram-positive aerobic bacteria. As periodontal disease progresses along the root surface and periodontal pockets form, the subgingival bacterial flora changes to a more gram-negative anaerobic population. This is also true in both dogs and cats.[5] (See chapter 3 for a complete discussion of periodontal bacteria.)

Another consideration for selection of the appropriate drug is the ability of that drug to get to where the bacteria reside. Plaque is a unique bacterial biofilm, and as such, delivery of the antibiotic directly to the bacteria can be difficult.[7] Some antibiotics such as clindamycin, clarithromycin, and azithromycin may be more effectively delivered to the plaque bacteria via their mode of action, and may have the ability to penetrate areas of active infection through uptake and delivery within inflammatory cells.[4,8,9] In most instances, plaque disruption via ultrasonic debridement, root planing, and subgingival curettage allows any antibiotic that is selected to be more effective.

Appropriate dosing and duration would ideally be determined by minimum inhibitory concentrations of those antibiotics that the oral pathogens were found to be susceptible to. Again, this is problematic since culture and sensitivity testing of periodontal pathogens is not routinely performed in veterinary medicine. In most instances, we rely on past calculations to choose the antibiotic dosage. Unfortunately, as bacteria evolve we may be selecting dosages that are insufficient to eliminate the targeted pathogens. The result is underdosing of antibiotics to effectively kill bacteria, a practice that can lead to bacterial resistance.

Indications for antibiotic therapy in periodontal disease

Few if any veterinary studies have focused on the benefits of antibiotics post-SRP, but there have been many human studies that tout gains in attachment of periodontal tissues following SRP with antibiotics versus SRP alone.[10,11] The rationale is that by reducing the bacterial load in the healing periodontal pocket, the bacterial degradation enzymes and inflammatory mediators would subsequently be reduced. In turn, this could positively influence the healing of the periodontal pocket. At this point, the administration of postoperative antibiotic therapy for periodontal disease in companion animals is controversial.

Nieves et al. found bacteremia was a common sequela following ultrasonic scaling in anesthetized dogs, and as such, concern was generated over this release of bacteria into the bloodstream during these procedures.[12] Considering these findings, concern grew for those patients with pre-existing cardiac disease and the potential development of endocarditis. A clinical case of endocarditis that resulted in death was subsequently reported following a dental prophylaxis procedure, giving more credibility to the need for antibiotic protection during dental procedures.[13] A recent retrospective study with more than 50,000 patients suggested periodontal disease was associated with endocarditis and cardiomyopathy.[14] Other recent human publications have suggested tooth brushing could create similar bacteremia and called for consideration of the clinical significance of this consequence.[15] However, further retrospective studies on endocarditis in dogs did not support a relationship between infective endocarditis and dental procedures, and called for re-evaluation of recommendations of antibiotic usage with dental procedures.[16] Retrospective findings of a collaborative effort of the American Dental Association and the American Heart Association came to similar conclusions.[17] More studies are needed in veterinary dentistry to quantify the significance of the bacteremia elicited during dental procedures. Other suggested indications for antibiotic administration during dental procedures include:[6]

1. Cases in which the local tissues around teeth are severely infected, which necessitates either periodontal surgery or extractions. These patients may benefit from decreased inflammation and more rapid healing if the infection is controlled at the time of the procedure. Administration of the preferred antibiotic (based on the degree of alveolar bone involvement) should commence at least 24–48 hours prior to the procedure.
2. Cases in which the periodontal infection has progressed to osteomyelitis and despite treatment with extractions or root planing, deep-seeded bone infection will remain. In these circumstances, starting antibiotics several days prior to the procedure and continuing for 10–14 days postoperative is advocated.

3. Cases involving severe ulceration and loss of oral mucosal integrity as in canine or feline stomatitis. Usually these patients are managed with other treatments such as extractions, dental cleaning, and meticulous homecare.
4. Cases involving patients that are immunocompromised such as those with feline immunodeficiency virus or those concurrently receiving radiation or chemotherapy.
5. Cases involving patients who have received a splenectomy.
6. Cases involving patients with prostheses such as an ocular prosthesis, total hip replacement, or cruciate repair using a non-absorbable material.
7. Cases involving patients with other metabolic derangement such as hepatic, renal, cardiac, pancreatic, or adrenal disease. As mentioned earlier, endocarditis may not be as much of a risk during dental procedures as once thought. These guidelines are being reviewed, but others have yet to be investigated fully and more studies are needed.
8. Patients receiving sterile surgeries in other areas, such as dermatologic surgeries.

It should be noted that most patients undergoing routine dental cleaning do not warrant antibiotic coverage for the resulting bacteremia. Healthy patients should be able to eliminate these bacteria via the reticuloendothelial system without consequence. Clinical judgments need to be made in every circumstance as to the need for adjunctive antibiotic therapy, and discretion is warranted. If antibiotics are chosen, the clinician must consider an appropriate dose for the expected bacteria involved and an adequate amount of administration time.

Local delivery of antibiotics

Some of the concerns regarding systemic administration of antibiotics include the need for high doses of certain drugs given systemically to achieve adequate levels within periodontal pockets, exposure of some beneficial bacteria to these antibiotics, inadequate levels of antibiotic reaching other areas of the body predisposing development of bacterial resistance, and finally questions regarding the need for a systemic medication in the treatment of a focal disease. Recent advances in delivery technology have allowed for placement of a sustained-release antibiotic directly into the location of the periodontal disease. These "local delivery" antibiotics help avert many of the concerns of systemic antibiotics and allow for selective targeting of the periodontopathogens in their specific locations. There is a veterinary-approved local delivery antibiotic[A] that utilizes the antibacterial properties and anticollagenase effect of doxycycline to assist periodontal healing and prevent further periodontal tissue loss following scaling and root planing.[18,19] (See chapter 12 for a detailed discussion of local antibiotic usage.)

Potential alternative uses of antibiotics

The anticollagenase activity of the tetracycline group of antibiotics may prove useful in the future of veterinary dentistry as another tool for the prevention of periodontal tissue loss. At low doses (below both the antimicrobial dose and level that would allow resistance), doxycycline may be used for prevention in the breakdown of collagen. One human product[B] is a 20 mg tablet given twice daily that has been approved by the FDA for this use in people.[4] Azithromycin has also been found to help in the treatment of gingival hyperplasia induced by the administration of cyclosporine.[20] While long-term use of azithromycin cannot be advocated, it may be used as an adjunct to help prevent gingival overgrowth in some cases, and thus help in the prevention of periodontal disease. (See chapter 20 for a complete discussion of host modulation agents.)

Box 14.2 Key points

- Antibiotics are not a monotherapy for periodontal disease. They are used as an adjunctive measure along with professional care and homecare.

Indications for antibiotics in dentistry include:
  - Pretreatment in cases of severe infection requiring extensive extractions or periodontal surgery to decrease inflammation. This should be continued postsurgery.
  - Osteomyelitis.
  - Ulcerative disease (such as caudal stomatitis).
  - Immune compromised and splenectomized patients.
  - Patients with prostheses such as eye, total hip joints, or TPLOs.
  - Systemically compromised patients such as those with renal, hepatic, and heart disease.
  - Patients having sterile surgical procedures performed concurrent with dental procedures.
- Most patients undergoing routine dental cleaning do not need antibiotic coverage.
- The antibiotic regimen must be broad spectrum and include an anaerobic spectrum due to the types of bacteria seen in periodontal disease.

Notes

A. Doxyrobe Gel, Pfizer Animal Health.
B. Periostat, Collagenex Pharmaceutical Inc.

References

1. Socransky SS, Haffajee AD. The bacterial etiology of destructive periodontal disease: Current concepts. J Periodontol. 63:322, 1992.
2. Lindhe J, Hamp SE, Loe H. Plaque induced periodontal disease in beagle dogs: A 4-year clinical, roentgenographical and histometrical study. J Periodontal Res. 10(5):243–255, 1975.
3. Williams RC. Understanding and managing periodontal diseases: A notable past, a promising future. J Periodontol. 79(8):1557, 2008.
4. Jolkovsky DL, Ciancio S. Chemotherapeutic agents. In: Carranza's Clinical Periodontology. St. Louis: Saunders, 2006, pp. 798–812.
5. Harvey CE, Thornsberry C, Miller BR, Shofer FS. Antimicrobial susceptibility of subgingival bacterial flora in dogs with gingivitis. J Vet Dent. 12(4):151–155, 1995.
6. Harvey CE, DuPont G. Little mouth, big problems: What is the safest, most effective approach. In: Antimicrobial Use: Results Speak Loudest of All. Wilmington, DE: Gloyd Group, 2003, pp. 35–50.
7. DuPont GA. Understanding dental plaque: Biofilm dynamics. J Vet Dent. 14(3):91–94, 1997.
8. Burrell RC, Walters JD. Distribution of systemic clarithromycin to gingival. J Periodontol. 79(9):1712–1718, 2008.
9. Zetner K, Thiemann G. The antimicrobial effectiveness of clindamycin in diseases of the oral cavity. J Vet Dent. 10(2):6–9, 1993.
10. Ciancio SG. Systemic medications: Clinical significance in periodontics. J Clin Periodontol. 29(Suppl 2):17–21, 2002.
11. Page RC. The microbiological case for adjunctive therapy for periodontitis. J Int Acas Periodontol. 6(Suppl 4):143–149, 2004.
12. Nieves MA, Hartwig P, Kinyon JM, Riedesel DH. Bacterial isolates from plaque and blood during and after routine dental procedures in dogs. Vet Surg. 26(1):26–32, 1997.
13. Tou SP, Adlin DB, Castleman WL. Mitral valve endocarditis after dental prophylaxis in a dog. J Vet Intern Med. 19(2):268–270, 2005.
14. Glickman LT, Glickman NW, Moore GE, Goldstein GS, Lewis HB. Evaluation of the risk of endocarditis and other cardiovascular events on the basis of the severity of periodontal disease in dogs. JAVMA 234(4):486–494, 2009.
15. Lockhart PB, Brennan MT, Sasser HC, Fox PC, Paster BJ, Bohrani-Mougeot FK. Bacteremia associated with toothbrushing and dental extraction. Circulation 117(24):3118–3125, 2008.
16. Peddle GD, Drobratz KJ, Harvey CE, Adams A, Sleeper MM. Association of periodontal disease, oral procedures, and other clinical findings with bacterial endocarditis in dogs. JAVMA 234(1):100–107, 2009.
17. Wilson W, Taubert KA, Gewitz M, Lockhart PB, Baddour LM, Levison M, Bolger A, Cabell CH, Takahashi M, Baltimore RS, Newburger JW, Strom BL, Tani LY, Gerber M, Bonow RO, Pallasch T, Shulman ST, Rowley AH, Burns JC, Ferrieri P, Gardner T, Goff D, Durack DT. Prevention of infective endocarditis: Guidelines from the American Heart Association: A guideline from the American Heart Association Rheumatic Fever, Endocarditis and Kawasaki Disease Committee, Council on Cardiovascular Disease in the Young, and the Council on Clinical Cardiology, Council on Cardiovascular Surgery and Anesthesia, and the Quality of Care and Outcomes Research Interdisciplinary Working Group. J Am Dent Assoc. 139(3):253, 2008.
18. Polson AP, et al. Periodontal pocket treatment in beagle dogs using subgingival doxycycline from a biodegradable system. J Periodontol. 67:1176–1184, 1996.
19. Zetner K, Rothmueller G. Treatment of periodontal pockets with doxycycline in beagles. Vet Ther. 3(4):441–452, 2002.
20. Kim JY, Park SH, Cho KS, Kim HJ, Lee CK, Park KK, Choi SH, Chung WY. Mechanism of azithromycin treatment on gingival overgrowth. J Dent Res. 87(11):1075–1079, 2008.

SECTION 4

Periodontal surgical techniques

15

Gingival surgery

Introduction

Gingival surgery consists of two separate types of procedures: gingival curettage and gingivectomy/plasty. *Gingival curettage* is the technique of debriding the pocket epithelium from the periodontal pocket, without decreasing the pocket depth. G*ingivectomy* is the resection of attached gingiva. *Gingivoplasty* is related to gingivectomy, except it is a mild recontouring of the gingiva as opposed to its wholesale removal.[1]

Most veterinarians think of any scaling performed below the gingival margin as "subgingival" curettage; however, this is not quite correct. *Gingival* curettage is defined as debriding the internal lining of the pocket down to the level of the epithelial attachment (nadir of the pocket). *Sub*gingival curettage is defined as debridement of the connective tissue apical to the pocket, down to the level of the alveolar crest (Figure 15.1). Current periodontal pocket therapy has moved away from performing only gingivectomy without some sort of flap procedure. That being said, gingival resection is a required step in many flap designs and still has indications for pocket reduction. In addition, gingival enlargement is a fairly common presentation in dogs, and therefore gingivectomy/gingivoplasty is still commonly used in these cases.[2]

Gingival curettage

Gingival curettage is performed to remove the chronically infected soft tissue lining from the periodontal pocket. This diseased tissue contains areas of chronic infection and commonly contains bacterial colonies and pieces of calculus. The granulation tissue is lined by epithelium, which acts as a barrier to reattachment.

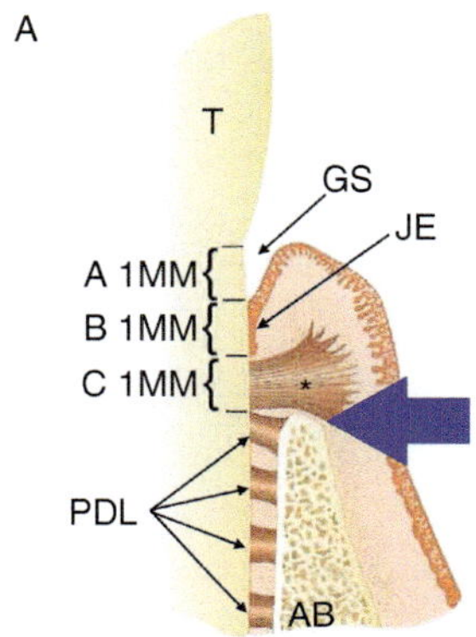

Figure 15.1 Medical illustration depicting the periodontal anatomy to show the alveolar crest (blue arrow). Reprinted with permission, J Vet Dent. 25(2):86–95, 2008.

True "intentional" gingival curettage is rarely performed today. This is partly due to the fact that some curettage will always accompany scaling and root planing, and this is termed *inadvertent curettage*. In addition, proper root planing/scaling has been shown to eliminate the majority of bacteria, allowing the patient's immune defenses to control what remains. Furthermore, the effectiveness of curettage in complete removal of the diseased tissue is questionable,[3,4] and the consequence of inadvertent removal of the junctional epithelium may result in gingival recession. Most importantly, however, it has been shown in numerous studies that intentional curettage beyond what accompanies scaling and root planing does not appear to provide any additional benefit.[5] Finally, it is important to note that curettage alone is insufficient for infection control and therefore must be performed with SRP.

Veterinary Periodontology, First Edition. Brook A. Niemiec.

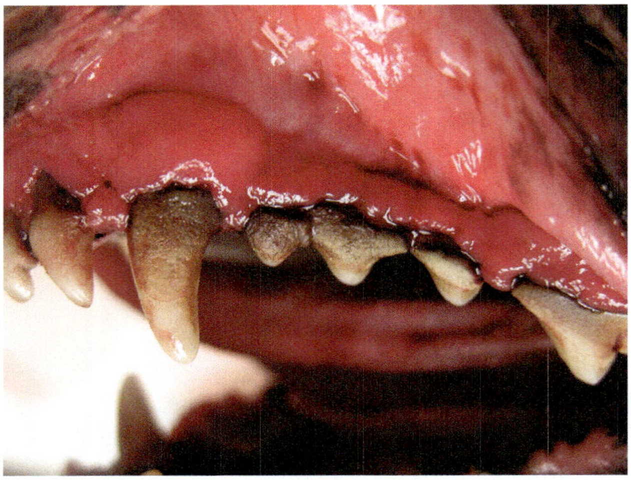

Figure 15.2 Intraoral picture of the maxillary left of a dog with significantly inflamed gingiva. Note that it affects the entire attached gingiva.

The very limited indications for intentional gingival curettage include[5]

1. Deep intrabony pockets where new attachment is planned without a flap. These exceedingly rare cases would include areas between maxillary molar teeth where access and exposure would be challenging.
2. As a "compromise procedure" when periodontal flaps or extraction are not possible due to financial or health concerns (or client wishes). Note, this is less than ideal therapy and should not be recommended.
3. Significant hypertrophic inflammatory gingiva in a mild (<6 mm) periodontal pocket (Figure 15.2).

However, the high likelihood of lack of complete debridement[4] as well as swift recurrence of the pocket makes intentional gingival curettage a poor choice. Rather, extraction or periodontal flap surgery should be encouraged.

The proper technique for gingival curettage is as follows:[5] Select a curette that will place the working edge against the pocket. A universal curette can be used, or more correctly, a Gracey 13–14 for mesial surfaces and 11–12 for distal surfaces. The instrument is placed in the sulcus to the bottom of the pocket and pulled out along the edge of the pocket, more or less horizontally (Figure 15.3a). Ideally, the gingiva is supported with a finger (Figure 15.3b). The procedure will remove the epithelial lining (pocket epithelium) but not the junctional epithelium.

During *sub*gingival curettage, the diseased pocket epithelium is removed *along with* the junctional epithelium to the level of the alveolar crest. This is performed by placing the curette deep into the pocket and cutting down to the bone in a scooping motion (Figure 15.4). This degree of denudation requires that the gingiva be readapted with 2–3 minutes of finger pressure against the tooth, and occasionally interdental sutures may be indicated.

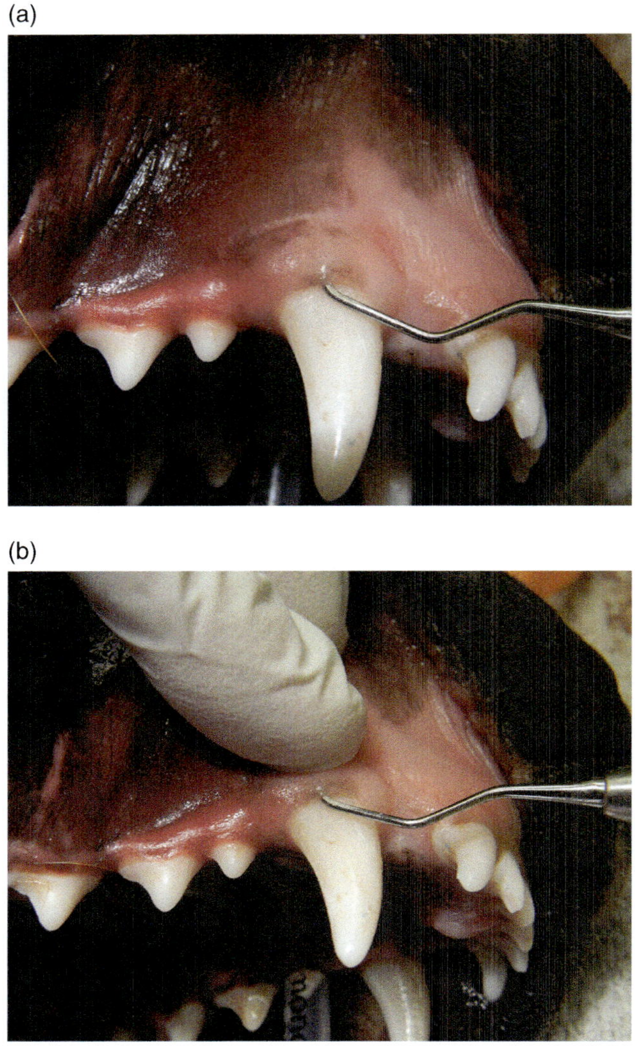

Figure 15.3 Gingival curettage. (a) Intraoral picture of the correct placement of the curette under the gingival margin and parallel to the long axis of the tooth. (b) Intraoral picture of placing a finger over the gingiva for support during the curettage.

Variations on curettage include ultrasonic and chemical techniques. With proper instrument selection and technique, ultrasonic debridement has been found to be as effective as mechanical curettage with less inflammation and removal of underlying connective tissue.[6,7] In fact, inadvertent ultrasonic curettage is likely performed during ultrasonic subgingival scaling (as mentioned above). A fine periodontal tip is the typical choice for this procedure. Chemical techniques have been around a long time but are generally not recommended due to

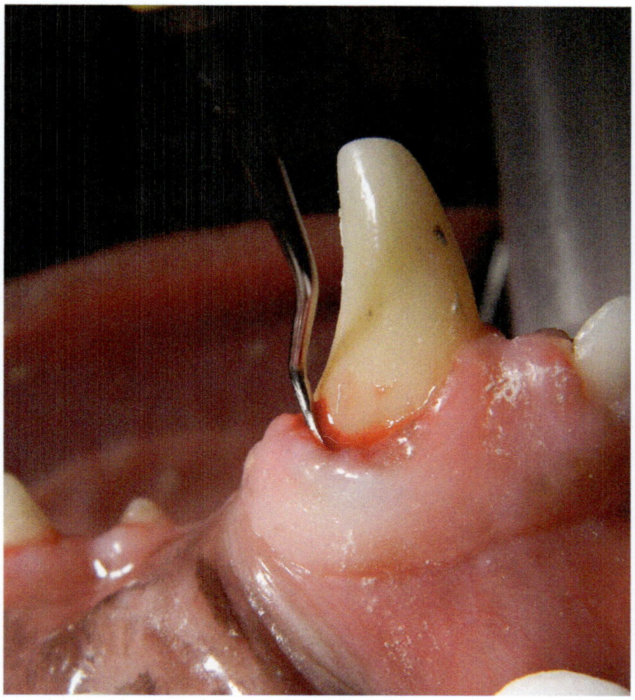

Figure 15.4 Subgingival curettage: The curette has been placed deep into the periodontal pocket and is being used to "scoop" the diseased tissue.

their ineffectiveness, the degree of inflammation they produce, and the lack of control they afford.[8,9]

One other variation of gingival curettage is called the *excisional new attachment procedure* (ENAP).[10] It is a complete subgingival curettage performed with a knife or blade.

ENAP technique

1. An internal bevel incision is made from the gingival margin apically to below the bottom of the pocket (Figure 15.5).[5]
2. The incision is carried interdentally mesially and distally, maintaining as much interdental tissue as possible to remove the pocket epithelium circumferentially around the tooth (Figure 15.6).
3. The excised tissue is removed with a curette and careful root planing is performed (Figure 15.7).
4. The incised edges are approximated and interdental sutures are placed (Figure 15.8). If the edges do not meet easily, careful bone recontouring may be necessary.

There are minimal indications for true gingival curettage other than the small amount of *inadvertent curettage* that occurs with scaling/root planing. In most cases, periodontal flap surgery or extraction is a far better choice. This author uses this technique primarily in cases where there is significant inflammatory granulation

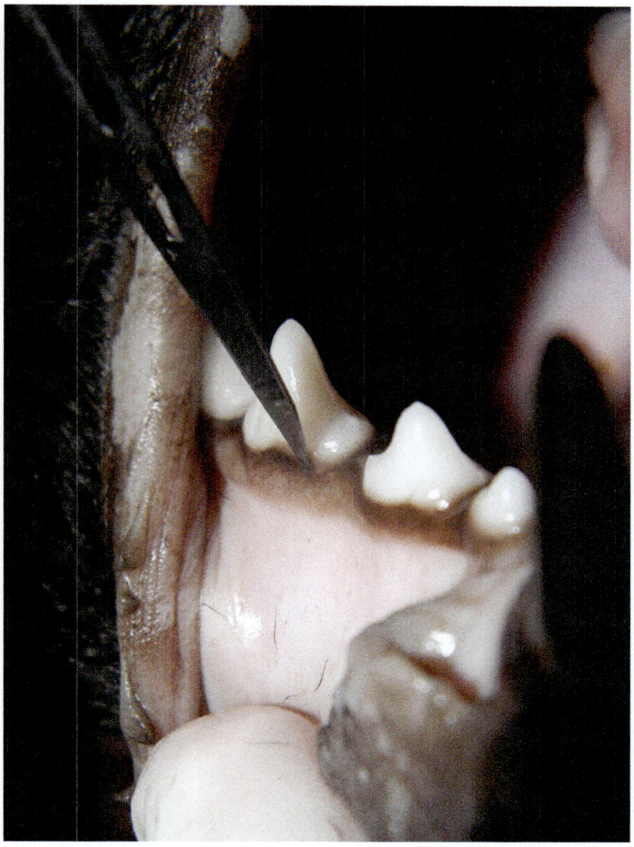

Figure 15.5 Internal bevel incision.

tissue in a relatively shallow periodontal pocket (< 6 mm) that does not cross the mucogingival junction (i.e., periodontal flap surgery is not necessarily indicated). If this extends along most or all of an arcade, the ENAP procedure may be of benefit.

Gingivectomy

Gingivectomy is defined as excision of the gingiva.[1] As a periodontal pocket therapy, it is performed to reduce pocket depth, provide visibility and accessibility for proper cleaning and smoothing, and provide a proper environment for healing and better anatomy for homecare. Although gingivectomy was widely used in the past for periodontal pocket therapy, it is used only sparingly now. There are two indications for gingivectomy in the treatment of periodontal disease,[11] both of which are rare in veterinary medicine. One is for reduction of suprabony pockets[1] with fibrous gingiva (which would not likely respond favorably to conservative therapy), and the other is for management of suprabony periodontal abscesses.

Gingival hyperplasia/enlargement is a benign lesion but can have a similar appearance to neoplasia. There is a documented case where both benign gingival hyperplasia and malignant lesions were found in

(a) (b) (c)

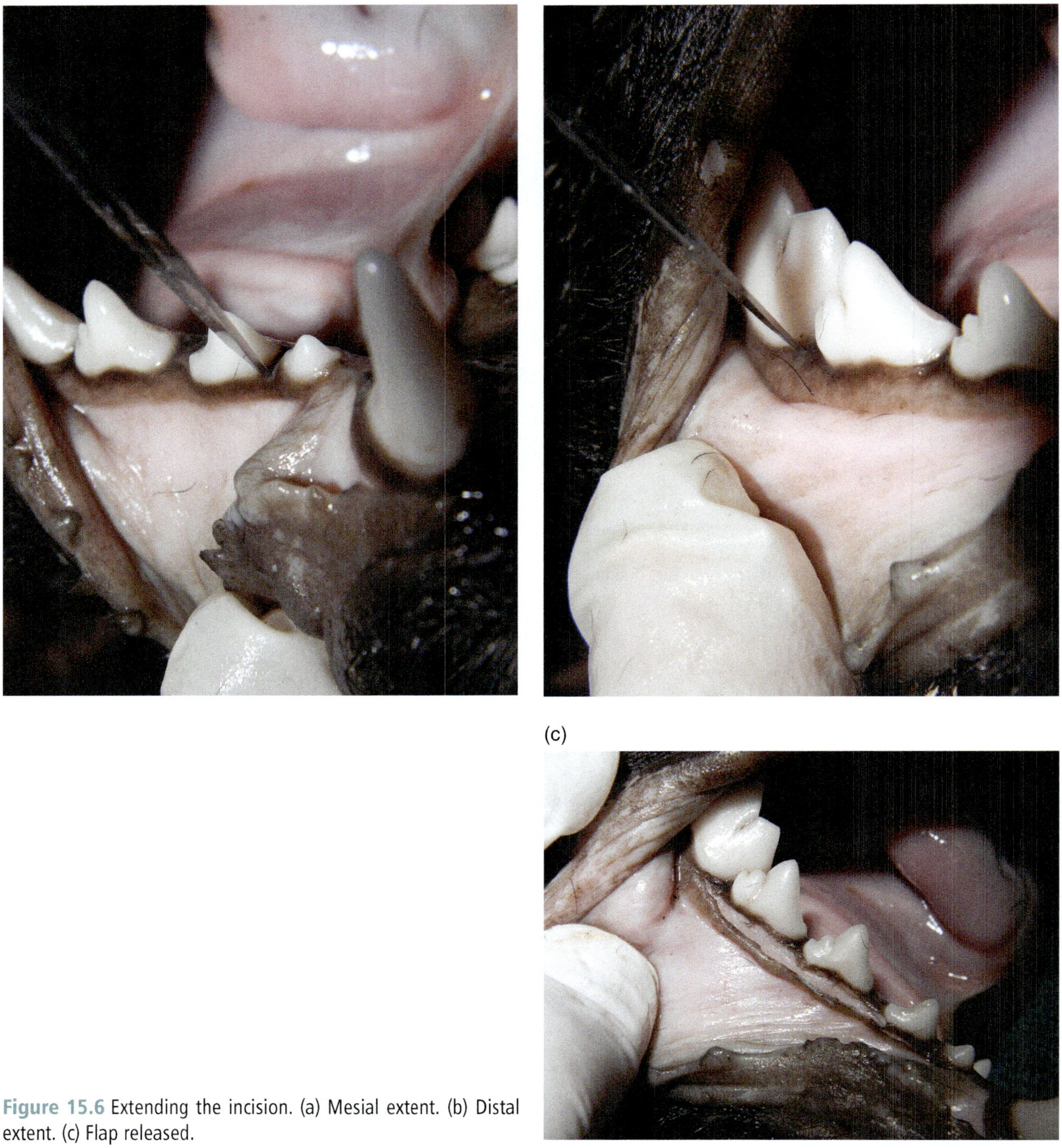

Figure 15.6 Extending the incision. (a) Mesial extent. (b) Distal extent. (c) Flap released.

the same patient.[20] Therefore, any suspect gingival enlargements should be sampled and submitted for histopathologic evaluation. Additionally, dental radiographs should be made to evaluate the underlying bone prior to initiating the surgical procedure.[12] If the radiographs reveal bony changes that raise the index of suspicion for neoplasia (Figure 15.10), an incisional biopsy (including some bone) should be performed prior to planning definitive surgery.[21]

With generalized gingival enlargement, the gingival tissue grows thicker and may cover part of or the entire crown (especially the mandibular incisors) (Figure 15.11). This overgrowth often creates pseudopockets that hinder plaque control (natural as well as homecare), resulting in increased plaque and calculus formation.[2] Consequently, gingival enlargement may result in early onset of periodontal disease (see Figure 2.7). Therefore, it is important to remove

(a) (b)

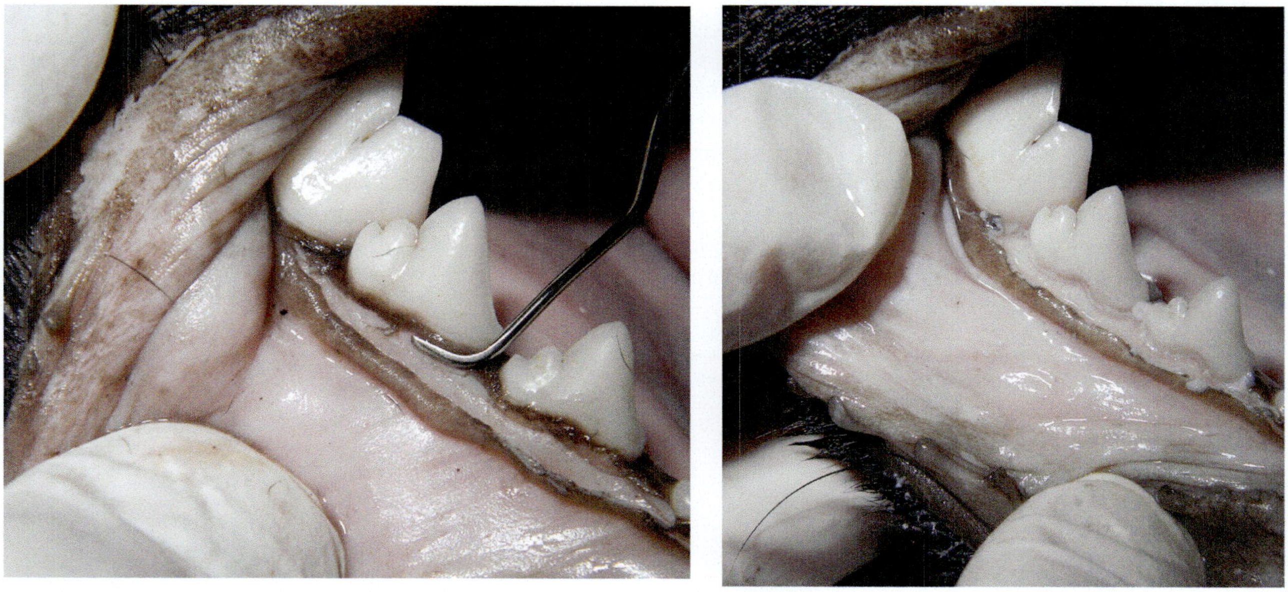

Figure 15.7 Removal of excised tissue with a curette. (a) Preoperative. (b) Postoperative.

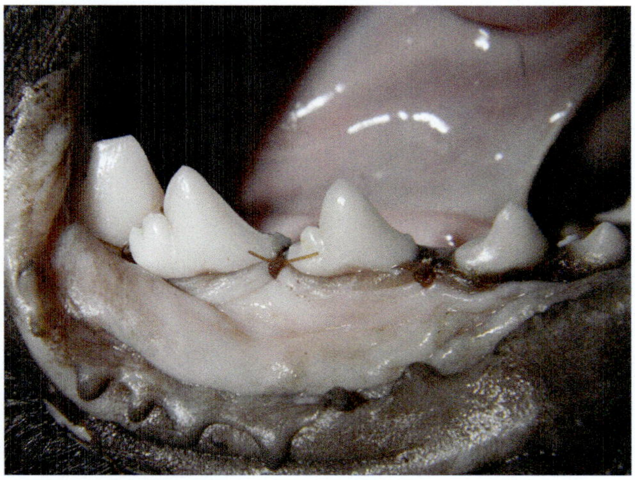

Figure 15.8 Closure.

the excess gingival tissue and restore normal physiological contours (gingivoplasty).

Gingival enlargement can affect the entire mouth or present as either single (localized) or multiple nodular lesions.[12,13] The principles of surgery are the same for treating small areas of focal hyperplasia and cases where the whole mouth is affected. Proper case selection and technique are critical. The most important detail is that there must be a minimum of 2 mm of attached gingiva remaining at the end of the procedure.[22]

Gingivectomy is *contraindicated* if less than 2 mm of attached gingiva will remain after the procedure, if the defect extends below the muco-gingival junction, or if osseous examination or surgery is necessary.[1] In these cases, alternative types of periodontal surgery (such as apical repositioned flaps) or extraction should be considered.

Note that the 2 mm of attached gingiva has been the recommendation for decades; however, recent publications have put that requirement into question.[23,24] The basis for this is long-term stability of teeth without this amount. However, these are reports from human dentists, where homecare is generally much more effective, and thus these compromised teeth will have a much better chance of long-term health. In veterinary patients, 2 mm should still be maintained, especially in gingivectomy cases.

Treatment and management of gingival enlargement

In cases that may be drug induced, the offending medication should be discontinued or changed, if possible. This alone may result in the resolution of the hyperplasia. If changing the medication regimen is not possible, the gingival enlargement is likely to recur after the surgical treatment.

Control of oral inflammation is very important, especially after surgery. This should include daily tooth brushing (and/or chlorhexidine rinses) and regular professional cleaning. Non-responsive or recurrent cases of gingival enlargement may need to be periodically retreated with a gingivectomy.

Gingivectomy equipment options

There are several equipment options for this procedure, including scalpels/knives, electrocautery, lasers, and

Box 15.1 Gingival enlargement

By far the most common indication for gingivectomy in small animal veterinary patients is gingival enlargement (GE) (Figure 15.9).[12] This condition was previously known as gingival *hyperplasia;* however, this is a histologic diagnosis. GE is a common disease in dogs[13] and is defined as a proliferation of normal cellular components of the gingiva, especially the connective tissue.[2] It occurs more often in certain breeds, such as Boxers and Collies, in which it may have a familial tendency.[2,14] GE has a higher prevalence in males, possibly due to the presence of testosterone receptors within the gingiva.[15] It can also be caused by either acute or chronic inflammation of the gingiva.[13] Finally, it is known to be a drug reaction associated with several oral medications including immunosuppressants, anticonvulsants, ACE inhibitors, amlodipine, and calcium channel blockers.[16,17] The immunosuppressant cyclosporine has been implicated more frequently in recent years due to its increased use as a treatment for atopic dermatitis.[18,19]

(a) (b)

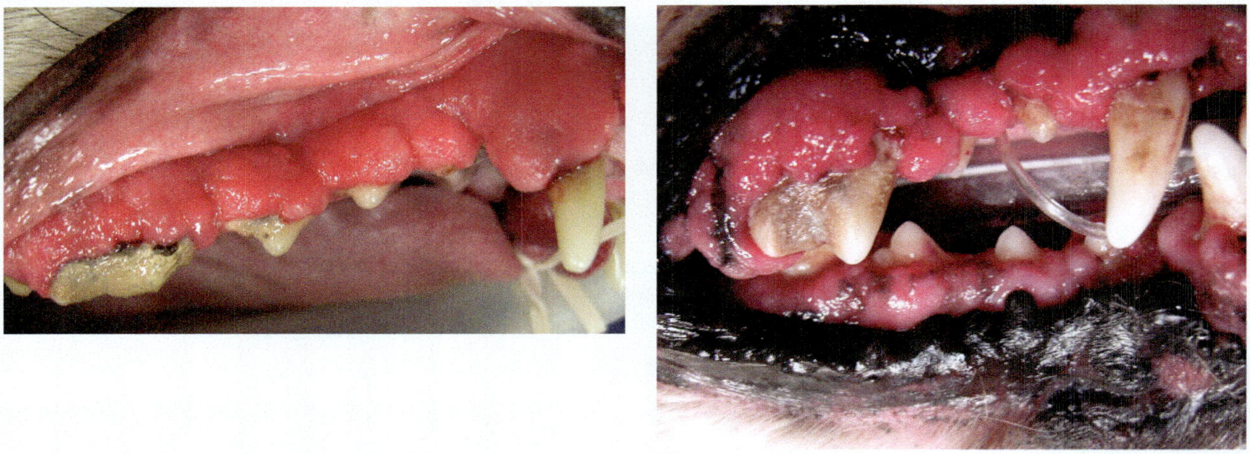

Figure 15.9 Gingival enlargement. (a) Intraoral picture of a dog with gingival enlargement secondary to phenobarbital therapy. (b) Intraoral picture of the maxillary right in a dog with extreme gingival enlargement secondary to cyclosporine administration.

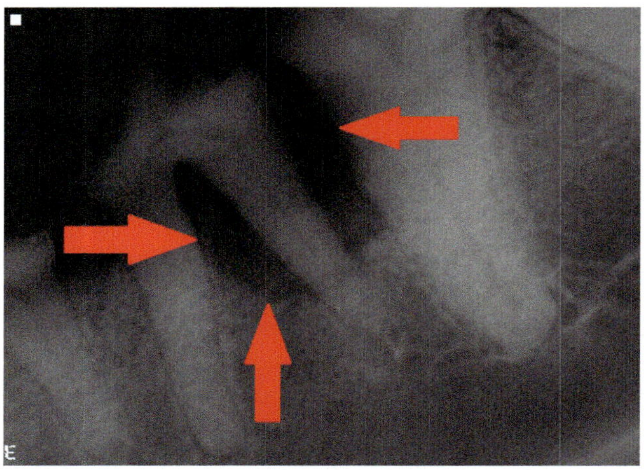

Figure 15.10 Intraoral dental radiograph of the left mandibular fourth premolar (308) of a patient with suspect gingival enlargement. The image reveals significant bony destruction, which is suspicious for a neoplastic process. This was confirmed histopathologically as fibrosarcoma.

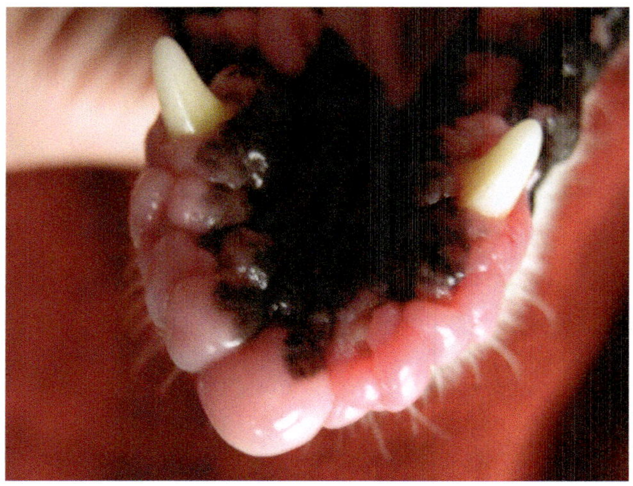

Figure 15.11 Intraoral picture of a canine patient with severe gingival enlargement. The mandibular incisors are completely overgrown by the gingiva.

chemicals. Currently, knives/blades are the equipment of choice for many veterinary dentists; however, lasers and radiosurgery are favored by some.[1,25]

Using electrocautery as a surgical instrument provides the major advantage of hemostasis, which allows superior visualization.[26] Some researchers report favorable results with the use of electrocautery;[27,28] however, there are several potential complications that can occur if it is used improperly.[1] If the root is touched with the instrument, areas of cementum may burn and undergo thermal necrosis.[29] In addition, if the bone is touched, irreparable damage can occur.[5] In fact, there are more complications associated with the improper use of electrocautery as compared to knives/blades, especially when these instruments are used in close proximity to the bone. These complications can include delayed healing, increased gingival recession, bone injury, furcation exposure, bone necrosis/sequestration, and tooth mobility.[30–33] Therefore, the use of electrocautery is discouraged for inexperienced operators or for any procedures expected to come close to the bone. When performing radiosurgery, it is important to use the proper power setting on the radiosurgery unit. Too much power results in thermonecrosis of the tissue, while inadequate power causes the electrode loop to drag through the tissue. It is important to keep the electrode tip moving, as prolonged application of the current can cause tissue destruction.[22] Furthermore, cutting should be done at intervals, with 5–10 seconds allowed for cooling in between applications, as this significantly reduces the heat buildup.[22] The use of a large loop (Figure 15.12) facilitates leaving a properly beveled edge to the gingiva.

Lasers can also be used to perform gingivectomies. There are several advantages to laser therapy including hemostasis, minimal wound contraction, and a bactericidal effect.[34,35] However, several studies show that healing is delayed with laser usage compared to scalpel gingivectomies.[36,37] In addition, the procedure time required to treat cases of generalized gingival enlargement is significantly longer if performed with a laser. Therefore, lasers are not currently recommended for widespread gingivectomies,[5,38] but recent developments in lasers (especially the erbium group) show promise for periodontal therapy.[39] Practitioners are encouraged to continually review this rapidly changing field.

Chemical techniques were used in the past and involve the application of caustic products to the gingiva. These products include paraformaldehyde and potassium hydroxide.[40,41] They are not recommended due to the lack of control and delayed healing associated with their use.

Gingivectomy techniques

There are two main options for the gingivectomy procedure, standard and surgical flap.[1,5,12,26,42] The standard technique is faster and easier but is best suited for small areas, as the raw/beveled edge of gingiva will need to heal by secondary intention. Furthermore, this technique causes increased loss of keratinized tissue, increased patient discomfort, and increased bleeding compared to the surgical flap technique.[12] When using the standard surgical technique, postsurgical homecare must be delayed to allow for healing, whereas homecare can be instituted sooner with the surgical flap technique.[43]

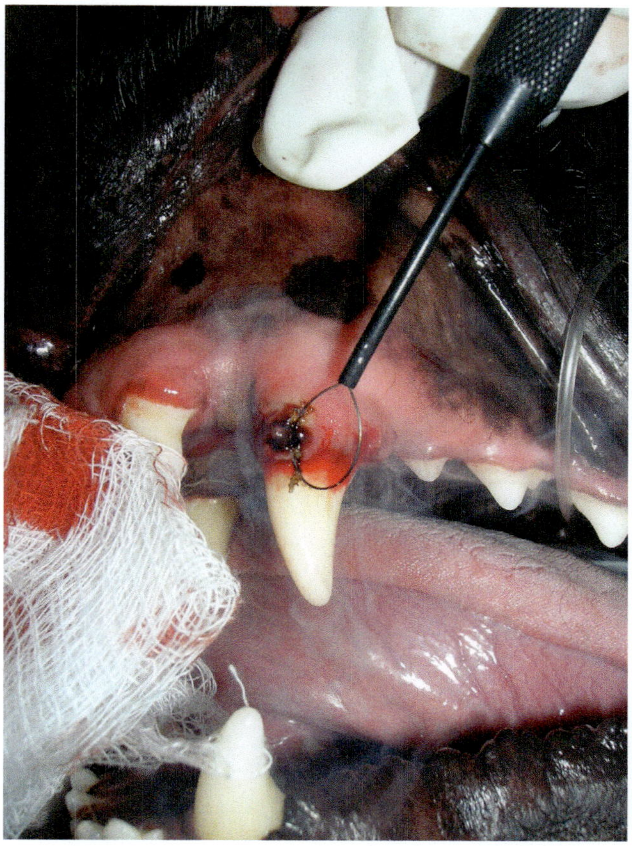

Figure 15.12 Electrocautery with a large wire loop used for a surgical gingivectomy. Notice the smoke being produced.

In cases that require large areas to be treated, or if minimal attached gingiva will remain, the surgical flap technique should be utilized. Also, if the entire attached gingiva is affected (as is typical with the hereditary form), the flap technique allows proper thinning/beveling of the resultant tissue and gives a superior result. Finally, the flap technique should be used in cases where osseous surgery will or may be necessary.

Procedure for standard gingivectomy

1. Measure the depth of the pocket in several areas on each tooth and note the buccal surface of the gingiva at the base of the pocket.[1,26,42] Then, mark a bleeding point 3 mm coronal to the base of the pocket (Figure 15.13). This can be done with a standard periodontal probe and needle but is more accurate and efficient if a periodontal pocket marker is used (Figure 15.14). The 3 mm allows for 1 mm of gingival recession following surgery "die back" and 2 mm of physiological pocket depth. When accomplished, the contour of the defect will be outlined (Figure 15.15).

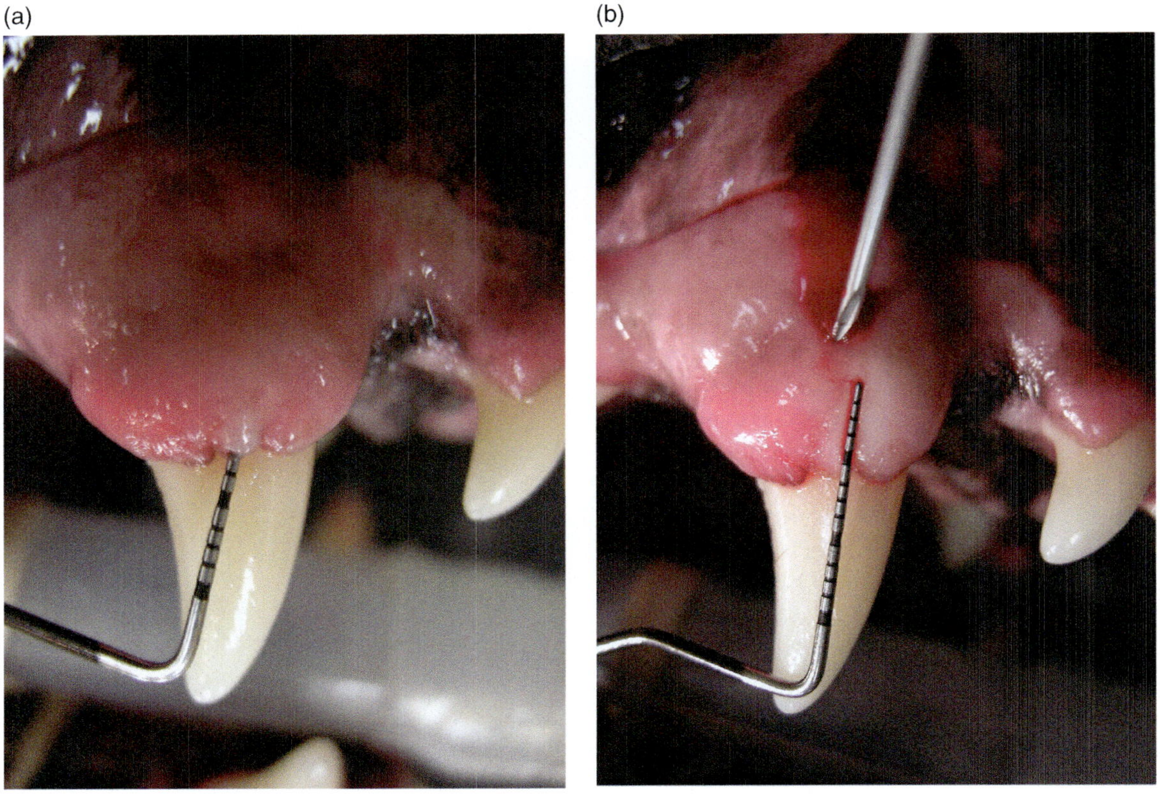

Figure 15.13 (a) Measuring the amount of hyperplasia with a periodontal probe. In this case, the depth is approximately 9 mm. (b) Marking the "bleeding point" with a needle approximately 3 mm coronal to the base or approximately 6 mm from the margin. Note: this author finds it challenging to mark right at the probe and therefore will hold the probe a few mm above the mark for the bleeding point.

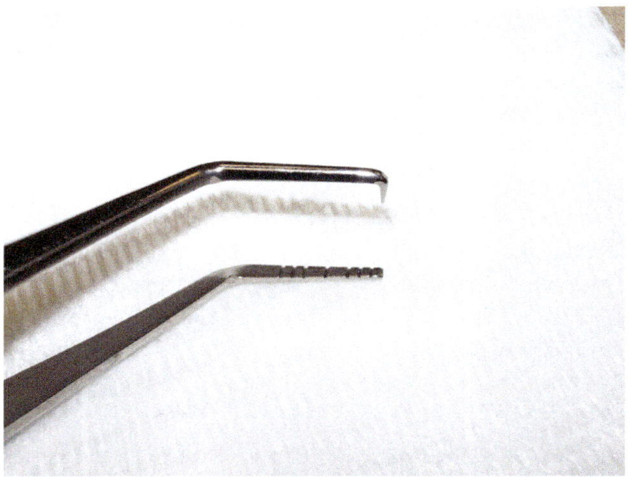

Figure 15.14 Gingivectomy marking tool.

2. The gingivectomy incision(s) are made. These can be performed with a Kirkland or Orban knife or with a #11 or #15 scalpel blade used on a scalpel handle. The incision can be continuous and thus connecting the teeth or discontinuous and around each tooth. The incision is started apical to the mark and carried coronally at a 45-degree bevel to

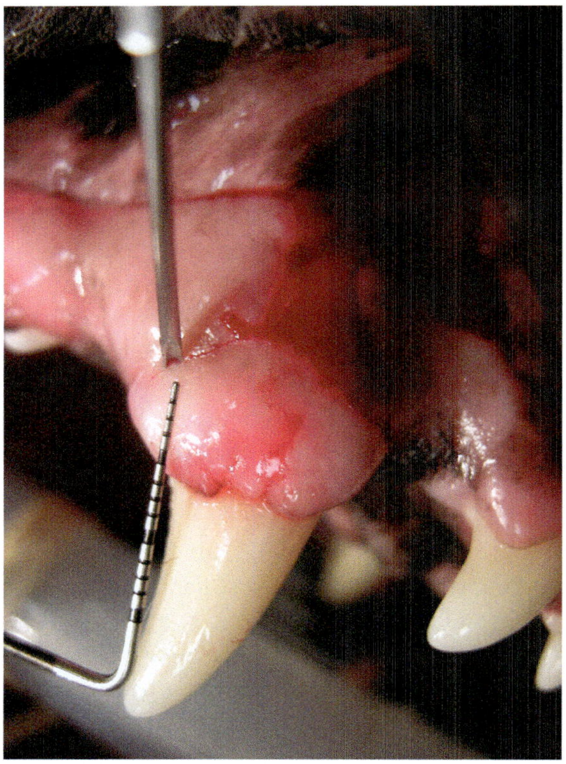

Figure 15.15 Bleeding points combined to outline the defect for proper incision.

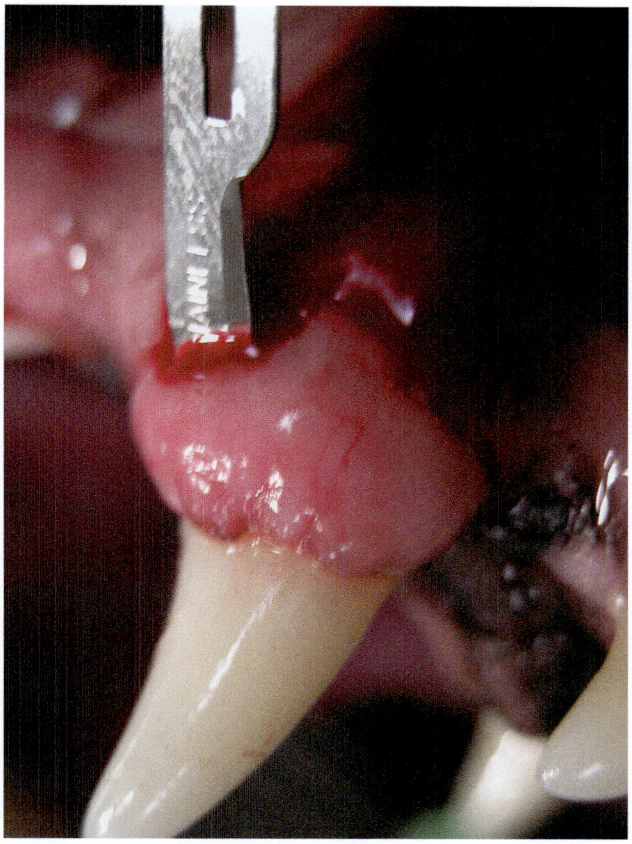

Figure 15.16 Initial incision with a #15 scalpel blade angle 45 degrees to create a thin margin.

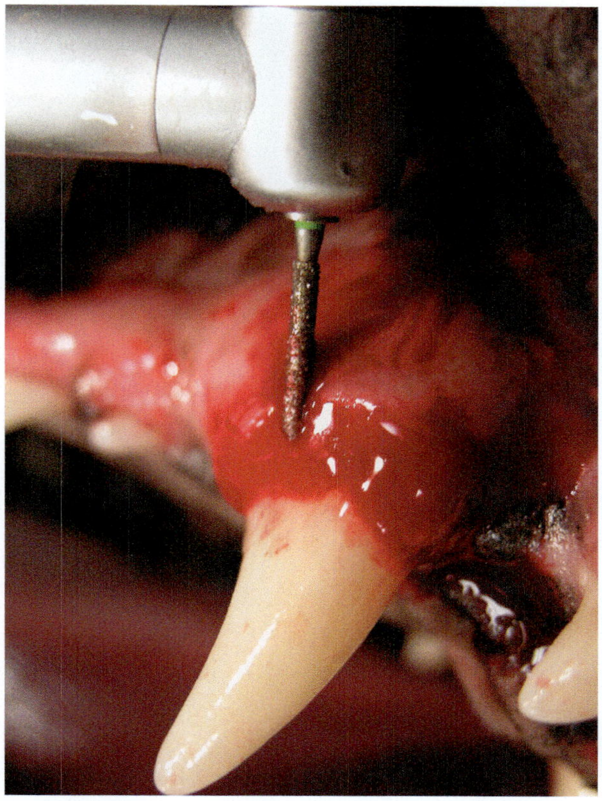

Figure 15.17 Gingivoplasty with a coarse diamond bur.

just below the bleeding point line, making sure that the incision starts at least 2 mm coronal to the MJG[5] (Figure 15.16). Proper beveling restores an anatomically natural contour, speeds recovery, and avoids a blunt gingival margin that would promote plaque accumulation.

3. Remove the excised gingiva with a sharp curette and clean the exposed root surfaces and granulation tissue with a combination of ultrasonic and hand scaling. (See chapters 10 and 11.)
4. If indicated, gingivoplasty can be performed to remove any uneven areas and to accomplish final contouring of the gingiva. Knives, blades, lasers, and cautery can be used for this technique, but this author prefers coarse tapered diamond or 12-fluted finishing burs (Figure 15.17).[2,25,30] When shaping with the diamond bur, follow the underlying bony contours.
5. Gingival bleeding (perhaps significant) can be expected. Bleeding generally stops on its own, but several minutes of direct pressure with moistened gauze may speed hemostasis. Electrocautery or hemostatic solutions can be used if necessary (Figure 15.18).

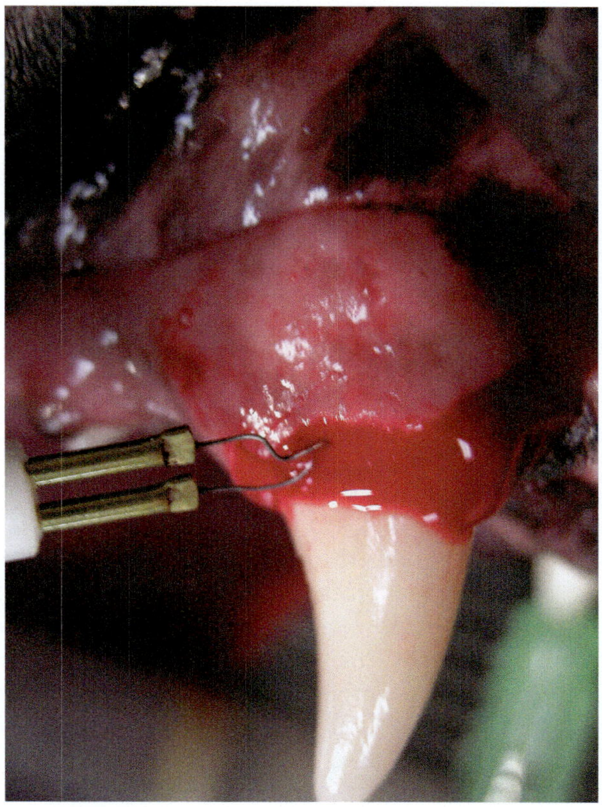

Figure 15.18 "Spot" electrocautery for small areas of hemorrhage.

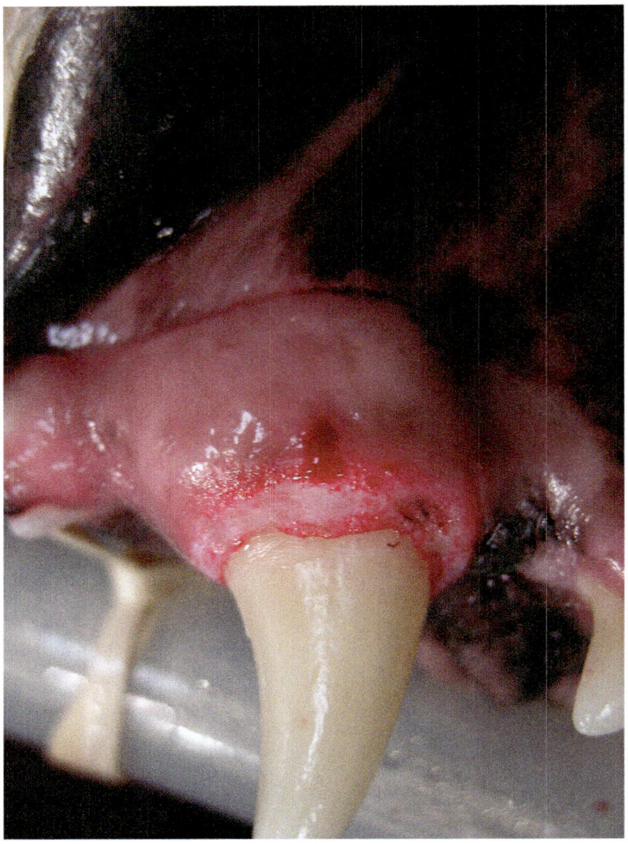

Figure 15.19 Postoperative picture demonstrating a smooth and regular margin that is nicely beveled.

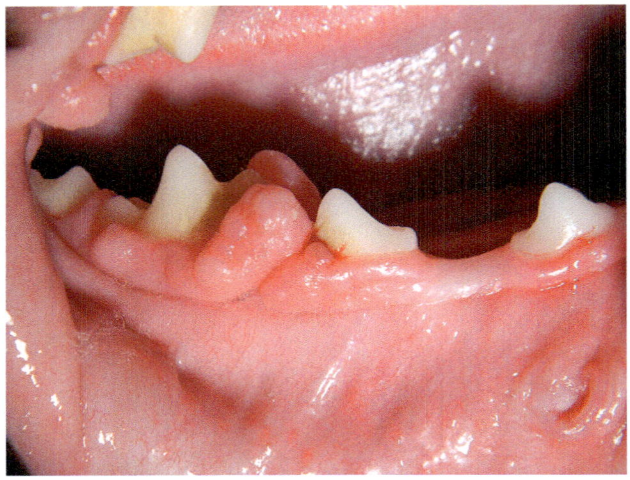

Figure 15.20 Preoperative picture of significant gingival enlargement over the right mandibular fourth premolar and first molar (408 and 409) in a dog. In this case, it is fairly obvious where the attachment should be.

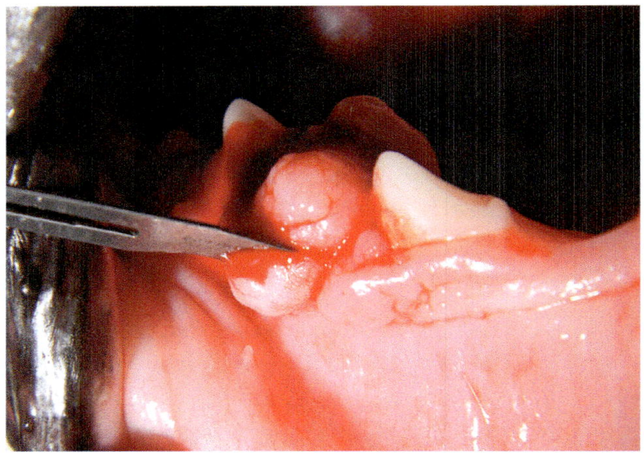

Figure 15.21 Internal "reverse" bevel incision performed with a #15 scalpel blade.

6. Ideally, a periodontal pack is applied to the surgical site(s). However, lack of patient acceptance and difficulty maintaining these products are issues with veterinary patients. One product that does appear to work better than most is a light-cured liquid dam.[26,A]
7. Re-evaluate the surgical site for smoothness (Figure 15.19).

Periodontal flap method

The flap technique[12] for treating gingival enlargement is very similar to the envelope flaps utilized for periodontal flap surgery.

1. Measure the depth of the pocket/overgrowth in several areas on each tooth and mark the buccal surface of the gingiva at the base of the pocket (as above). This can be done with a standard periodontal probe and needle but is more accurate and efficient if a periodontal pocket marker is used. When accomplished, the contour of the defect will be outlined. Experienced surgeons may skip this step in areas where the physiologic attachment level is well known (Figure 15.20).
2. The initial *internal* bevel incision is made a minimum of 3 mm above the muco-gingival margin with a #15 blade. This incision should be scalloped and should recreate the interdental papilla (Figure 15.21).
3. Next, the scalpel blade is used to thin the gingiva by removing the interior aspect of the tissue (Figure 15.22). This will return the gingiva to a normal physiologic width. Subsequently, the interdental areas are cut with a blade or knife and the excess gingiva is removed (Figure 15.23).
4. The soft tissue tabs are trimmed with LaGrange scissors and the roots scaled and planed.

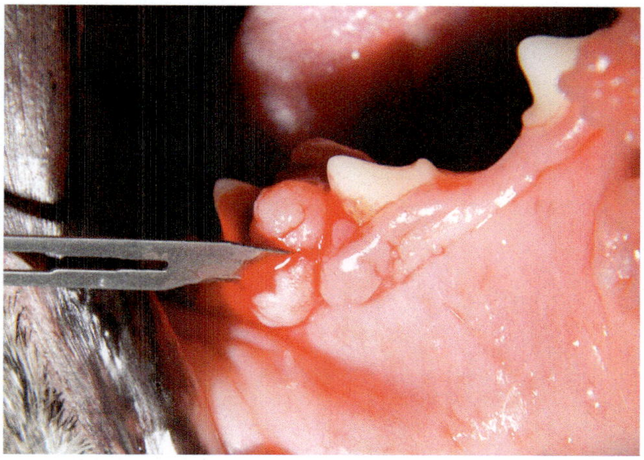

Figure 15.22 Thinning the excess gingival tissues to a normal width from the inside, thus leaving the external surface of the keratinized tissue intact for faster healing.

(a)

(b)

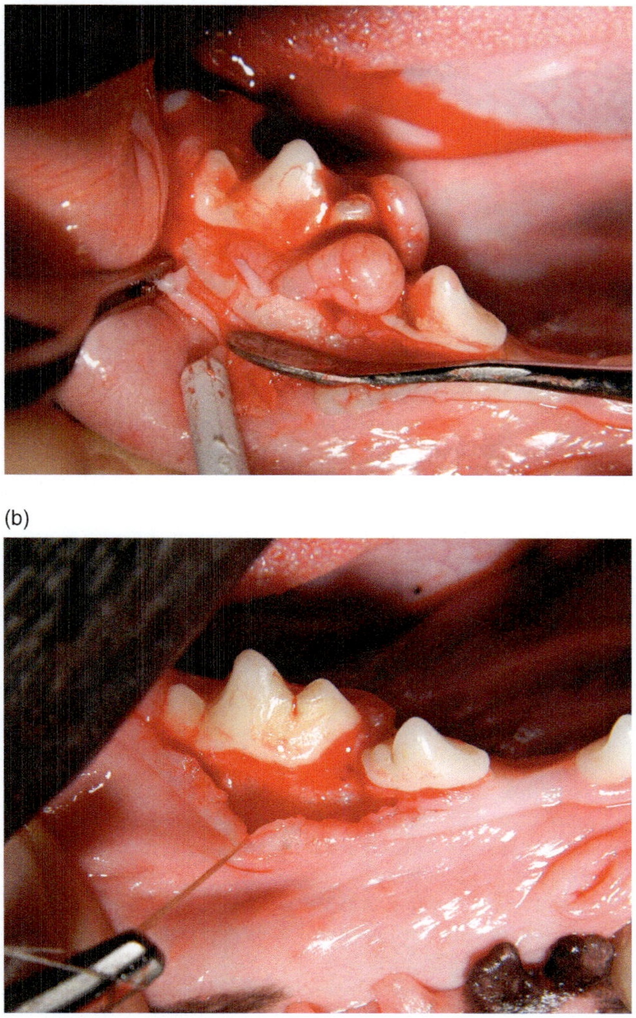

Figure 15.23 Removing the excess tissue. (a) Reflecting the created flap of tissue. (b) Excised area after removal with knife. Note the thin marginal edge with intact keratinized tissue.

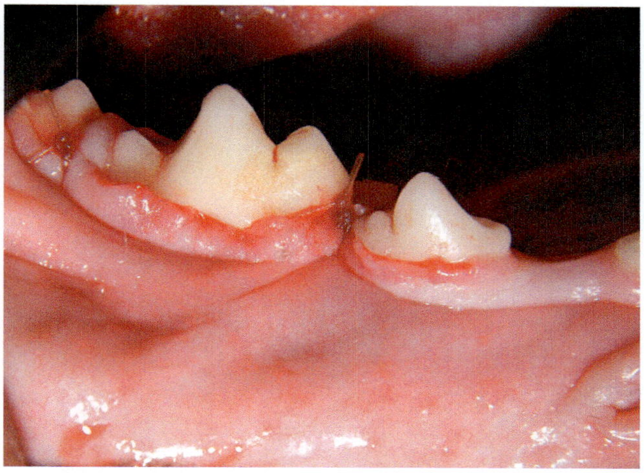

Figure 15.24 Flap is closed interdentally with simple loop sutures. Note the thin marginal edge with intact keratinized tissue.

5. The flap is replaced and if necessary trimmed to fit the tooth/bone interface correctly.
6. Interdental sutures are used to close the flaps (Figure 15.24).

Conclusions

Gingivectomy was commonly used in the past as a means of pocket reduction. However, current thoughts on the biology of periodontal disease and the need to maintain keratinized tissues with other surgical methods (primarily flaps and regenerative techniques) have greatly reduced its role in pocket reduction. The most common indication for gingivectomy in veterinary medicine is generalized gingival enlargement. Standard gingivectomy technique utilizes a standard bevel incision to create an anatomically appropriate margin. The flap technique, while significantly more technical, achieves similar if not superior results without the significant hemorrhage and long healing time associated with the standard method (Figure 15.25).

Box 15.2 Key points

- Gingivectomy is most commonly used for cases of gingival enlargement.
- Periodontal flap procedures are preferred in cases of deep periodontal pockets.
- While radiosurgery and lasers have been utilized, most veterinary dentists prefer using scalpel blades or knives.
- Gingivectomy is contraindicated if there will be less than 2 mm of attached gingiva remaining after surgery.
- The surgical gingivectomy, while more technical, is less painful and allows a quicker return to function/homecare.

(a)

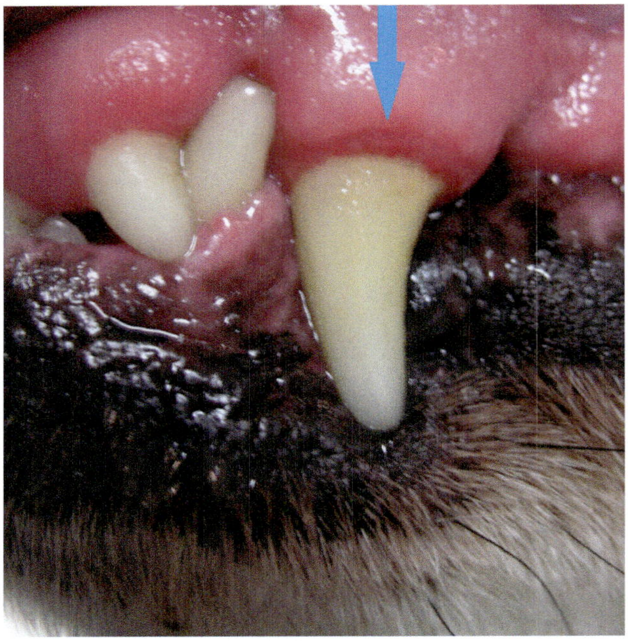

(b)

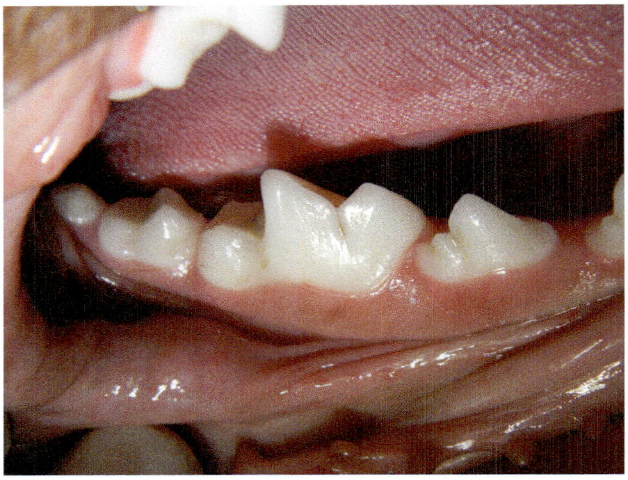

Figure 15.25 Recheck pictures of gingivectomy procedures demonstrating more rapid healing time with the periodontal flap surgical technique in contrast to the standard gingivectomy technique. (a) 3-week recheck picture of the patient in Figures 15.12–15.19 . Note the significant inflammation to the incised gingival margin (blue arrow) after a longer period of time. Homecare efforts were still producing hemorrhage. (b) 2-week recheck picture of the patient in Figures 15.20–15.24. Notice the gingiva is completely healed with no evidence of inflammation.

Note

A. Paint on Dam, Den-Mat Corp.

References

1. Wiggs RB, Lobprise HB. Periodontology. In: Veterinary Dentistry, Principles and Practice. Philadelphia: Lippincott-Raven, 1997, pp. 186–231.
2. Debowes LJ. Problems with the gingiva. In: Small Animal Dental, Oral and Maxillofacial Disease, a Color Handbook (Niemiec BA ed.). London: Manson, 2010, pp. 159–181.
3. Waerhaug J. Microscopic demonstration of tissue reaction incident to removal of subgingival calculus. J Periodontol. 26:26, 1955.
4. Stone S, Ramfjord SP, Waldron J. Scaling and gingival curettage: A radioautographic study. J Periodontol. 37:415, 1966.
5. Takei HH, Carranza FA. Gingival surgical techniques. In: Carranza's Clinical Periodontology. St. Louis: Saunders, 2006, pp. 909–917.
6. Zach I, Cohen G. The histologic response to ultrasonic curettage. J Dent Res. 40:751, 1961.
7. Sanderson AD. Gingival curettage by hand and ultrasonic instruments: A histologic comparison. J Periodontol. 37:279, 1966.
8. Glickman J, Patur B. Histologic study of the effect of antiformin on the soft tissue wall of periodontal pockets in humans. J Am Dent Assoc. 51:420, 1955.
9. Beube FE. An experimental study of the use of sodium sulphide solution in treatment of periodontal pockets. J Periodontol. 10:49, 1939.
10. Yukna RA. A clinical and histological study of healing following the excisional new attachment procedure in rhesus monkeys. J Periodontol. 47:701, 1976.
11. Glickman I. The results obtained with the unembellished gingivectomy technique in a clinical study in humans. J Periodontol. 27:247, 1956.
12. Camargo PM, et al. Treatment of gingival enlargement. In: Carranza's Clinical Periodontology. St. Louis: Saunders, 2006, pp. 918–925.
13. Wiggs RB, & Lobprise HB. Veterinary Dentistry, Principles and Practice. Philadelphia: Lippincott-Raven, 1997, p. 116.
14. Burstone MS, Bond E, Litt CR. Familial gingival hypertrophy in the dog (boxer breed). AMA Arch Pathol. 54(2):208–212, 1952.
15. Davan D, Kozlovsky A, et al. Castration prevents channel blocker-induced gingival hyperplasia in beagle dogs. Hum Experimental Toxicology 17(7):396–402, 1998.
16. Lafzi A, Farahani RM, Shoja MA. Phenobarbitol-induced gingival hyperplasia. J Contemp Dent Pract. 8(6):50–56, 2007.
17. Eggerath J, English H, Leichter JW. Drug-associated gingival enlargement: Case report and review of aetiology, management and evidence-based outcomes of treatment. J NZ Soc Periodontol. 88:7–14, 2005.
18. Nam HS, McAnulty JF, et al. Gingival overgrowth in dogs associated with clinically relevant cyclosporine blood levels: Observations in a canine renal transplantation model. Vet Surg. 37(3):247–253, 2008.
19. Nishikawa S, Nagata T, et al. Pathogenesis of drug-induced gingival overgrowth. A review of studies in the rat model. J Periodontol. 67(5):463–471, 1996.
20. Sitzman C. Simultaneous hyperplasia, metaplasia, and neoplasia in an 8 year-old boxer dog: A case report. J Vet Dent. 17(1):27–30, 2000.
21. Carranza FA, Hogan EL. Gingival enlargement In: Carranza's Clinical Periodontology. St. Louis: Saunders, 2006, pp. 279–294, 582–583.

22. Lewis JR, Reiter AM. Management of generalized gingival enlargement in a dog-case report and literature review. J Vet Dent. 22(3):160–169, 2005.
23. Tackas VJ. Root coverage techniques: A review. J West Soc Periodontol Periodontal Abstr. 43(1):5–14, 1995.
24. Wolf HF, Rateitschak EM, Rateitschak KH, Hassell TH. Color Atlas of Dental Medicine: Periodontology 3rd ed. Stuttgart: Thieme, 2005.
25. Force J, Niemiec B. Gingivectomy and gingivoplasty for gingival enlargement. J Vet Dent. 26(2):132–137, 2009.
26. Holmstrom SE, Frost PF, Eisner ER. Periodontal therapy and surgery. In: Veterinary Dental Techniques for the Small Animal Practitioner. 3rd ed. Philadelphia: Saunders, 2004, pp. 233–290.
27. Fisher SE, Frame JW, Browne RM, et al. A comparative histological study of wound healing following CO_2 laser and conventional surgical excision of the buccal mucosa. Arch Oral Biol. 28:287, 1980.
28. Malone WF, Eisenmann D, Kusck J. Interceptive periodontics with electrosurgery. J Prosthet Dent. 22:555, 1969.
29. Wilhelmsen NR, Ramfjord SP, Blankenship JR. Effects of electrosurgery on the gingival attachment in Rhesus monkeys. J Periodontol. 47:160, 1976.
30. Pope JW, Gargiulo AW, Staffileno H, et al. Effects of electrosurgery on wound healing in dogs. Periodontics 6:30, 1968.
31. Kalkwarf KL, Freici RF, et al. Histological evaluation of gingival response to an electrosurgical blade. J Oral Maxillofac Surg. 45(8):671–674, 1987.
32. Azzi R, Kenney EB, Tsao TF, et al. The effect of electrosurgery upon alveolar bone. J Periodontol. 54:96, 1983.
33. Glickman I, Imber LR. Comparison of gingival resection with electrosurgery and periodontal knives: Biometric and histologic study. J Periodontol 41:242, 1970.
34. Ando Y, Aoki A, Watanabe H, Ishikawa I. Bacteriocidal effect of erbium YAG laser on periodontopathic bacteria. Lasers Surg Med. 19:190, 1996.
35. Yamaguchi H, Kobayashi K, Osada R, et al. Effects of irradiation of an erbium:YAG laser on root surfaces. J Periodontol. 68:1151, 1997.
36. Pogrel MA, Yen CK, Hanser LS. A comparison of carbon dioxide laser, cryosurgery, and scalpel wounds in healing. Oral Surg Oral Med Oral Path. 69:269, 1990.
37. Loumanen M. A comparative study of healing of laser and scalpel incision wounds in rat oral mucosa. Scand J Dent Res. 95:65, 1987.
38. Goultschin J, Gasit D, et al. Changes in teeth and gingiva of dogs following laser surgery: A block surface light microscope study. Lasers Surg Med. 8(4):402–408, 1988.
39. Ishikawa I, Aoki A. Lasers in periodontics. In: Carranza's Clinical Periodontology. St. Louis: Saunders, 2006, pp. 1035–1037.
40. Loe H. Chemical gingivectomy: Effect of potassium hydroxide on periodontal tissues. Acta Odontol Scand. 19:517, 1961.
41. Orban B. New methods in periodontal treatment. Bur. 14:116, 1942.
42. Force J, Niemiec B. Gingivectomy and gingivoplasty for gingival enlargement. J Vet Dent. 26(2):132–137, 2009.
43. Carmargo P, Melnick P, Pirih F, et al. Treatment of drug induced gingival enlargement: Aesthetic and functional considerations. Periodontol 2000 27:131, 2001.

16

Periodontal flap surgery

Introduction

The goals of periodontal flap surgery are the reduction or elimination of pathologic periodontal pockets while improving the client's ability to perform homecare and maintain a disease-free state. Ideally, the pocket reduction will be via regeneration, but it is commonly necessary to perform resection or apical repositioning. Consequently, periodontal flaps are performed to.[1,2]

1. Establish direct root visualization and improved accessibility for effective cleaning during the procedure, at future treatments, and for homecare.
2. Allow access to the hard tissues for reshaping in order to create a healthier surface.
3. Eliminate the pathologic pocket walls.
4. Cover exposed surfaces (i.e., lateral sliding flap/free gingival grafts).

Visualization and hard tissue access are possible with a modified Widman flap. If reduction of pocket depth is a goal, an undisplaced or apically repositioned flap is necessary (see below).[1]

An additional indication for periodontal flaps is improved aesthetics.[3] While aesthetics is currently much more important in human dentistry, future generations of veterinary dentists will likely be asked to perform these "cosmetic" surgeries. For example, free gingival grafting for root coverage of rostral teeth is a common cosmetic surgery in humans.

After the flap is created, the first step is to remove the infection from the root surface. Following this, the root surface is smoothed, root conditioning performed, and the incisions are closed. It is critical to note that the most important step of any periodontal surgery is the complete cleaning of the root surface. If this step is not performed correctly, the effectiveness of the flap will be greatly diminished.[4] (See chapter 17 for a detailed discussion regarding treatment of the exposed root surface.) Performing a periodontal flap surgery including the above steps allows for gingival reattachment and thus a decrease in pocket depth (at least by shrinkage). These are advanced procedures but can be learned by general practitioners. For a list of hands-on training classes, please see appendix 4.

It is important to clarify that while periodontal surgery is very effective for regaining attachment and salvaging teeth, the maintenance of the reduced pocket is a critical part of the periodontal therapy.[2,3,5] Therefore, without a commitment to regular periodontal care (consistent homecare and professional cleanings), these surgeries will ultimately fail. This should be communicated to the client *prior* to performing surgery.

Indications

As pockets deepen, cleaning becomes increasingly difficult and surface irregularities increase, thus complicating closed periodontal therapy.[6–8] Periodontal pockets greater than 5–6 mm (Figure 16.1) *require* direct root visualization for effective cleaning,[2,9] owing to the fact that residual calculus after closed root planing is seen with regularity in pockets greater than 6 mm.[10] In humans, this is known as the "*5 mm standard*."[11,12] In addition to deep pockets, periodontal flap surgery is indicated for teeth with even moderate alveolar bone loss (Figure 16.2), furcation exposure level II and III (Figures 16.3 and 16.4), and inaccessible areas (Figure 16.5).[3] Also, areas with deep bone craters or irregular bone contours should be treated surgically.[3]

Veterinary Periodontology, First Edition. Brook A. Niemiec.

(a) (b) (c)

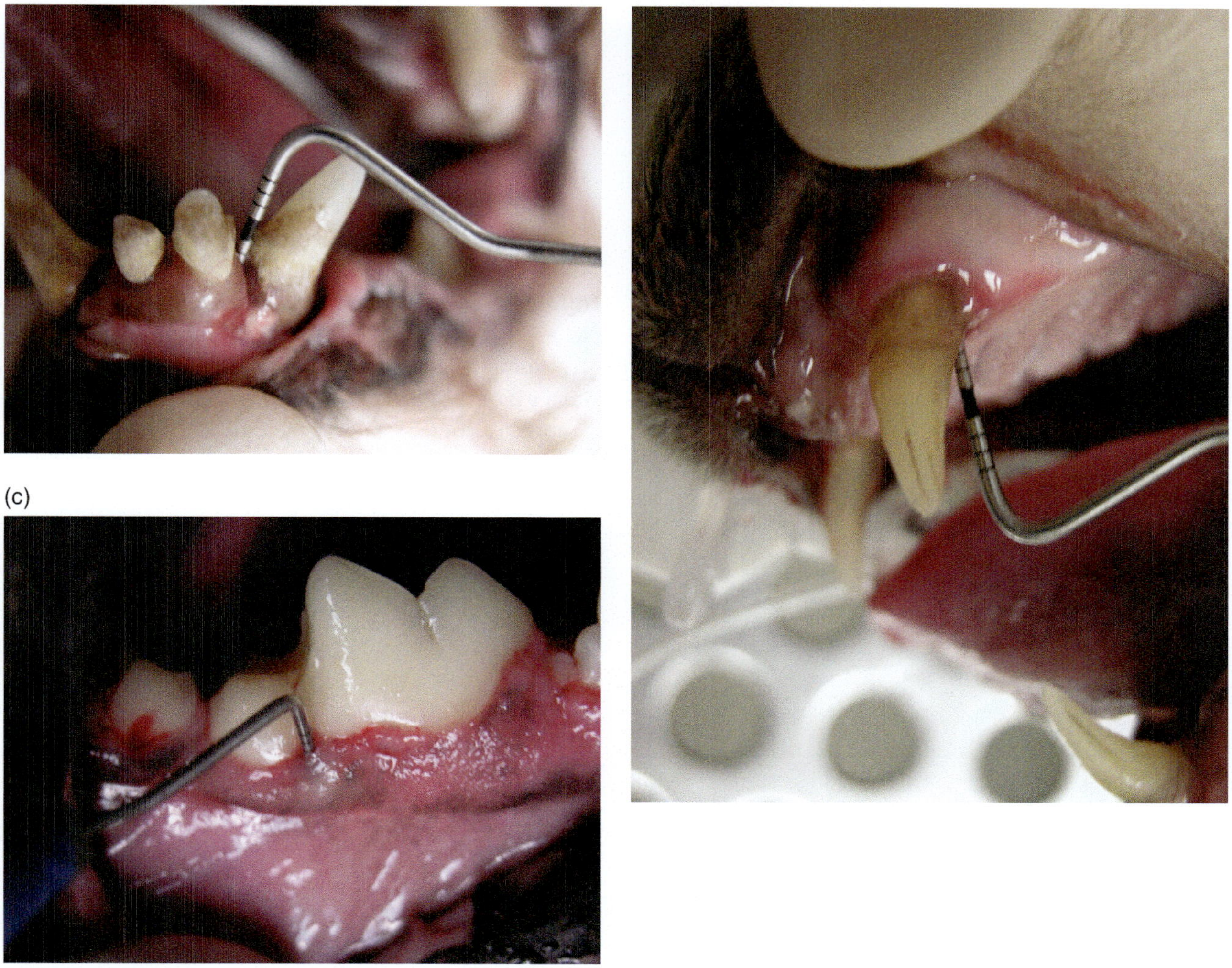

Figure 16.1 Deep periodontal pockets are an indication for periodontal surgery. (a) Intraoral dental picture of the left mandibular canine (304) in a dog. This tooth has a 9 mm periodontal pocket on the mesial surface. (b) Intraoral dental picture of the left maxillary canine (204) in a cat. This tooth has a 7 mm periodontal pocket on the palatal surface. (c) Intraoral dental picture of the left mandibular first molar (309) in a dog. This tooth has a 13 mm periodontal pocket on the mesial surface. Each of these pockets require direct visualization (via a periodontal flap) for complete cleaning.

Finally, any area that has not responded favorably to conservative treatment (closed scaling/root planing) should be treated surgically.[3]

Results of pocket therapy

The ultimate goal of any periodontal therapy (including surgery) is the elimination of the pathologic pocket. This will occur only with meticulous scaling/root planing (open or closed).[4] Shallow pockets can be returned to a relatively normal state via closed root therapy. However, conservative treatment (i.e., closed root planing) of deep pockets will generally result in reduction of pocket depth via a long junctional epithelium. While this results in an elimination of current infection, this form of attachment is generally considered tenuous at best. Animal patients may be more resistant to reinfection,[13] but further research is required before we rely on this structure to maintain periodontal health. Moreover, in human patients, strict homecare and regular professional therapy *may* be able to maintain this arrangement,[4,14] but this level of care is exceedingly rare in veterinary patients today.

Consequently, it is recommended to more permanently reduce pocket depth in animal patients. This is ideally achieved by regeneration techniques (guided tissue regeneration), which at the time of this writing can only be performed in select cases (see chapter 18).

Therefore, pocket reduction is generally accomplished by resection techniques (gingivectomy or ideally apical repositioning flaps). If the result of the initial therapy or surgery is less than ideal, these techniques should be considered.

Equipment needs

Incisions for periodontal surgery are best accomplished with a number 11, 15, 15 c, or 12 d scalpel blade.[5,15,16] These small blades are best for the fine incisions required in tight, interdental areas. A wide selection of *sharp* periosteal elevators and curettes should be available. Gentle tissue handling is critical; therefore 1 x 2 forceps should *not* be utilized. Less traumatic 7 x 7 or DeBakey tissue forceps are preferred. Small, fine (iris) scissors should also be available,[16] and this author prefers LaGrange scissors. Finally, small needle holders should be utilized, ideally Castroviejo. These basic instruments have been packaged for convenience and are commercially available (see chapter 22).[A] It is recommended to have this minimal set of instruments, as well as a sharpening stone, in a sterile pack. Additional equipment that should be considered includes gingivectomy/interdental knives, heavy curettes/sickles (e.g., Pritchard), and chisels (for a complete discussion of periodontal hand instruments please see chapter 22).

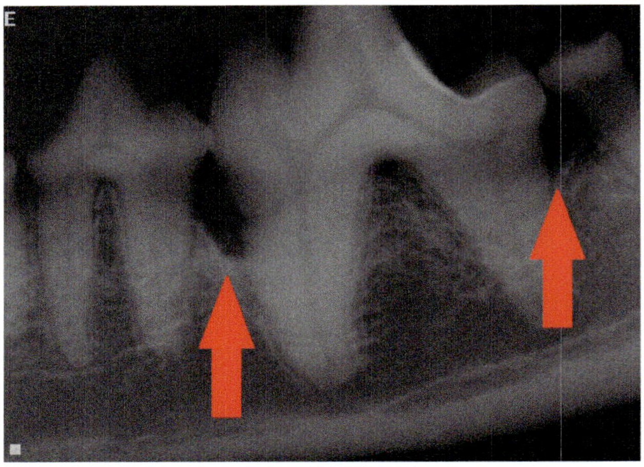

Figure 16.2 Intraoral dental radiograph of the left mandibular first molar (309) in a dog. There is moderate angular bone loss (red arrows) to both the mesial and distal aspects of this tooth (red arrows). (See chapter 9 for a discussion of radiographic diagnosis of periodontal disease.) Periodontal surgery is indicated for this case, as well as guided tissue regeneration (see chapter 18).

Suture should always be swedged on, preferably on a *reverse* cutting needle,[17] unless the tissue is exceedingly friable, in which case a taper needle may be best. Any absorbable material is acceptable,[5] but monofilament is preferable as it avoids the "wicking" effect of the braided material.[17,18] In humans, the minimum coaption time is approximately 5 days;[58] and thus quick-dissolving materials are ideal. Chromic cat gut, polyglecaprone,[B] polyglactin 910,[C] and polyglycolic acid[D] are all well suited materials.[17,19] Recently, an antibiotic impregnated suture has become available[E] that was shown to decrease bacterial infection.[20,21] The suture should be very fine (4-0 to 6-0) to minimize the trauma to the delicate periodontal tissues.[17]

(a) (b)

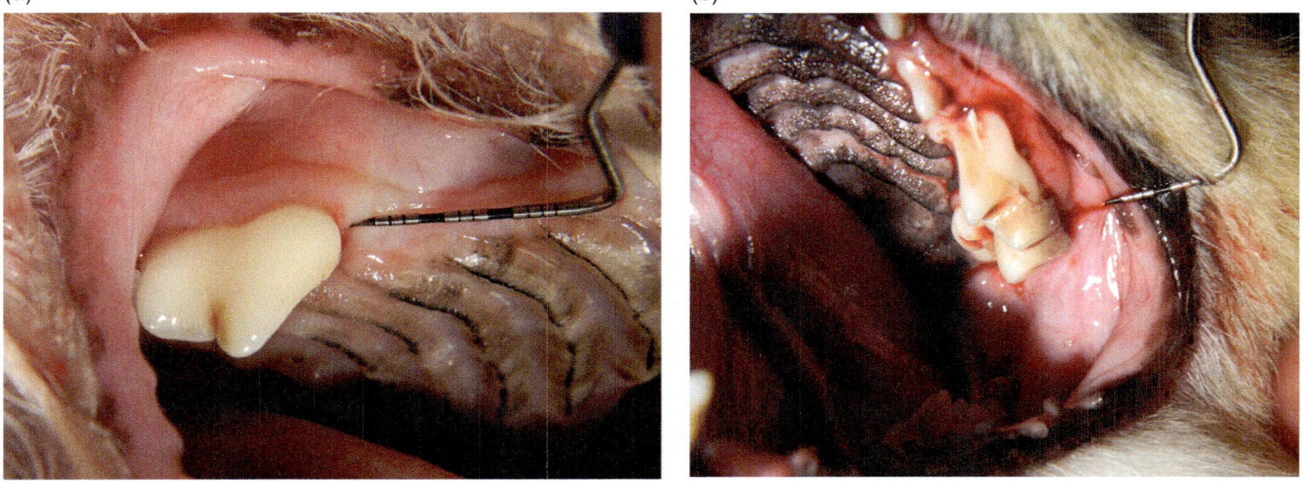

Figure 16.3 Furcation exposure level II is an indication for periodontal flap surgery. (a) Intraoral dental picture of the right maxillary fourth premolar (108) in a dog. This tooth has a grade II furcation exposure on the mesial surface. This pocket requires direct visualization (via a periodontal flap) for complete cleaning. Note the location of the furcation is unusual, as well as the lack of gingival inflammation, confirming the importance of a complete oral exam in all cases. (b) Intraoral dental picture of the left maxillary first molar (109) in a dog. This tooth has a grade II furcation exposure on the buccal surface. This area requires direct visualization (via a periodontal flap) for complete cleaning.

(a)

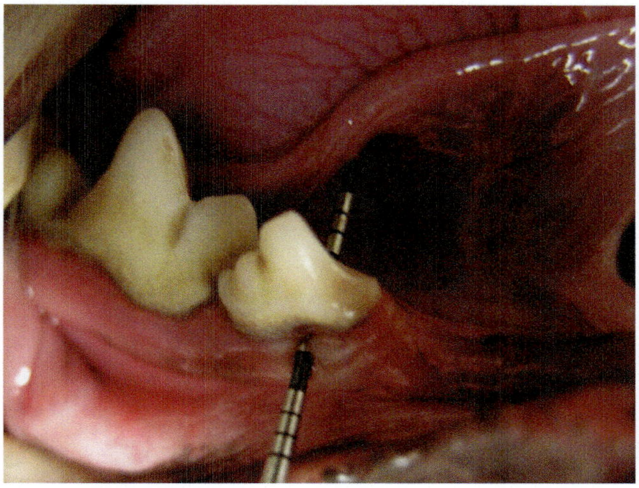

(b)

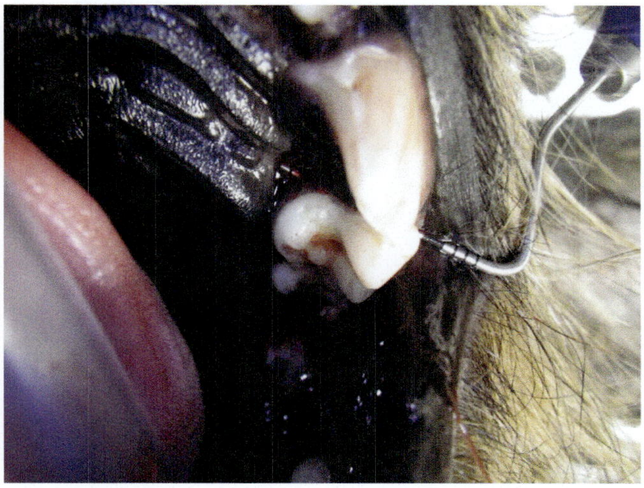

Figure 16.4 Furcation exposure level III is an indication for periodontal flap surgery. (a) Intraoral dental picture of the right mandibular fourth premolar (408) in a dog. This tooth has a grade III furcation exposure. This area requires direct visualization (via a periodontal flap) for complete cleaning. (b) Intraoral dental picture of the left maxillary first molar (209) in a dog. This tooth has a grade III furcation exposure. This area requires direct visualization (via a periodontal flap) for complete cleaning. Extraction should also be considered for this case.

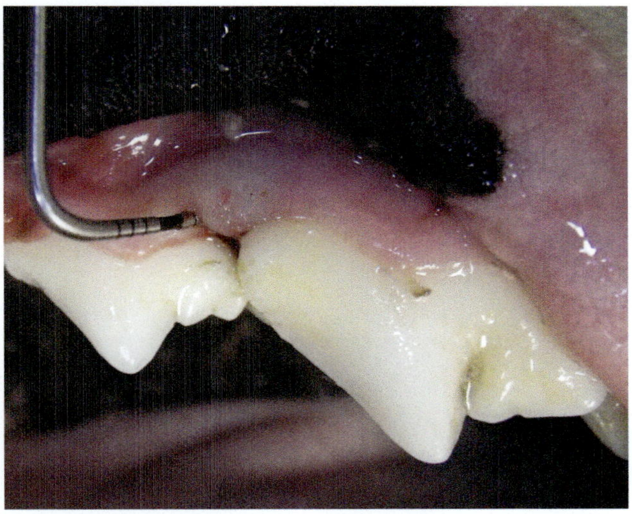

Figure 16.5 Inaccessible areas are an indication for periodontal flap surgery. Intraoral dental picture of the left maxillary third and fourth premolars (207 and 208) in a dog. There is a deep periodontal pocket between the teeth with a very tight contact. This would limit the effectiveness of closed root planing. This area is best treated with direct visualization (via a periodontal flap) for complete cleaning. Extraction of 207 should also be considered as part of the treatment plan.

Additional materials should include an absorbable barrier membrane such as polyglactin 910 knitted mesh,[F] cross-linked bovine type I collagen, ossifflex, doxirobe, or PGLA. Finally, a bone augmentation particulate that may be natural[G] or synthetic[H] should be part of the armatairum. (See chapter 18 for a detailed discussion of these products.)

Proper lighting and magnification are strongly recommended for periodontal surgery, to provide the visualization necessary for meticulous plaque and calculus removal. Lighting can be achieved with "spot" surgical lights or head lights. There are numerous manufacturers of head loupes, and these are very helpful. A new product that combines both light and magnification in one package works well for this author.[I]

Surgical suction is strongly recommended for periodontal surgery;[15] this too will help provide the appropriate visualization necessary for surgical procedures and proper calculus removal.[15] With oral procedures, hemorrhage is often significant due to both the high vascularity of the periodontal tissues and the inflammation that accompanies periodontal disease. In addition, a thorough debridement of granulation tissue (which is highly vascular) is necessary for proper healing.

A selection of hemostatic agents should be available in the event of hemorrhage. Periodontal surgery requires the creation of gingival/periodontal flaps that are often in the area of significant vessels (e.g., the infraorbital and mental arteries). The reader is directed to chapter 1 to review important structures prior to initiating surgery. Identifiable vessels should be ligated if possible,[15] or alternatively *carefully* treated with electrocautery (Figure 16.6).[22] Generalized oozing can usually be controlled with direct pressure (ideally with a cold pack) or the application of a vasoconstrictor (e.g., epinephrine).[15,22] If this is ineffective, hemostatic agents may be utilized, such as absorbable gelatin sponges,[J,K] oxidized

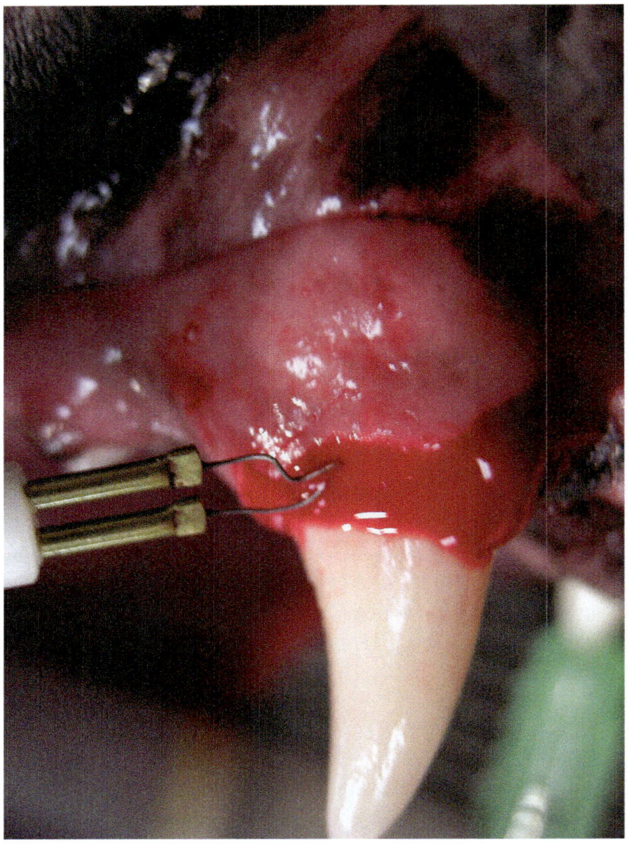

Figure 16.6 Intraoral dental picture of a handheld electrocautery unit on the gingiva of the maxillary right canine (104) in a dog.

regenerated cellulose,[L] micorfibrillar collagen,[M] or thrombin.[N,15,22]

Surgical preparation

All periodontal surgical procedures should start with a complete dental prophylaxis (including closed root planing/scaling) to decrease oral contamination. Ideally, this is performed as a separate procedure 2–4 weeks prior to the surgical treatment, and followed by oral hygiene ± chemotherapeutics.[15,23,24] This protocol will reduce inflammation, resulting in less friable tissue, and may even resolve some lesions entirely.[15,25,26] In addition, it allows the practitioner to fully discuss the therapy and future care necessary for success. It also allows for proper scheduling, and more importantly shorter anaesthetic time, which may be in the patient's best interest. Many owners may be resistant to the additional cost, but proper client education can be very effective.

Prior to initiating surgery, a complete oral exam with careful periodontal probing is performed (see Box 10.4).[2,15,27] *Sounding* should be performed by utilizing the periodontal probe, not in the sulcus/pocket, but on the surrounding tissues (Figure 16.7). By

(a)

(b)

(c)

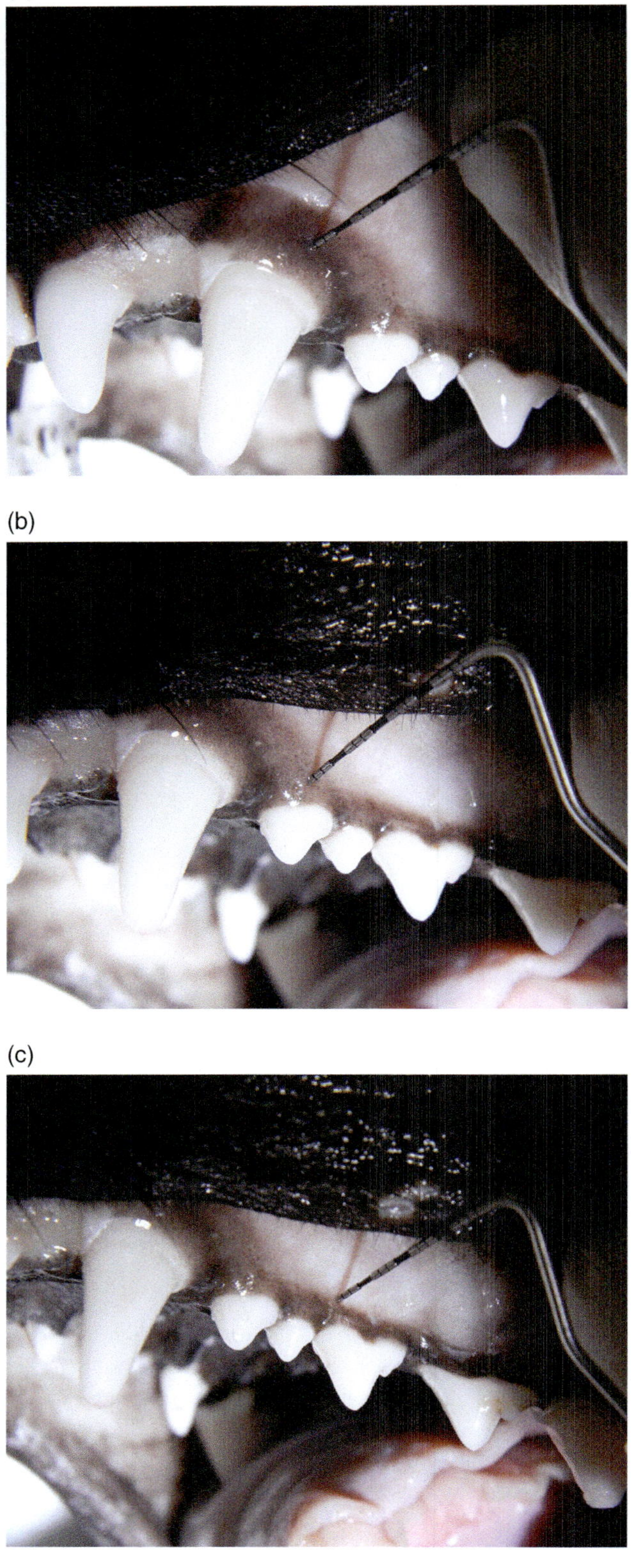

Figure 16.7 (a–c) Sounding the maxillary left of a dog.

pressing on the tissues, the operator can get a sense as to the extent and configuration of the intrabony component of the pocket and furcational defects.[28,29] Next, a

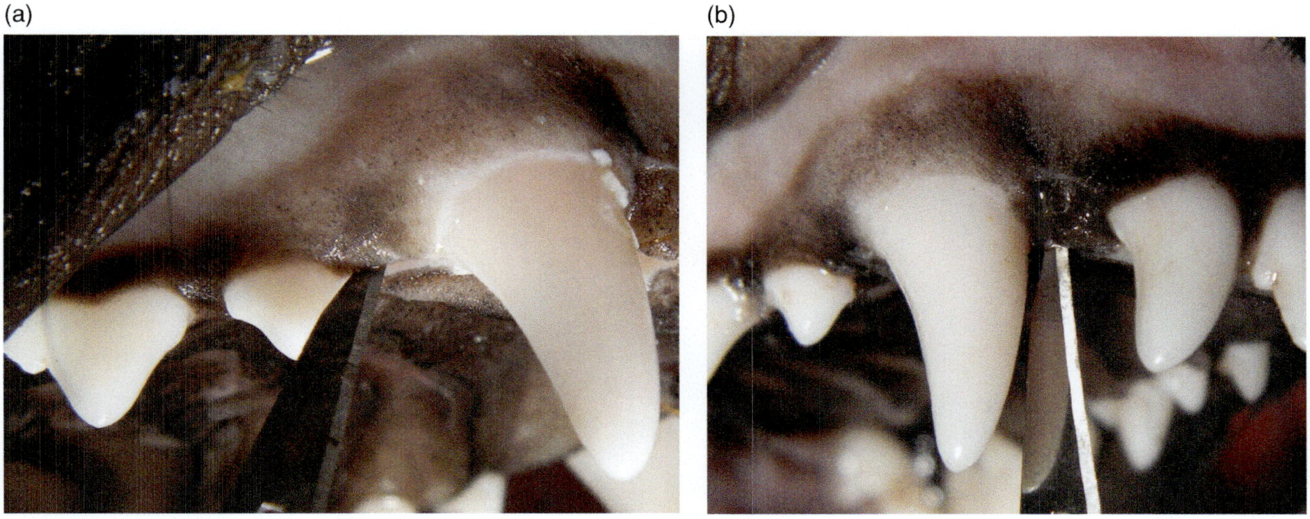

Figure 16.8 Carrying the incision (a) distal and (b) mesial to the target tooth for additional visualization.

dental radiograph should be exposed of the surgical area to document attachment levels.[5,30] Once the surgical site is determined, proper pain and antimicrobial (if indicated) management is administered. (See chapters 14 and 19, respectively, for complete information on these subjects.)

The entire surgical procedure (including bone augmentation and closure) should be planned prior to making the initial incision. This gives the practitioner the greatest chance of successful treatment while minimizing surgical trauma.

Flap types

There are numerous options for flap design, depending on the clinical presentation. The most common flap used in veterinary oral surgery approximates a full flap, or one with vertical releasing incisions.[2] This allows for increased exposure but is somewhat more invasive. Another commonly used flap for periodontal surgery is the envelope flap. This is created along the arcade, without vertical incisions. Less common flap designs include the lateral sliding flap, palatine flap, and flaps for regenerative surgeries, which are subsets of the above types. The initial incision is the same for all flaps but the incision point will vary slightly (as detailed below).

Periodontal flaps are typically made *full thickness*, which means the periosteum is released from the underlying hard tissue and kept with the flap.[5,19] However, any flap design can be created as *partial thickness*, which leaves the periosteum attached to the underlying alveolar bone.[19] This is typically done to avoid leaving an area of bone uncovered and is most common with lateral sliding flaps or free gingival grafts.[5]

The sulcal incision (creation of an envelope flap)

The initial incisions (three in total) for the periodontal flap are the most critical part of the surgery, as the sulcal incision[15,19] is different from any other incision used in the oral cavity (or veterinary medicine in general). This is because these initial incisions not only release the gingiva from the underlying hard tissues but also excise the diseased pocket epithelium and granulation tissue. Furthermore, the sum of these incisions creates a sharp marginal edge of the resulting flap, which allows for superior apposition when it is replaced. There are three distinct cuts that comprise the sulcal incision, which will be detailed below.

Prior to creating the incision, the extent of the flap should be determined. All involved teeth in the area should be involved from the beginning, to allow for a smooth incision. In most cases, carrying the incision a little mesial and distal of the target tooth is necessary for adequate visualization and access (Figure 16.8).

The initial or "first" incision is created reverse (or internal) bevel as opposed to the standard bevel used in gingivectomies.[2,5] The incision is initiated in the healthy attached gingiva at or near the gingival margin and directed toward the alveolar crest (Figure 16.9). The incision should curve around the tooth or teeth to create a scalloped appearance, allowing for superior adaptation (Figure 16.10).

After the initial incision is made across the area to be treated, the crevicular incision is performed. A delicate blade (e.g., 12D) is directed parallel and adjacent to the buccal or lingual/palatal aspect of the tooth down into the pocket to end at the alveolar crest, just inside the first incision (Figure 16.11). These two incisions will create a

(a) (b)

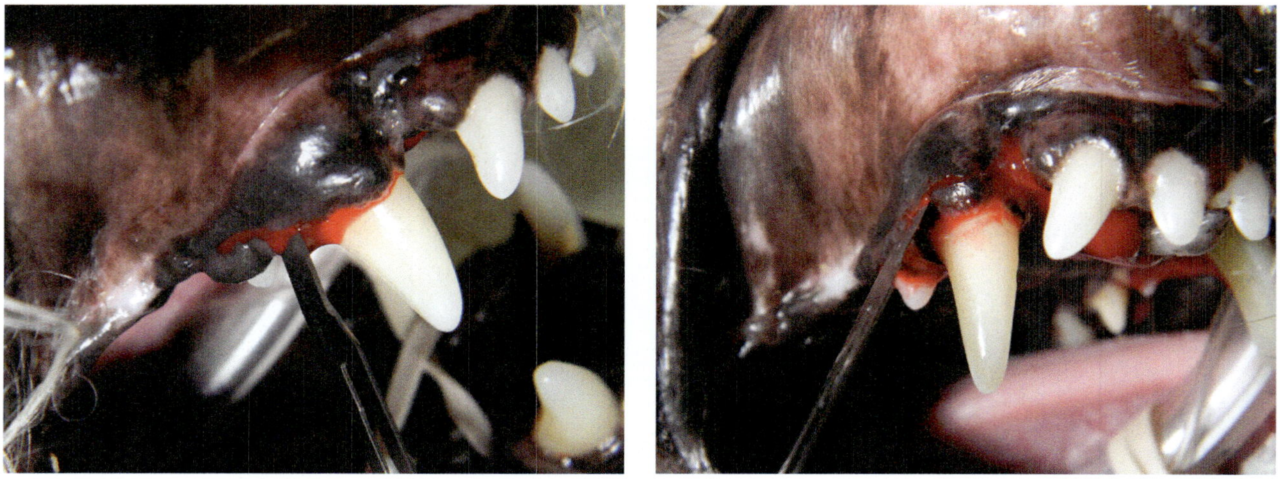

Figure 16.9 (a and b) The initial (first) 45-degree internal bevel incision.

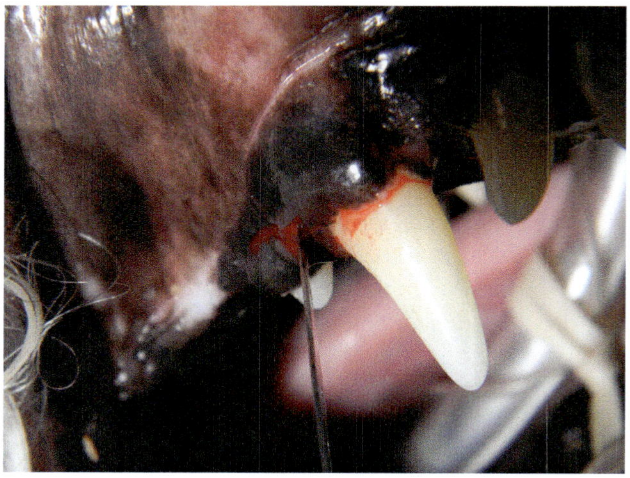

Figure 16.10 Scalloping the incision along the tooth.

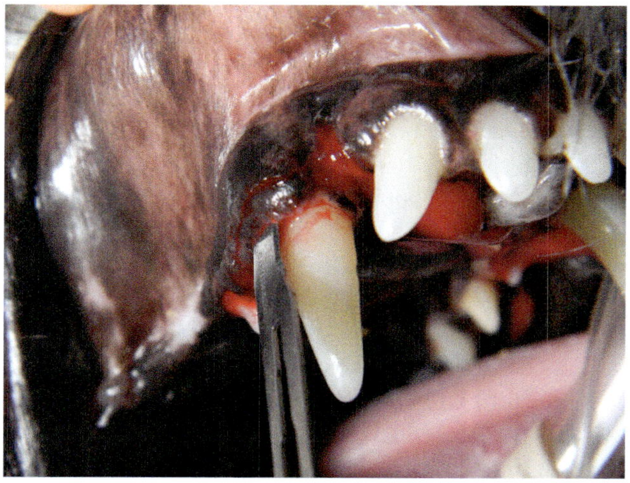

Figure 16.11 The crevicular (second) incision. The blade is directed parallel and adjacent to the buccal aspect of the tooth down into the pocket to end at the alveolar crest, just inside the first incision.

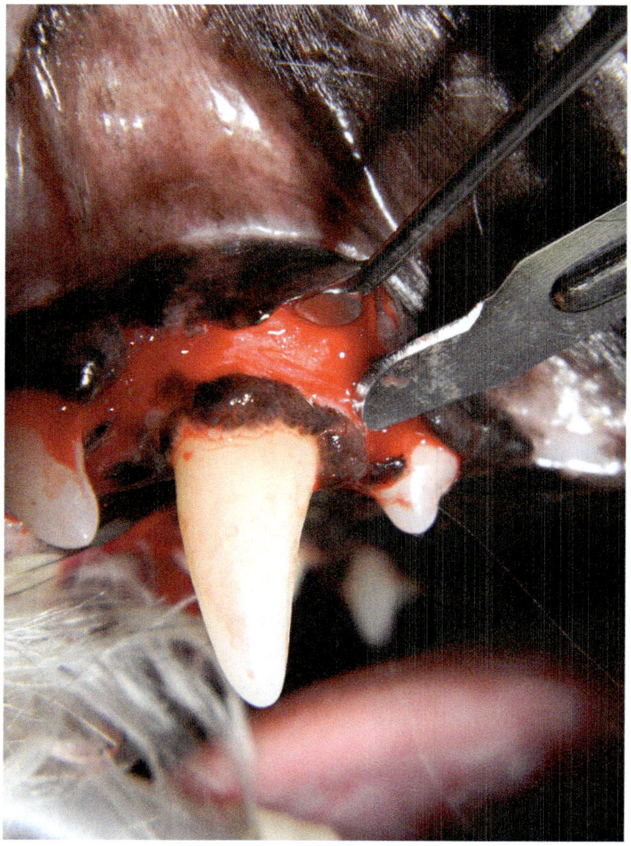

Figure 16.12 The "third" incision. Releasing the wedge of infected tissue with a scalpel blade.

wedge of infected tissue (pocket epithelium and granulation tissue).

A periosteal elevator is then utilized to reflect the healthy flap tissue from the alveolar bone. Once these steps are accomplished, the surgeon will have excellent visibility of the infected area.

The next step involves removing the wedge of infected tissue by releasing it from the bone/teeth with a scalpel blade or Orban knife (third incision) (Figure 16.12). Finally, the wedge of tissue is removed, usually with a curette (Figure 16.13).

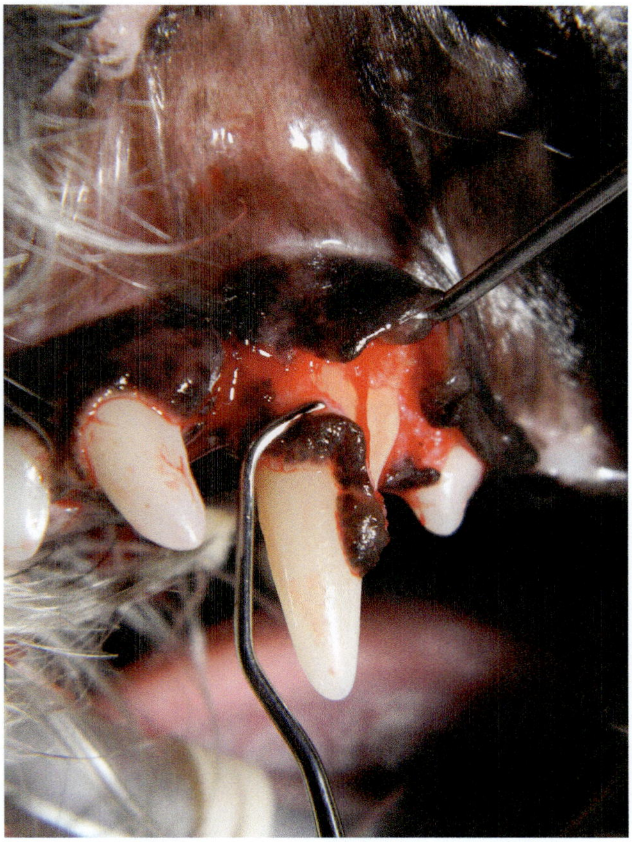

Figure 16.13 Removing the infected tissue with a curette.

The traditional interdental incision splits the interdental papilla in the middle, causing half of the papilla to stay with the buccal flap and the other half with the lingual/palatal flap (Figure 16.14). Recently, the papilla-sparing flap has been recommended as a superior alternative in interdental areas for non-displaced flaps.[1] With this technique, the interdental incisions are made in the gingival crevice so that all of the papilla stays with one side of the flap (Figure 16.15). This is less important in animal patients as true papillae are only really seen in tight contact areas such as the incisor and molar teeth.

The sulcal incisions above basically create a horizontal (*envelope*) flap[5] (Figure 16.16). In most instances, this is sufficient exposure to properly clean and treat the root surface. Following therapy (see chapters 17 and 18), the flap is replaced (without tension) and sutured interdentally. If further visualization is required or repositioning is planned, vertical incisions will be necessary to create a full flap (see below).

Full flap

The full flap is created when further exposure is necessary or the flap is to be repositioned (coronally, apically, or laterally).[5] It is a more invasive procedure with increased complication potential (e.g., hemorrhage and dehiscence) and therefore should not be performed when an envelope flap is sufficient.

The full flap is initiated by creating the same three sulcal incisions as listed for the envelope flap above. Once accomplished, vertical or oblique releasing incisions are created mesial and/or distal to the target teeth. The incisions must not be made over the root or through the papilla in tight occlusal areas (such as between the

(a) (b)

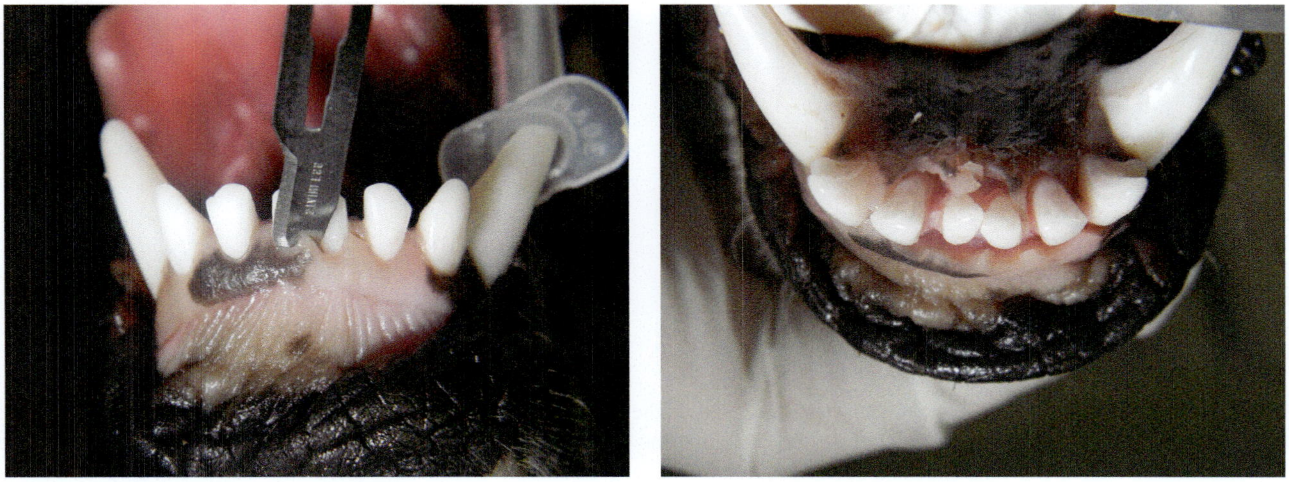

Figure 16.14 (a and b) Traditional papilla splitting technique on the mandibular incisors of a dog.

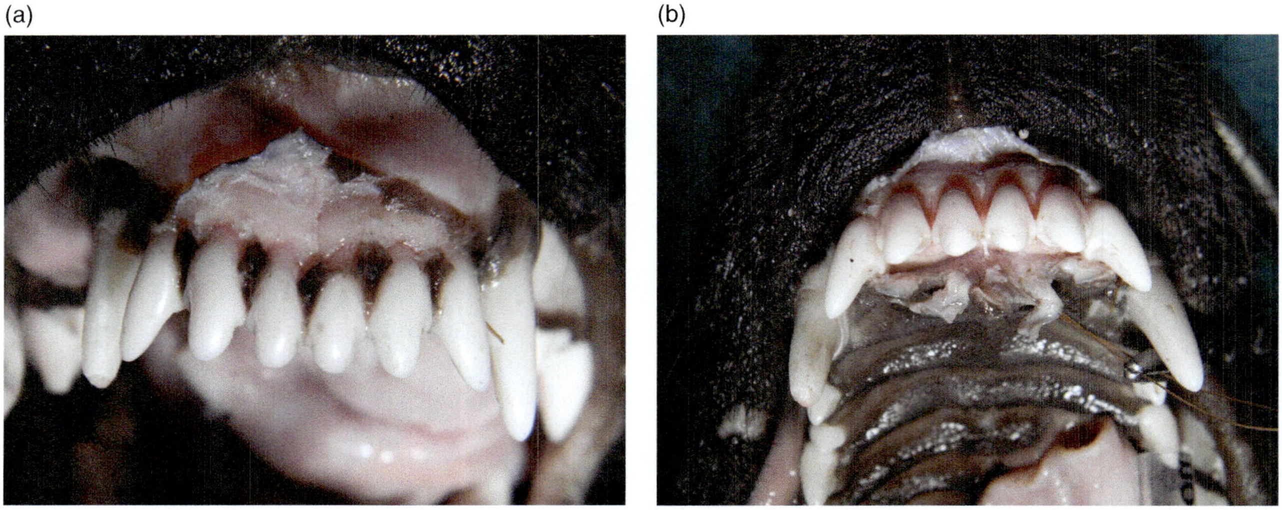

Figure 16.15 (a and b) Papilla-sparing technique. Note the papilla stays with the palatal aspect of the flap. (See below.)

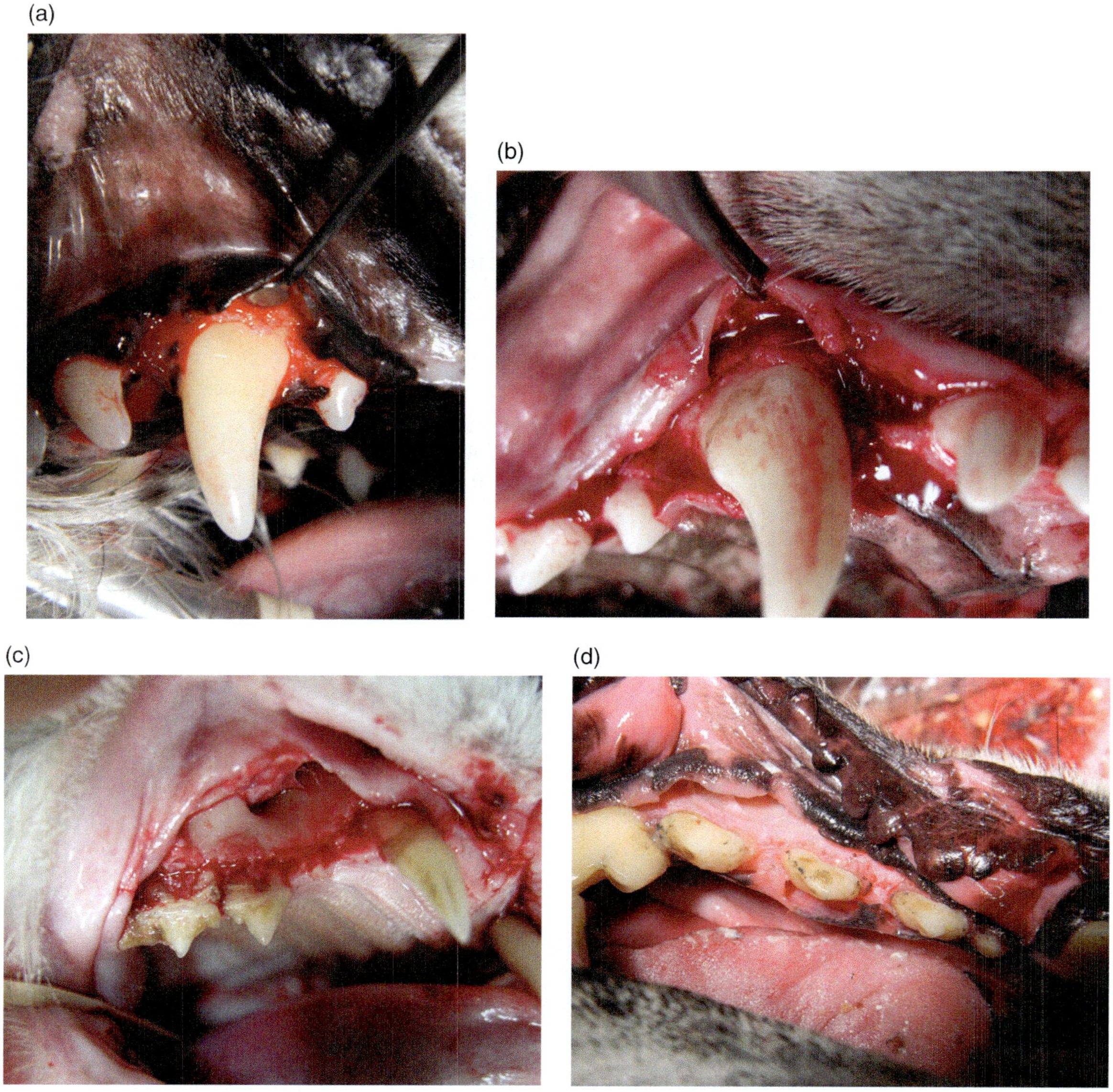

Figure 16.16 Envelope flaps created. (a) Postoperative picture of the patient in Figure 16.8. (b) Postoperative picture of an envelope flap on the maxillary right canine of an additional patient. Note that the incision is carried to healthy adjacent teeth for increased exposure. (c) Postoperative picture of an envelope flap over the entire maxillary right quadrant of a cat. (d) Postoperative picture of an envelope flap over several mandibular left premolars of a dog.

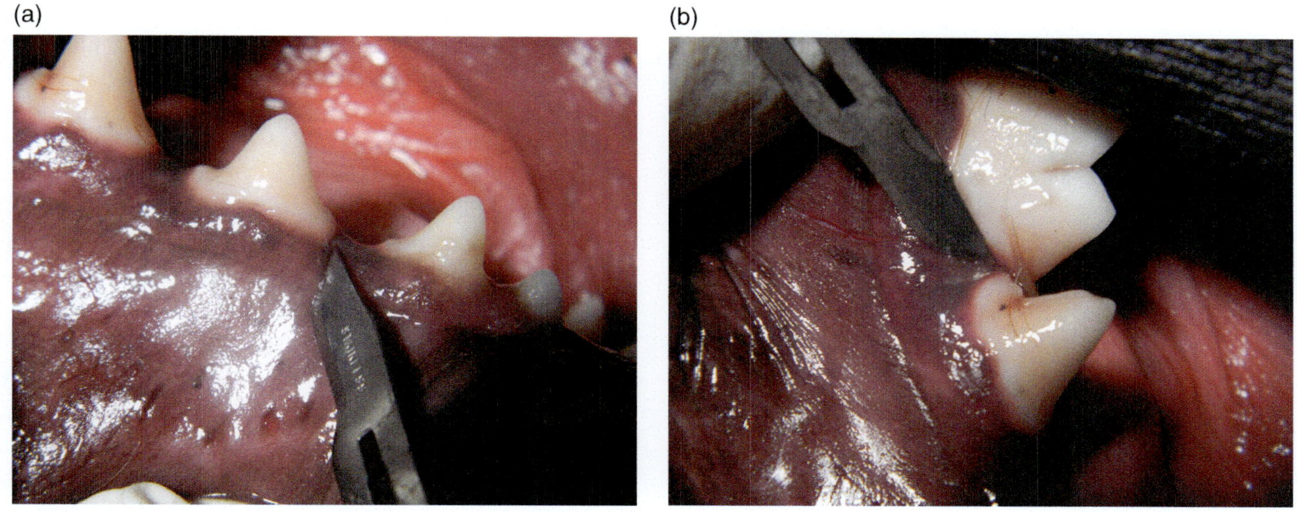

Figure 16.17 Creation of a "full" flap. Intraoral dental picture of the mandibular right of a dog. Vertical releasing incisions are created on the (a) mesial line angle of the third premolar (407) and (b) distal line angle of the fourth premolar (408).

molar and incisor teeth) as this will damage the periodontal attachment. Rather, the incisions should be created on line angles of the target teeth, or one mesial and distal to the target tooth (teeth)[2,19,31] (Figure 16.17). It is important for these incisions to either avoid or include the papilla completely. Line angles are theoretic lines where two edges of a tooth meet.[5,32] If there is a diastema between the teeth (most notable around the canine teeth) an interdental incision may be preferred[32] (Figure 16.18) These incisions should be made very slightly divergent (so that the base is slightly wider than the gingival area) to maintain blood supply[22] (Figure 16.19).

After the extent of the flap is created, it is elevated from the alveolar bone (as the envelope flap above). In general, flaps are created full thickness, which means keeping the periosteum attached to the flap and completely denuding the alveolar bone. This elevation is performed bluntly with a periosteal elevator (Figures 16.20 and 16.21), and if performed carefully is fairly easy to master. The main disadvantage of a full thickness flap is that when the bone is stripped of its periosteum, a small amount of marginal bone will be lost.[33]

Partial thickness (split) flaps

These flaps[19] are created by sharply dissecting the epithelium and a small amount of underlying connective tissue away from the alveolar bone, leaving it covered with a thin layer of connective tissue and periosteum.[5] These flaps are more challenging than the bluntly created full thickness flaps above. The major advantage to partial thickness flaps is that they leave

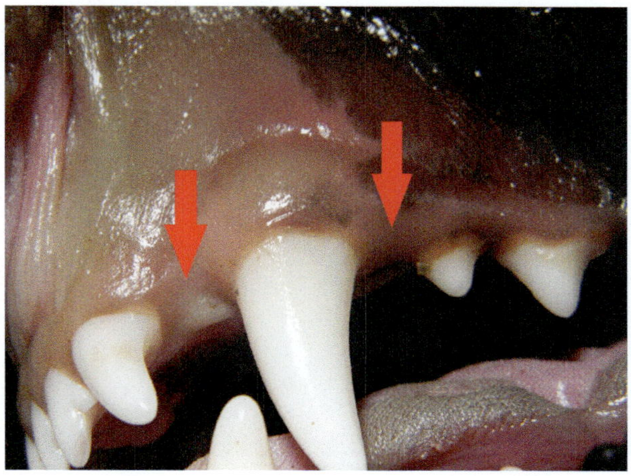

Figure 16.18 Intraoral picture of the left canine (204) showing the wide diastemas (red arrows). Creating the vertical incisions here is preferable to line angles, as less trauma is created on the periodontal ligament and attached gingiva. These areas should be used when possible.

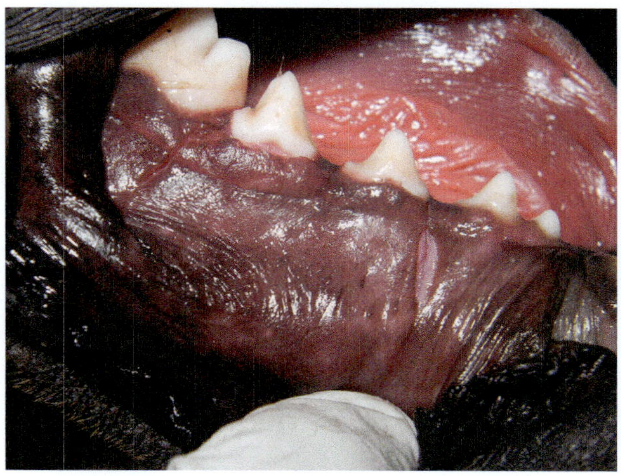

Figure 16.19 Slightly divergent full thickness incisions.

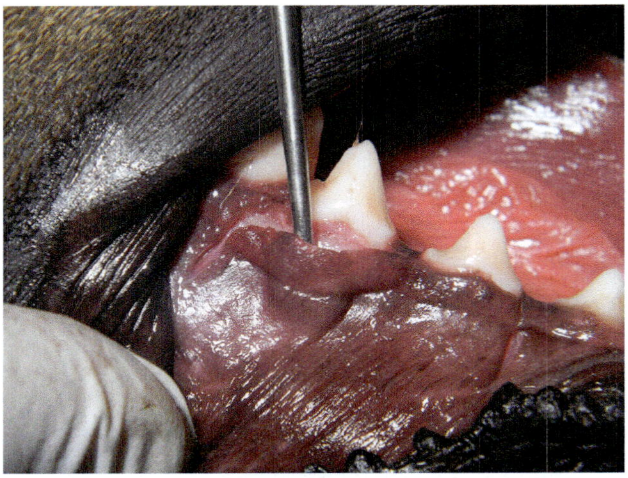

Figure 16.20 *Bluntly* releasing the flap with a periosteal elevator.

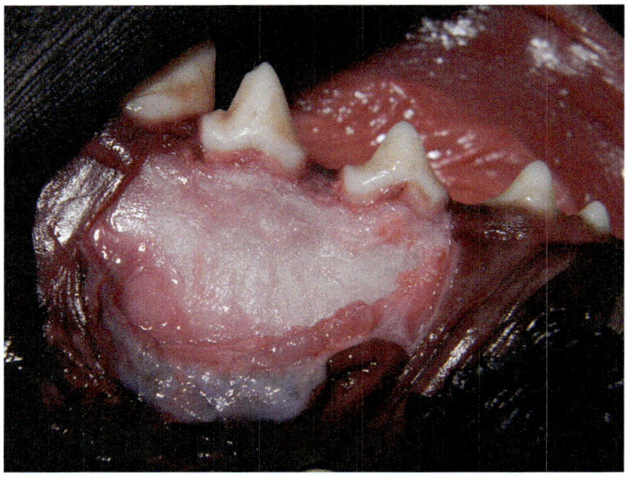

Figure 16.21 Flap reflected, revealing exposed bone.

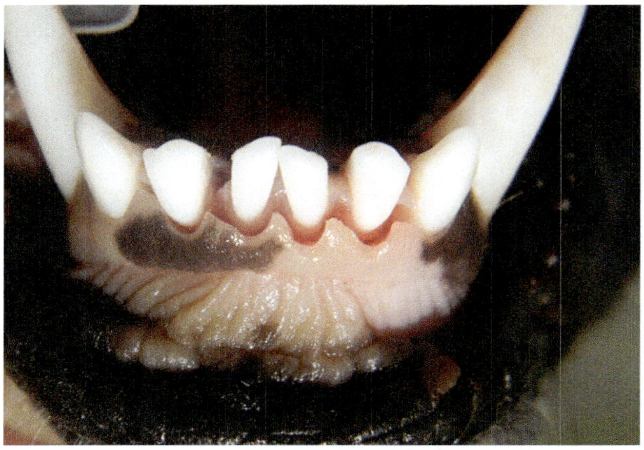

Figure 16.22 Creation of a "split thickness" flap. Intraoral dental picture after the initial three incisions are made and the wedge of tissue removed.

the alveolar bone covered in soft tissue, which allows for faster healing and decreases the loss of marginal bone as compared to the full thickness flap above.[34] This is because full thickness flaps (i.e., where the bone is exposed) will result in approximately 1 mm of bone loss.[33]

Partial thickness flaps can be performed in any case where bone reconturing/augmentation is not planned. However, they are definitely indicated when the surgeon plans on leaving bone exposed (e.g., apical repositioning, lateral sliding, free gingival grafts).[2,5] Split thickness flaps are created by sharp dissection (generally with scissors or a scalpel) between the periosteum and the alveolar mucosa. This is a tedious procedure and often results in tearing (therefore, practice with this technique is recommended prior to performing on a patient).

Technique

1. The standard initial incisions are made to remove the packet wall (Figure 16.22).
2. The vertical incisions are created as above, but are *shallower* and should not go all the way to the bone (Figure 16.23).
3. The flap is sharply dissected from the underlying tissue (Figures 16.24 and 16.25).
4. This leaves the periostium intact (Figure 16.26).

Specific flap types

Modified widman flap

This flap[1] is designed to provide access for proper root instrumentation with immediate/direct closure of the surgical area. This type of flap has been utilized for decades and was originally called the "unrepositioned mucoperiosteal flap".[35] It is the most conservative flap, as it is not designed to remove the periodontal pocket wall but just the lining, while allowing adequate access for cleaning as well as good coaptation of tissues postoperatively.[36] This type of flap will not directly reduce the pocket depth, other than by long junctional epithelium. Despite this, studies have shown this conservative method (without pocket elimination and aggressive bone contouring) to be equal or superior to the more aggressive surgeries for maintaining attachment height and shallow pocket depth.[26,37] Since the pocket wall is not to be removed, the initial internal bevel incision is made very close to the gingival margin.

(a)

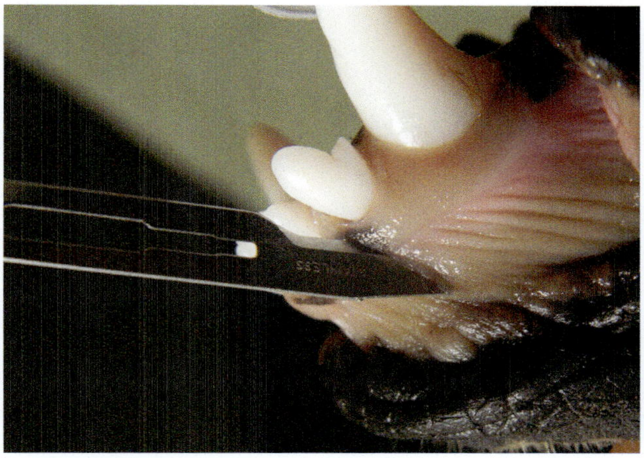

(b)

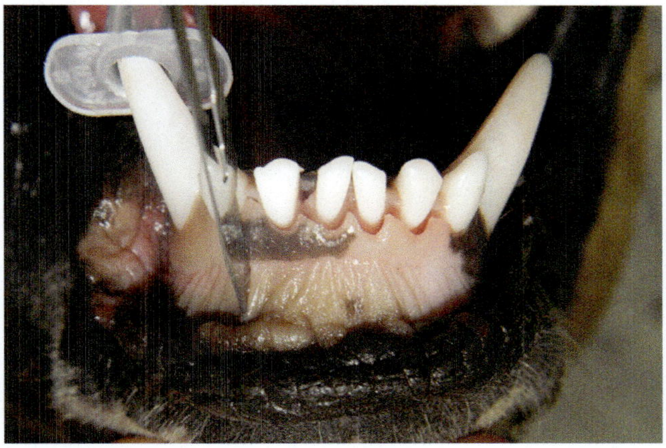

Figure 16.23 (a and b) Shallow vertical incisions are created at the extent of the flap area.

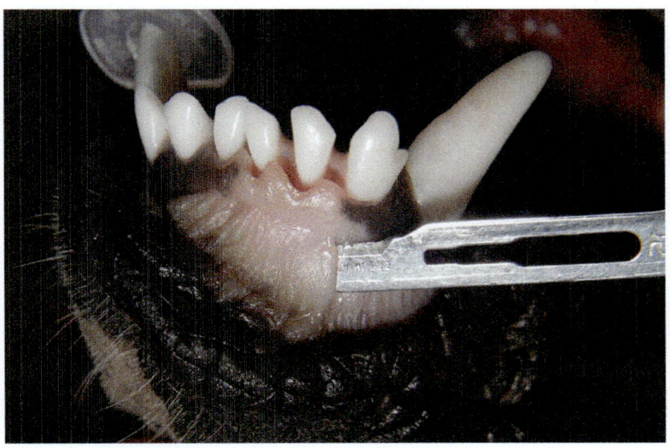

Figure 16.24 The flap is *sharply* dissected from the underlying periosteum with a scalpel.

(a)

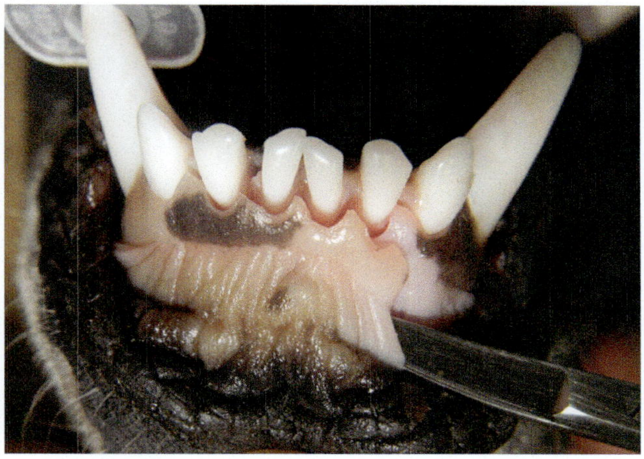

(b)

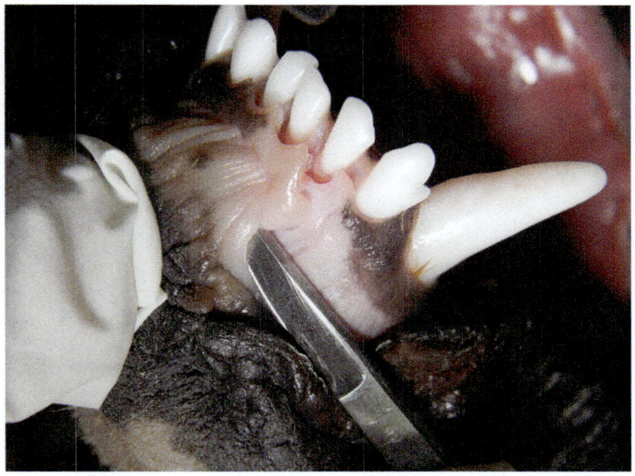

Figure 16.25 (a and b) The flap is *sharply* dissected from the underlying periosteum with a LaGrange scissors.

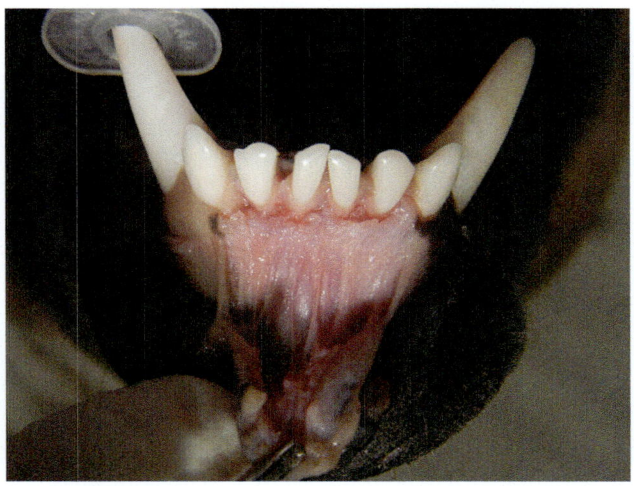

Figure 16.26 Postoperative flap. Note the bone is still covered with connective tissue and periosteum.

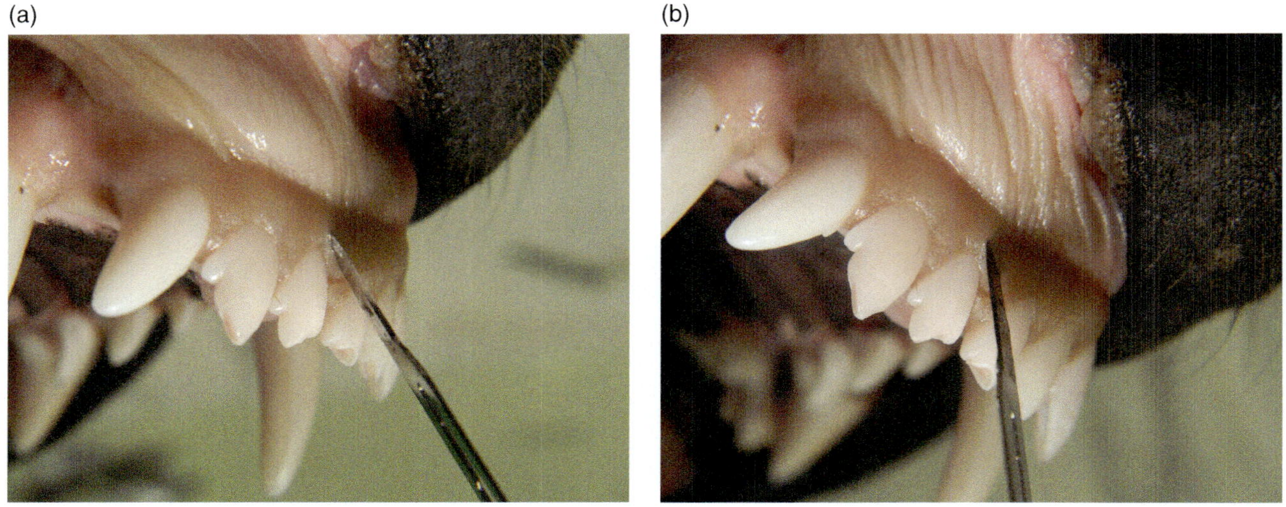

Figure 16.27 (a and b) Modified Widman flap of the maxillary incisors of a dog. Initial incision that is started very near the free gingival margin and created very steeply (almost parallel to the tooth).

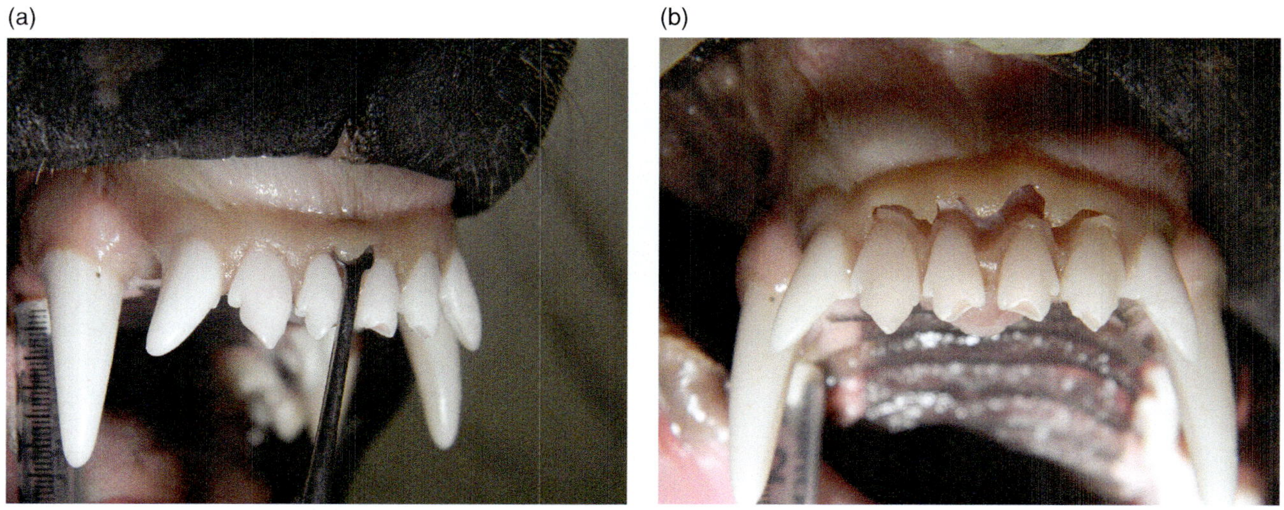

Figure 16.28 (a and b) The flap is *bluntly* dissected with a periosteal elevator.

Technique

1. The initial incision is made very steep starting close to the gingival margin (0.5–1 mm) (Figure 16.27) and scalloped around the tooth to maintain the proper anatomy. The incision should split the papilla. However, it should be created in such a way that the gingival thickness in the area of the papilla is the same as the remainder of the flap (i.e., the majority of the papilla is left with the lingual/palatal gingiva). *It is critical to maintain a minimum of 2 mm of attached gingiva.*
2. The gingiva is reflected with a periosteal elevator (Figure 16.28) and the crevicular incision created from the bottom of the pocket to the bone (Figure 16.29). This creates a triangular wedge of tissue that contains the diseased pocket epithelium.
3. The third incision is made in the interdental area to separate the gingival collar and it is removed (Figure 16.30).
4. The teeth are thoroughly scaled and planed, and any granulation tissue is removed ± root conditioning (see chapter 17) (Figure 16.31).

(a)

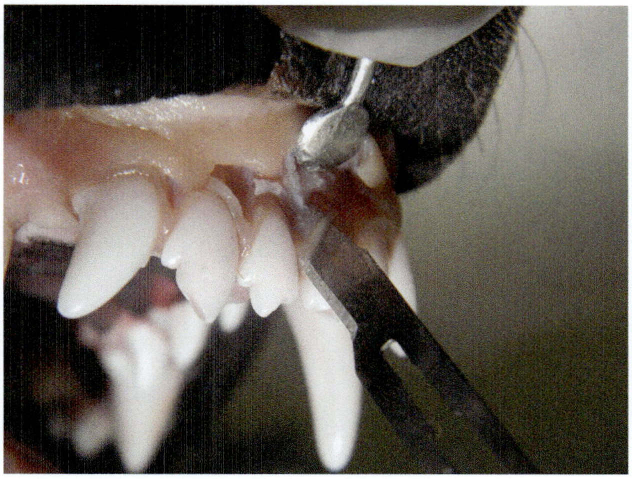

(b)

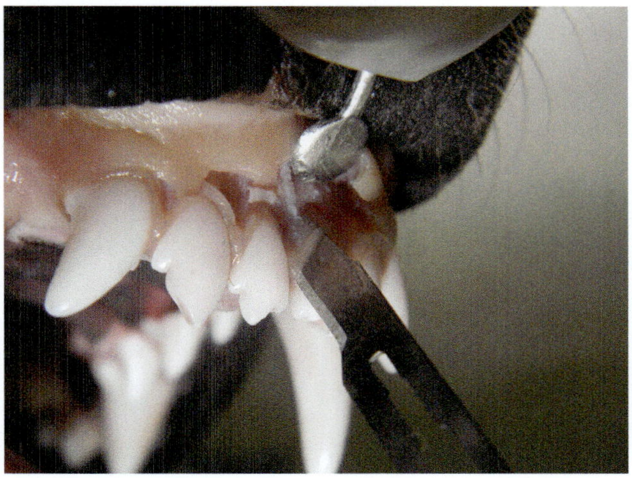

Figure 16.29 (a and b) The crevicular incision is created with a scalpel blade.

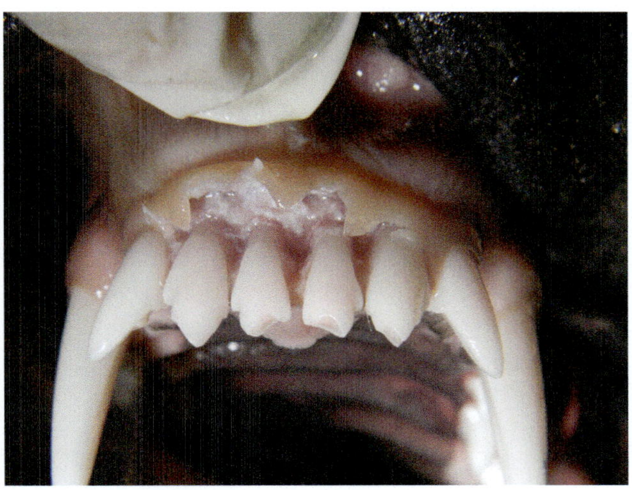

Figure 16.30 The wedge of tissue has been removed.

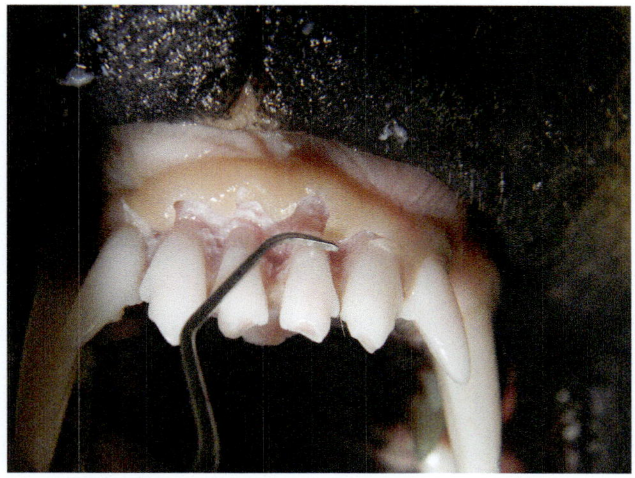

Figure 16.31 Scaling the exposed root surfaces.

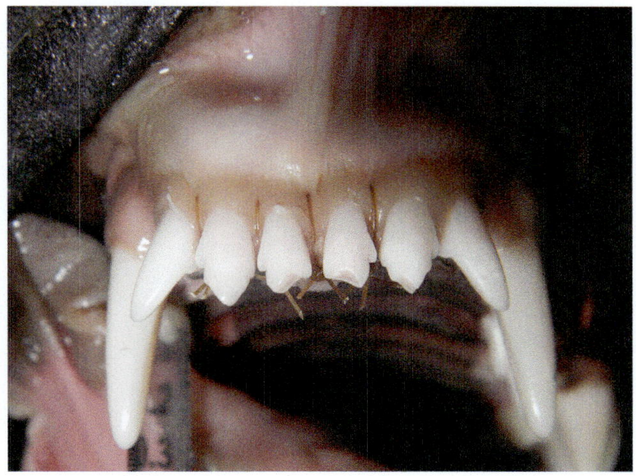

Figure 16.32 The flap is closed interdentally. Note the knots are tied *off* (palatal to) the incision line.

5. Minimal to no bone contouring is performed, unless it is required for proper flap adaptation.
6. The flaps may be thinned if necessary, to allow proper adaptation of the flap to the tooth around its entire circumference as well as to each other interdentally.
7. Interrupted sutures are placed interdentally (see below), so that no bone is left exposed (Figure 16.32).

Undisplaced flap

This[1] is the most aggressive periodontal flap as it is designed to completely remove the periodontal pocket. In essence, it is a combination of gingivectomy

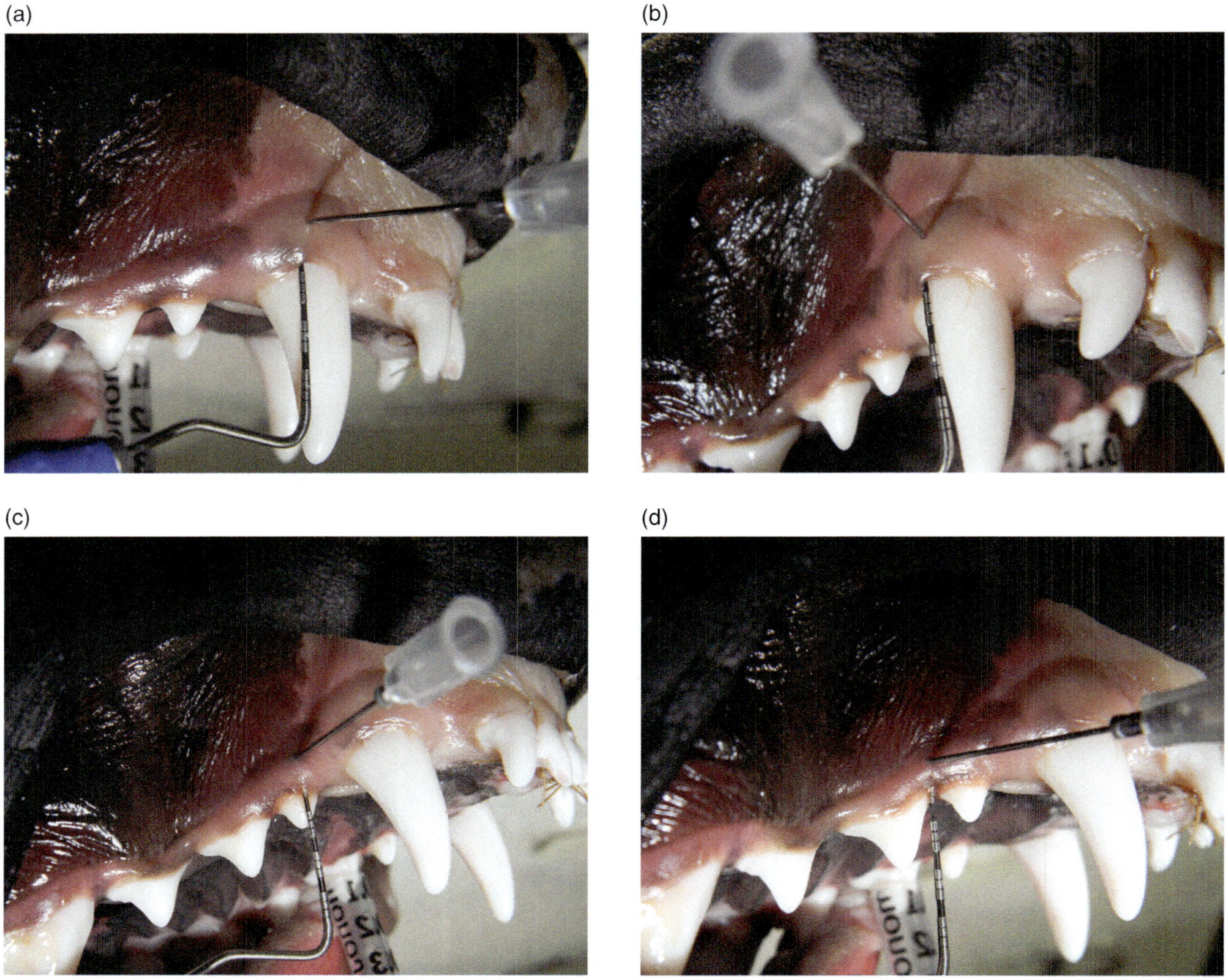

Figure 16.33 (a–d) Undisplaced flap on the maxillary right of a dog. Measuring pocket depth and creating bleeding points with a needle.

and periodontal flap. Despite the significant sacrifice of attached gingiva, this is currently the most common flap utilized in human periodontology. Prior to performance of this procedure, the practitioner must ensure that a minimum of 2 mm of attached gingiva will remain after the surgery. If not, a different flap must be selected (or the tooth extracted). Note that the 2 mm of attached gingiva has been the recommendation for decades; however, recent publications have put that requirement into question.[38,39] The basis for this is long term stability of teeth without this amount of attached gingiva. However, these are reports from human dentists, where homecare is generally much more effective, and thus these compromised teeth will have a much better chance of long-term health. In veterinary patients, 2 mm is still recommended.

Technique

1. Using a periodontal probe, the pocket depths are measured and bleeding points marked on the buccal surface of the gingiva at the apical extent of the pocket (Figure 16.33).
2. The internal bevel incision is made following the scalloping of the teeth along the bleeding points (Figure 16.34). It is important to note that this scalloping is generally carried to a point apical to the alveolar crest. Furthermore, the thicker the gingiva, the deeper the scallop. If thinning of the flap is desired for proper adaptation, it should be performed at this time.
3. The crevicular incision is created to separate the flap from the gingival collar (Figure 16.35). A full thickness flap is created via blunt dissection with a periosteal elevator (Figure 16.36).

(a) (b)

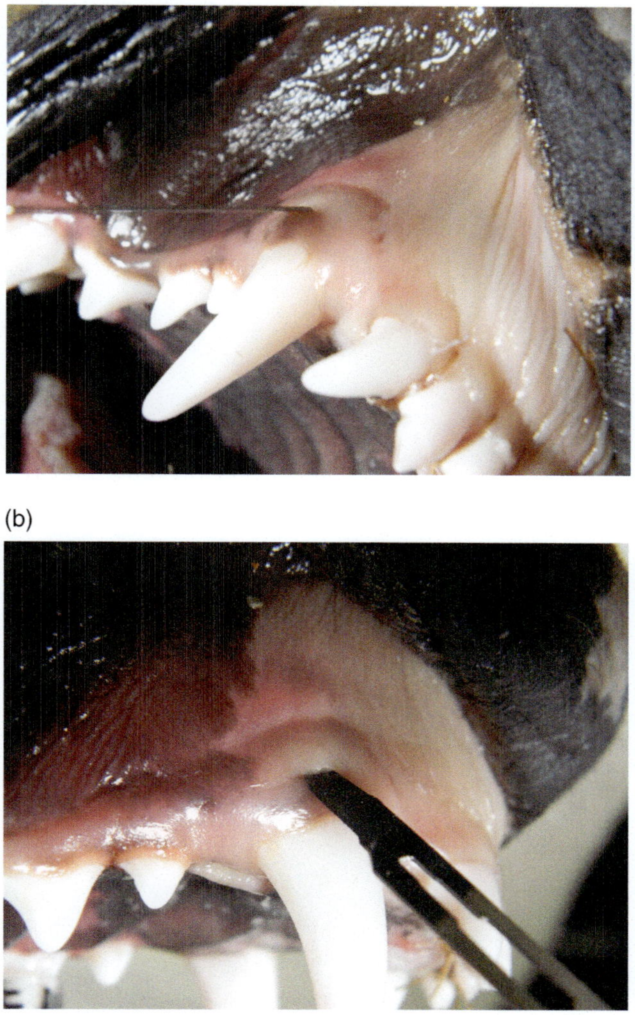

Figure 16.34 (a and b) The initial internal bevel incision is created.

(a) (b)

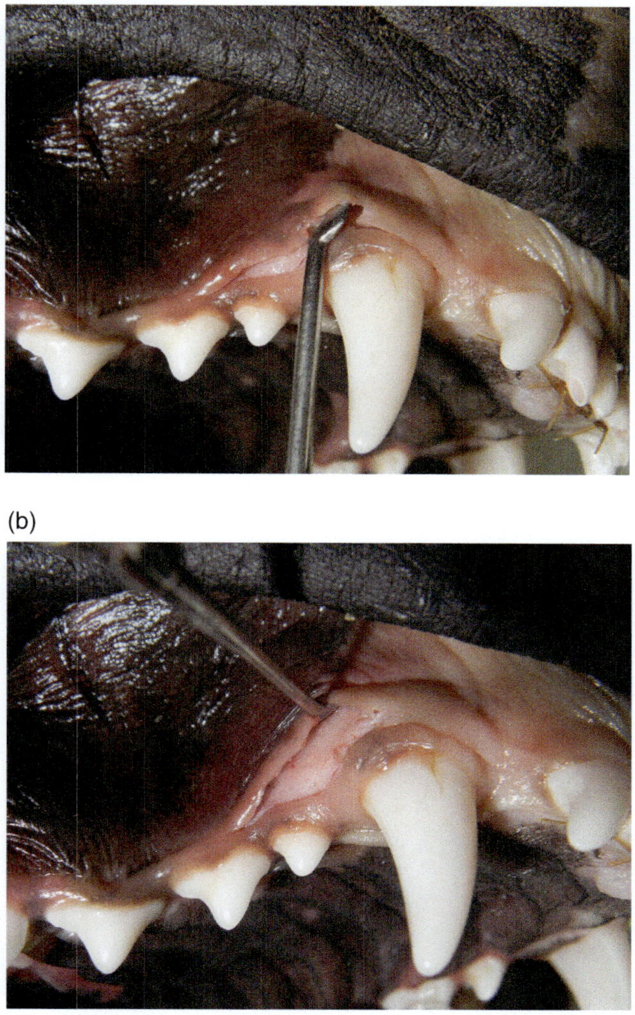

Figure 16.36 (a and b) The flap is *bluntly* dissected with a periosteal elevator.

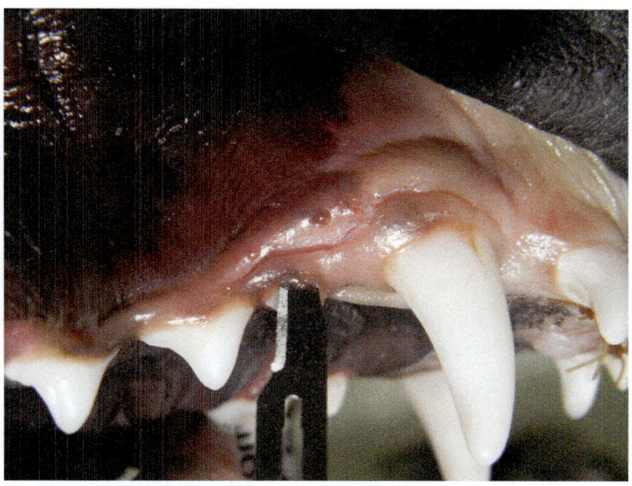

Figure 16.35 The second or crevicular incision is created parallel to the tooth.

4. The gingival collar is separated from the bone with a sharp instrument (knife or blade) (Figure 16.37).
5. The teeth are thoroughly scaled and planed and any granulation tissue is removed ± root conditioning (see chapter 17) (Figure 16.38).
6. After cleaning and osseous surgery (if indicated), the flap should rest at the bone/tooth junction (Figure 16.39). If not, further scalloping/trimming is recommended to allow for proper attachment.
7. A continuous sling suture (see below) is utilized to maintain the flap in proper position at the root/bone interface. *Note* that this will result in the interproximal bone being denuded. This will heal over time, but the area should be protected with a periodontal pack.

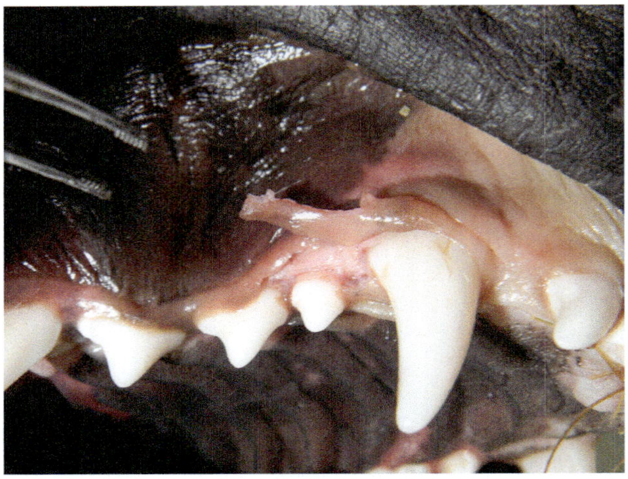

Figure 16.37 The third incision is made and the gingival collar removed.

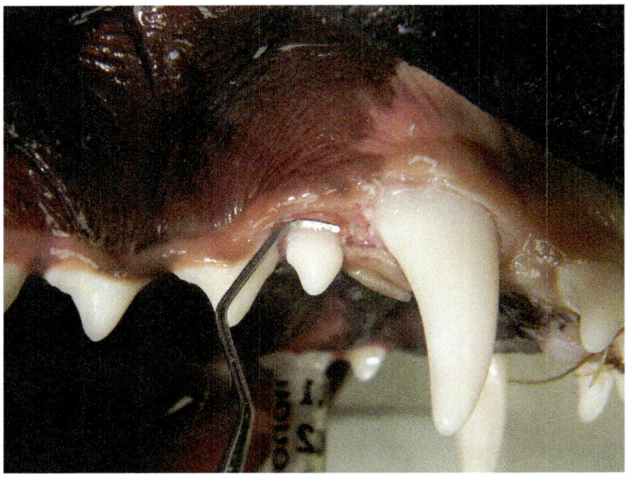

Figure 16.38 The roots are thoroughly scaled, and other root and bone treatments performed as necessary.

(a)

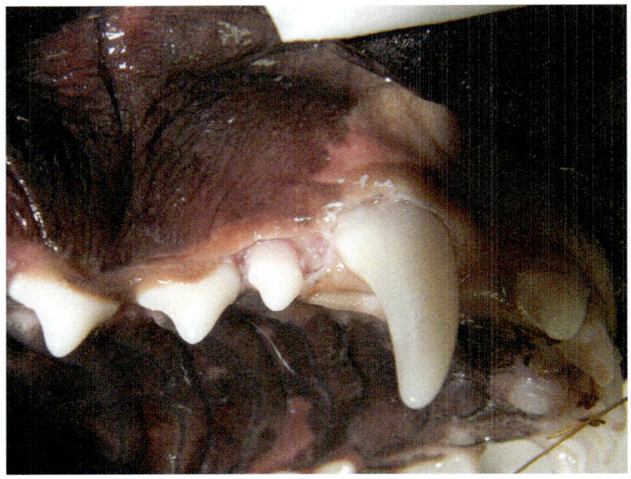

(b)

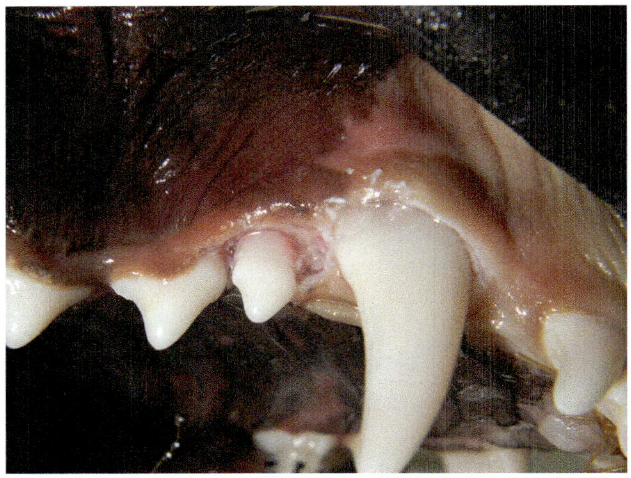

Figure 16.39 (a and b) The flap should rest at the tooth/bone interface.

Apically displaced flap

Periodontal flaps can also be sutured at different levels on the tooth. Apical repositioned flaps[1] are utilized to move the gingival attachment apically. This reduces pocket depth while maintaining the vital attached gingiva. This results in easier care of the diseased areas and decreased infection. These flaps are generally used in areas with horizontal bone loss where regeneration of the lost bone is not currently possible. This is most common in the mandibular incisor area. However, an additional indication is in areas of grade III furcational defects. This procedure lowers the gingival height, allowing for superior homecare in the furcational area. These flaps can also be used to widen the zone of attached gingiva. This technique requires a technical and time-consuming split thickness flap to be created in order to maintain the periosteum over the bone to be exposed. This allows for the regeneration of gingival tissues above the repositioned flap.

Technique

1. The internal bevel incision is similar to that for a modified Widman flap.[1] However, since it is designed to preserve as much of the attached gingiva as possible, it should be started no more than about 1 mm from the gingival margin and directed steeply toward the alveolar crest (Figure 16.40). The incision should follow but not accentuate the natural scalloping.
2. The crevicular incisions are made, followed by the interdental incisions to remove the pocket wall.
3. Vertical incisions are then made mesial and distal to the flap. It is important for these incisions to cross the mucogingival junction (MGJ) (red arrows) to allow repositioning of the flap (Figure 16.41).
4. The flap is then elevated from the underlying bone.
   a. If a full thickness flap is planned, this is accomplished via blunt dissection with a periosteal elevator.

(a)

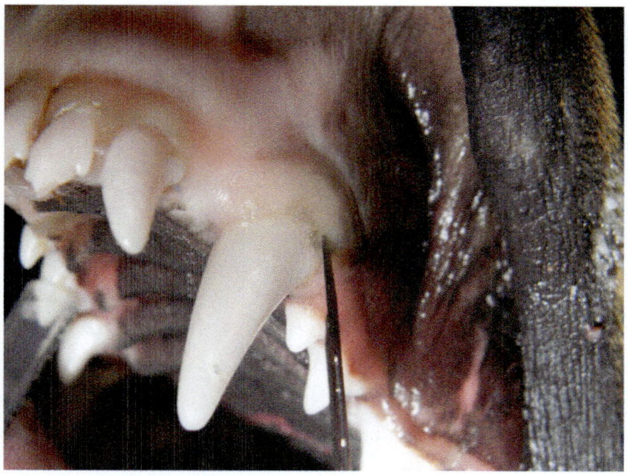

(b)

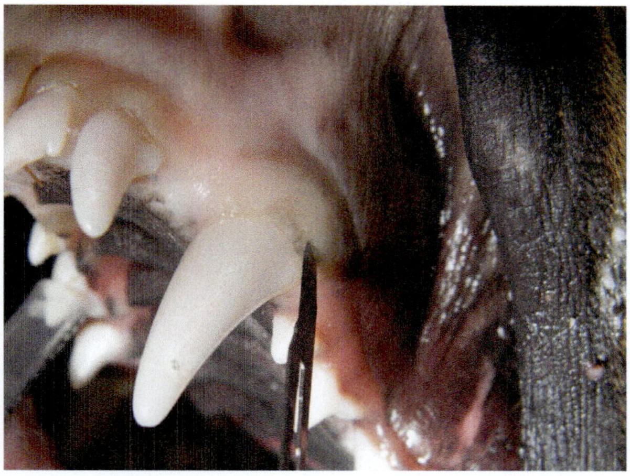

Figure 16.40 (a and b) Apical repositioning flap, cadaver specimen. Initial internal bevel incision.

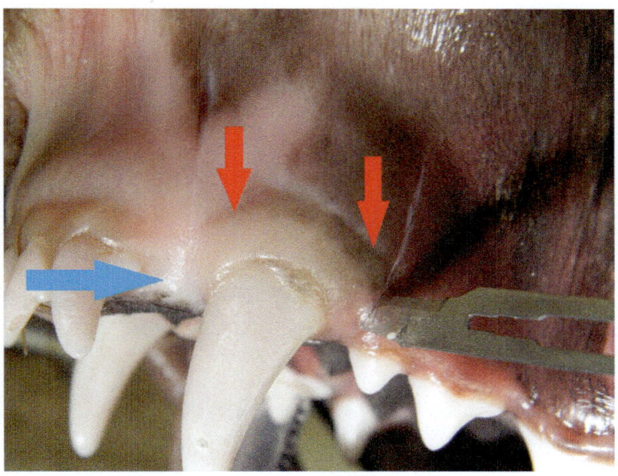

Figure 16.41 Vertical incisions created slightly divergent mesial (blue arrow) and distal to the target tooth. Note the mesial incision is in the diastema, and the distal incision on the mesial line angle of the first premolar. Finally, the incisions must cross the MGJ (red arrows).

(a)

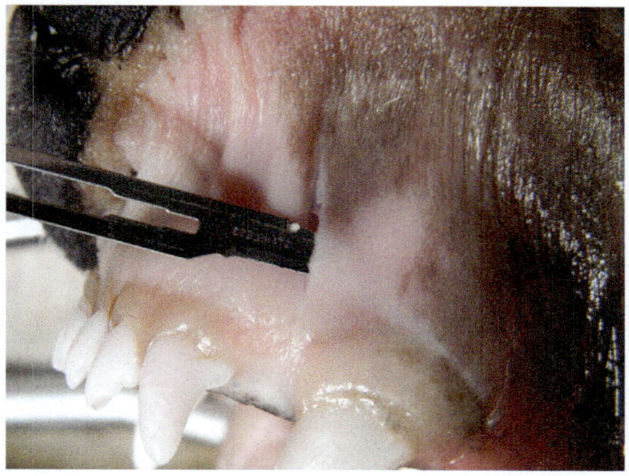

(b)

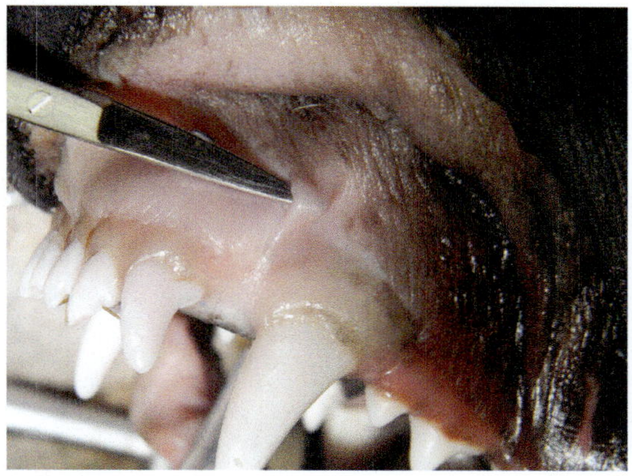

(c)

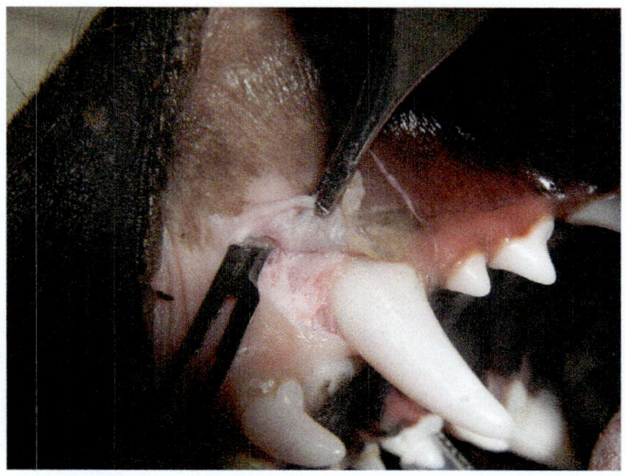

Figure 16.42 Sharp dissection with a (a) scalpel blade and (b) a LaGrange scissors. (c) Continued careful elevation of the flap with a scalpel blade.

b. In cases where a split thickness flap is necessary, it is performed with a blade or knife to leave the periosteum attached to the bone (Figures 16.42 and 16.43).

5. After cleaning and osseous surgery (if indicated) (Figure 16.44), the flap should rest at the bone/tooth junction.
6. The flap is then sutured into place at the root/bone interface (Figure 16.45).

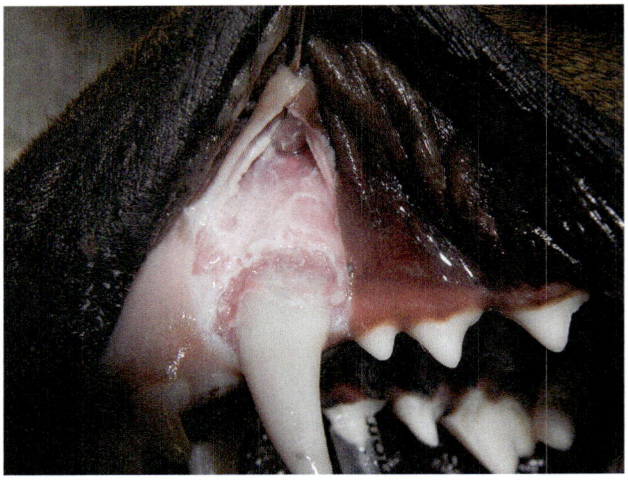

Figure 16.43 The split thickness flap.

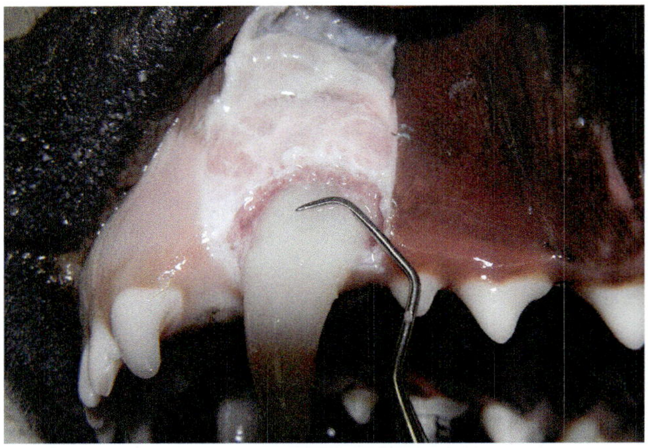

Figure 16.44 Scaling the exposed root surface.

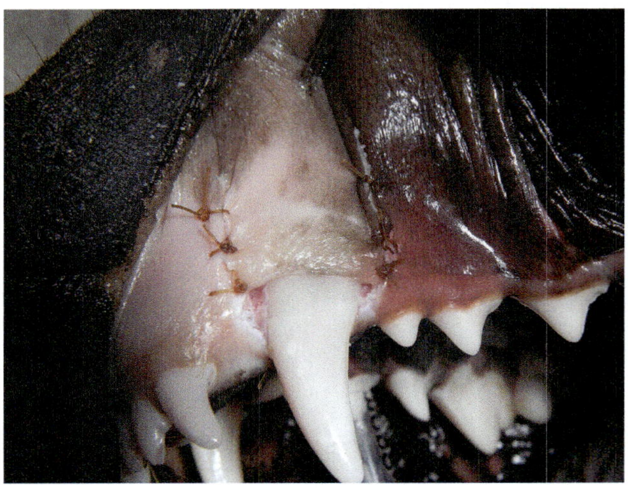

Figure 16.45 The flap is moved and sutured apically to reduce pocket depth.

a. If a full thickness flap is elected, a sling suture should be used to keep the flap from moving apically (see below).
b. If a split thickness flap is elected, it can be sutured to the periosteum with a direct loop or a combination loop-anchor suture. (See also Figures 16.46 through 16.48.)

Coronally displaced flaps

Coronal repositioning flaps are designed to move the gingival attachment coronally on the tooth to gain additional attachment. This procedure is often performed in combination with guided tissue regeneration to gain new bone.[2] It can also be used in areas of gingival recession to gain soft tissue attachment. If performed

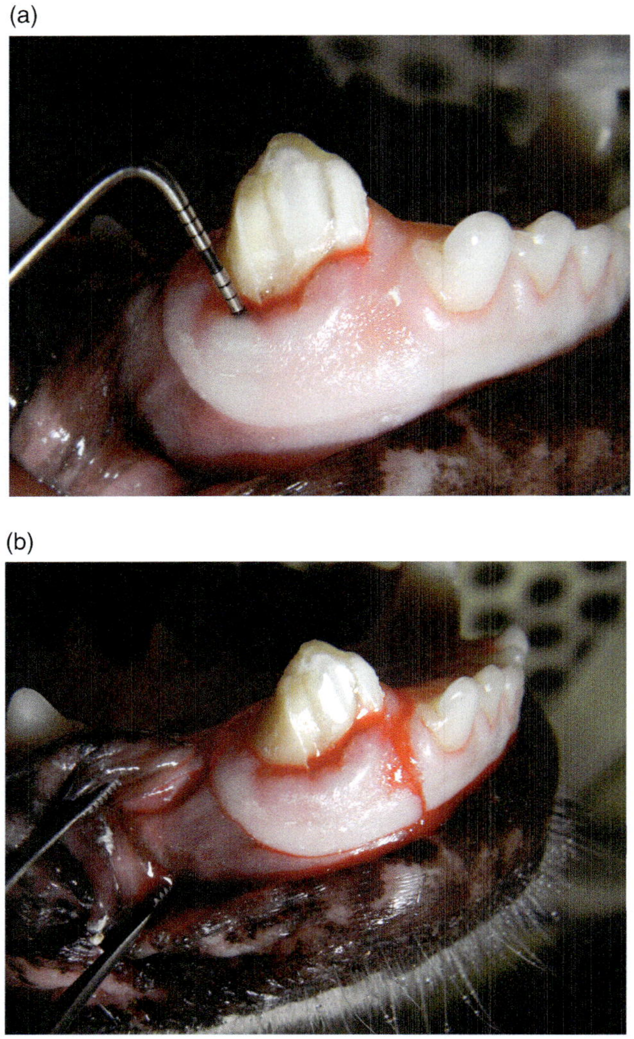

Figure 16.46 Treatment of a complicated crown root fracture of a right mandibular canine (404) of a dog (standard endodontic therapy was also performed). Note the 10 mm periodontal pocket that has resulted from the subgingival fracture (a). (b) Vertical incisions created slightly divergent mesial and distal to the target tooth. Both incisions are created in the diastema and cross the MGJ.

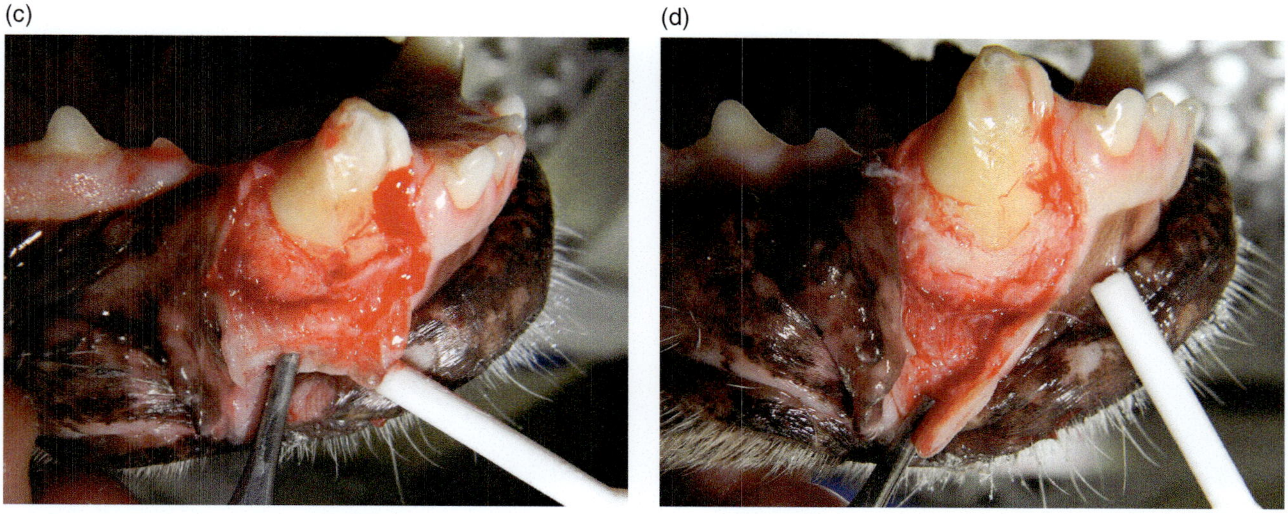

Figure 16.46 (cont'd) (c) The full thickness flap is elevated. (d) Following scaling and osteoplasty (to give a sharp and smooth alveolar crest).

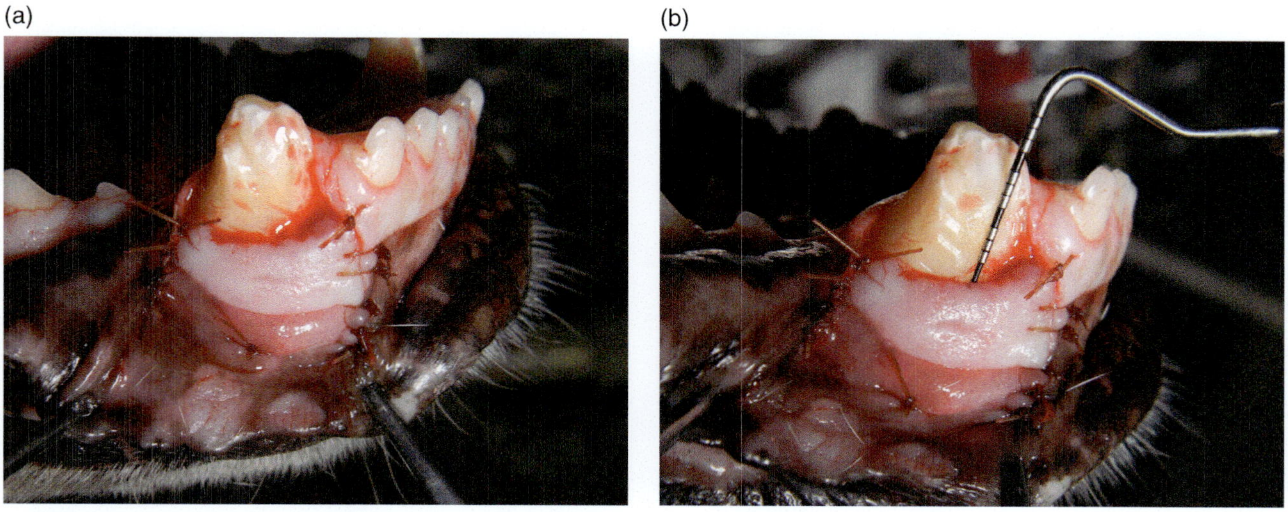

Figure 16.47 Closure. (a) Apical repositioning and closure. (b) Note that the pocket is only 4 mm deep postoperatively.

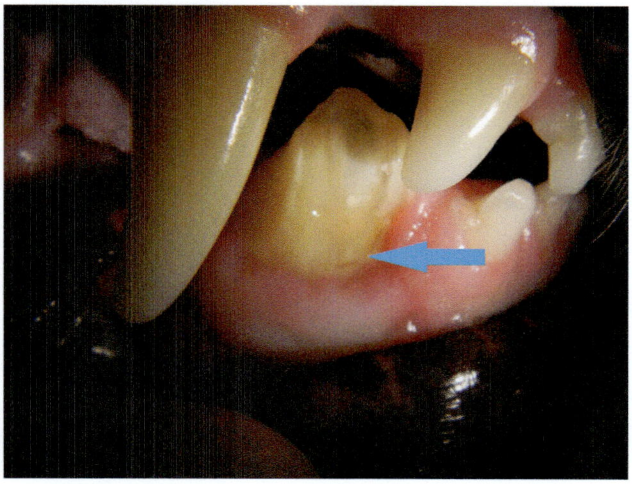

Figure 16.48 Two-week recheck picture. Note the excellent healing and lack of inflammation. Additionally, the gingival margin is now below the fracture, allowing for pocket reduction.

properly, this procedure can result in increased attachment,[40] but if ineffective may also result in increased pocket depth.

Technique

1. Two vertical incisions are created to delineate the flap, making sure to carry them *beyond* the mucogingival junction[41] (Figures 16.49a).
2. A conservative reverse bevel incision is then made to the base of the pocket to remove the diseased pocket epithelium (Figure 16.49b).
3. A *split* thickness flap is carefully created using sharp dissection technique (Figure 16.49c).
4. The exposed root surface is carefully scaled and planed (Figure 16.49d).

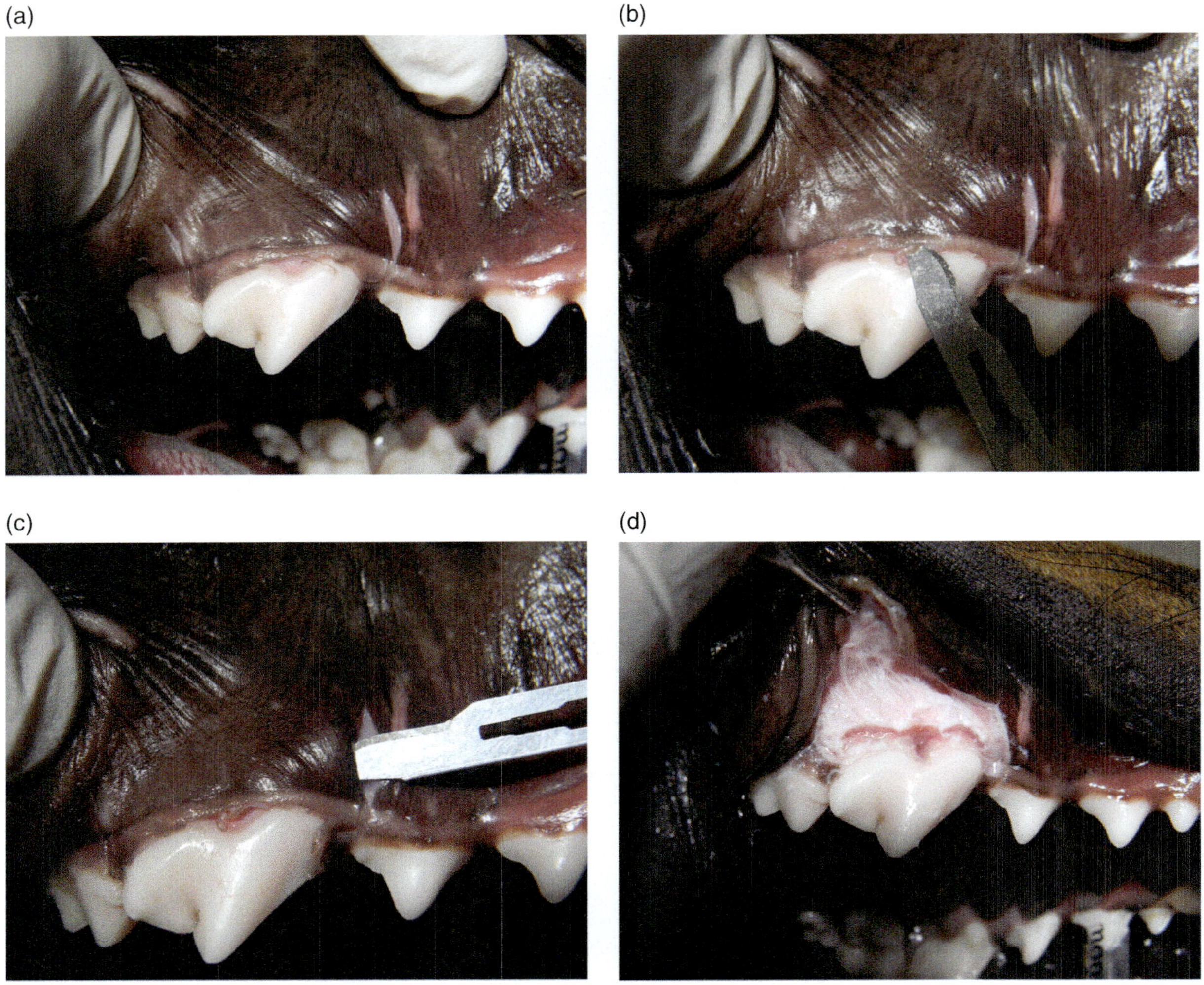

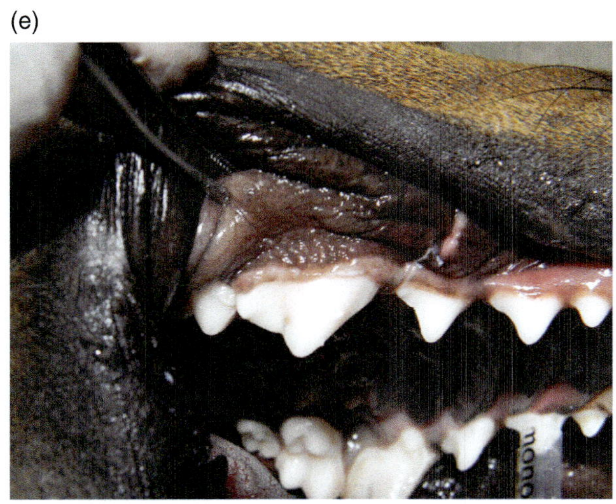

Figure 16.49 Coronally displaced flap on a maxillary fourth premolar with gingival recession and class II furcation exposure. (a) Slightly divergent vertical releasing incisions are created mesial and distal to the target tooth. Note the gingival recession and furcation exposure to the tooth. (b) Conservative internal bevel incision to maintain as much attached gingiva as possible. (c) Sharp dissection to create a ***split*** thickness flap. (d) Partial thickness flap is elevated for scaling. Note the intact periosteum covering the exposed bone. (e) Flap is moved coronally on the tooth to cover the defect.

5. Citric acid therapy should be performed (see chapter 17).
6. The flap is repositioned *without tension* more coronal on the tooth surface (Figure 16.49e) and sutured in place.

The standard coronally positioned flap can be very effective in increasing keratinized gingiva, but these flaps are not always successful due to insufficient amounts of attached gingiva.[42] Therefore, on occasion, the addition of a free gingival graft is necessary (see below).

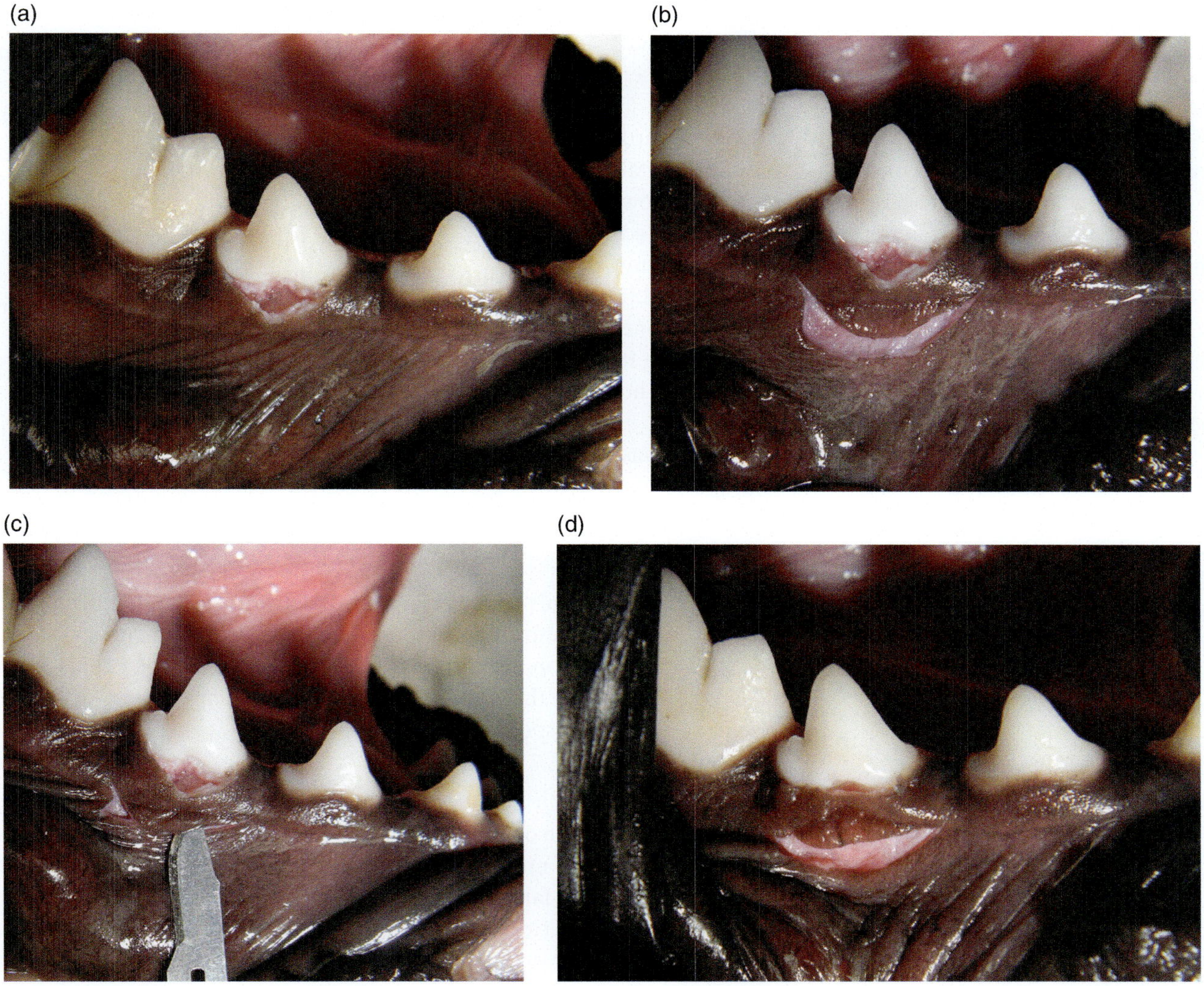

Figure 16.50 Semilunar flap to increase the keratinized attached gingiva. (a) Gingival recession on a mandibular fourth premolar. (b) The semilunar incision is created following the curvature of the receded gingival margin, stopping 2–3 mm apical to the papillae. (c) A split thickness flap is created by using sharp dissection coronally under the flap. (d) After release, the flap slides naturally into place.

Semilunar flap

An alternate form of coronally positioned flap has been devised called the *semilunar flap*.[43]

Technique

1. A semilunar incision is created following the curvature of the receded gingival margin.[41] This *must* stop 2–3 mm apical to the papillae to ensure continued blood supply to the flap. The incision may extend to the alveolar mucosa if necessary (Figures 16.50b).
2. A split thickness flap is created by using sharp dissection coronally under the flap (Figure 16.50c).
3. Once fully released from the periosteum, the flap will naturally slide coronally into position (Figure 16.50d).
4. Hold the flap in place for a few minutes to allow healing to begin; no sutures are necessary. The denuded area (covered by periosteum) will heal by secondary intention.

Palatine flaps

The palate is a unique area for periodontal surgery since it is composed of inelastic/keratinized tissue.[1] Therefore, it cannot be displaced nor can a split thickness flap be created.[1] Since the palatal flap cannot be displaced to properly adapt to the root bone interface, the initial incision is critical for proper flap placement. This flap must be created in such a way that it adapts well around the entire portion of the tooth. In general, the edges are too thick for proper attachment and must be thinned prior to closure. Thick palatine tissue will not adapt well and often separates from the tooth, delaying and complicating wound healing. A thin and sharp margined papilla that adapts well to the tooth is critical for proper healing.

If the tissue is not excessively thick, a standard internal bevel can be used. For thick areas, a horizontal gingivectomy will thin the tissue sufficiently to allow proper attachment. If this is not done or is performed insufficiently, it is best to trim the flap prior to releasing from the underlying bone, as it is easier to work with when attached. If thinning is necessary, it can be done by holding the flap with Adson forceps and thinning it with a sharp, small blade tapering to the tip of the papilla.

It is best to anticipate whether significant osseous surgery will be necessary. Probing for defects (sounding) along with careful radiographic review will assist with proper flap creation. If no osseous surgery is planned, the internal bevel incision can be placed near the gingival margin (as Widham above). If significant bone work is planned, the incision should be made more apical.

Vertical incisions are rarely indicated, as repositioning is not possible on the palate. In fact, they should be avoided if possible, due to the pain they create and the difficulty of closing this inelastic tissue. Finally, these flaps must be performed carefully and conservatively to avoid the palatine vessels.

Flaps for regenerative surgery

Owing to the advances in human periodontology, bone regrowth (guided tissue regeneration) is now possible. If the clinical presentation is compatible with the procedure, this is the preferred method of pocket reduction. (For a discussion of indications, materials, and techniques, see chapter 18.)

Flaps for regenerative surgery procedures should be designed to maintain the maximum amount of attached gingiva. Therefore, the initial internal bevel incision is *not* performed in this case, only the second (crevicular) incision is made to release the flap. These flaps are typically made full thickness, and either envelope or full flap designs can be used. In addition, these flaps should result in primary closure over the membrane/graft. Finally, papilla-sparing techniques should be utilized when there is sufficient interdental space.

Papilla preservation flap

This type of flap keeps the papilla in place and allows for superior healing. It is of most value in the incisor region, as true papillae are only seen there and also in the molar region. These flaps are a challenge in the molar region due to tight contacts that do not allow the papilla to be kept intact.

Technique

1. The initial incision is made circumferentially around each tooth and the interdental spaces are "reverse scalloped" to avoid the papillae entirely. The papillae can be left with either side of the flap; however, they are typically left on the lingual/palatal flap (Figure 16.51a).
2. A sharp instrument (typically an Orban knife) is introduced into the incision and used to carefully dissect the flap off the underlying bone (Figure 16.51b).
3. The papillae are reflected with the flap (Figures 16.51c and d).
4. The flaps are not thinned but rather should maintain as much attached gingiva and thickness as possible.

Conventional flap

This is performed similarly to the above papilla preservation flap technique but with only the crevicular incision performed. In this case, however, the papilla is split in the middle. The halves are then reflected with their respective flap.

Flaps to increase/replace attached gingiva

On occasion, patients will present with areas of minimal to no attached gingiva, while the remainder of the tooth is fairly healthy. This can occur secondary to standard periodontal disease but is more common due to trauma or toxic injuries. The most definitive treatment for these teeth is extraction. However, there are other therapeutic options to cover these areas and salvage the teeth. These types of procedures can also be used to increase the level of attached gingiva for aesthetic reasons. Affected areas can be treated via three different surgeries: free gingival autograft, free connective tissue autograft, and lateral sliding (or pellicle) flap. For all of these flaps (as well as any periodontal flap) the critical steps are a thorough scaling and root planing in addition to the removal of any pocket epithelium (see chapters 11 and 17).

Classically, the incisions for these types of flaps are created split thickness, leaving a layer of periosteum.[2,5] However, recent studies have shown that placing the graft directly on the bone leads to less postoperative mobility, decreased swelling and hemorrhage,[44] and significantly less shrinkage of the flap.[45,46] In addition, the bluntly dissected full thickness flap is much easier to create. The main disadvantage of this technique is that healing may be delayed,[47,48] which is more of concern in animal patients because we cannot control their oral activity.

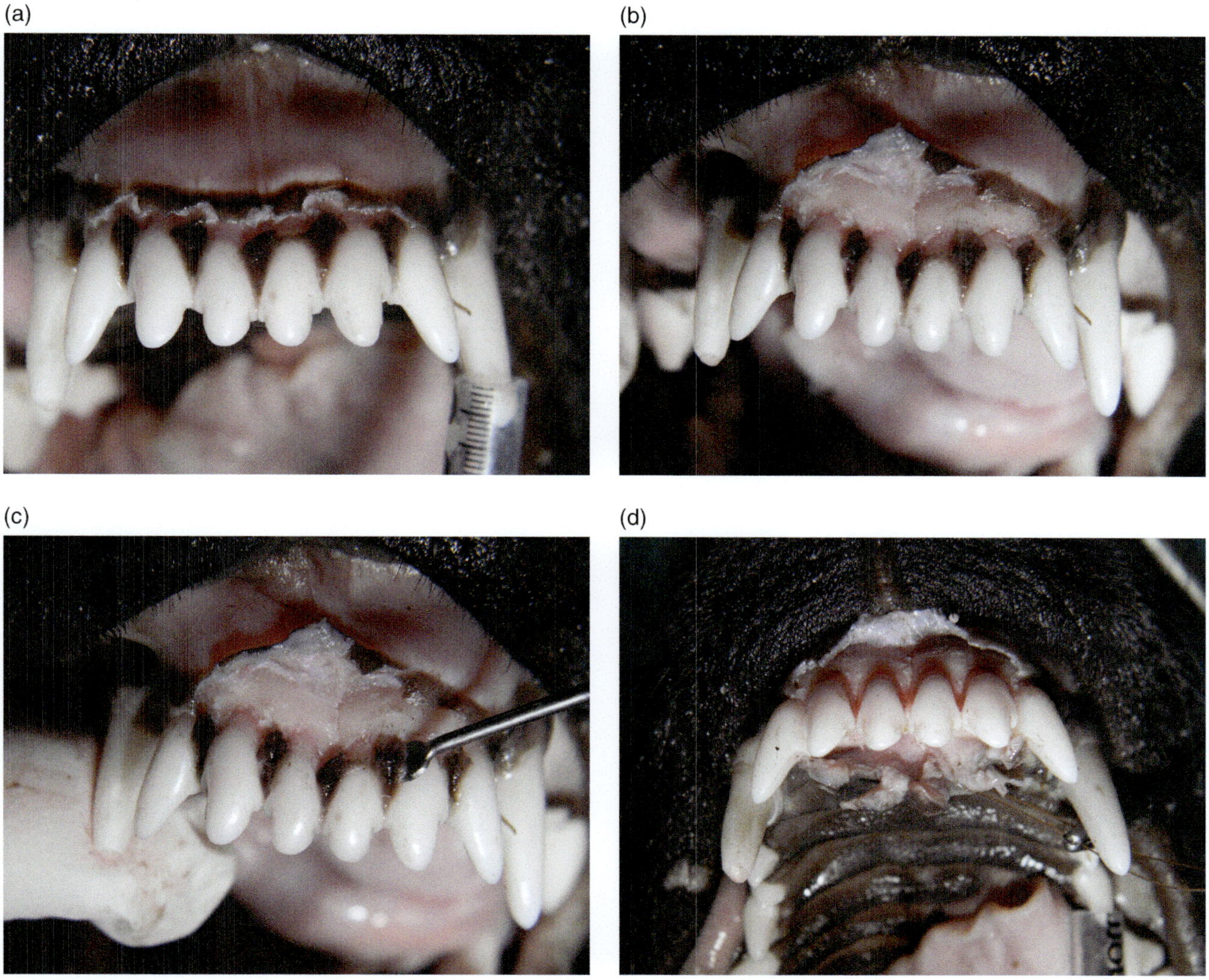

Figure 16.51 Papilla preservation flap on the maxillary incisors of a dog. (a) The incision is made circumferentially and the interdental spaces "reverse scalloped" to avoid the papillae entirely. In this case, the papillae will be left with the palatal flap. (b) Buccal flap released. (c) Papillae carefully raised to stay with the palatine flap. (d) Flap created. Note the papillae are intact and attached to the palatine flap.

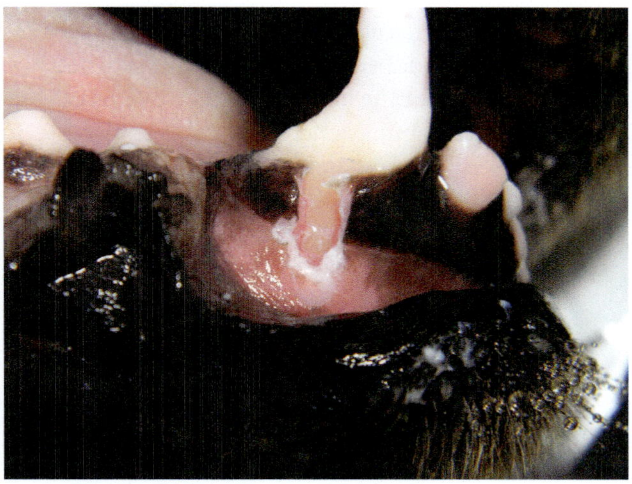

Figure 16.52 Deep gingival cleft beyond the MGJ on the right mandibular canine (404) of a dog.

Free gingival autograft

This technique was first described in 1963 and has been improved and modified since that time.[49] Autografts are used to increase the width of the keratinized attached gingiva where the defect extends very close to or beyond the mucogingival junction (Figure 16.52). This technique is typically employed in areas where there is insufficient adjacent gingival tissue (to utilize a lateral sliding flap).

Technique

1. Prepare recipient site.
   a. Create a bed for grafting by marking a 3–4 mm area and removing the soft tissue. The area should be approximately twice the size of the defect to allow for 50% contraction during healing (Figure 16.53).

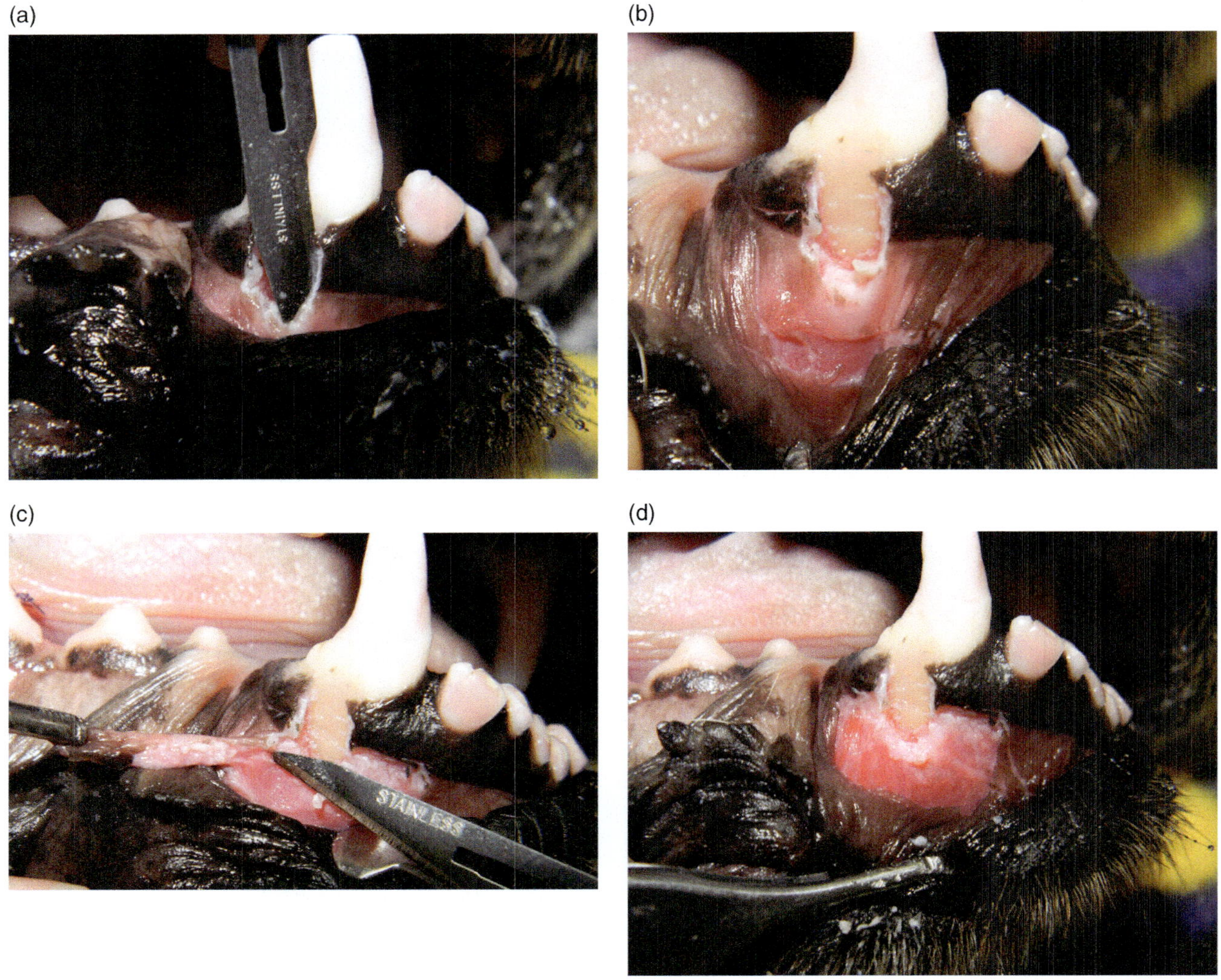

Figure 16.53 (a) Preparing the recipient site by debriding the edges of the lesion. (b) Shallow incisions are made to define the edges of the recipient bed. (c) The site is created *split* thickness with sharp dissection. (d) Prepared recipient site.

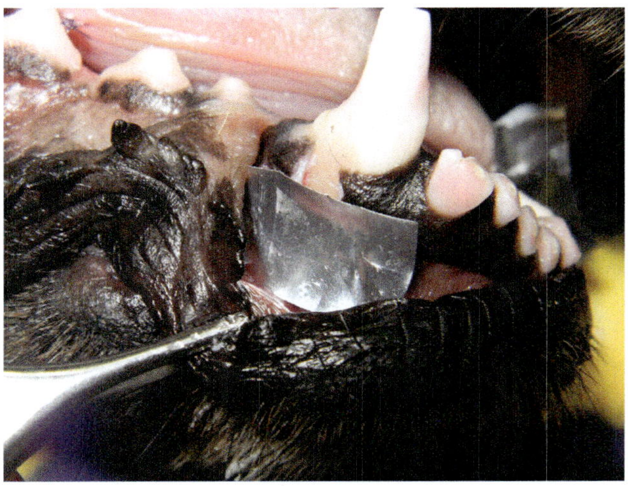

Figure 16.54 Placing tinfoil over the site and cutting to match the prepared bed.

  b. Using sterile tinfoil, create a template for the recipient bed, which will help guide the incisions for the donor site (Figure 16.54).
  c. Place a moistened sponge over the site to keep it moist and help control hemorrhage.
2. Obtain graft from the donor site.
  a. Select the donor area that has enough attached gingiva to supply the graft while maintaining 2–3 mm of remaining attached gingiva coronal to the graft. The maxillary canine and mandibular first molar are the most commonly used places in veterinary patients.
  b. Place the template over the graft site (Figure 16.55).
  c. Carefully make shallow incisions to outline the graft.

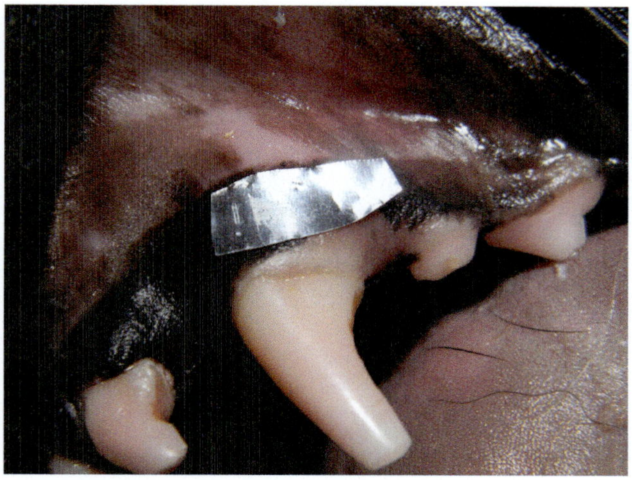

Figure 16.55 Tinfoil is placed over the maxillary canine.

d. Carefully create a split thickness graft that maintains the periosteum over the donor site. It is best to start elevation on the corner and using a fine suture to hold the corner, use sharp dissection to free the graft (Figure 16.56). ***This is very tedious and should be performed using very fine/sharp instruments and with the aid of magnification.*** The graft should be 1.0–1.5 mm thick.[50] Note that the thickness of the graft is critical to successful healing. A graft that is too thin risks necrosis, and if too thick makes diffusion of nutrients and new circulation to the superficial layer challenging, thus also risking failure.[41] If the obtained graft is too thick it can be carefully thinned with a blade.

3. Transfer and immobilize the graft.
   a. Use extreme care when handling the graft, as it will be very sensitive to any injury.
   b. Remove the sponge and any excess clot (as a thick clot can interfere with healing).[51]
   c. Place the graft onto the recipient site and place pressure down onto the bone for 3–5 minutes. This step helps to remove any air or blood that may be creating deadspace and also initiates healing.
   d. Inspect the edges of the graft for any clots or loose tissue.
   e. Suture with fine (5-0 to 6-0) swedged on suture with a simple interrupted pattern every 2 mm (Figure 16.57). Care must be taken not to move the graft during suturing.
   f. Consider adding a sling or cruciate suture over the recipient site (anchored on both sides in native tissue) to help stabilize the graft.

(a)

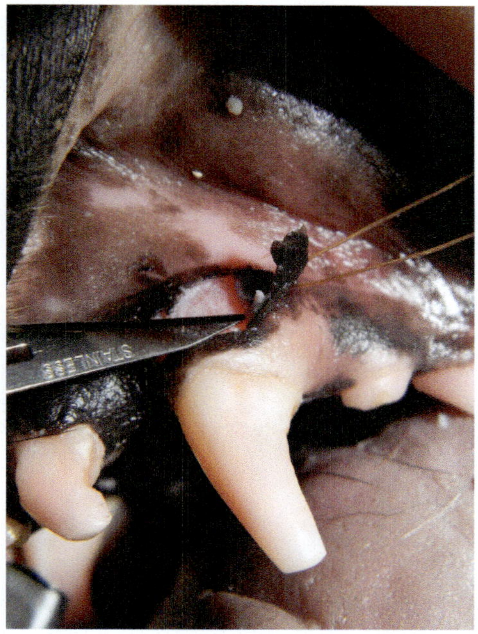

(b)

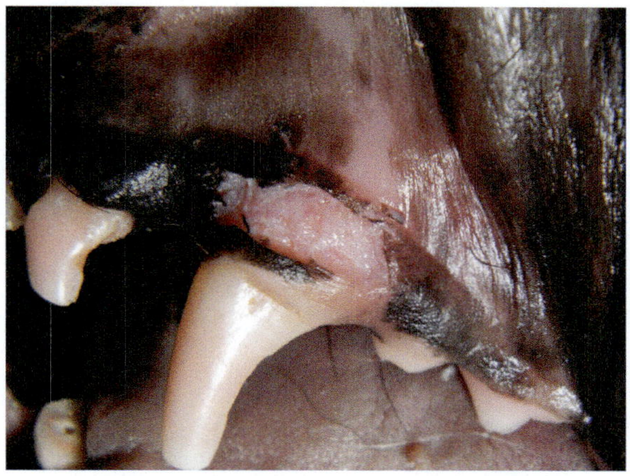

Figure 16.56 (a and b) *Sharply* dissecting the graft from the donor site, making sure to leave a layer of periosteum.

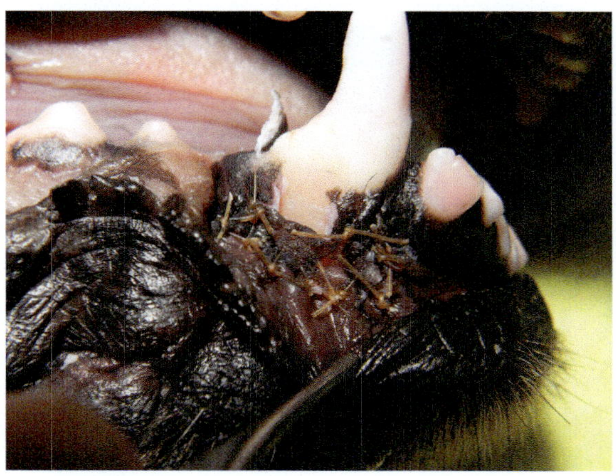

Figure 16.57 Transfer graft to recipient bed and close with simple interrupted sutures of a fine material.

Free connective tissue autograft

This procedure[41] was first described by Edel in 1974.[52] It is a variant on the free gingival graft above. It takes advantage of the fact that connective tissue from keratinized sites carries the genetic message to become keratinized. The major advantages of this technique are provided by the fact that the graft is taken from the underside of the palatine tissue. This allows for a much larger selection of donor sites, as well as significantly decreases postoperative pain and complications because the donor site can be closed primarily. The only disadvantage is that this type of graft cannot easily be measured with a template. Therefore a slightly larger graft piece should be harvested and subsequently trimmed to size.

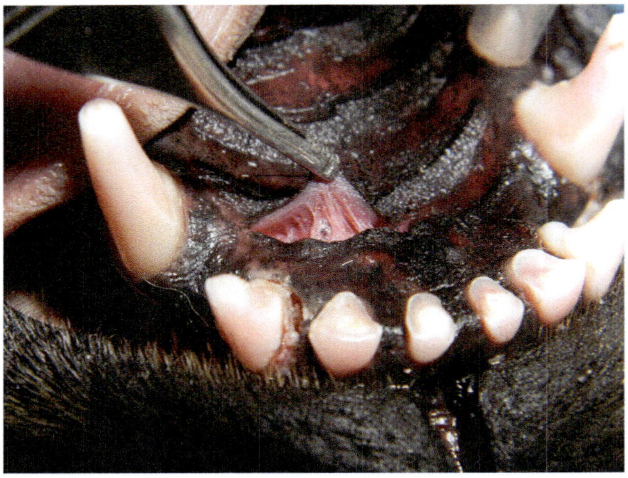

Figure 16.58 Harvesting a connective tissue graft. Making an elliptical incision in the palate in a relatively avascular area.

The preparation of the recipient site and transport/securing of the graft is the same as for free gingival graft above. To harvest the free connective tissue autograft:

1. Make an elliptical incision in the palate in a relatively avascular area that ideally does not have significant rugae (Figure 16.58).
2. Carefully elevate the flap and harvest the connective tissue (Figure 16.59).
3. Close the incisions with simple interrupted sutures (Figures 16.60 and 16.61).

(a) (b) (c)

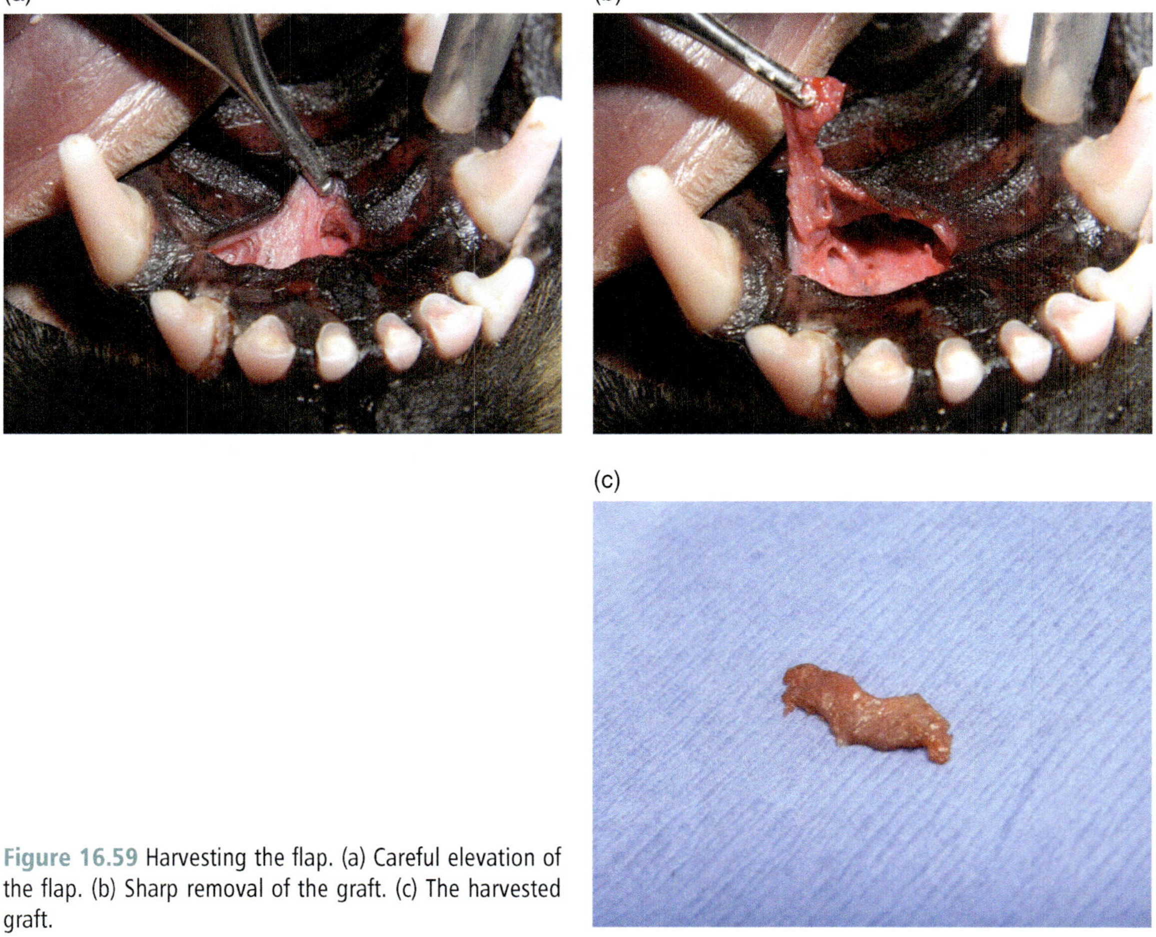

Figure 16.59 Harvesting the flap. (a) Careful elevation of the flap. (b) Sharp removal of the graft. (c) The harvested graft.

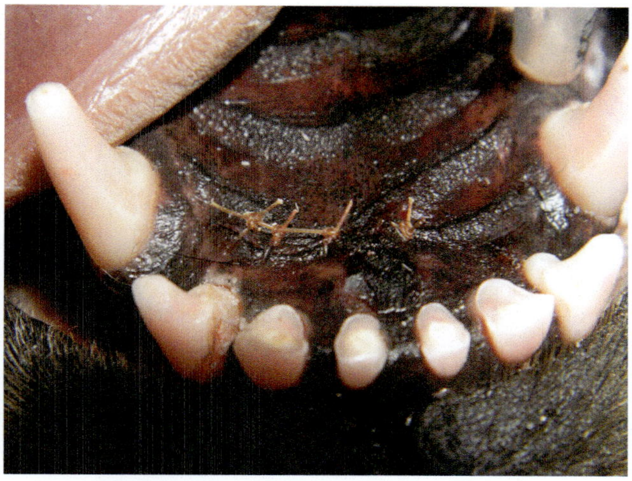

Figure 16.60 Primary closure of the site.

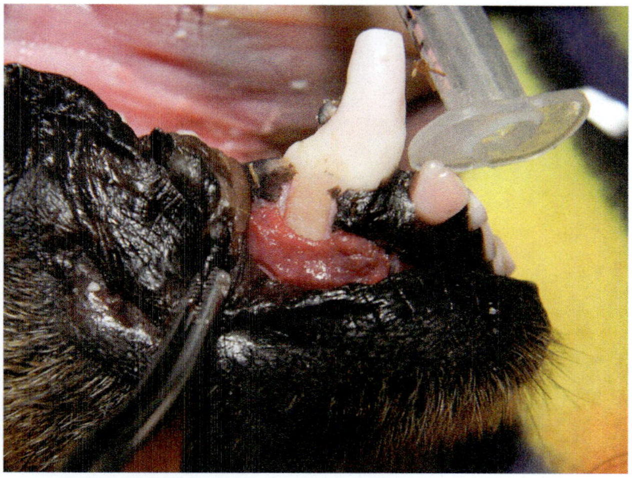

Figure 16.61 Graft placed in defect.

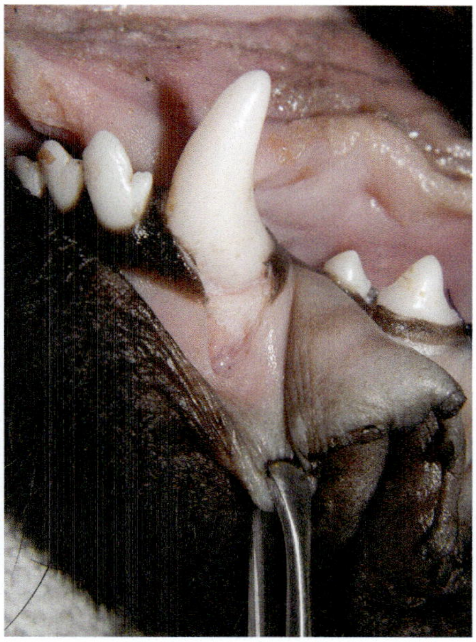

Figure 16.62 Lateral sliding flap for a deep gingival cleft beyond the MGJ on the mandibular left canine (304) of a dog.

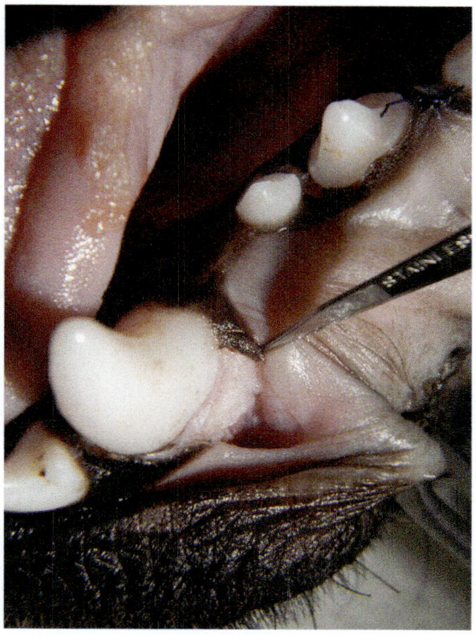

Figure 16.63 Creating an external bevel on the side away from the graft.

Lateral sliding (pedicle) flap

This flap[2,5,41,53,54] can also be used to cover denuded areas of root. It has been utilized since the 1950s and is very effective in the correct situation. The main indication for this type of flap is an area of denuded bone with sufficient healthy attached gingiva directly adjacent to it (Figure 16.62). (Note that inflamed/infected tissue will not function well as a graft.) Ideally, the donor site is edentulous (i.e., the diastema behind the canine teeth). However, for mandibular incisors, the frenulum can become an issue with tension; therefore taking the graft apical to the mandibular incisors is recommended.

1. Preparation of recipient site: Create bevelled incisions along the defect. The recipient side (away from the graft) is bevelled externally (Figure 16.63) and the graft side internally (Figure 16.64), to create a greater surface area for healing.
2. Flap preparation:
    a. Lateral sliding flaps can be made split or full thickness. Full thickness flaps are easier and may allow for superior healing of the graft site but result in longer healing times and a potential for lost crestal bone at the donor site. Therefore, the combined approach is recommended (see below).

    Starting halfway down the attached gingiva, create a *partial thickness* vertical incision. The incision should be made 1.5 times the distance from the near edge of the defect as the defect is wide (Figure 16.65). This incision

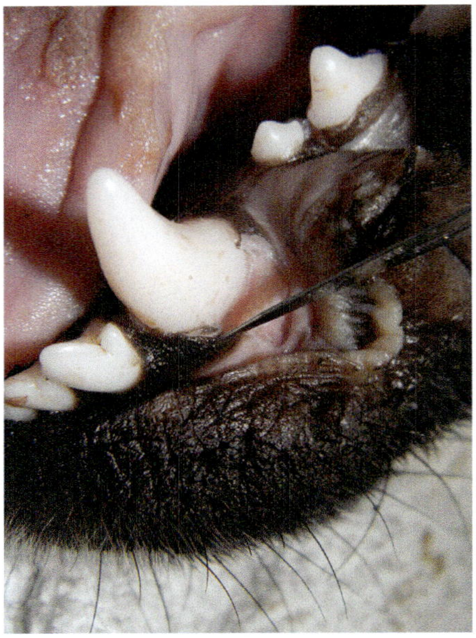

Figure 16.64 Creating an internal bevel on the side of the graft that faces the defect.

should be carried past the MGJ to the same point apically as the defect (Figure 16.66).

 b. Make a split thickness horizontal incision from the defect edge to the vertical incision (Figure 16.67).
 c. Elevate the flap starting full thickness at the defect edge (Figure 16.68), switching to split thickness once the area to be left denuded is reached (Figure 16.69).
 d. Fenestrate the periosteum at the base of the flap to release tension (if necessary).

3. Transfer and closure of the flap, and protection of the donor site:
 a. Transfer the flap to the recipient site and match edge to edge (Figure 16.70).
 b. Ensure that no tension is present.
 c. Place finger pressure on the flap for 3–5 minutes to initiate healing and force out any air or clots that might delay healing.
 d. Close with simple interrupted sutures placed 1.5–2.0 mm apart (Figure 16.71).
 e. Place a cruciate suture over the site anchored into normal tissue (Figure 16.72).
 f. Consider a periodontal or aluminium foil dressing (especially if a full thickness flap was used).

Frenectomy and frenotomy

The frenulum is a muscular fold of tissue that attaches lips and cheeks to the gingiva or alveolar mucosa and underlying periosteum.[2,5,41] The dog has three primary

(a)

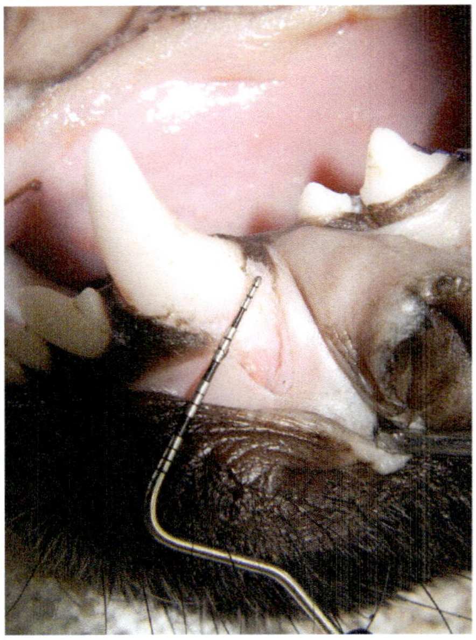

(b)

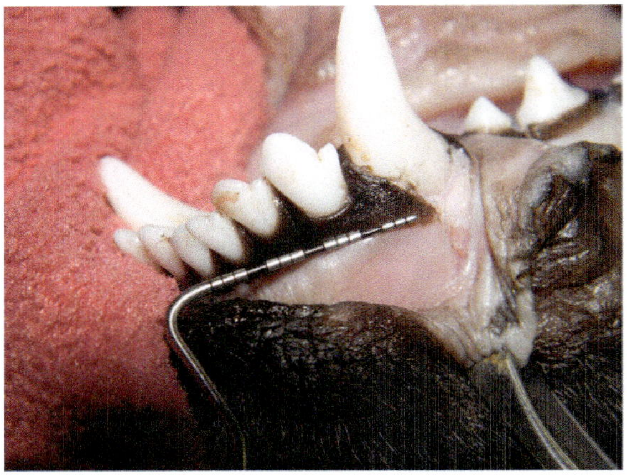

Figure 16.65 Measuring the width of the defect. (a) Measuring the defect with a periodontal probe. (b) Determining and marking the width of graft necessary.

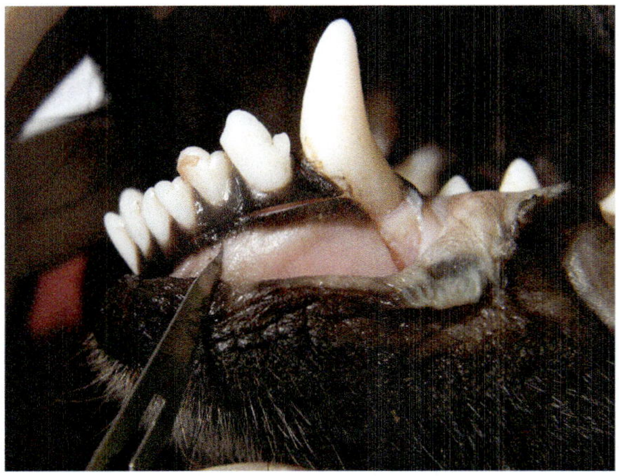

Figure 16.66 Vertical incision at the point determined by measuring. This incision crosses the MGJ and is shallow to allow for split thickness harvesting.

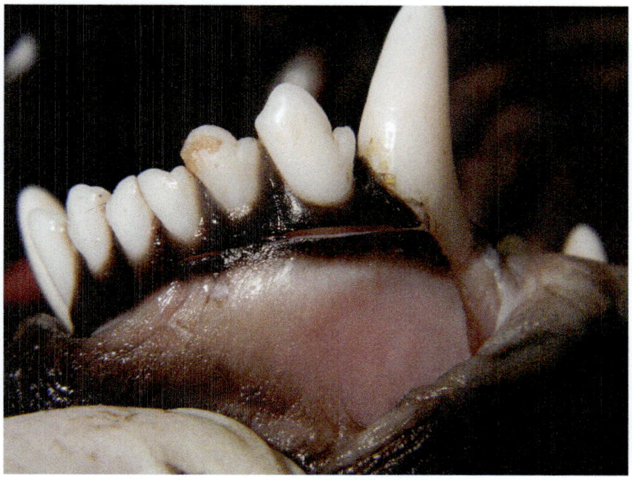

Figure 16.67 Split thickness horizontal incision.

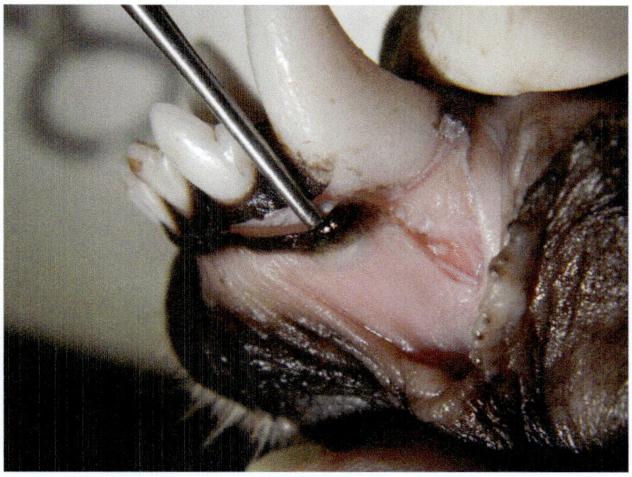

Figure 16.68 *Bluntly* dissecting the area of the graft that will cover the defect. This is done to keep a periosteal attachment with the graft.

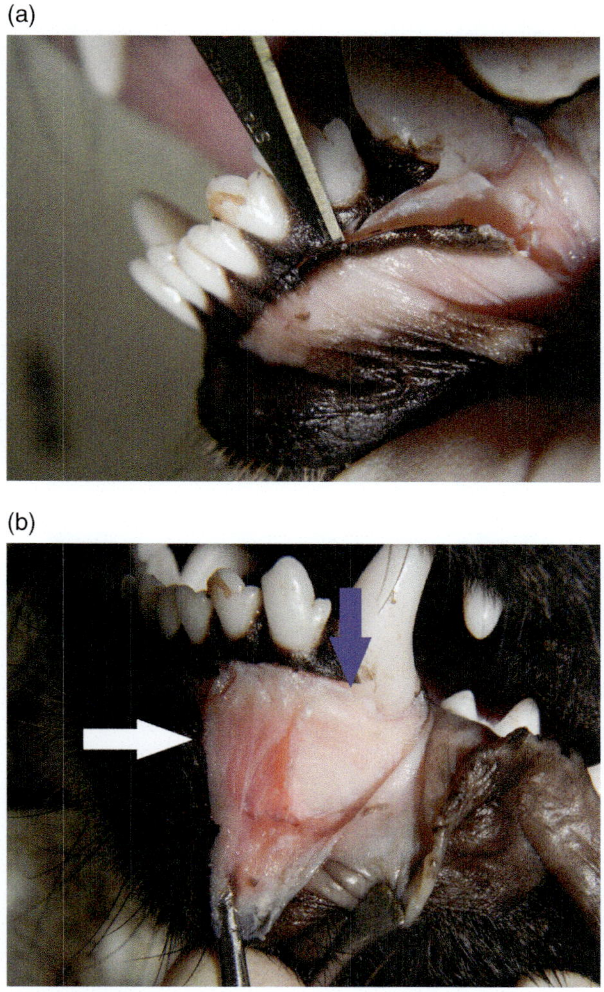

Figure 16.69 *Sharply* dissecting part of the graft away from the defect to create a split thickness graft. This is the area that will be left denuded. (a) Sharp dissection. (b) Graft harvested. Note the area toward the defect is completely denuded revealing bare bone (blue arrow), while the area away from the graft (which will be left uncovered) retains a soft tissue covering (white arrow).

frenula, one maxillary and two mandibular.[55] The maxillary frenulum runs from the lip to the gingiva just apical to the first incisors (Figure 16.73). The mandibular frenula arise from the mandibular lip and extend to the level of the mandibular canine teeth (Figure 16.74). The latter are much more important in periodontal disease and surgery.

The goal of these procedures is to release the tension from the frenulum, which may contribute to attachment loss, as well as to remove a potential food trap. It is generally performed when there is significant periodontal disease to the mandibular canine, and therefore is often performed at the same time as other flap surgeries in this area.

The two procedures are similar in intent and approach and differ in extent. *Frenotomy* incises the muscular

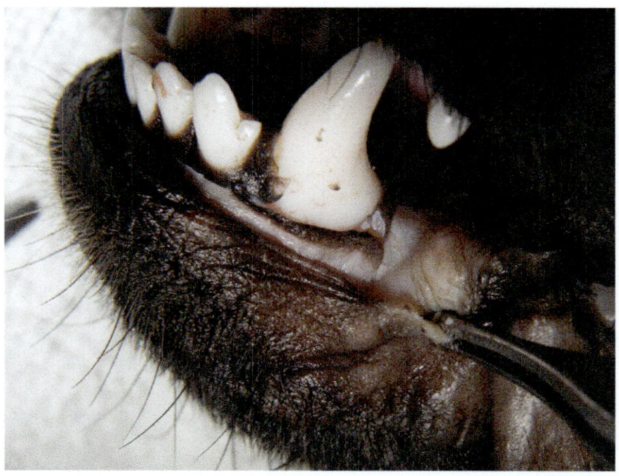

Figure 16.70 Graft is rotated to cover the defect and trial fit to ensure no tension is present.

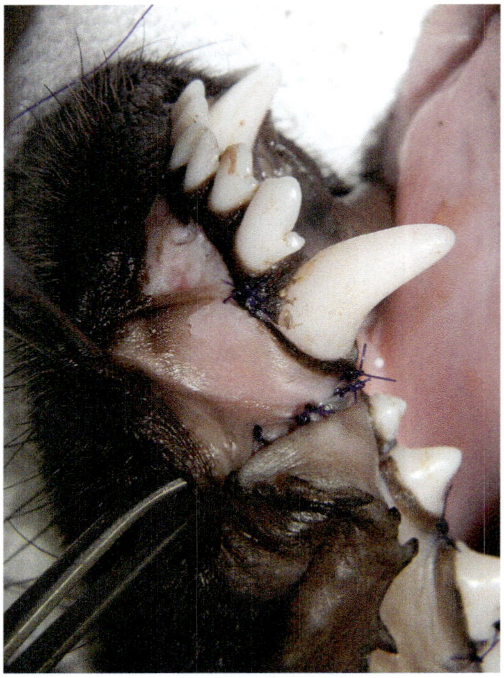

Figure 16.71 Closure with simple interrupted sutures.

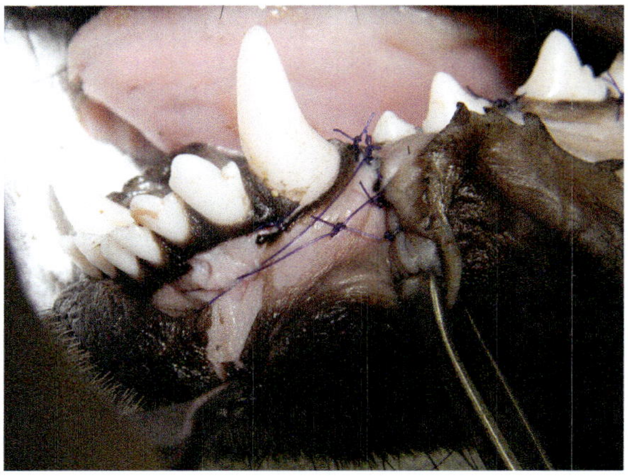

Figure 16.72 Cruciate suture placed over the site.

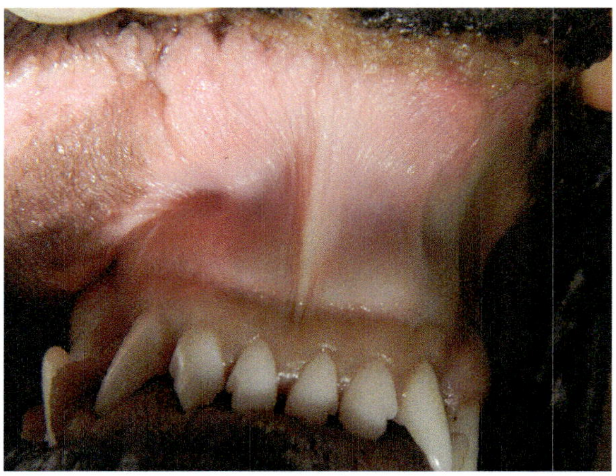

Figure 16.73 Maxillary frenulum.

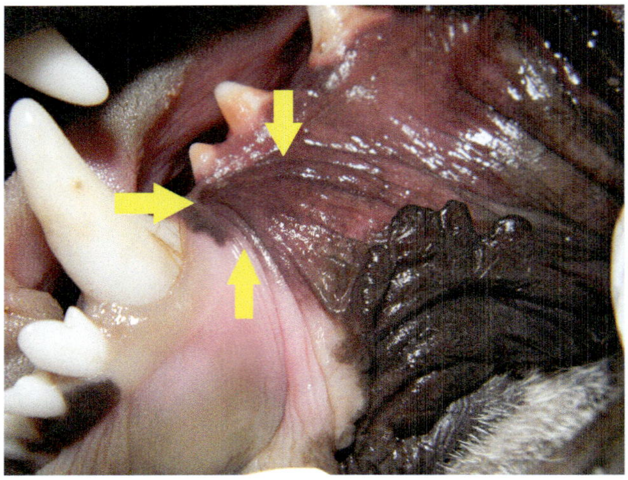

Figure 16.74 Mandibular frenulum (yellow arrows).

frenulum, whereas a *frenectomy* completely removes it. For periodontal purposes, a frenotomy should suffice and will be presented here.

Technique

1. Using a blade or ideally LaGrange scissors, cut the frenulum horizontally close to its attachment at the gingiva (Figure 16.75).
2. Using sharp/blunt dissection, incise the frenulum to relieve the muscular attachments (Figure 16.76a). Once this is performed, the lip should hang freely. This will create a diamond-shaped defect (Figure 16.76b).
3. Using a simple interrupted pattern, suture from mesial to distal (Figure 16.77).

Suture patterns for periodontal surgery

Following thorough root cleaning ± osseous surgery (see chapters 17 and 18), the flap is replaced.[19] It is critical to ensure that there is *no tension* on the incision line. If tension is present, the incision line will likely dehisce and the flap will fail. This can lead to disastrous results for the treated teeth, potentially necessitating extraction. The tension should be tested prior to any suturing. If tension has been sufficiently released, the flap should temporarily stay in place without sutures (Figure 16.78). If the flap pulls back at all (Figure 16.79), tension is present and must be eliminated before suturing.

Tension can be released by fenestrating the periosteum.[22,56,57] This is done by pulling up on the flap gently and carefully incising the thin layer of periosteum on the underside at the base of the flap. This can be done with

(a) (b)

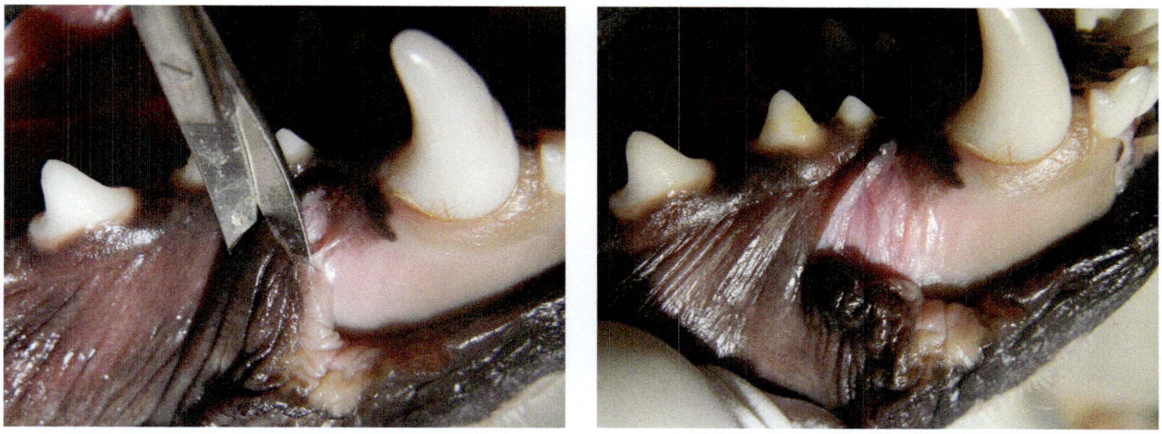

Figure 16.75 Frenotomy of the mandibular frenula. (a) Horizontal incision of the frenula with a LaGrange scissors. (b) Flap created.

(a)

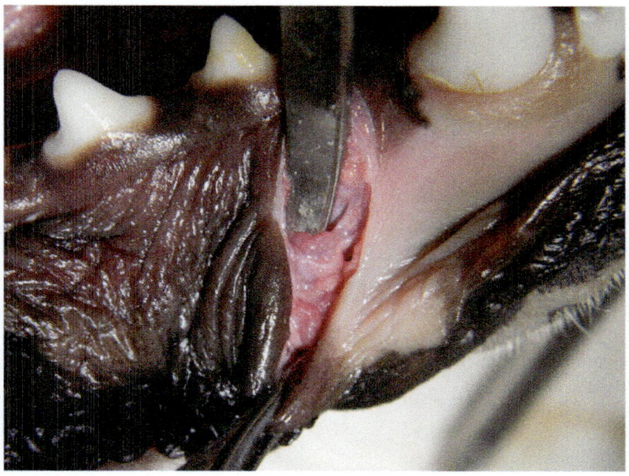

(b)

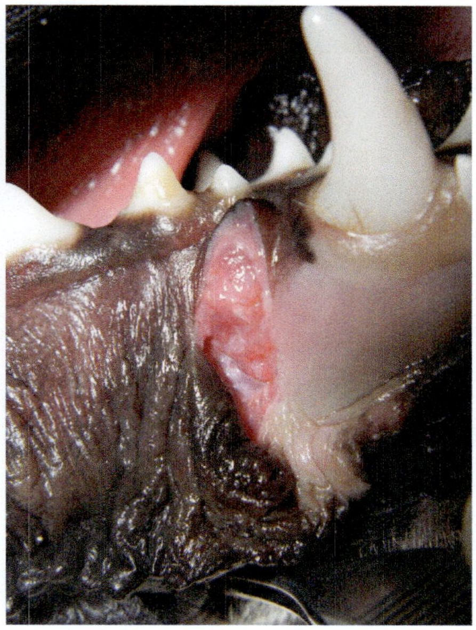

Figure 16.76 (a) Sharp/blunt dissection to relieve the muscular attachments. (b) Frenula hanging loose.

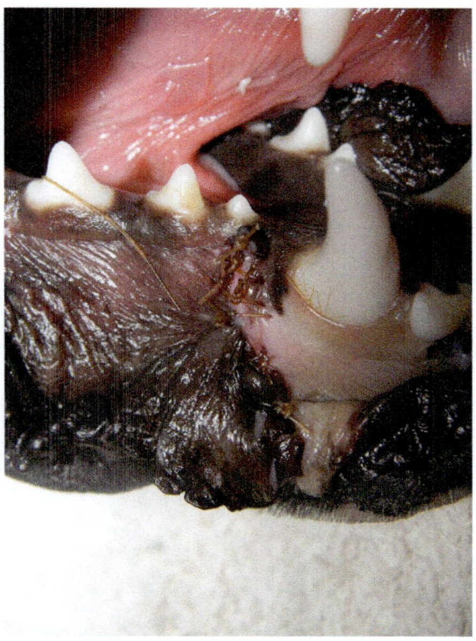

Figure 16.77 Horizontal closure.

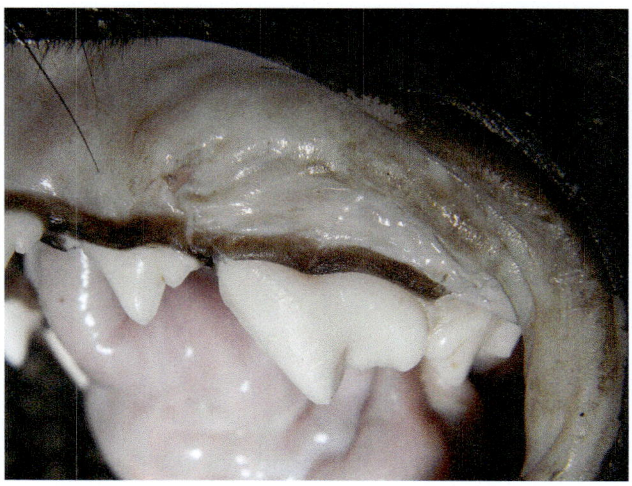

Figure 16.78 Intraoral picture of a maxillary fourth premolar that has received periodontal flap therapy. The flap has been preplaced to ensure that there is no tension. The flap stays in position, indicating that tension has been released and the flap can be sutured.

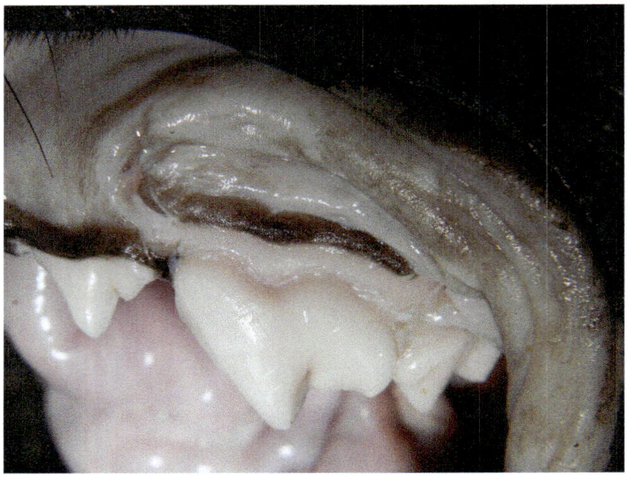

Figure 16.79 Flap with tension present. When the flap was placed in position, it pulled apically, indicating that tension is still present. If the flap is sutured at this point, it will dehisce and fail. The tension must be released *prior* to closure.

a scalpel blade (Figure 16.80), but this author prefers sharp/blunt dissection with a LaGrange scissors (Figure 16.81). Once lack of tension is assured, the flap is replaced and held in position for a few minutes to initiate healing.

The gingiva is very friable compared to skin and must be sutured precisely to ensure healing. Imprecise or rough suturing techniques that may be adequate for healing in other oral procedures will likely have untoward effects in periodontal surgery. Therefore, special care should be taken when securing the gingival flaps.

When suturing the gingiva, ensure that the needle enters the tissue at a right angle and at a distance of at least 2–3 mm from the margin[19] (Figure 16.82). If the interdental papilla is part of the suture, make sure to pierce the tissue below where the papilla begins narrowing.[19] The initial suture bite should be on the flap (or unattached) side,[57] which is usually the buccal side. This

(a) (b) (c)

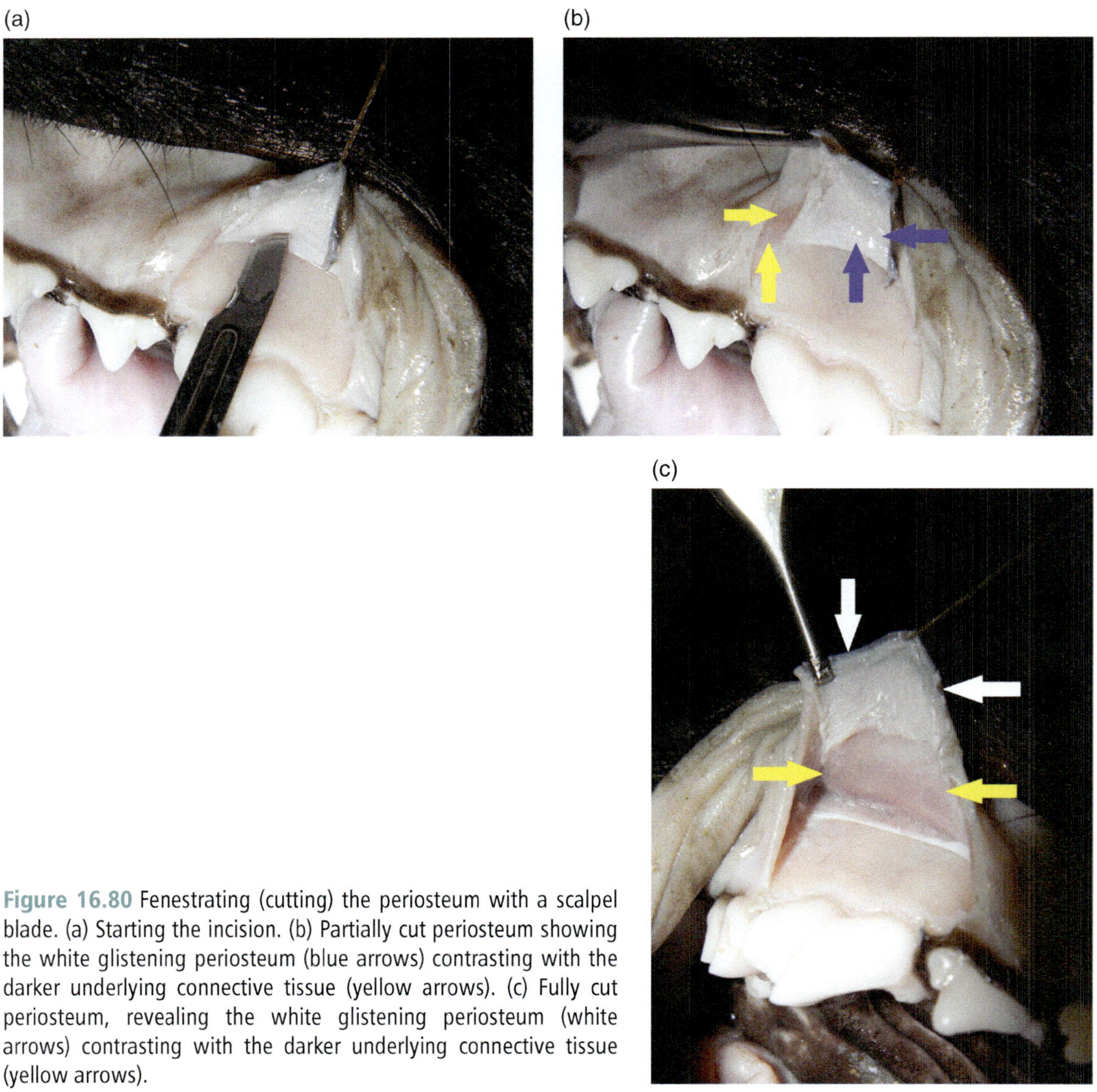

Figure 16.80 Fenestrating (cutting) the periosteum with a scalpel blade. (a) Starting the incision. (b) Partially cut periosteum showing the white glistening periosteum (blue arrows) contrasting with the darker underlying connective tissue (yellow arrows). (c) Fully cut periosteum, revealing the white glistening periosteum (white arrows) contrasting with the darker underlying connective tissue (yellow arrows).

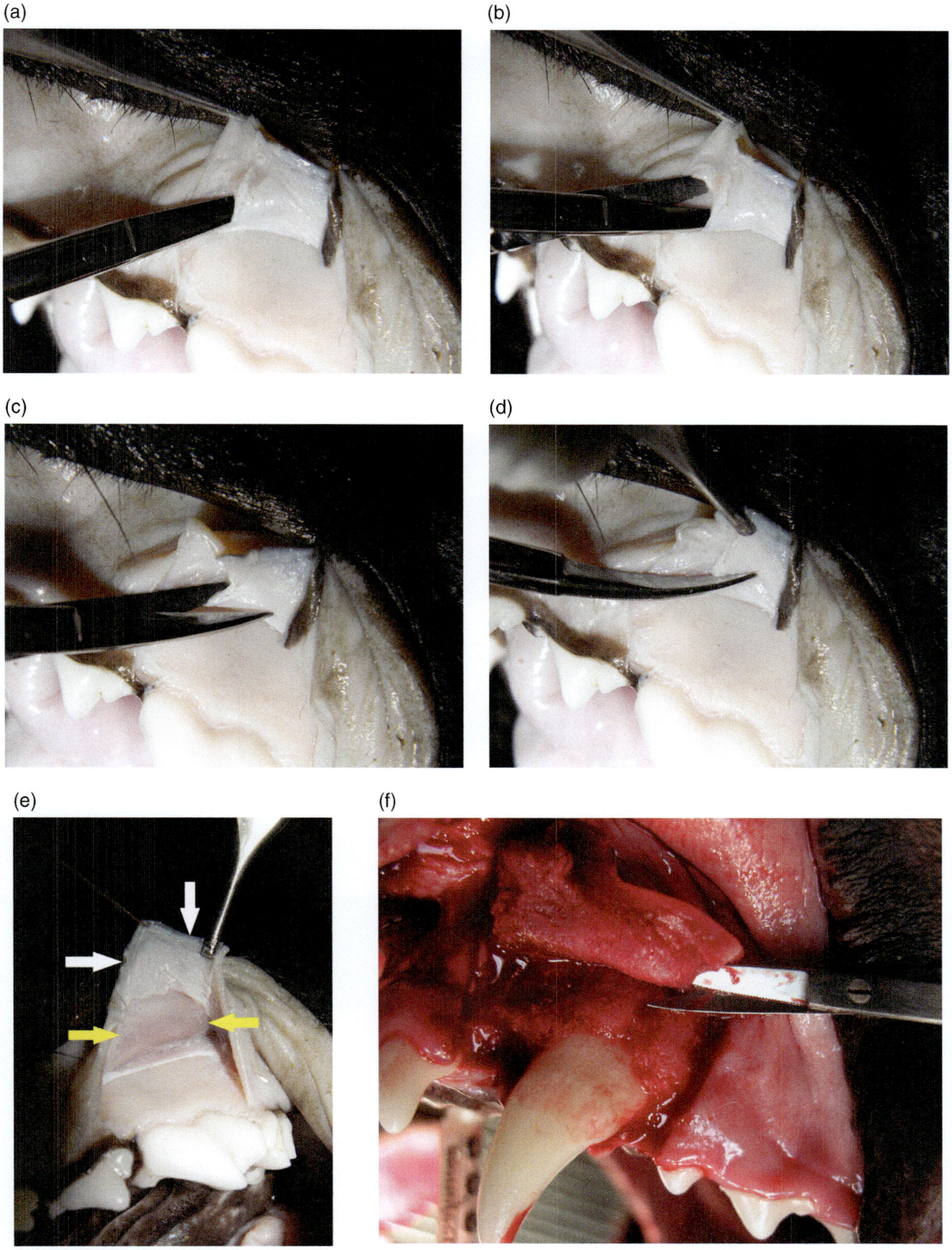

Figure 16.81 Fenestrating (cutting) the periosteum with a LaGrange scissors. (a) Bluntly inserting the closed scissors between the periosteum and the buccal mucosa. (b) Separating the scissors to create a space between the two tissue layers. (c) Opening the scissors and placing one blade in the created space and one above. Make sure that the lower blade is *between* the two layers so that both are not cut. (d) Cutting the periosteum. (e) Fully cut periosteum, revealing the white glistening periosteum (white arrows) contrasting with the darker underlying connective tissue (yellow arrows). (f) Fenestrating the periosteum in a clinical case with a LaGrange scissors.

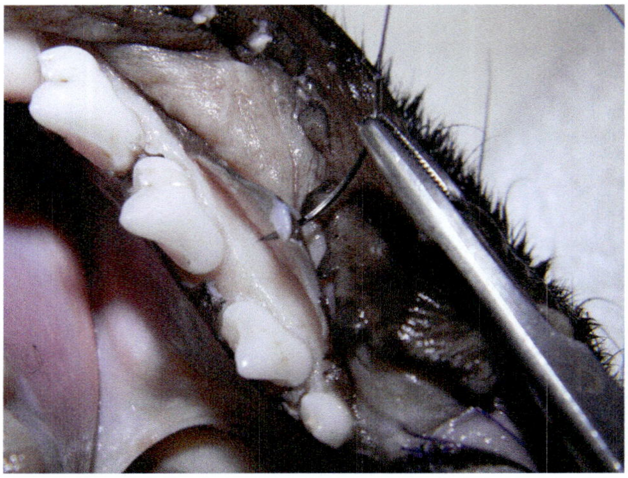

Figure 16.82 Correct first bite when suturing the gingiva. The needle enters the tissue from the buccal aspect, at a right angle, and at a distance of at least 2–3 mm from the margin.

is done to avoid placing pressure on the flap during subsequent sutures, as the needle dulls during numerous passes through the tough attached gingiva. Since cutting needles are generally used, it is critical to advance the needle through the tissue using wrist motion to follow the curve of the needle. The suture should be advanced completely through the initial side prior to piercing the other side. This helps to avoid tearing the flap with increased drag. Finally, the knots should be tied off the incision line[19] with one throw over manufacturer's recommendation (to account for tongue motion).[57]

The most common and simplest suture patterns for periodontal surgery are interdental ligations. However, sling sutures are also used and are valuable because they are less likely to buckle the flaps and are better at distributing masticatory tension. These are complicated patterns and should be practiced prior to attempting them in a patient.

Interdental ligation

The most basic suture is the *direct loop suture*, which is very similar to the simple interrupted pattern (Figure 16.83). This is generally utilized in cases where the gingival tissue can be directly opposed without tension. This is the most correct form of closure and should be used whenever possible.

A variation of this pattern that is useful for tight interdental contacts, such as between maxillary fourth premolars/first molars as well as between mandibular molar teeth, is the "Niemiec" pattern. With this technique, the needle is passed backwards through the interdental space (Figure 16.84) to pierce the lingual/palatal side first (Figure 16.85) and then pass interdentally and finally

(a)
(b)
(c)

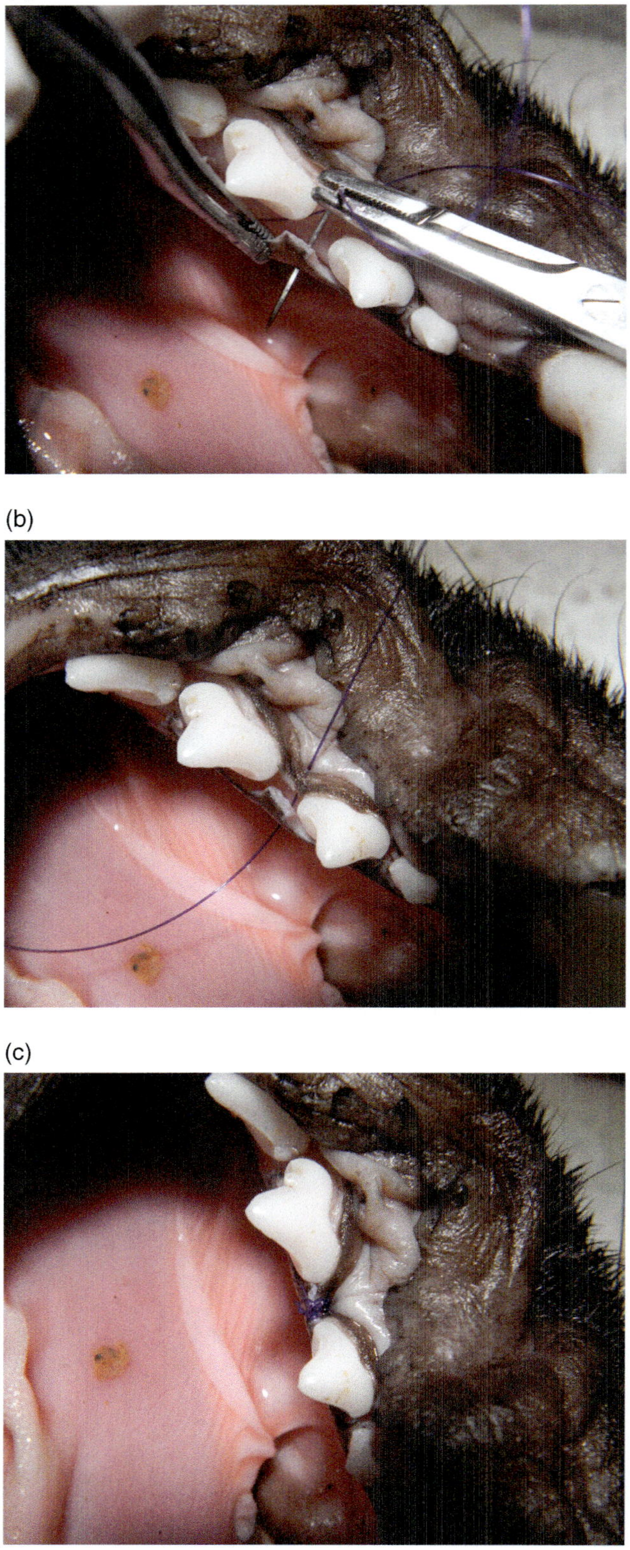

Figure 16.83 Direct loop suture. See Figure 16.82 for the first step: needle is passed through the buccal mucosa. (a) Needle is passed through the lingual side of the flap from the inside. (b) Suture is pulled carefully through the tissue. (c) The suture is tied. One throw over manufacturer's recommendation is advised.

(a) (b)

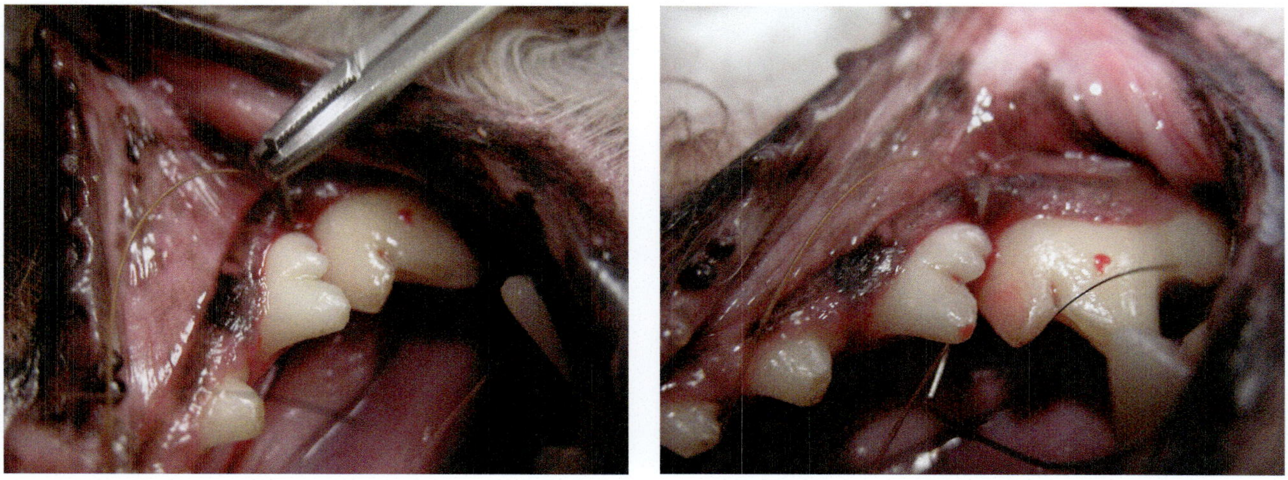

Figure 16.84 (a and b) "Niemiec" stitch in the tight occlussal space between the mandibular fourth premolar and first molar. Needle is passed "backward" or blunt end first through the interproximal space.

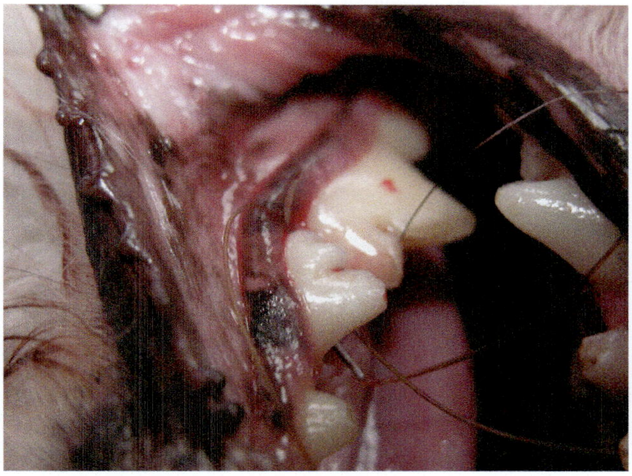

Figure 16.85 Needle pierces through the lingual mucosa from the lingual aspect and then through the interproximal space.

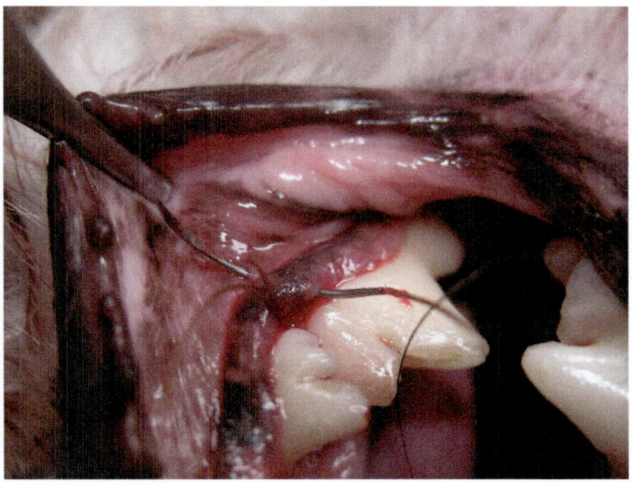

Figure 16.86 Buccal mucosa is pierced from the "inside" connective tissue side.

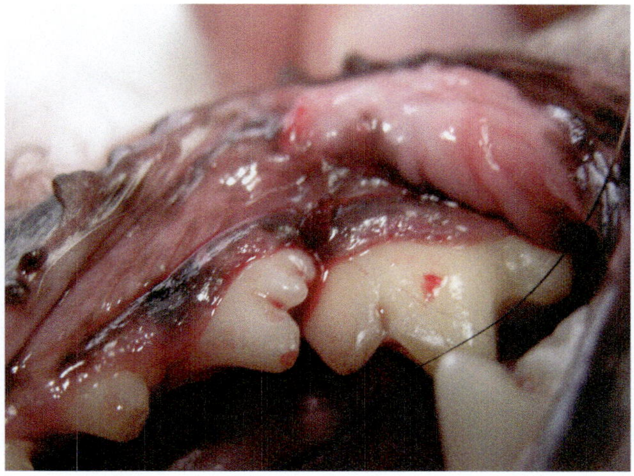

Figure 16.87 The suture is tied. One throw over manufacturer's recommendation is advised.

pierce the buccal side (Figure 16.86). Finally it is tied normally (Figure 16.87).

Another type of suture pattern is the "*figure-8*," which puts the suture between the flap edges. This pattern is used when the flap edges cannot be directly opposed, which is most commonly encountered with apical repositioning flaps (Figure 16.88).

For wide interdental spaces, a horizontal mattress suture can be utilized. This suture pattern adapts both the mesial and distal edges of the papilla snug against the bone and tooth.

Sling ligation patterns

Sling ligation patterns have the advantage of using the tooth as an anchor for the flap, rather than relying on the

(a) (b)

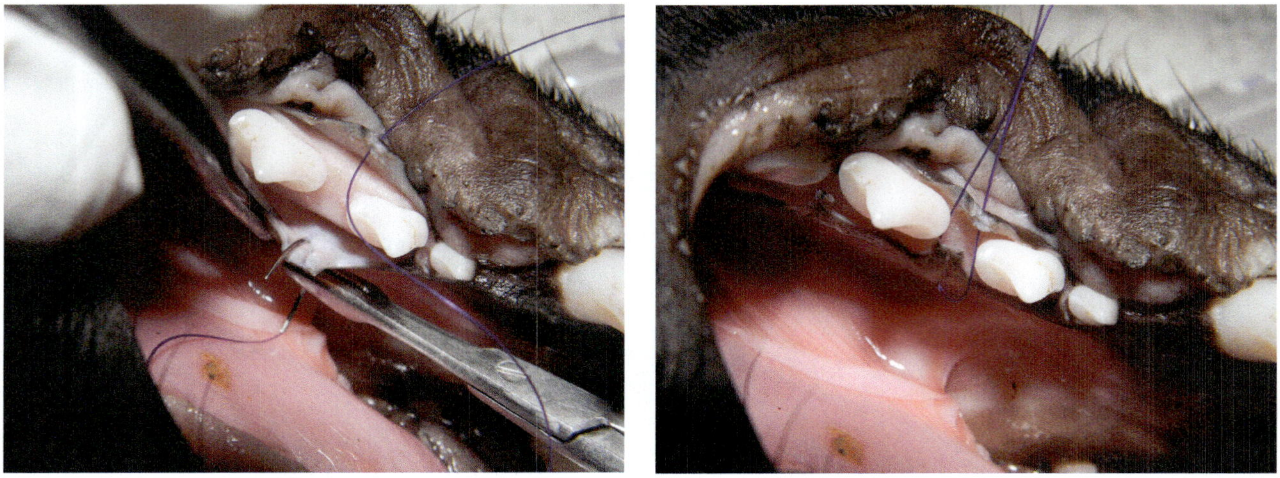

(c)

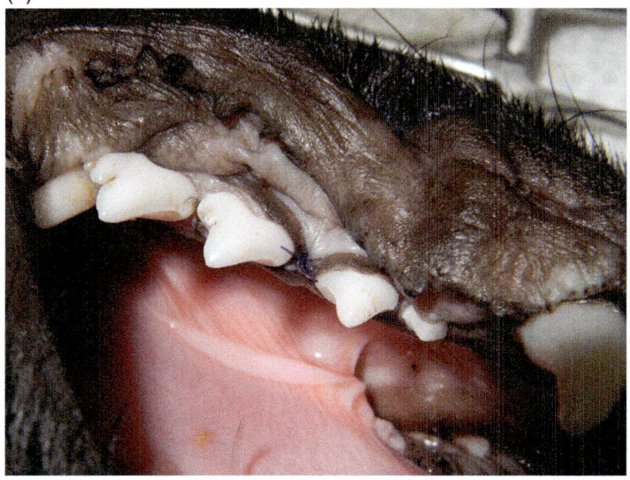

Figure 16.88 Figure-8 suture. See Figure 16.82 for the first step: needle is passed through the buccal mucosa. (a) Needle is reversed and passed through the lingual gingiva from the lingual aspect. (b) Suture is pulled carefully through the tissue. (c) The suture is tied. One throw over manufacturer's recommendation is advised.

gingival sutures. Sling ligations are typically used when large flaps are created both lingually and bucally, as well as when the edges are not designed to touch. They are especially valuable on the maxillary arcade, as the palatine tissue is fibrous and the buccal tissues are more elastic. These suture patterns do not attach the wound edges together (although the edges can touch) but use the teeth as anchors for the sutures. They can be done in an interrupted or continuous pattern.

The *interrupted* sling pattern (Figures 16.89 and 16.90) is initiated by passing through the outer edge of the gingiva and then through the interdental area and around the tooth. Once in the next interdental area, the gingiva is again pierced from the outside and passed around the tooth to return to the initial area and the knot is tied.

The *continuous sling suture* pattern is initiated at the mesial interdental space and carried distally, as it is easier to place the knot in this position. The initial suture bite through the gingiva is placed from the outside of the gingiva and passed through the interdental space (Figure 16.91), and then around the tooth and back out bucally in the next distal interproximal space. Next, the needle is reversed and passed back through the gingiva from the outside (Figure 16.92a). This is continued (Figures 16.92b and c) until the last tooth, at which point the suture is anchored around the tooth immediately distal to the flap (Figure 16.93). This suture is carried to the palatal/lingual side and the process is repeated mesially (Figure 16.94). The suture is then anchored around the tooth immediately mesial to the flap and tied (Figure 16.95).

The *anchor suture* (Figure 16.96) pattern is used on the ends of the flaps when there is no tooth distal to the flap. This pattern can be used with either continuous or interrupted sling sutures. This technique starts with passing the needle through the outer edge of the facial flap. Next, the tooth is encircled and the lingual/palatal flap pierced from beneath. Finally, the knot is tied.

(a) (b)

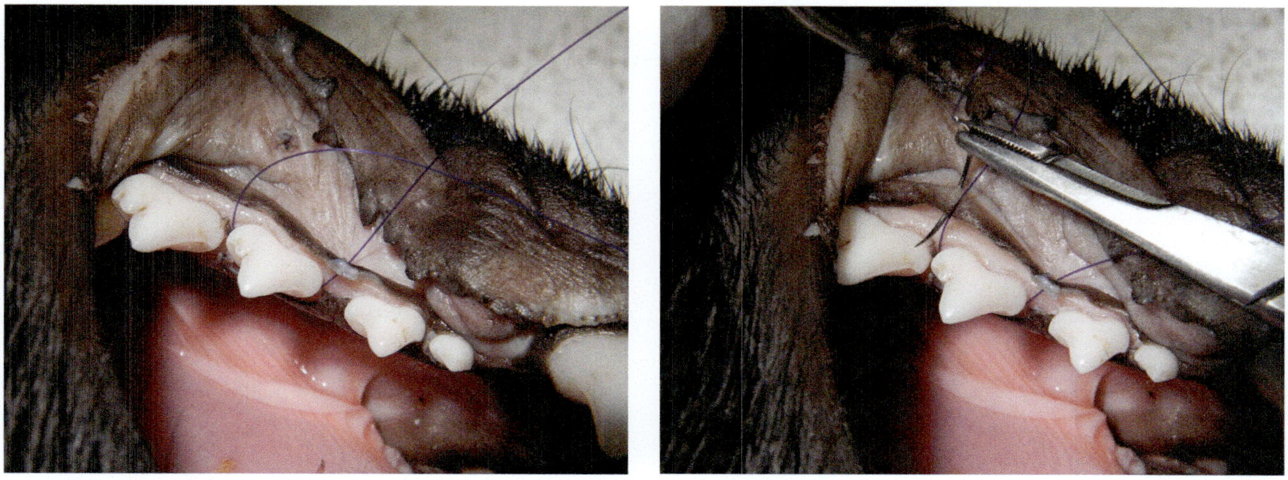

Figure 16.89 *Interrupted* sling suture pattern. See Figure 16.82 for the first step: needle is passed through the buccal mucosa. (a) Next, the needle is passed through the interdental area and around the tooth. (b) The needle is reversed and passed again through the buccal side of the buccal mucosa.

(a) (b)

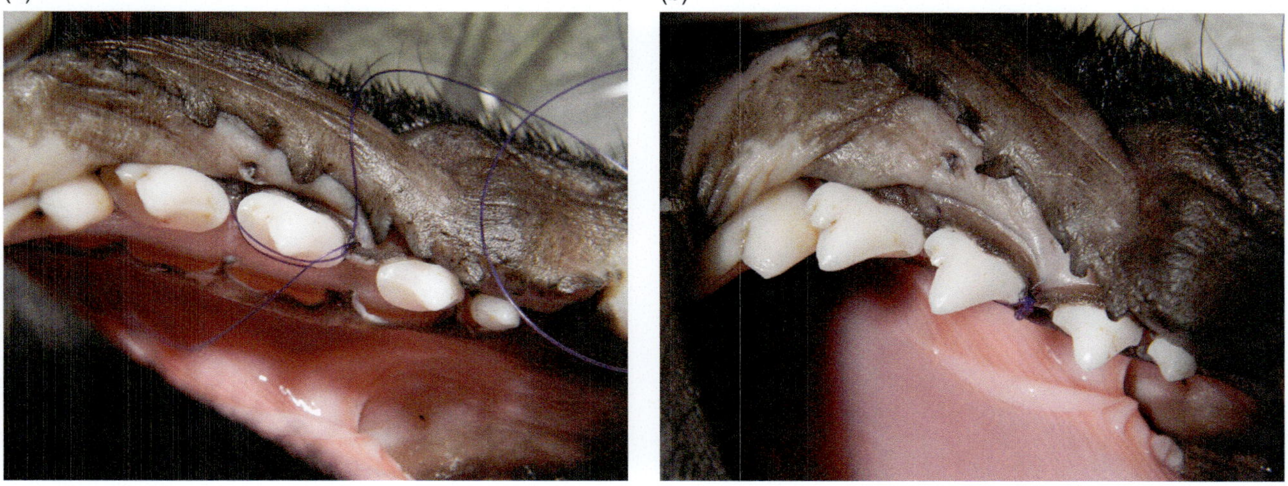

(c)

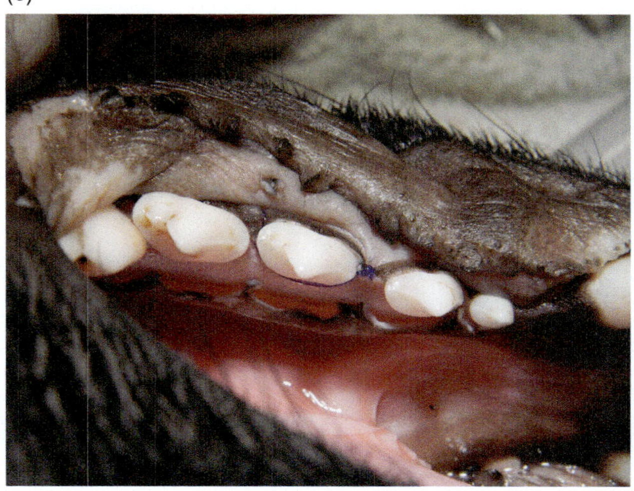

Figure 16.90 (a–c) The suture is passed back around the lingual aspect of the tooth and the knot is tied. One throw over manufacturer's recommendation is advised.

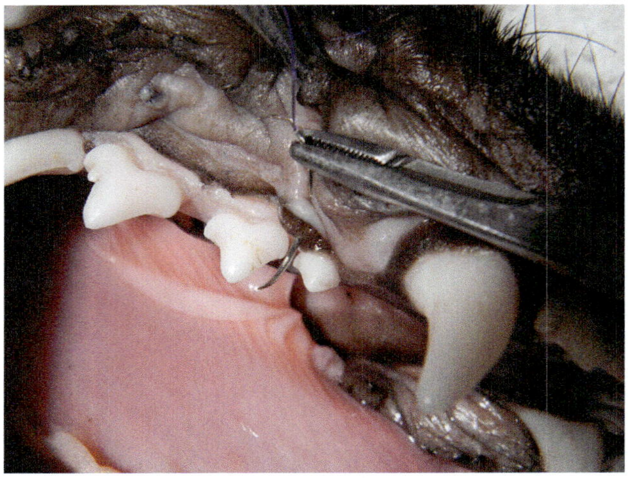

Figure 16.91 *Continuous* sling suture pattern. Needle is passed through the buccal mucosa (as in Figure 16.82 above).

A more challenging variation of this knot is the *closed anchor*. It is used to close flaps that have an edentulous area on one or both ends. The closed anchor requires tying a direct suture to close the proximal flap followed by carrying one of the sutures around the tooth to anchor the tissue against the tooth, and finishes by tying the two ends of suture.

For vertical incisions, wide diastemas, or edentulous areas, simple interrupted sutures should be used, placed 2–3 mm apart[2] (Figure 16.97). However, practitioners should be familiar with several other suture patterns that may be useful in various situations.

Postoperative care

In primates, initial healing of the flap starts within 24 hours as a blood clot forms. Within 1 week there is an epithelial attachment to the tooth, and at 2 weeks new

(a)

(b)

(c)

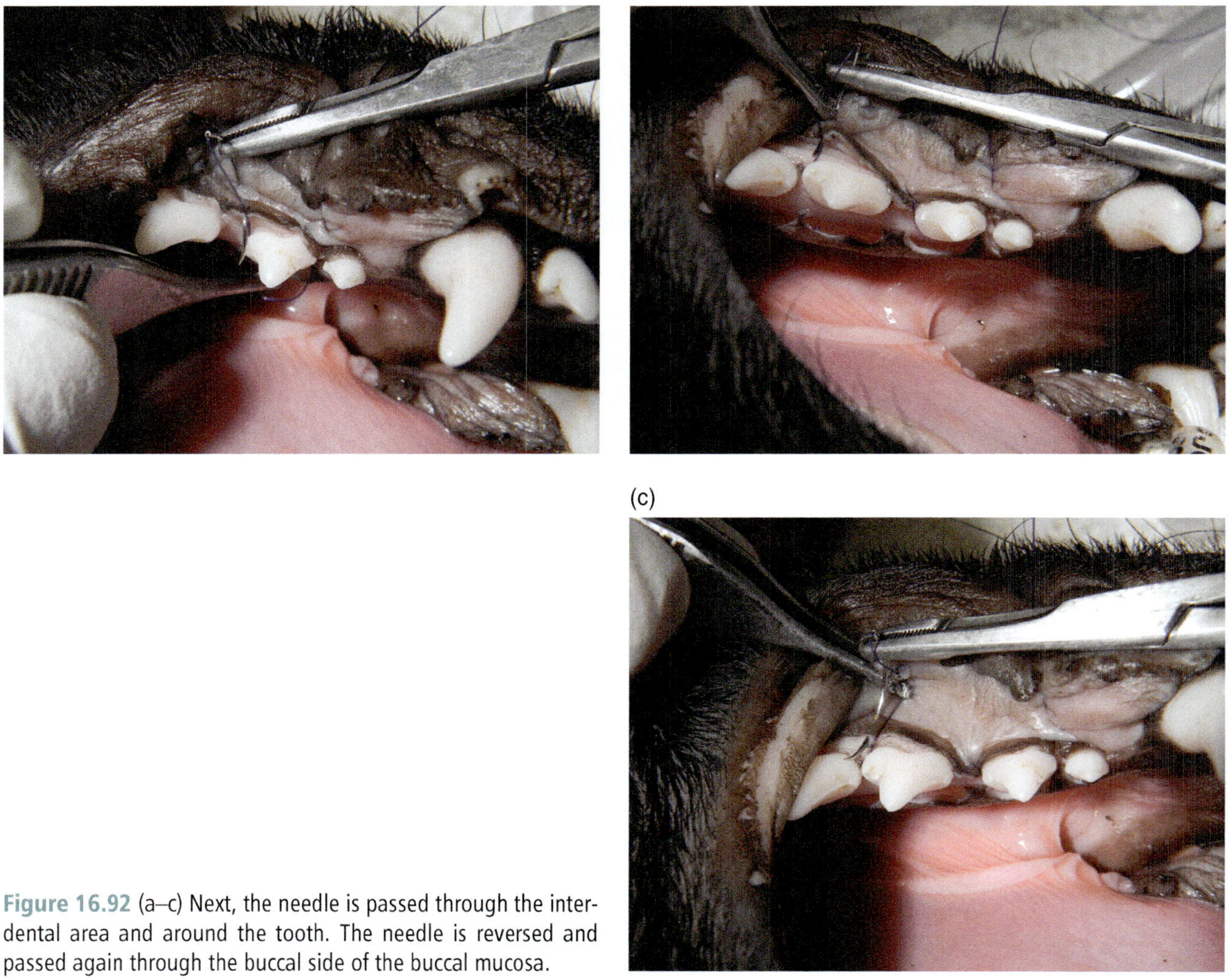

Figure 16.92 (a–c) Next, the needle is passed through the interdental area and around the tooth. The needle is reversed and passed again through the buccal side of the buccal mucosa.

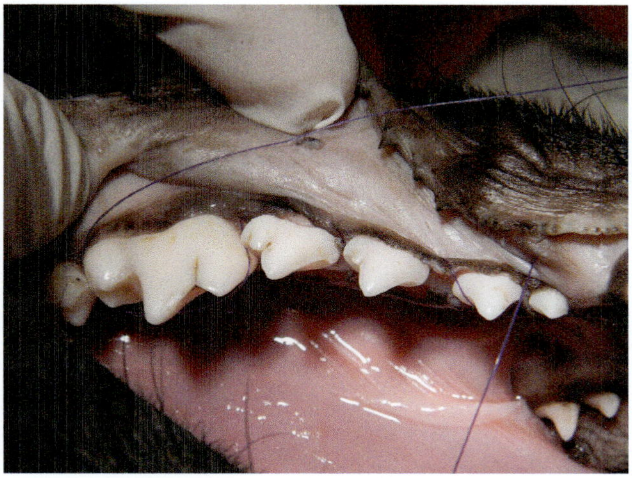

Figure 16.93 Anchoring the suture around the first molar, which is the tooth immediately distal to the flap.

collagen fibers begin to appear.[33] However, the attachment at this point is still weak due to the presence of immature collagen fibers. Complete healing does not occur (at least in primates) until 1 month following surgery. Therefore, the patient should be placed on soft food (and no hard toys) for a minimum of 2 weeks. Brushing should also be avoided during this time to minimize trauma to the sutures and/or wound dehiscence. Alternate plaque control strategies should be used for the initial 2 weeks postoperatively (such as barrier sealants or antiseptic rinses).

Postoperative medications, such as antibiotics and pain medications, should be prescribed as indicated. (See chapters 14 and 21 for details.)

Patients should be rechecked in 2 weeks to evaluate soft tissue healing, followed by an anesthetized exam and radiographs scheduled at 6–9 months postop and regularly thereafter to evaluate the success of the procedure and the degree of infection.

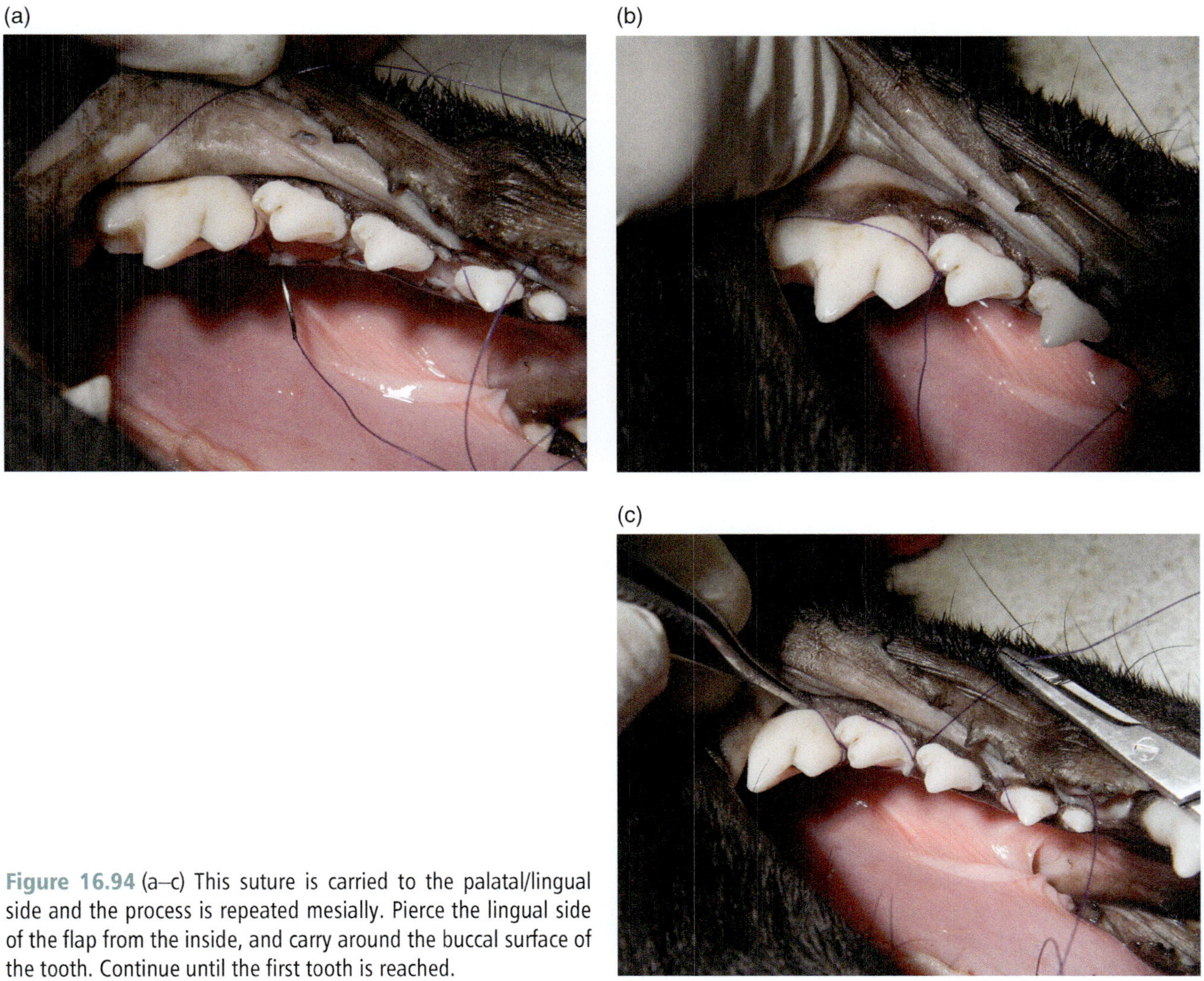

Figure 16.94 (a–c) This suture is carried to the palatal/lingual side and the process is repeated mesially. Pierce the lingual side of the flap from the inside, and carry around the buccal surface of the tooth. Continue until the first tooth is reached.

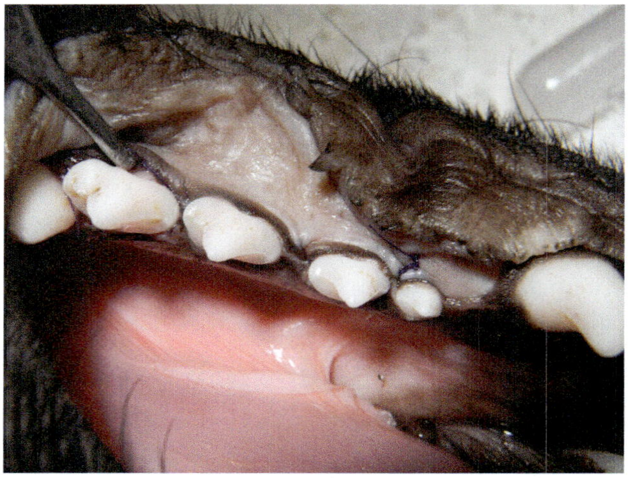

Figure 16.95 The knot is tied. One throw over manufacturer's recommendation is advised.

(a)

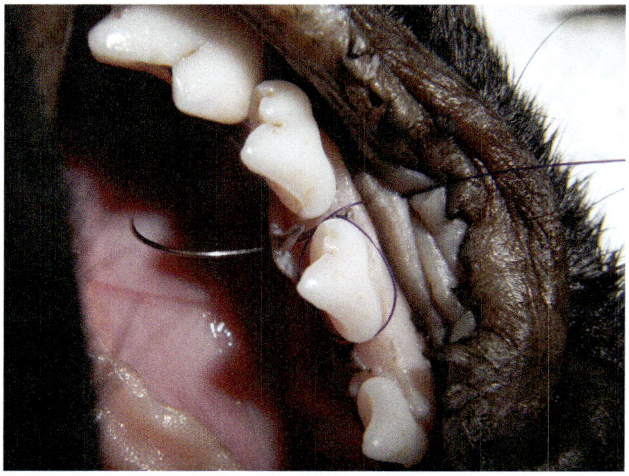

(b)

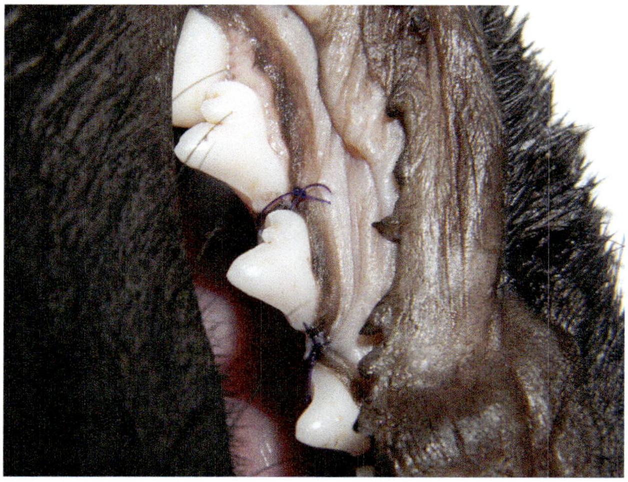

Figure 16.96 Anchor suture pattern. See Figure 16.82 for the first step: needle is passed through the buccal mucosa. (a) The tooth is encircled and the lingual/palatal flap pierced from beneath. (b) The knot is tied. Note this image also has a suture from a separate flap.

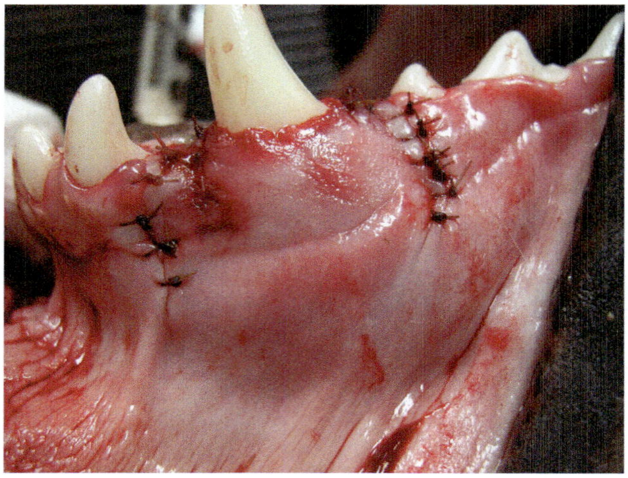

Figure 16.97 Simple interrupted sutures closing a full flap.

Box 16.1 Key points

- Periodontal surgery is indicated for pockets greater than 5–6 mm or with furcation exposure level II or III.
- The use of proper instruments greatly improves the efficiency and speed of periodontal procedures as well as the therapeutic outcome.
- Periodontal flaps can be created with or without vertical releasing incisions.
- Periodontal pockets with alveolar bone loss are ideally treated with regenerative techniques.
- The efficacy and benefit of periodontal surgery should be questioned in the absence of homecare.

Notes

A. Diplomate Periodontal surgery kit, Dentalaire.
B. Monocryl, Ethicon, Novartis Animal Health.
C. VICRYL RAPIDE, Ethicon, Novartis Animal Health.
D. Hu-Friedy Mfg. Co.
E. MONOCRYL* Plus, Ethicon, Novartis Animal Health.
F. Vicryl Mesh, Ethicon, Johnson and Johnson.
G. Osteoallograft, Veterinary Transplant Services.
H. Consil, Nutramax.
I. Perioptix.
J. Vetspon, Ethicon, Novartis Animal Health.
K. Gelfoam, Pfizer.
L. Surgicel, Ethicon, Johnson and Johnson.
M. Collaplug, Zimmer Dental.
N. Thrombostat, Parke-Davis, Pfizer.

References

1. Carranza FA, Takei HH. The flap technique for pocket therapy. In: Carranza's Clinical Periodontology. St. Louis: Saunders, 2006, pp. 937–949.
2. Wiggs RB, Lobprise HB. Periodontology. In: Veterinary Dentistry, Principles and Practice. Philadelphia: Lippincott-Raven, 1997, pp. 186–231.

3. Carranza FA, Takei HH. Phase II periodontal therapy. In: Carranza's Clinical Periodontology. St. Louis: Saunders, 2006, pp. 881–886.
4. Hill RW, Ramfjord SP, et al. Four types of periodontal treatment compared over 2 years. J Periodontol. 52:655–662, 1981.
5. Holmstrolm SE, Frost P, Eisner ER. Periodontal therapy and surgery. In: Veterinary Dental Techniques. 2nd ed. Philadelphia: Saunders, 1998, pp. 167–213.
6. Rabbini GM, Ash MM, Caffesse RG. The effectiveness of subgingival scaling and root planing in calculus removal. J Periodontol. 52:119, 1981.
7. Greensteifi G. Contemporary interpretation of probing depth assessment: Diagnostic and therapeutic implications, a literature review. J Periodontol. 68:1194,1997.
8. Waerhaug J. Healing of the dentoepithelialjunction following subgingival plaque control, II, as observed on extracted teeth. J Periodontol. 40:119, 1978.
9. Bellows J. Equipping the dental practice. In: Small Animal Dental Equipment, Materials, and Techniques, a Primer. Ames, IA: Blackwell, 2004, pp. 13–55.
10. Caffesse RG, Sweeney PL, Smith BA. Scaling and root planing with and without periodontal flap surgery. J Clin Periodontol. 13(3):205–210, 1986.
11. Perry DA, Schmid MO, Takei HH. Phase I periodontal therapy. In: Carranza's Clinical Periodontology. St. Louis: Saunders, 2006, pp. 722–727, 2006.
12. Zetner K, Rothmueller G. Treatment of periodontal pockets with doxycycline in beagles. Vet Ther. 3(4):441–452, 2002.
13. Magnusson I, Runstad L, Nyman S, et al. A long junctional epithelium: A locus minoris resistentiae in plaque infection. J Clin Periodontol. 10:333, 1983.
14. Philstrolm BL, Ortiz Campos C, McHugh RB. A randomized 4 year study of periodontal therapy. J Periodontol. 52:227, 1981.
15. Klokkevold PR, Takei HH, Carranza FA. General principles of periodontal surgery. In: Carranza's Clinical Periodontology. St. Louis: Saunders, 2006, pp. 887–901.
16. Bellows J. Periodontal equipment, materials, and techniques. In: Small Animal Dental Equipment, Materials, and Techniques, a Primer. Ames, IA: Blackwell, 2004, pp. 115–173.
17. Silverstein LH, Kurtzman GM. A review of dental suturing for optimal soft-tissue management. Compend Contin Educ Dent. 26(3):163–166, 169–170, 2005.
18. Manor A, Kaffe I. Unusual foreign body reaction to a braided silk suture: A case report. J Periodontol. 53:86–88, 1981.
19. Takei HH, Carranza FA. The periodontal flap. In: Carranza's Clinical Periodontology. St. Louis: Saunders, 2006, pp. 926–936.
20. Ming X, Nichols M, Rothenburger S. In vivo antibacterial efficacy of MONOCRYL plus antibacterial suture (Poliglecaprone 25 with triclosan). Surg Infect (Larchmt). 8(2):209–214, 2007.
21. Ming X, Rothenburger S, Yang D. In vitro antibacterial efficacy of MONOCRYL plus antibacterial suture (Poliglecaprone 25 with triclosan). Surg Infect (Larchmt). 8(2):201–208, 2007.
22. Holmstrolm SE, Frost P, Eisner ER. Exodontics. In: Veterinary Dental Techniques. 2nd ed. Philadelphia: Saunders, 1998, pp. 215–254.
23. Morrison EC, Lang NP, et al. Effects of repeated scaling and root planning and/or controlled oral hygiene on periodontal attachement level and pocket depth in beagle dogs. I. Clinical findings. J Periodontal Res. 14:428–437, 1979.
24. Grove TK. Treatment of periodontal disease. Vet Clin North Am Small Animal Pract. 28:1147–1164, 1998.
25. Greensteifi G. Contemporary interpretation of probing depth assessment: Diagnostic and therapeutic implications. A literature review. J Periodontol. 68:1194, 1997.
26. Shoukry M, Ali B, Naby MA, Soliman A. Repair of experimental plaque-induced periodontal disease in dogs. J Vet Dent. 24(3):152–165, 2007.
27. Huffman LJ. Oral examination. In: Small Animal Dental, Oral and Maxillofacial Disease, a Color Handbook (Niemiec BA ed.). London: Manson, 2010, pp. 39–61.
28. Measley BL, Beybayer M, Butzin CA, et al. Use of furcal bone sounding to improve the accuracy of furcation diagnosis. J Periodontol. 65:649, 1994.
29. Easley J. Methods of determining alveolar osseous form. J Periodontol38:112, 1967.
30. Debowes LJ. Problems with the gingiva. In: Small Animal Dental, Oral and Maxillofacial Disease, a Color Handbook (Niemiec BA ed.). London: Manson, 2010, pp. 159–181.
31. Carr GB. Surgical endodontics. In: Pathways of the Pulp (Cohn S, Burns RC eds.). 6th ed. St. Louis: Mosby, 1994, pp. 535–536.
32. Smith MM. Line angle incisions. J Vet Dent. 20(4):241–244, 2003.
33. Caffesse RG, Ramfjord SP, Nasjleti CE. Reverse bevel periodontal flaps in monkeys. J Periodontol. 39:219, 1968.
34. Carranza FA, Carro JJ. Effect of removal of periosteum on postoperative result of mucogingival surgery. J Periodontol. 34:223, 1963.
35. Morris ML. The unrepositioned mucoperiosteal flap. Periodontics 3:147, 1965.
36. Ramfjord SP. Present status of the modified Widman flap procedure. J Periodontol. 48:558, 1977.
37. Ramfjord SP, Nissle RR. The modified Widman flap. J Periodontol. 45:601, 1974.
38. Tackas VJ. Root coverage techniques: A review. J West Soc Periodontol Periodontal Abstr. 43(1):5–14, 1995.
39. Wolf HF, Rateitschak EM, Rateitschak KH, Hassell TH. Color Atlas of Dental Medicine: Periodontology. 3rd ed. Stuttgart: Thieme, 2005.
40. Stahl SS, Froum SJ. Human suprabony healing responses following root demineralization and coronal flap anchorage. J Clin Periodontol. 18:685, 1991.
41. Takei HH, Azzi RR, Han TJ. Periodontal plastic and esthetic surgery. In: Carranza's Clinical Periodontology. St. Louis: Saunders, 2006, pp. 1005–1029.
42. Hall WB. Pure Mucogingival Problems: Etiology, Treatment, and Prevention. Chicago: Quintessence, 1984.
43. Tarno DP. Semilunar coronally repositioned flap. J Clin Periodontol. 13:182, 1986.
44. Donnenfeld OW, Marks R, Glickman I. The apically repositioned flap: A clinical study. J Periodontol. 37:381–387, 1964.
45. James WC, McFall WT Jr, Burkes EJ. Placement of free gingival grafts on denuded alveolar bone. Part I: Clinical evaluations. J Periodontol. 49(6):283–290, 1978.
46. James WC, McFall WT Jr, Burkes EJ. Placement of free gingival grafts on denuded alveolar bone. Part II: Microscopic observations. J Periodontol. 49(6):291–300, 1978.
47. Caffesse RG, Burgett FG, Nasjleti CE, Castelli WA. Healing of free gingival grafts with and without periosteum. Part I. Histologic evaluation. J Periodontol. 50(11):586–594, 1979.
48. Caffesse RG, Burgett FG, Nasjleti CE, Castelli WA. Healing of free gingival grafts with and without periosteum. Part II. Radioautographic evaluation. J Periodontol. 50(11):595–602, 1979.
49. Bjorn H. Transplantation of gingiva propia. Sveriges Tandlak T. 22:684, 1963.
50. Mörmann W, Schaer F, Firestone AR. The relationship between success of free gingival grafts and transplant thickness. Revascularization and shrinkage—a one year clinical study.

51. Nabers JM. Free gingival grafts. Periodontics 4(5):243–245, 1966.
52. Edel A. Clinical evaluation of free connective tissue grafts used to increase the width of keratinised gingiva. J Clin Periodontol. 1(4):185–196, 1974.
53. Beckman BW. Lateral sliding pedicle flap for gingival cleft at the maxillary canine tooth. J Vet Dent. 22(4):282–285, 2005.
54. Rawlinson JE, Reiter AM. Repair of a gingival cleft associated with a maxillary canine tooth in a dog. J Vet Dent. 22(4):234–242, 2005.
55. Wiggs RB, Lobprise HB. Oral anatomy and physiology. In: Veterinary Dentistry, Principles and Practice. Philadelphia: Lippincott-Raven, 1997, pp. 55–103.
56. Wiggs RB, Lobprise HB. Oral surgery. In: Veterinary Dentistry, Principles and Practice. Philadelphia: Lippincott-Raven, 1997, pp. 232–228.
57. Niemiec BA. Extraction techniques. Top Companion Anim Med. 23(2):97–105, 2008.
58. Wound Closure Manual. Somerville, NJ: Ethicon Inc. 1985, pp. 1–101.

17

Treatment of the exposed root surface

Introduction

The goal of periodontal surgery is to create a smooth and clean tooth surface for reattachment.[1] This is facilitated with the visualization afforded by the periodontal flap procedure (Figure 17.1). Once the root surface is clean and smooth, additional therapies such as root conditioning and guided tissue regeneration may be indicated.

Root scaling/planing

As with non-surgical periodontal therapy, the key to successful periodontal surgery is to produce a clean and smooth root surface.[1] This allows for reattachment of the periodontal tissues. Therefore, the first and most important step of the treatment of the dental hard tissues is a thorough SRP.[2–4] This is best performed with a combination of ultrasonic and hand scaling.[4] Start with an ultrasonic scaler (on a low power setting) on the root surface to remove the vast majority of the plaque and calculus (Figure 17.2). Following this, a sharp curette is used to plane the exposed root surface to as smooth as possible a finish (Figure 17.3). Alternatively, a fine scaler may be used in these cases since the flap has greatly decreased the chance of soft tissue laceration. (See chapter 11 for a complete discussion of SRP.)

Bone treatment (osteoplasty)

Uneven or jagged edges of alveolar bone (Figure 17.4) will hinder healing and therefore periodontal reattachment.[3,5] Therefore, these surfaces should be treated to promote maximum patient benefit. The purpose of osteoplasty is to return the remaining alveolar bone to a knife-sharp edge (Figure 17.5). Additionally, the bone

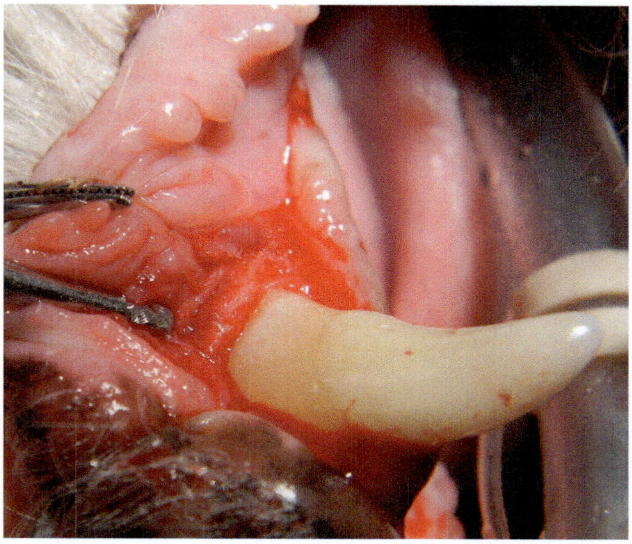

Figure 17.1 Horizontal "envelope" flap created for visualization of the root surface.

should be scalloped around the tooth, as this allows for superior flap apposition.[3] It should be noted, however, that due to the sacrifice of some alveolar bone, this concept is not universally accepted.[6]

There are several equipment options for this step.[6] Classically, it was performed by hand with bone chisels or periosteotomes. Today, however, a fine diamond or finishing bur is more expedient and may result in a superior finish. However, the speed and relative lack of control of powered instruments as well as the potential for heat production can make these more dangerous. Regardless, rotary methods appear to be the recommended technique in veterinary texts.[3,7] (See chapter 18 for a complete discussion of osseous surgery.)

Veterinary Periodontology, First Edition. Brook A. Niemiec.

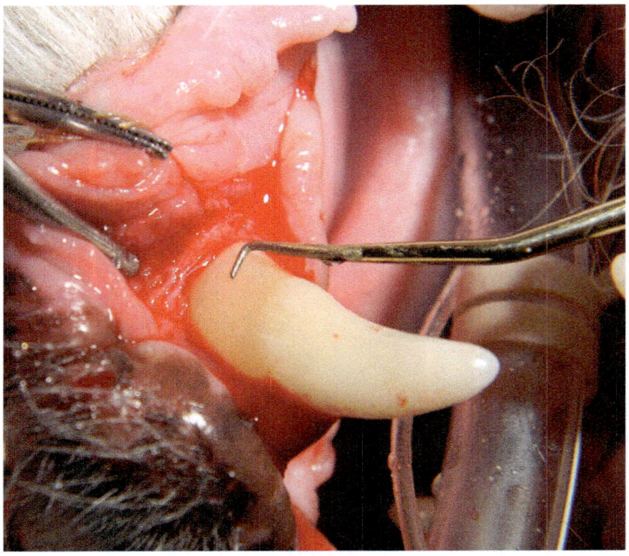

Figure 17.2 Ultrasonic debridement of the exposed root surface with a periodontal (subgingival) tip on low power.

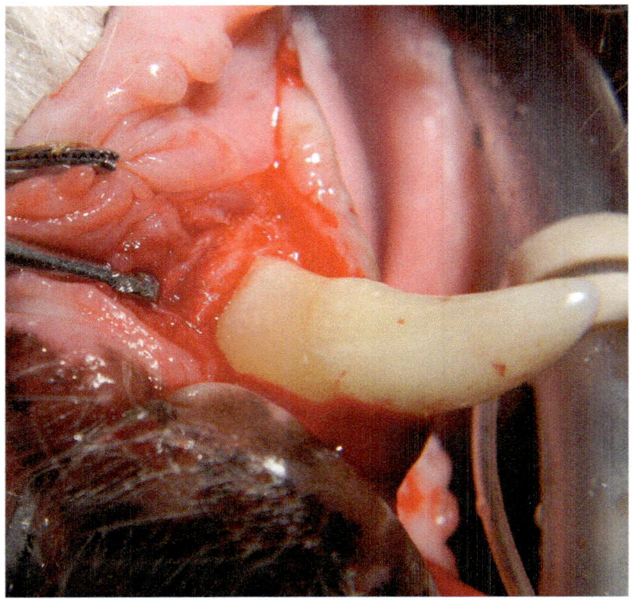

Figure 17.4 Postscaling: surface is smooth and clean.

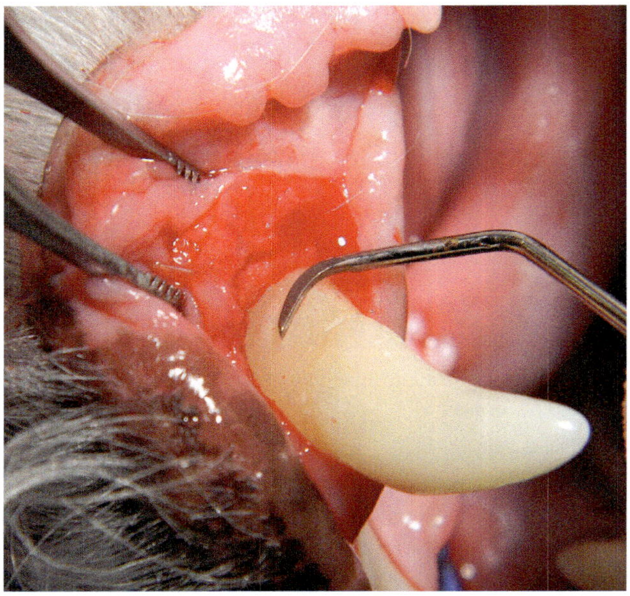

Figure 17.3 Hand scaling of the exposed root surface with a Gracey curette.

Root conditioning (biomodification of the root surface)

The goals of root conditioning are to enhance the cleaning effects of root planing, speed healing, and improve the chances of gaining new attachment. There are several major benefits associated with root conditioning.[8] The first is the removal of any remaining diseased tissue, bacterial infection, and endotoxins from the root surface.[9,10] Second, root conditioning products remove the smear layer from the root surface and expose more dentinal tubules.[11] ***The smear layer is a thin layer with small crystalline characteristics that appears on the surface of teeth that have undergone dental instrumentation and interferes with reattachment.*** Finally, they slightly demineralize the root surface and expose a collagen fiber matrix.[12] These properties have been shown to improve fibroblast reattachment in several in vitro studies.[13–15] One additional effect of chemical root conditioning is that the dentinal tubules become wider and more funnel shaped; however, it is not yet known whether this is a beneficial effect or not.[16,17]

Root conditioning has largely fallen out of favor on the human side due to inconsistent in vivo results.[18–23] However, it has shown positive results in the studies performed in dogs.[24–26] This is especially true in the case of citric acid conditioning in furcational defects.[27,28]

There are many products that have been or can be used for this step. Classically it has been performed with citric acid.[7,A] This product has shown to consistently achieve the biomodification goals listed above.[14,24,29] However, the operator must be careful not to allow this product to contact the gingival tissues, as it can have a necrotizing effect.[30]

Recently an EDTA solution has been promoted as the best product,[13] but most studies still support citric acid as the correct choice.[29,31,32]

Tetracycline has also been touted as a good choice for root conditioning, as it does remove the smear layer and expose dentinal tubules.[33,34] It is superior to the other medicants in its class (doxycycline, minocycline).[34,35] However, it has not been shown to consistently detoxify the root surface and is not as effective as citric acid or EDTA.[32,36]

(a) (b)

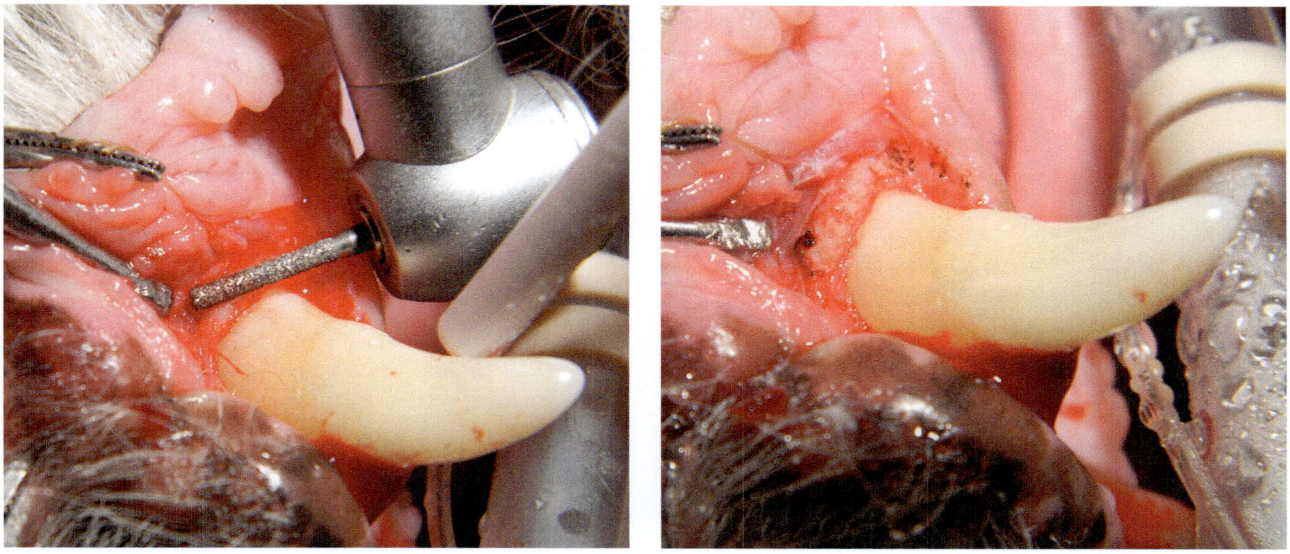

Figure 17.5 (a) Osteoplasty of the bony ledge with a coarse diamond bur on a water-cooled, high-speed hand-piece. (b) Resultant bony edges that are smooth and tapered coronally.

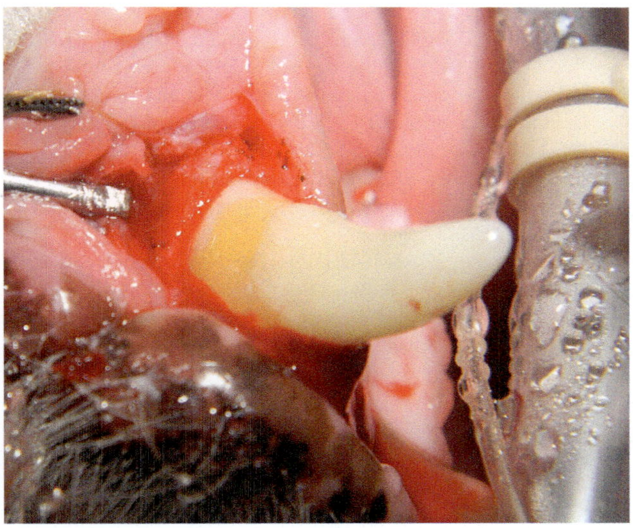

Figure 17.6 Application of the citric acid etchant to the tooth. A thin layer is placed, avoiding the soft tissues.

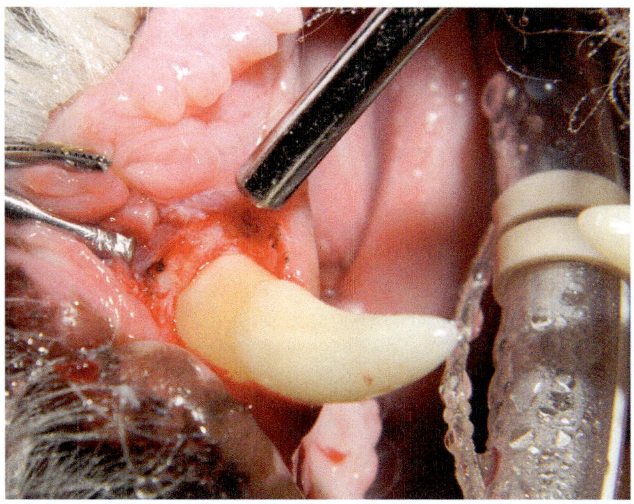

Figure 17.7 Thorough rinsing of the etch.

Based on the above, this author recommends citric acid biomodification of the root surface during periodontal flap procedures. This is especially true when performing guided tissue regeneration for furcational defects.

Root conditioning technique:[8] Following the manufacturer's recommendations, the selected product is carefully placed on the scaled and planed root surface with an applicator or cotton pledgets (Figure 17.6). It is important to avoid contact with the healthy periodontal tissues, especially if utilizing citric acid. The product is allowed to sit in contact with the root surface for the prescribed time. The ideal time appears to be 4 minutes for EDTA,[13] 2–3 minutes for tetracycline,[37] and 2–5 minutes for citric acid.[8] After the prescribed time, it is thoroughly rinsed from the root surface (Figure 17.7).

In the future, laser irradiation may prove to be a superior means of root conditioning. This may be expected because laser therapy reliably removes the smear layer, opens the dentinal tubules, and exposes collagen in a similar manner to citric acid. However, laser therapy does not affect the shape of (i.e., it does not widen) the tubules.[17,38] One in vitro study showed that

CO_2 laser irradiation for 1 second provided superior attachment to either EDTA, citric acid, or H_2O_2.[39] Further studies are needed to evaluate the clinical application of this technology.

Box 17.1 Key points

- Meticulous scaling and root planing is the most important part of any periodontal surgical procedure.
- Scaling is best performed using a combination of mechanical and hand instrumentation.
- Smoothing and shaping of the remaining alveolar bone (osteoplasty) improves healing.
- Root conditioning is an additional aid to maximize reattachment, especially in furcational defects.

Note

A. Citric-etch, Ellman International.

References

1. Hill RW, Ramfjord SP, et al. Four types of periodontal treatment compared over 2 years. J Periodontol. 52:655–662, 1981.
2. Shoukry M, Ali B, Naby MA, Soliman A. Repair of experimental plaque-induced periodontal disease in dogs. J Vet Dent. 24(3): 152–165, 2007.
3. Holmstrom SE, Frost P, Eisner ER. Periodontal therapy and surgery. In: Veterinary Dental Techniques. 2nd ed. Philadelphia: Saunders, 1998, pp. 167–213.
4. Pattison AM, Pattison GL. Scaling and root planning. In: Carranza's Clinical Periodontology. St. Louis: Saunders, 2006, pp. 749–797.
5. Easley J. Methods of determining alveolar osseous form. J Periodontol. 38:112, 1967.
6. Sims TN, Ammons W. Resective osseous surgery. In: Carranza's Clinical Periodontology. St. Louis: Saunders, 2006, pp. 950–967.
7. Wiggs RB, Lobprise HB. Periodontology. In: Veterinary Dentistry, Principles and Practice. Philadelphia: Lippincott-Raven, 1997, pp. 186–231.
8. Carranza FA, Takei HH, Cochran DL. Reconstructive periodontal surgery. In: Carranza's Clinical Periodontology. St. Louis: Saunders, 2006, pp. 968–990.
9. Daly CG. Anti-bacterial effect of citric acid treatment of periodontally diseased root surfaces in vitro. J Clin Periodontol. 9(5):386–392, 1982.
10. Fine DH, Morris ML, Tabak L, Cole JD. Preliminary characterization of material eluted from the roots of periodontally diseased teeth. J Periodontal Res. 15(1):10–19, 1980.
11. Babay N. Comparative SEM study on the effect of root conditioning with EDTA or tetracycline Hcl on periodontally involved root surfaces. Indian J Dent Res. 11(2):53–57, 2000.
12. Garrett JS, Crigger M, Egelberg J. Effects of citric acid on diseased root surfaces. J Periodontal Res. 13(2):155–163, 1978.
13. Gamal AY, Mailhot JM. The effects of EDTA gel conditioning exposure time on periodontitis-affected human root surfaces: Surface topography and PDL cell adhesion. Int Acad Periodontol. 5(1):11–22, 2003.
14. Chandra RV, Jagetia GC, Bhat KM. The attachment of V79 and human periodontal ligament fibroblasts on periodontally involved root surfaces following treatment with EDTA, citric acid, or tetracycline HCL: An SEM in vitro study. J Contemp Dent Pract. 7(1):44–59, 2006.
15. Zaman KU, Sugaya T, Hongo O, Kato H. A study of attached and oriented human periodontal ligament cells to periodontally diseased cementum and dentin after demineralizing with neutral and low pH etching solution. J Periodontol. 71(7):1094–1099, 2000.
16. Polson AM, Frederick GT, Ladenheim S, Hanes PJ. The production of a root surface smear layer by instrumentation and its removal by citric acid. J Periodontol. 55(8):443–446, 1984.
17. Ito K, Nishikata J, Murai S. Effects of Nd:YAG laser radiation on removal of a root surface smear layer after root planing: A scanning electron microscopic study. J Periodontol. 64(6): 547–552, 1993.
18. Mariotti A. Efficacy of chemical root surface modifiers in the treatment of periodontal disease. A systematic review. Ann Periodontol. 8(1):205–226, 2003.
19. Sculean A, Berakdar M, Willershausen B, Arweiler NB, Becker J, Schwarz F. Effect of EDTA root conditioning on the healing of intrabony defects treated with an enamel matrix protein derivative. J Periodontol. 77(7):1167–1172, 2006.
20. Parashis AO, Tsiklakis K, Tatakis DN. EDTA gel root conditioning: Lack of effect on clinical and radiographic outcomes of intrabony defect treatment with enamel matrix derivative. J Periodontol. 77(1):103–110, 2006.
21. Kersten BG, Chamberlain AD, Khorsandi S, Wikesjö UM, Selvig KA, Nilvéus RE. Healing of the intrabony periodontal lesion following root conditioning with citric acid and wound closure including an expanded PTFE membrane. J Periodontol. 63(11):876–882, 1992.
22. Kassab M, Cohen RE. The effect of root modification and biomodification on periodontal therapy. Compend Contin Educ Dent. 24(1):31–37, 2003.
23. Blomlöf L, Bergman E, Forsgardh A, Foss L, Larsson A, Sjöberg B, Uhlander L, Jonsson B, Blomlöf J, Lindskog S. A clinical study of root surface conditioning with an EDTA gel. I. Nonsurgical periodontal treatment. Int J Periodontics Restorative Dent. 20(6):560–565, 2000.
24. Register AA, Burdick FA. Accelerated reattachment with cementogenesis to dentin, demineralized in situ. J Periodontol. 47(9):497–505, 1975.
25. Register AA, Burdick FA. Accelerated reattachment with cementogenesis to dentin, demineralized in situ. I. Optimum range. J Periodontol. 646–655, 1975.
26. Caffesse RG, Holden MJ, Kon S, Nasjleti CE. The effect of citric acid and fibronectin application on healing following surgical treatment of naturally occurring periodontal disease in beagle dogs. J Clin Periodontol. 12(7):578–590, 1985.
27. Crigger M, Boyle G, Nilveus R, et al. The effect of topical citric acid application on the healing of experimental furcation defects in dogs. J Periodontal Res. 13(6):538–549, 1978.
28. Nilvéus R, Bogle G, Crigger M, Egelberg J, Selvig KA. The effect of topical citric acid application on the healing of experimental furcation defects in dogs. II. Healing after repeated surgery. J Periodontal Res. 15(5):544–550, 1980.
29. Ruggeri A Jr, Prati C, Mazzoni A, Nucci C, Di Lenarda R, Mazzotti G, Breschi L. Effects of citric acid and EDTA conditioning on exposed root dentin: An immunohistochemical analysis of collagen and proteoglycans. Arch Oral Biol. 52(1):1–8, 2007.

30. Blomlöf JP, Blomlöf LB, Lindskog SF. Smear removal and collagen exposure after non-surgical root planing followed by etching with an EDTA gel preparation. J Periodontol. 67(9):841–845, 1996.
31. Pant V, Dixit J, Agrawal AK, Seth PK, Pant AB. Behavior of human periodontal ligament cells on CO2 laser irradiated dentinal root surfaces: An in vitro study. J Periodontal Res. 39(6):373–379, 2004.
32. Balos K, Bal B, Eren K. The effects of various agents on root surfaces (a scanning electron microscopy study). Newsl Int Acad Periodontol. 1(2):13–16, 1991.
33. Lafferty TA, Gher ME, Gray JL. Comparative SEM study on the effect of acid etching with tetracycline HCl or citric acid on instrumented periodontally-involved human root surfaces. J Periodontol. 64(8):689–693, 1993.
34. Shetty B, Dinesh A, Seshan H. Comparative effects of tetracyclines and citric acid on dentin root surface of periodontally involved human teeth: A scanning electron microscope study. J Indian Soc Periodontol. 12(1):8–15, 2008.
35. Madison JG 3rd, Hokett SD. The effects of different tetracyclines on the dentin root surface of instrumented, periodontally involved human teeth: A comparative scanning electron microscope study. J Periodontol. 68(8):739–745, 1997.
36. Chandra RV, Jagetia GC, Bhat KM. The attachment of V79 and human periodontal ligament fibroblasts on periodontally involved root surfaces following treatment with EDTA, citric acid, or tetracycline HCL: An SEM in vitro study. J Contemp Dent Pract. 7(1):44–59, 2006.
37. Ishi EP, Dantas AA, Batista LH, Onofre MA, Sampaio JE. Smear layer removal and collagen fiber exposure using tetracycline hydrochloride conditioning. J Contemp Dent Pract. 9(5): 25–33, 2008.
38. Misra V, Mehrotra KK, Dixit J, Maitra SC. Effect of a carbon dioxide laser on periodontally involved root surfaces. J Periodontol. 70(9):1046–1052, 1999.
39. Pant V, Dixit J, Agrawal AK, Seth PK, Pant AB. Behavior of human periodontal ligament cells on CO2 laser irradiated dentinal root surfaces: An in vitro study. J Periodontal Res. 39(6): 373–379, 2004.

18

Osseous surgery and guided tissue regeneration

Brook A. Niemiec and Robert Furman

Introduction

Osseous surgeries are the procedures by which the alveolar bone is managed following periodontal flap creation. In other words, these are procedures that remove, reshape, or repair defects in the alveolar bone caused by periodontal disease. Gingival tissues respond best to bone with proper architecture, and thus recreating this form allows for optimized pocket management.[1] Furthermore, irregular bone architecture may result in periodontal pocket recurrence.[2] Osseous surgery can be broken down into two basic types, regenerative and resective. Resective (subtractive) surgery is the selective removal of alveolar bone to recreate normal architecture.[1] Regenerative (additive) osseous surgery (guided tissue regeneration) is intended to recreate the periodontal tissues and regain attachment. This type of procedure should be used whenever possible. Resective surgery should be used sparingly, as maintenance of alveolar bone is ideal. This chapter will cover both types of osseous surgery, including the indications and contraindications, rationale, necessary equipment and materials, techniques, and follow-up. In addition, normal bone architecture and periodontal defects will be discussed as a means of determining proper therapy.

Alveolar bone architecture

Across species lines (dog, cat, and human) for healthy alveolar bone,[2] the interproximal areas should be more coronal in relation to the facial/lingual/palatal surfaces. In addition, the tooth form affects the interdental form in that the more tapered the tooth, the more pyramidal the interdental space will be. Finally, the more distal the tooth, the more flat the transition between the buccal or lingual/palatal and interdental will be (Figure 18.1 a). Conversely, the mesial teeth (canines and incisors) will have more defined scalloping (Figure 18.1 b).

Ideal osseous form is as described above, where the bone is of a similar height across the arcade and the interdental bone is consistently higher than the facial/lingual surfaces with gentle transitions between the two (Figure 18.1 c).

Positive osseous form is similar to the ideal form, where the interdental bone is coronal to the radicular bone. In this type, however, the overall height may not be equal and the transitions not ideally smooth (Figure 18.1 d).

Negative osseous form is where the interdental bone is apical when compared to the facial or palatal-lingual bone (Figure 18.1e).

Flat osseous form is where the height is similar across the arcade (Figure 18.1 f).

Patterns of bone loss

Alveolar bone loss[3–6] is broken down into two broad categories, horizontal and vertical (or angular). *Horizontal bone loss* is diagnosed when the loss of bone is at approximately the same level across the arcade (or a section of it) (Figure 18.2 a). *Vertical (angular)* bone loss is where the loss of bone in one area and the surrounding bone is more coronal (Figure 18.2 b). In reality however, these two types rarely occur separately; bone loss is typically a combination of these two patterns in varying degrees (Figure 18.2 c).

Alveolar bone loss is further defined in regards to the number of bony walls surrounding the defect. True horizontal bone loss is known as a zero-walled pocket, where all the bone is at the same height. A one (1) walled pocket exists where there is no interdental

Veterinary Periodontology, First Edition. Brook A. Niemiec.

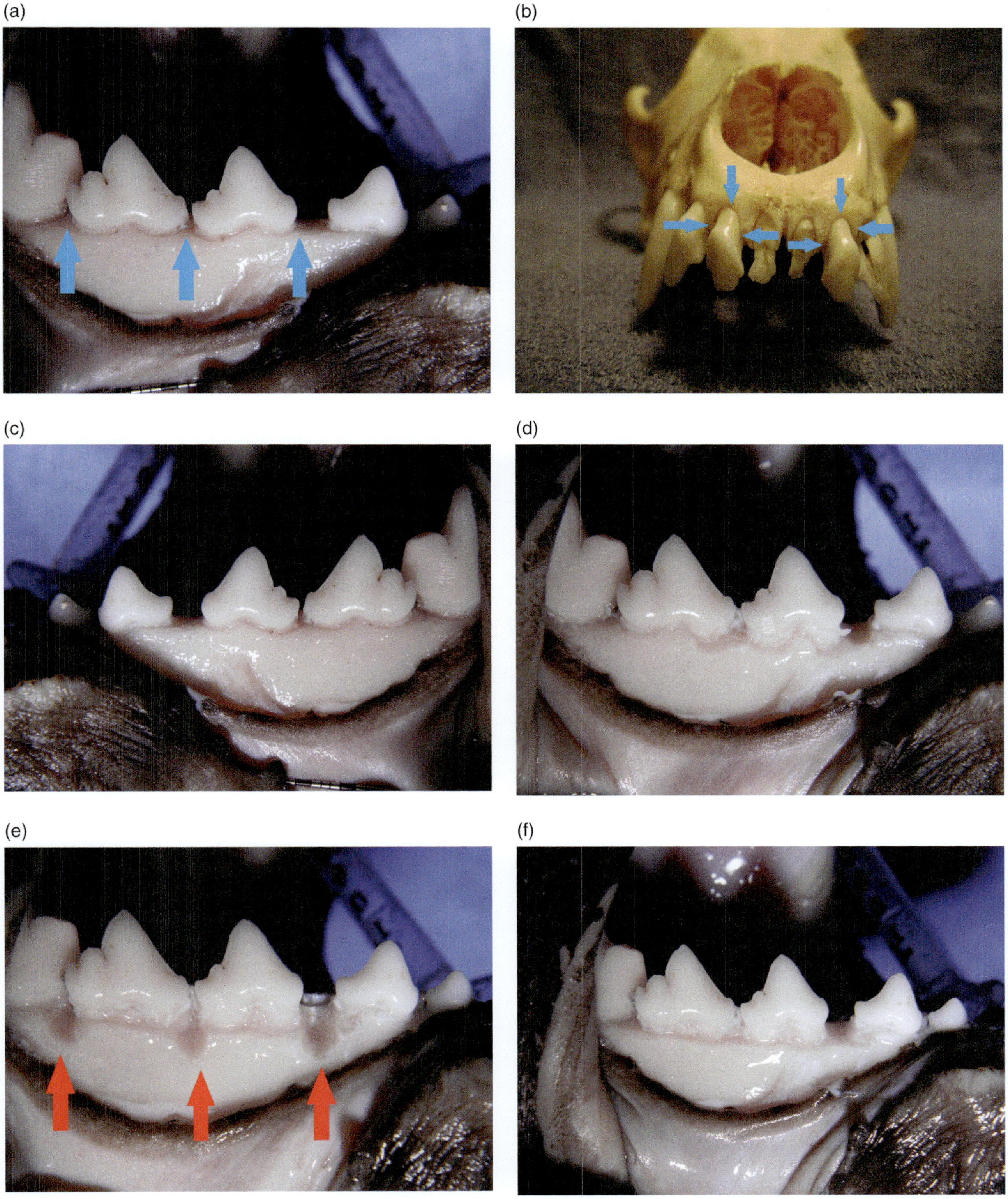

Figure 18.1 Alveolar bone architecture. (a) Distal teeth (premolars): Flat transition between buccal or lingual/palatal and interdental areas (blue arrows). (b) Mesial teeth (incisors): More defined scalloping (blue arrows). (c) Ideal osseous form: Bone is of a similar height across the arcade and the interdental bone is consistently higher than the facial/lingual surfaces with gentle transitions. (d) Positive osseous form: Interdental bone is coronal to the radicular bone, but overall height may not be equal and the transitions not smooth. (e) Negative osseous form: The interdental bone is apical when compared to the facial or palatal-lingual bone (red arrows). (f) Flat osseous form.

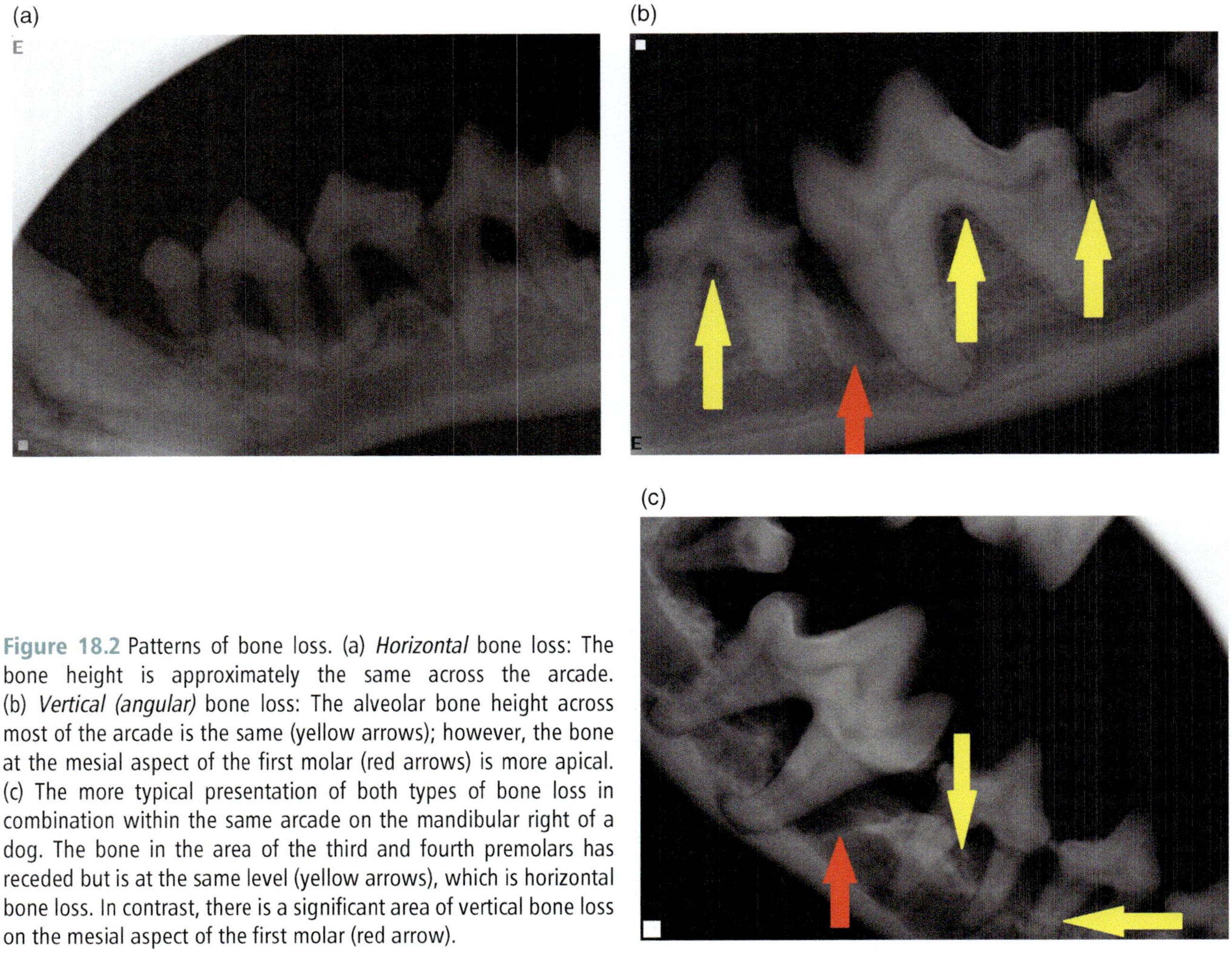

Figure 18.2 Patterns of bone loss. (a) *Horizontal* bone loss: The bone height is approximately the same across the arcade. (b) *Vertical (angular)* bone loss: The alveolar bone height across most of the arcade is the same (yellow arrows); however, the bone at the mesial aspect of the first molar (red arrows) is more apical. (c) The more typical presentation of both types of bone loss in combination within the same arcade on the mandibular right of a dog. The bone in the area of the third and fourth premolars has receded but is at the same level (yellow arrows), which is horizontal bone loss. In contrast, there is a significant area of vertical bone loss on the mesial aspect of the first molar (red arrow).

bone between two teeth and one of the facial/lingual-palatal bone plates is also lost. Two (2) walled pockets most commonly appear as "crater" defects in the interdental space, where the facial/lingual-palatal walls are present, but the interproximal area is more apical. This is the most common infrabony pocket in veterinary[7] and human[1] patients. These pockets can also exist where there is interproximal bone, but nothing interdental, and one of the facial/lingual-palatal walls is also missing. Three (3) walled pockets are seen where there is bone interdentally and both the palatal-lingual and facial walls are present. In addition, this type of pocket can exist on the radicular surface of the teeth, with no interproximal involvement. In veterinary patients, 3-walled pockets are most commonly diagnosed on the palatine surface of the maxillary canines (Figure 18.3). This defect is especially prevalent in chondrodystrophic patients (i.e., Dachshunds and Basset Hounds) and is the precursor of oronasal fistulas.[8,9] Four (4) walled pockets are defects in the bone not directly associated with a root surface. In this way, they do not directly impact the periodontium and are therefore not truly periodontal lesions, rather are generally the result of trauma or foreign bodies. (See chapter 9 for a further discussion of patterns of bone loss.)

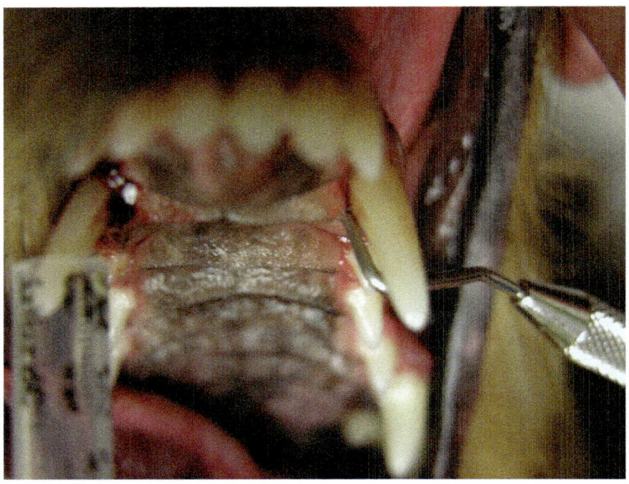

Figure 18.3 Intraoral picture of the left maxillary canine (204) in a dog with a deep 3-walled pocket on the palatal aspect.

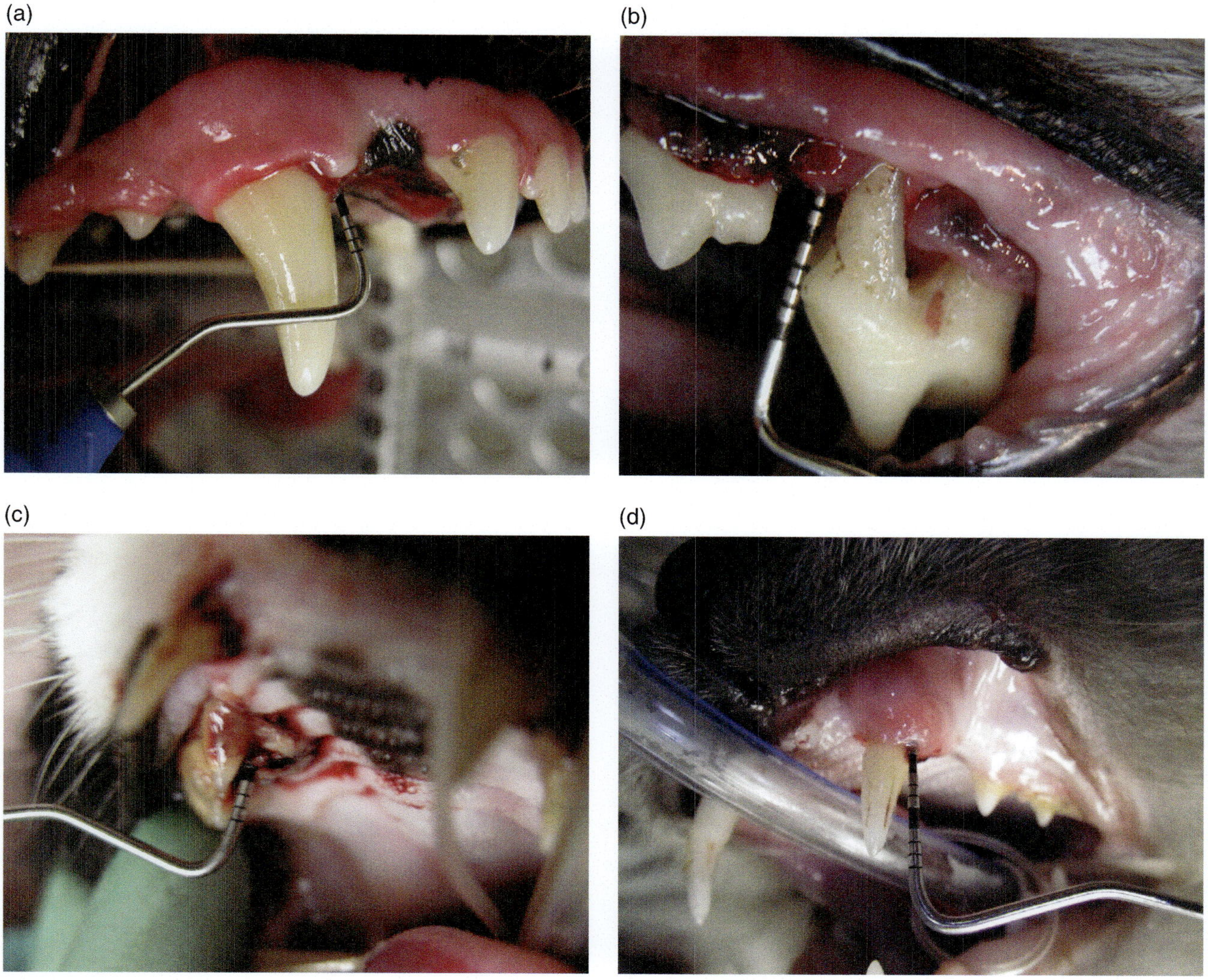

Figure 18.4 Periodontal probing. The tooth to be treated must be evaluated circumferentially to determine the attachment levels around the entire tooth. Intraoral dental pictures of the periodontal probe in action: (a) Right maxillary canine (104) in a dog with a 9 mm periodontal pocket on the mesio-palatal aspect. Note how healthy the gingiva appears. (b) Left maxillary fourth premolar (208) in a dog with a 6 mm periodontal pocket and 5 mm of gingival recession on the mesio-buccal aspect. This equals 11 mm of attachment loss. (c) Right maxillary fourth premolar (108) in a cat with a 10+ mm periodontal pocket on the palatal aspect. This has resulted in an oroantral fistula. (d) Left maxillary canine (204) in a cat with a 5 mm periodontal pocket on the buccal aspect.

Preoperative diagnostics

It is critically important to determine if a patient is a candidate for osseous surgery (and if so, what type) *prior* to commencing the periodontal flap procedure.[1] This is important because the type of osseous surgery (if any) will determine the proper flap design. This is challenging because the flap must be created "blind," meaning that the type of osseous surgery must be determined before the bone can be directly examined. The recommended types of flaps for the different surgeries will be delineated below, and detailed instructions for their performance listed in chapter 16.

There are three main diagnostic methods for evaluating the status of the alveolar bone prior to creating the initial incision. These methods are periodontal probing, transgingival probing (or *sounding*), and dental radiology.

Periodontal probing (Figure 18.4) is the cornerstone of periodontal diagnostics.[10,11] It is utilized to determine pocket depth, the location of the apical extent of the pocket in relation to the mucogingival junction (MGJ), as well as the presence and degree of furcation exposure (Figure 18.5). In addition, it can give a preliminary idea of the number of remaining walls.

Sounding is performed by utilizing the periodontal probe not in the sulcus/pocket, but on the surrounding tissues (Figure 18.6). By pressing on the tissues, the operator can get a sense as to the extent and configuration of the intrabony component of the pocket and furcational defects.[2,12] This can be critical information for the surgeon.

Dental radiographs should be made of all areas prior to surgery.[1] Radiographs are a critical piece of the diagnostic

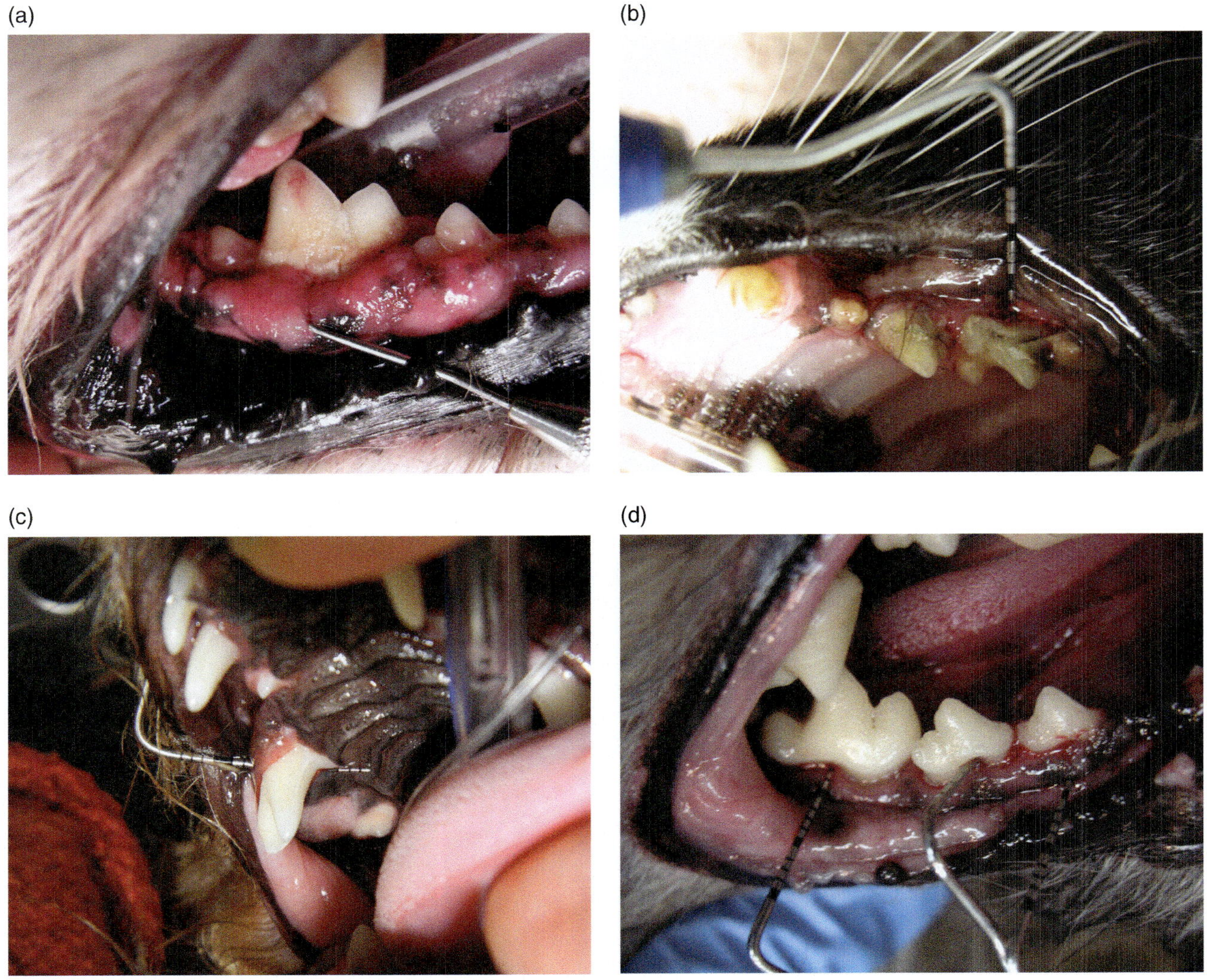

Figure 18.5 Furcational involvement. (a) Class III furcation involvement on the mandibular right first molar (409) in a dog. Note that there is no recession (and in fact there is enlargement) in the area. This issue would not have been found without the use of a periodontal probe. (b) Class II furcational involvement on the buccal aspect of the left maxillary fourth premolar (208) of a cat. (c) Class III furcation involvement on the right maxillary fourth premolar (108) in a dog. Note there is no recession and minimal inflammation in the area. This issue would not have been found without the use of a periodontal probe. (d) Class II furcational involvement on the buccal aspect of the right mandibular third and fourth premolars and first molar (407, 408, 409) of a dog.

puzzle but should not be relied on as the sole diagnostic tool. Properly made radiographs can help determine the amount of interproximal bone loss and presence of vertical (angular) bone loss (Figure 18.7), as well as root length and morphology. Additionally, they can elucidate root or other pathology that must be evaluated and/or treated as part of the periodontal surgery (Figure 18.8). Finally, radiographs can be used to monitor the success or failure of the therapy. It is important to note, however, that dental radiographs cannot provide an accurate image of the pocket, as they are a two-dimensional image of a three-dimensional area. In addition, they do not diagnosis periodontitis, nor document the number of remaining bony walls or the extent of bony deficits. Finally, due to the significant radiodensity and summation of the roots, they cannot be relied upon to accurately evaluate the facial or lingual/palatal bone or furcational loss between mesial roots (e.g., MB and MP roots of the maxillary P4) (Figures 18.9 through 18.14).

In summary, all three of these diagnostic modalities have certain strengths and weaknesses. Therefore, the practitioner is encouraged to learn the subtleties of each one and employ all of them to perform treatment planning. Finally, cone beam CT may provide superior imaging of this complicated space in the future.

Treatment planning and case selection

Treatment planning should encompass solutions for all active periodontal disease sites as well as correction of

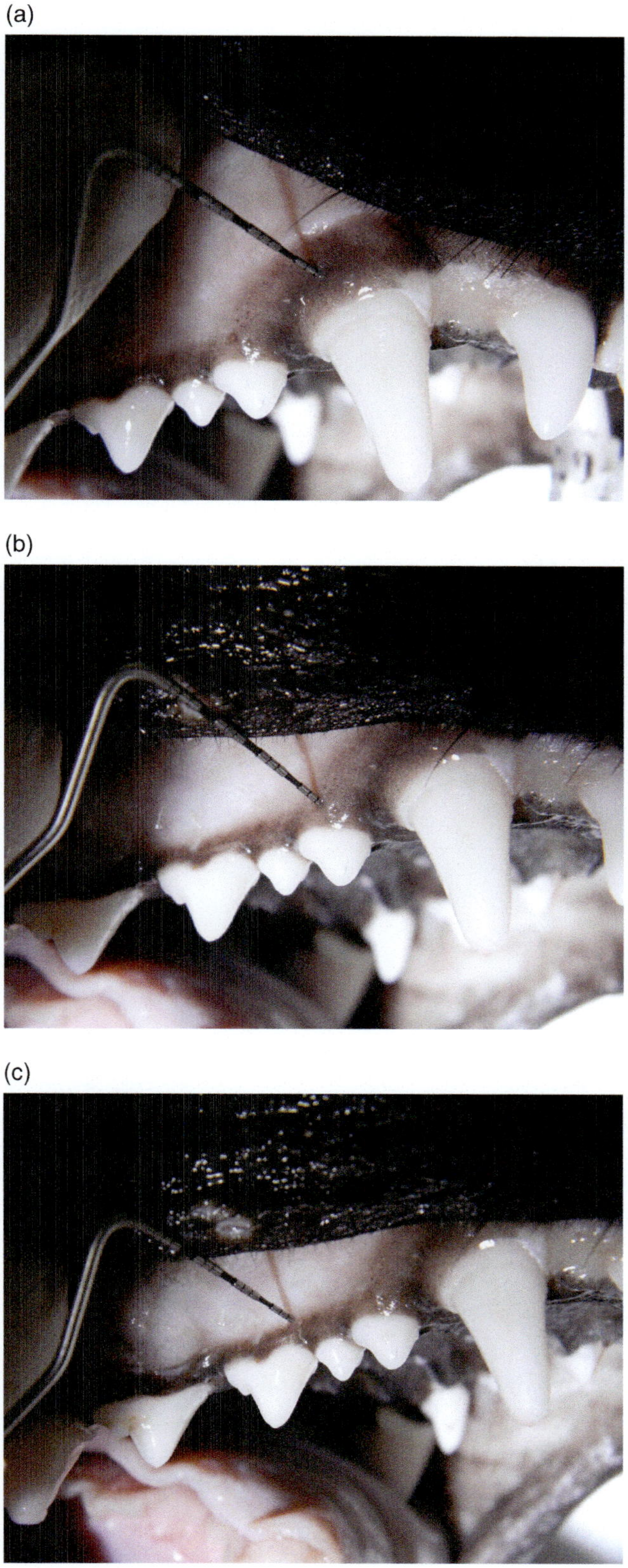

Figure 18.6 (a–c) Sounding the maxillary right of a dog.

bony deficits that may negatively affect the healing process or future plaque control.[1] In addition, the procedure should allow for treatment of any other problems in the area, such as root caries.

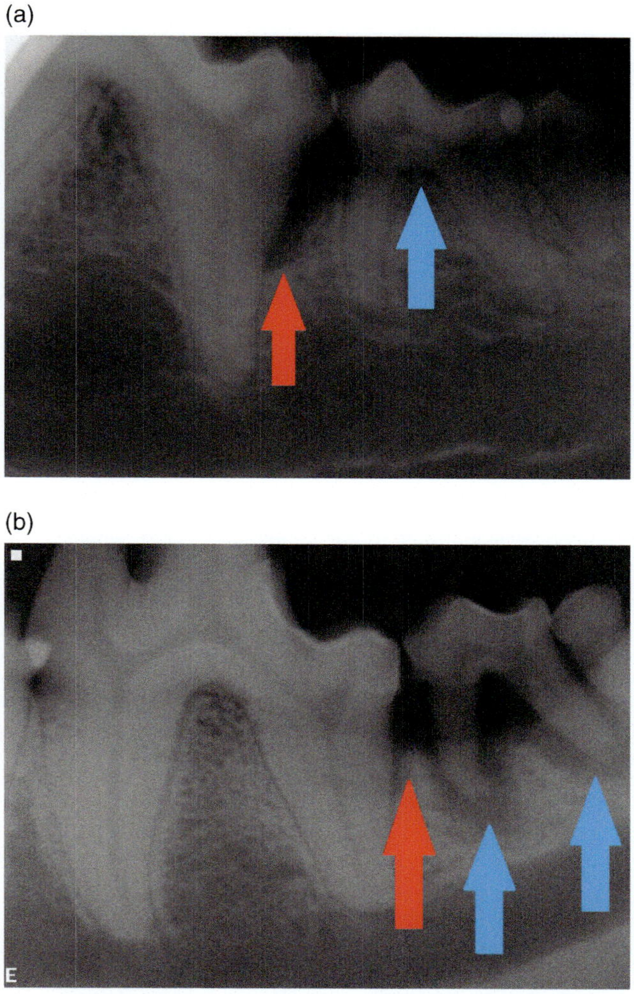

Figure 18.7 Intraoral dental radiographs of the mandibular left in two different canine patients. The physical exam (probing) of these two would be very similar; however, treatment would be different. (a) Deep periodontal pocket with significant vertical alveolar bone loss on the distal aspect of the first molar (309) (red arrow). However, the second molar is essentially normal (blue arrow). This is an excellent area for GTR. (b) The amount of bone loss is similar in the area between 309 and 310 (red arrow). However, the second molar is significantly involved and has a class II perio-endo lesion (blue arrows). This tooth must be extracted. (See chapter 6 for a discussion of perio-endo lesions.)

As previously stated, it is ideal to perform standard periodontal therapy, including closed root planing, prior to initiating periodontal surgery.[10] There are two main reasons for this. First, standard periodontal therapy may be sufficient to return pockets to healthy sulcal depth, thus negating the need for invasive surgery (Figure 18.15). In addition, it will decrease the inflammation, resulting in healthier tissue for surgery (i.e., minimized hemmorhage and improved visualization). Finally, without a client commitment to regular homecare, periodontal surgery is often doomed to failure, and therefore more definitive therapy (i.e., extraction) is

(a) (b)

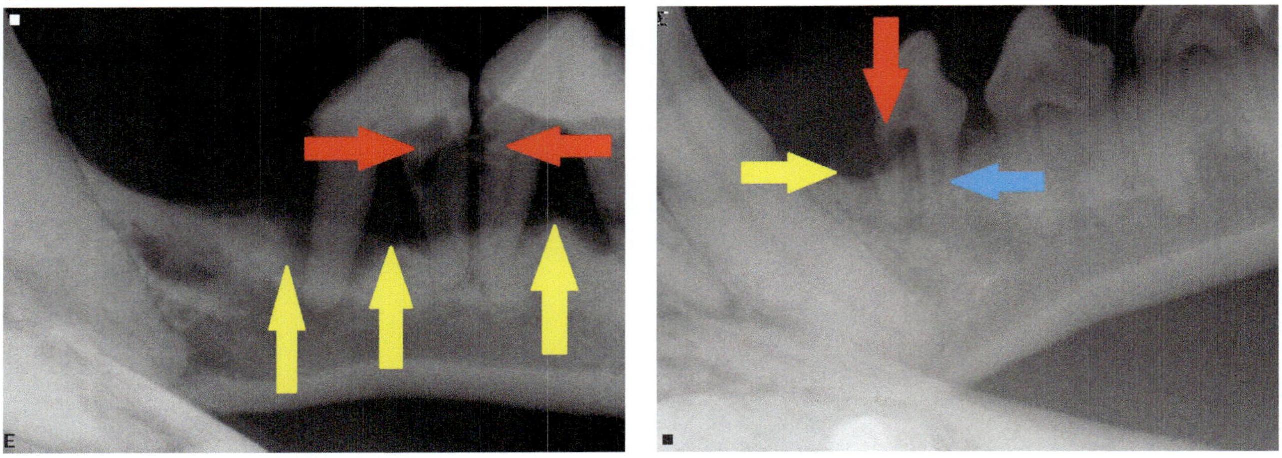

Figure 18.8 Intraoral dental radiographs of canine patient with significant periodontal disease as well as other conditions. Periodontal surgery, while indicated for the periodontal aspect, would be contraindicated due to the other pathology. Extraction is the only realistic option for these teeth. Obtaining this information *prior* to initiating surgery is critical. (a) Left mandibular second and third premolars (306, 307) in a dog with significant alveolar bone loss secondary to periodontal disease (yellow arrows) as well as tooth resorption (red arrows). (b) Left mandibular second premolar (307) in a dog with alveolar bone loss secondary to periodontal disease (yellow arrow) as well as a mesial root fracture (red arrow). This has resulted in its non-vitality, as evidenced by the larger endodontic space (blue arrow).

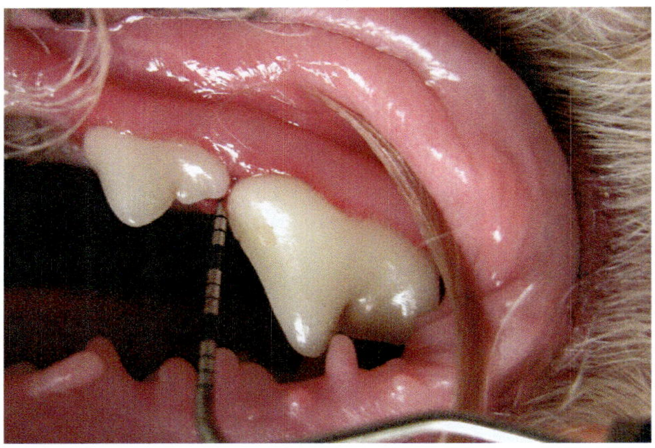

Figure 18.9 Intraoral dental picture of the left maxillary fourth premolar (208) of a dog with significant *focal* alveolar bone loss and secondary furcation level II exposure.

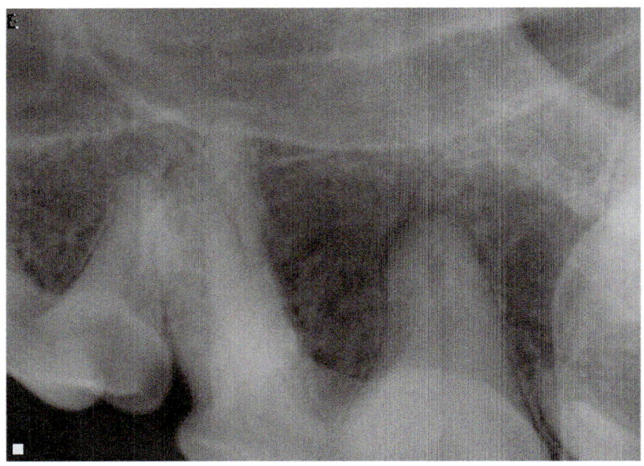

Figure 18.10 Corresponding dental radiograph that does not reveal any bone loss in the area. This is due to the superimposition of the mesio-buccal and mesio-palatine roots. The summation of these roots makes the furcation area exceedingly difficult to evaluate with dental radiographs.

typically recommended. However, this approach is controversial in veterinary patents due to the need for a second anesthesia.

The decision regarding what type of osseous surgery to perform (if any) is directed by the bony presentation. Factors included in this determination are the amount/degree of bone loss and number of walls remaining. Regenerative techniques are the ideal form of therapy and should always be attempted if a decent prognosis is present and the patient is a good candidate for future anesthesia for reevaluation.[13] Finally, patients with hypothyroidism or diabetes (especially if poorly controlled) are less than ideal candidates for periodontal surgery.

The combination of resective surgery and an apically repositioned flap is the most reliable method of pocket depth reduction.[14,15] However, this does sacrifice alveolar bone and is only indicated/recommended in shallow pockets (2–3 mm). In contrast, deep pockets that require extensive bone removal will likely result in an unacceptable amount of remaining bone. Therefore, regenerative techniques should be utilized wherever possible (see below), or the tooth should be extracted.

Prognosis for therapy

Three- and 4-walled pockets have a good to excellent prognosis[1,11,16] for regenerative surgery and this should be performed if at all feasible. Two-walled pockets

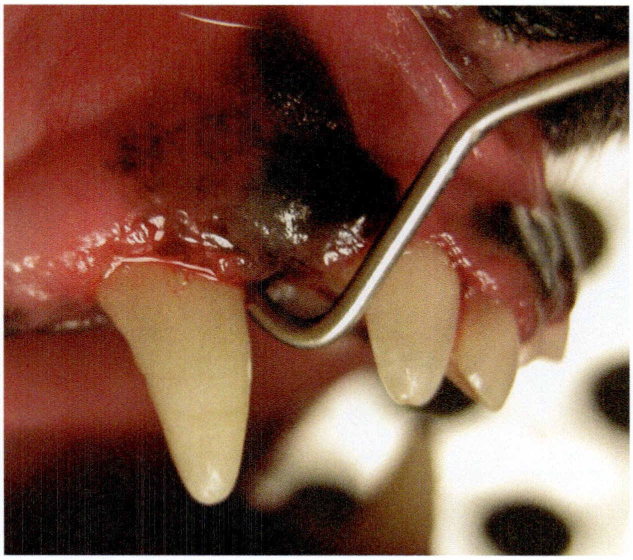

Figure 18.11 Intraoral dental picture of the right maxillary canine (104) of a dog with significant *focal* alveolar bone loss on the palatal aspect.

(a)

(b)

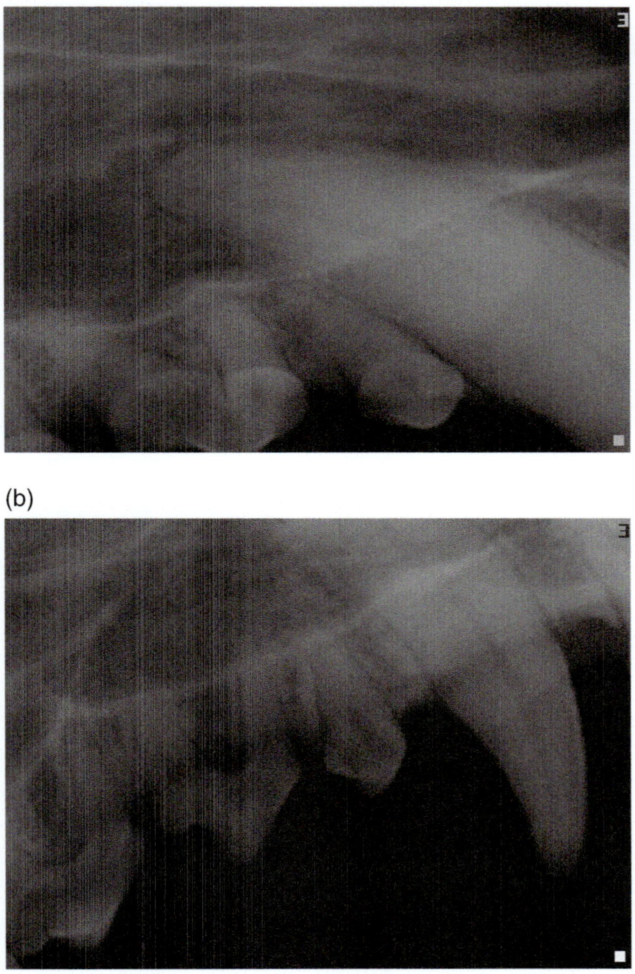

Figure 18.12 Corresponding dental radiographs of (a) the root and (b) the cervical area that do not reveal any bone loss in the area. This is due to the large root that overshadows the narrow area of loss.

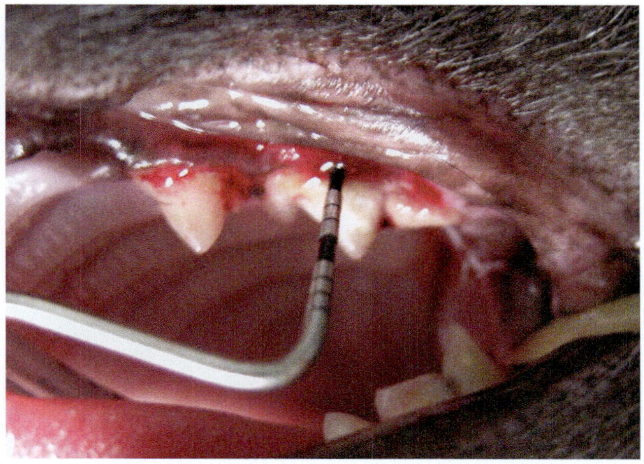

Figure 18.13 Intraoral dental picture of the left maxillary fourth premolar (208) of a cat with significant *focal* alveolar bone loss.

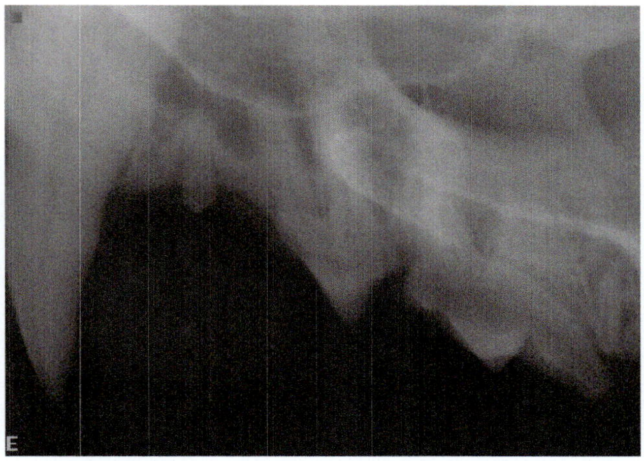

Figure 18.14 Corresponding dental radiograph that does not reveal any bone loss in the area. The area of bone loss is not seen on this view due to its small size and the zygomatic arch interference.

have a guarded to good prognosis for regenerative surgery, depending on presentation. "Crater" defects, which have both outer walls of bone with the interproximal bone missing, have a fairly good prognosis for regenerative surgery, and this should be attempted prior to considering resective techniques. Two-walled defects with one of the facial/lingual plates missing have a slightly worse prognosis, and resective techniques may be indicated depending on pocket depth. Regenerative therapy can be attempted on these 2-walled teeth, as long as the client is informed of the prognosis. One-walled pockets have a very poor prognosis for regenerative surgery, and therefore resective osseous surgery or extraction should be considered. Finally, zero-walled pockets do not require osseous surgery, other than possibly mild smoothing to achieve a proper architecture. (See chapter 9 for a complete discussion of walls.)

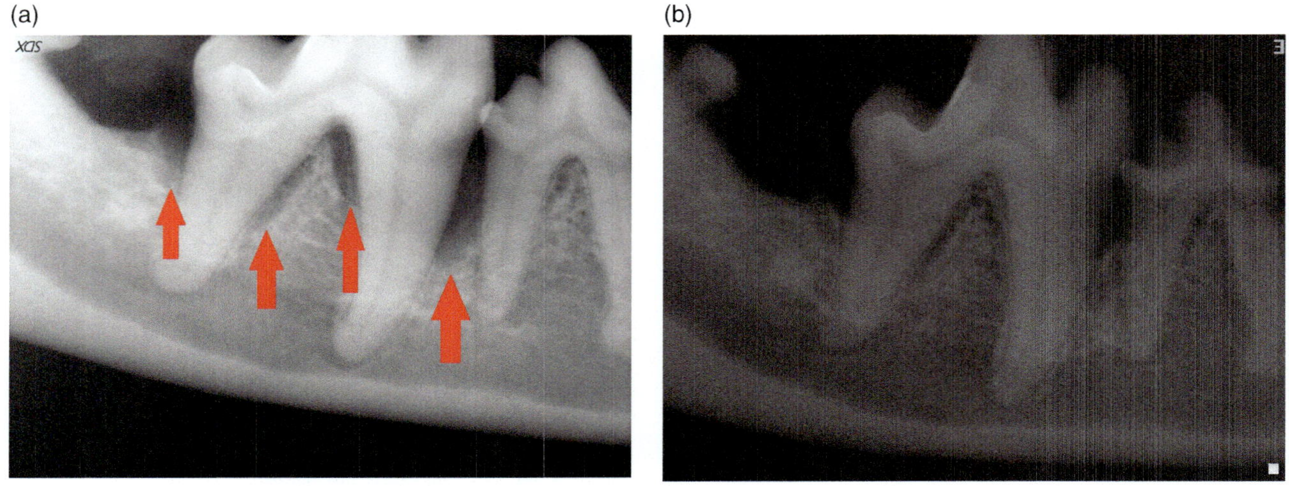

Figure 18.15 Response to conservative therapy. (a) Preoperative intraoral dental radiograph from a well-trained general practitioner. Note the significant alveolar bone loss (red arrows). The patient was treated with closed root planing and perioceutic and referred for periodontal surgery. (b) Recheck at a referral facility 6 weeks later. Note the significant amount of bone regeneration without advanced therapy.

Resective osseous surgery

Resective osseous surgery is best employed in areas of 1- to 2-walled pockets with mild bone loss (2–3 mm) and sufficient root length.[1] Patients with severe bone loss or 3- to 4-walled pockets should not be treated in this manner. Rather, teeth with 3- and 4-walled pockets should be treated with regenerative techniques, and those with severe bone loss (> 50%) should be extracted.

The goal of resective surgery is to create a steady and regular bone profile so that the soft tissues can predictably attach to the underlying bone in proper dimensions. The quality of the periodontal soft tissues that reattach following surgery depends on factors such as the bony architecture surrounding the tooth and the condition of the root surface, as well as the health of the periodontal tissues.[1] Ensuring the optimum condition of all these areas will allow for the best result. This being said, resective osseous surgery is an exceedingly precise technique.

Instrumentation

There are numerous options of instruments for this procedure. They can be broken down into two broad categories, rotary and hand. Some clinicians use only hand instruments, whereas some use a combination of both. Rotary instruments are suited for osteoplastic procedures. However, hand instruments are preferred for the delicate ostectomies. It is recommended that the surgeon have a good selection of both hand and rotary instrumentation. Regardless of the instrument chosen, extreme care is required to avoid root damage or excessive bone removal, as these are irreversible. Hand instruments include rongeurs, interproximal files, and chisels. Rotary instruments should include a good selection of carbide and diamond burs (see chapters 22 and 24 for details).

Technique

The first step in resective osseous surgery is the proper creation of an apical repositioning flap (see chapter 16). Following the flap creation and soft tissue removal, numerous presentations may be encountered such as ledges, craters, vertical defects, troughs, or combinations of these. The clinician must be prepared to handle any of these presentations correctly and potentially have his or her presurgical opinion changed, regardless of the amount of preoperative examination.

The following sequential steps are recommended for resective osseous surgery.[1] It should be noted that not all of these steps are necessary in every case, but by following the order listed below, the clinician can speed the procedure and avoid excessive bone removal. The first two steps are totally osteoplastic, inasmuch as they do NOT remove supporting bone. In contrast, ostectomy procedures (steps 3 and 4) remove alveolar bone that directly supports the tooth.

1. Perform vertical grooving (Figure 18.16).
   This is done to reduce the interproximal alveolar bone while providing relative prominence to the radicular areas. It is performed as the first step because it defines the general thickness of the bone as well as creates the shape of the alveolar housing. This step should be performed only where there is a very thick area of bone (i.e., areas with thin labial or buccal plates of bone should not be treated in this manner). Vertical grooving may be performed with rotary instruments such as carbide or diamond burs

(a)

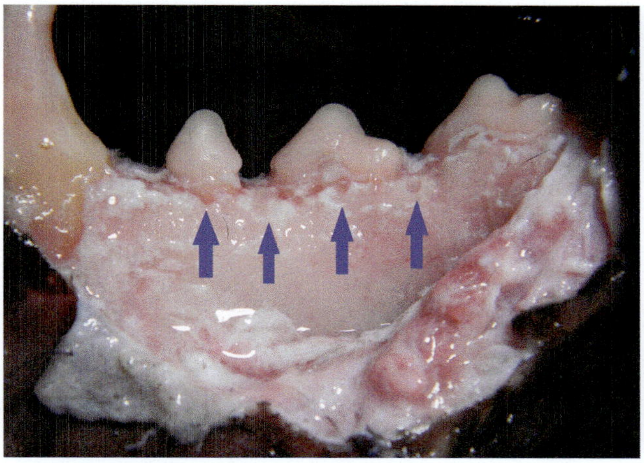

(b)

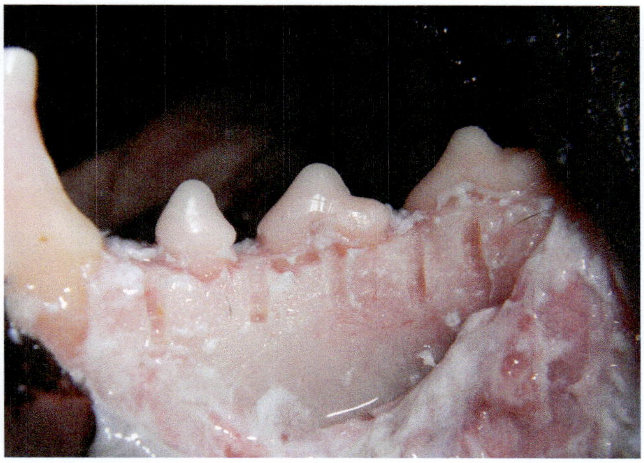

Figure 18.16 (a) Intraoperative dental picture of a patient with mild alveolar bone loss. A periodontal flap has been created for visualization. Note the jagged areas of bone (blue arrows), which will hinder healing and not allow for optimum dental health. (b) Vertical grooving.

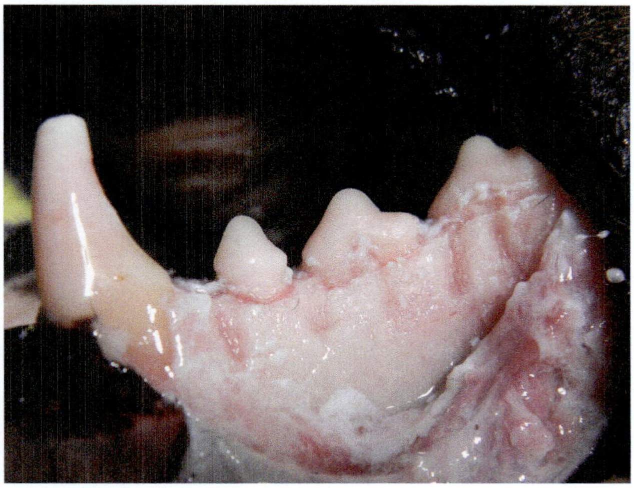

Figure 18.17 Radicular blending.

2. Radicular blending (Figure 18.17).
   This step is designed to create a gradual progression of the bony architecture from over the roots to the interdental areas. The goal is a smooth, gradual surface for superior flap adaptation. Again, this is only indicated for very thick labial plates of bone.
   The two steps listed above make up the vast majority of the osseous resective surgery procedure. In fact, thick osseous ledges, bony exostoses (Figure 18.18), class I and II furcations, and shallow craters can all be treated with these steps alone. The steps listed below are true ostectomy procedures and thus remove tooth-supporting bone. In other words, the instruments will come very close to the underlying roots. Damage to the root is a significant issue, and therefore it is recommended that these steps be performed with hand instruments such as files, curettes, and chisels.
3. Flatten the interproximal bone.
   This is the first step in which supporting bone is actively removed. It is generally indicated in situations where there is an incongruity of the interproximal bone on a facio-linguo aspect. This is most common in area of 1-walled interproximal pockets (hemiseptal). In this situation, it is performed to avoid increased pocket depths on the side where the bone is most apical.
   In addition, it is possible for this step to be used where there is a 1-walled pocket over a 3-walled pocket, in order to improve bony architecture. It is critical to note that this should only be performed in *shallow* defects, as significant discrepancies would entail removal of a significant amount of bone, thus excessively decreasing bony support. In these situations, less than ideal bony architecture is an acceptable alternative.
4. Gradualize the marginal bone.
   This step is also an ostectomy procedure, and therefore should be performed precisely to ensure the minimal amount of bone sacrifice. This small amount of bone reduction is necessary to provide a healthy, smooth surface for gingival attachment. Even small bony discrepancies on the gingival line angles (widow's peaks) will cause the gingival tissue to remain at higher levels than the bone can support in the interdental area. This results in incomplete pocket reduction. The removal of these small bony protuberances should be performed along with gradualization and blending of the radicular bone surface (Figure 18.19).

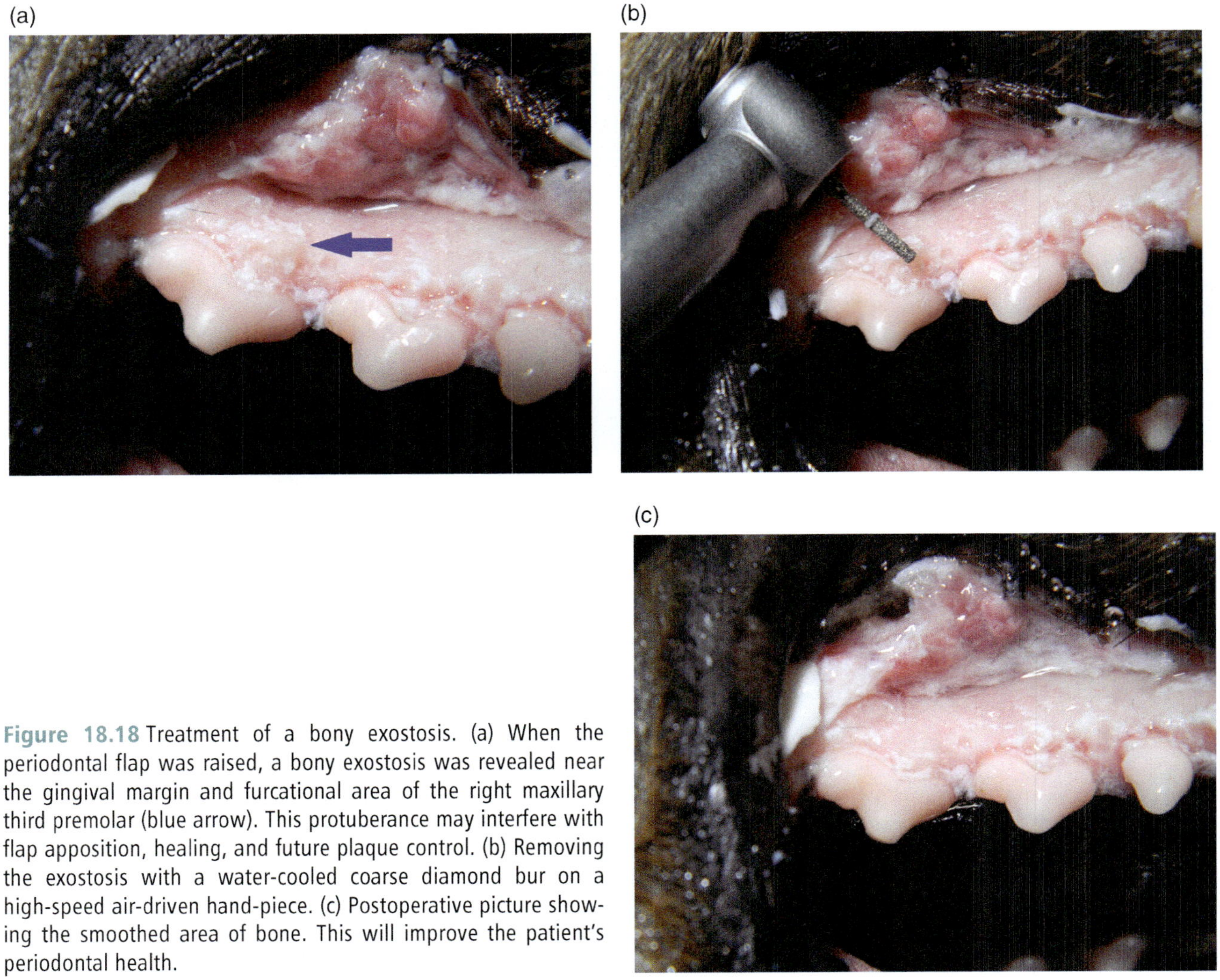

Figure 18.18 Treatment of a bony exostosis. (a) When the periodontal flap was raised, a bony exostosis was revealed near the gingival margin and furcational area of the right maxillary third premolar (blue arrow). This protuberance may interfere with flap apposition, healing, and future plaque control. (b) Removing the exostosis with a water-cooled coarse diamond bur on a high-speed air-driven hand-piece. (c) Postoperative picture showing the smoothed area of bone. This will improve the patient's periodontal health.

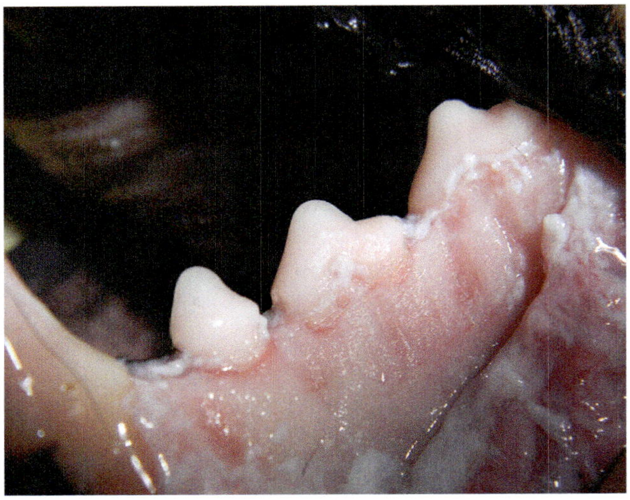

Figure 18.19 Postoperative picture of the patient in Figures 18.16 and 18.17 after flattening the interproximal bone and gradualizing the marginal bone. Note the fine margins and smooth transitions, which will optimize healing and long-term periodontal health.

Specific situations for osseous remodelling

Correction of 1-walled interproximal defects (hemiseptal) requires that all bone be reduced to the level of the most apical defect. If this is next to an edentulous area or a wide diastema, the bone in that area should be gradually lowered to the height of the defect.

Bony exostoses or ledges of bone (see Figure 18.18) are removed prior to any further osseous surgery. However, it is ideal to perform a degree of vertical grooving at the same time. In the absence of these ledges, the resection begins with the reduction of the interdental walls and the 1-walled component of angular defects, as well as moats and grooving into areas of early involvement.[14]

If the defect is a 2-walled crater and resection is elected over regenerative techniques, the surgical result may sacrifice the lingual, buccal, or both walls. The amount of bone removed should be the minimum to allow for:

1. Blending of the contours of the adjacent teeth.
2. Creating a satisfactory osseous form.
3. While preventing iatrogenic involvement of the furcations.

Ramping the bone to the palatal/lingual aspect via selective reduction to avoid the furcations has been recommended by several authors.[17,18]

Following the osseous surgery, the flap is replaced and sutured. Depending on the postoperative bone height, this can be either done at the original level or apically replaced.

Regenerative periodontal surgery

Creating new attachment via regeneration of the periodontal tissues is the ideal outcome of periodontal therapy, as it results in the reduction of the pocket as well as the recreation of normal periodontal attachment (alveolar bone, gingival connective tissue, cellular and acellular cementum, and a functionally oriented PDL).[19–21] Thus, the infection is treated and the pocket reduced without sacrificing attachment (as in resective techniques above). However, this is severely hampered by two critical factors.[22] First, periodontal regeneration requires the formation of at least three unique tissues. Second, the periodontium possesses a very limited endogenous regenerative ability. Consequently, true regenerative success is not consistent nor reliable with current techniques and materials.[20,21,23]

Healing may or may not occur with any of the techniques listed in this chapter. In fact, it is known that use of bone replacements or synthetic fillers will never achieve true periodontal regeneration.[22] Rather, it appears that the bone regrowth and attachment gain occurs via repair as opposed to true regeneration.[24] There has been, however, significant research and improvement in this area that is continually improving results. This has resulted in a much better prognosis, depending on the presentation (see below).

If healing does occur, it may take the form of long junctional epithelium (which can occur even in the presence of new bone) or ankylosis, which results in root resorption. If the procedure proves ineffective, it could lead to recurrence of the pocket or gingival recession. A combination of any or all of the above could occur; therefore clinical and radiographic follow-up is mandated in all cases of periodontal reconstruction.

Periodontal regeneration is exceedingly difficult in the presence of periodontal pathogens.[25,26] Therefore, homecare is a critical aspect of periodontal surgery. Homecare improves the prognosis for regeneration and is required for maintaining the regenerated bone. If there is no commitment to homecare, periodontal surgery is of dubious value, and therefore clients should be informed of this prior to pursuing therapy.

Periodontal regeneration

Periodontal regenerative surgery is designed to reconstruct the periodontal attachment (periodontal ligament, cementum, and alveolar bone). Only periodontal ligament cells (and possibly pluripotenet stem cells) have the ability to regenerate the periodontal attachment apparatus.[27,28] Gingival soft tissues recolonize faster than these periodontal structures, resulting in an attachment consisting of long junctional epithelium. While this does temporarily resolve the infection, it is generally not a lasting solution.[29] Therefore it is necessary to retard the downward growth of the gingival tissues and to allow the slower periodontal ligament/alveolar bone to regrow.[30,31] This procedure is called "guided tissue regeneration," because we are selecting the tissue that repopulates the site.[29] Guided tissue regeneration (GTR) has been shown to achieve greater attachment gains for infrabony pockets when compared to straight open flap debridement.[32–35] However, the only strong evidence of effectiveness is limited to infrabony and class II furcational defects.[29,35] Furthermore, most histopathologic studies show that current regenerative materials and methods result in repair of the defect as opposed to true regeneration of the periodontal apparatus.[35] This results in reattachment via ankylosis rather than periodontal ligament. Whether this is *clinically* important in our patients is debateable, but the more we can bring the tissues to their original form the better (see below).

GTR is performed by placing a barrier over the bony defect to allow for the alveolar bone and periodontal ligament to repopulate the defect rather than gingival tissues.[11,19] While there have been significant advances and research in the area of bone augmentation/grafting materials, in most cases, the barrier is the key therapeutic modality. This proves especially true with 3-walled pockets, where grafting does not necessarily increase attachment gains.[36,37] However, in 2-walled defects and furcational defects, the addition of a bone augmentation substance was shown to result in superior gains.[36] Finally, it appears that regeneration is more likely to occur with acute loss such as foreign bodies, gingival trauma, or abscesses.[38,39]

Barrier membranes

first generation membranes (non-resorbable)

The initial studies on GTR were performed with cellulose or Teflon membranes that showed regeneration of not only alveolar bone but also cementum and periodontal ligament.[40–45] Currently, the product of choice for non-resorbable membranes is expanded polytetrafluoroethylene (E-PTFE).[A] This product has also been shown to produce gains in attachment levels, but bone augmentation has not been consistently achieved.[46,47]

Non-resorbable membranes have to be removed following initial healing (3–6 weeks),[19] which presents even more of a problem in veterinary patients, as a second anesthesia is almost invariably required. Therefore resorbable membranes were developed. No statistically significant difference with respect to attachment gain has been demonstrated between the two types of membranes,[222] and thus the resorbable membranes are recommended.[223]

Second generation membranes (resorbable)

There are numerous options for bioresorbable membranes currently available. Studies on the early products that are no longer commercially available concluded that this type of membrane can be very effective in periodontal regeneration.[224,225]

The majority of bioresorbable membranes are prepackaged sheets that are cut to size for the defect. The combination of polyglycol acid, polylactic acid, and trimethylene carbonate[B] remains substantially intact for 16–24 weeks. A bovine Achilles tendon collagen[C] that resorbs in 4–18 weeks has also been proven effective. A bilayer porcine derived collagen,[D] which has been shown to be effective in regeneration of infrabony defects, is the easiest to use and generally the product of choice.[19,226,227]

Recently we have started looking at these membranes not only as a barrier to the downgrowth of gingival tissues but also as a delivery medium for substances that may improve attachment gains.[228] Similar to perioceutics[229] (see chapter 12), impregnating antibiotics (e.g., tetracyclines) and anti-inflammatories (e.g., flurbiprofen) into the membrane appears to further enhance the effects of GTR.[230,231] Additionally, adding a bone promotive material (e.g., hydroxyapatite) may improve attachment gain. Demineralized laminar bone sheets[E] have been tested and shown to be safe, resorbable, and as effective as standard first generation barriers at least in some cases.[232,233] Finally, there is now a layered product that combines the positive effects of the hydroxyapatite against the bone, a middle layer of polylactic acid (PLA), with a surface coating of metronidazole, which may combine the best of both of the above.[48]

The expense and challenge of customizing preformed membranes has resulted in the creation of flowable, customizable membranes. A polylactic acid gel[F] that is commercially available and approved as a barrier membrane has shown excellent results in most studies.[49–52] Furthermore, antibiotics and anti-inflammatories (as above) can be mixed into the product to take advantage of their additive properties. However, it should be noted that this product was found to be inferior to collagen membranes in some research.[227] Moreover, it has created foreign body reactions (occasionally significant) and may not be resorbed for more than 1 year.[53,54] Therefore, the positive attributes of this product must be viewed in light of the above research.

Finally, the resorbable base in the veterinary-labelled perioceutic[G] is very similar to the polylactic acid gel (above) and comes combined with doxycycline (see chapter 12) (Figure 18.20). It is not approved for this use and some argue that it does not last long enough to promote true tissue regeneration.[223] However, many veterinary dentists (including this author) have utilized the product for years with consistent clinical results (i.e., new bone formation and pocket depth reduction).

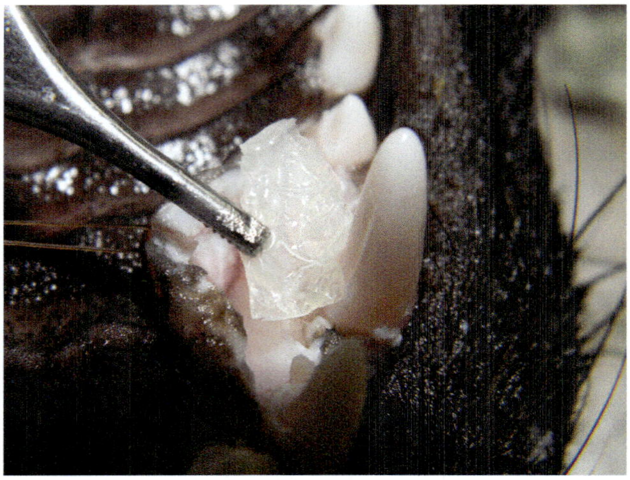

Figure 18.20 Prehardened and shaped Doxirobe membrane ready for placement.

Bone grafting materials

There has been significant interest in utilizing bone substitute products to increase the level of attachment gains with GTR. The ideal goal of a bone grafting material for periodontal disease is to regenerate the periodontium by reformation of the PDL and regrowth of lost bone in an effort to maintain tooth support. An ideal graft material is also expected to increase healing in fracture and extraction sites. Numerous studies have been performed with the various products listed below that have reported significant improvement in clinical parameters, including crestal bone height, clinical attachment level, and decreased probing depth over open flap debridement.[55–65] In addition, bone replacement grafts appeared to have a positive effect on the treatment of class II and III furcation exposure.[66,67] This gain is even more significant when combined with a barrier membrane.[68,69]

Comparison studies show that biologic grafts generally achieve better improvements than synthetic, nonanimal materials.[56,65,70] These effects were generally more favorable when combined with a barrier membrane.[35,71,223] Furthermore, to date, in long-term studies GTR has been enhanced significantly by the combination of bone graft and barrier membranes.[71]

In order to determine which bone augmentation substance to choose, one must first understand how new bone formation is achieved. There are three main categories of augmentation effects: osteogenesis, osteoinduction, and osteoconduction.[19,22] Osteogenesis refers to viable cells within the graft that lead to the synthesis of new bone. Osteoinduction is the process by which surrounding stromal or progenitor cells are converted into osteoblasts due to the release of growth factors and other mediators to produce native bone. This is a process of accelerated bone production (compared to normal bone remodelling) and a shortened healing period.[22] Osteoconduction is the formation of a scaffold that allows bone to grow into and around the affected site.[72,73] The importance of osteoinduction cannot be overstated, as it is a major contributor to the production of new bone. Many of the products listed blow (especially xenografts and *mineralized* allografts) are only osteoconductive and therefore do not recreate new bone.

There are three main types of bone-based grafting material (autografts, allografts, and xenografts) as well as non-animal-based bone substitutes. The following is an overview of the various options currently available.

Autografts

Autografts are bone material taken from the same individual. These grafts are generally harvested from elsewhere in the patient's mouth such as healing extraction sites, bone removed from osteoplasty or ostectomy, or edentulous areas such as the diastema distal to the canines.[19] The bone is obtained with a large round cutting bur that makes a coarse powder. It is important to ensure that the bone is not excessively heated during the burring, as high temperatures can inactivate osteoinductive proteins. Also, it is important not to use any type of suction during this procedure. The bone powder is collected and typically mixed with either the patient's blood or saline (in a dappen dish) and then placed into the bony defect where desired.[19]

Autografts have the best clinical outcome and are the gold standard that all other bone grafting materials are compared to.[74] This is because autografts have all three properties involved in new bone formation: osteogenesis, osteoconduction, and osteoinduction. The limitations of autografts are twofold. First, they are only available in small quantities and are therefore not adequate for repairing large deficits, and second, the harvesting of these grafts leads to morbidity in the patient.[74]

Allografts

Allografts are currently the most commonly used bone graft material. In humans, bone allografts have a nearly 40-year history of successful use in periodontal therapy.[71] This is bone material obtained from donors of the same species as the recipient. Samples are harvested from cadavers and then further processed in order to be stored and available when required.

The main advantages of allografts are that they are readily available and no additional patient morbidity is involved with their use. The disadvantage is that allografts are not osteogenic because they do not contain living cells; however, being comprised of natural bone with collagens and proteins, allografts inherently contain bone morphologic proteins present in all individuals.

While all allografts are osteoconductive, some allografts also have osteoinductive properties depending on their method of preparation.[19,72,73,75,76] It is traditionally held that mineralized allografts are osteoconductive only, and that demineralized allografts are both osteoinductive and osteoconductive.[19,70,71,73,75]

Allografts are prepared by processing and freezing or freeze-drying fresh bone obtained from cadaver donors. The freezing process leads to the loss of the majority of cells due to lysis or removal, which results in the loss of the graft's osteogenic properties and removes immunogenic concerns.

Allografts are most commonly prepared by decalcification (demineralization). This preserves the collagen and the acid-stable bone morphologic proteins (growth factors),[75] with collagen, proteins, and growth factors extracted. This is known as demineralized freeze-dried bone allograft (DFDBA).[75,76] Both mineralized and demineralized allograft products are effective due to their high osteoconductive effects, and freeze-dried products also have the advantage of a long shelf life.[72,75,77]

Bone morphogenic proteins (BMPs) are exposed within the underlying collagen during the demineralization process, thus providing immediate access to the BMPs when they are implanted.[75] This is an advantage over mineralized grafts (including autografts that are mineralized) because these require resorption of minerals to expose the BMPs. When implanted in to a vascular site, the BMPs recruit osteoblasts and this provides the beneficial effects for regeneration (see below).[78] Demineralized bone allografts have been shown to have the highest osteogenic potential and consistently create new attachment, which has been proven by histological evaluation.[35,75,79-81] *This product (DFDBA) currently appears to be the best choice for guided tissue regeneration.*[35] *Freeze-dried bone allografts are currently commercially available specifically for veterinary use*[H] (Figure 18.21).

One disadvantage of these products is the inability to see them radiographically in the postoperative setting (due to the lack of mineralization), and therefore confirmation of adequate filling of the defect is

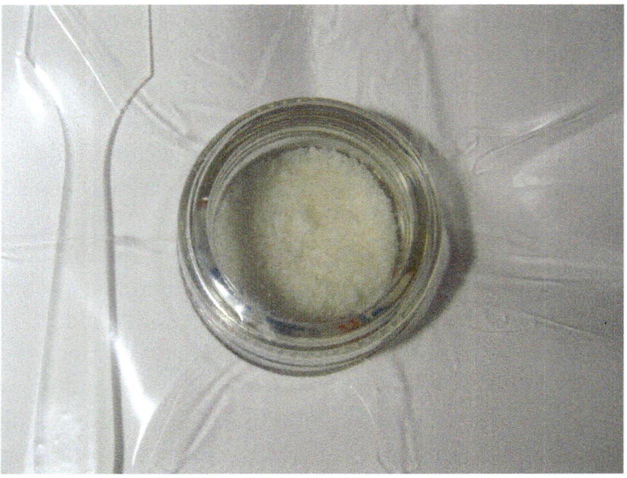

Figure 18.21 Osseoallograft bone particulate.

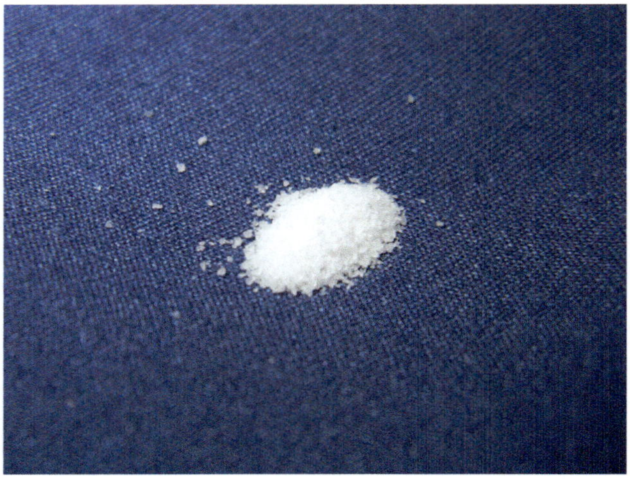

Figure 18.22 Consil, ceramic bone augmentation.

not possible. For this reason, some authors mix this with a more radiodense product; however, this may have the risk of reducing the concentration of BMPs in the site.

Xenografts

Xenografts are a bone grafting material commonly used in humans. Xenografts are bone or bone components obtained from a different species than the patient. Bovine is the species most commonly used for these grafts in human dentistry. The advantages of xenografts are that bovine bone is readily available and relatively inexpensive. Just like allografts, xenografts can be mineralized or demineralized and thus are osteoconductive, and because so many homologies in bone morphologic proteins exist between species, they may also have some osteoinductive activity.[19,82] In some cases, they have been shown to support periodontal regeneration.[83,84]

Non-animal products

Ceramic-based materials have been used for many years as a bone grafting substitute (Figure 18.22). Calcium phosphate, calcium sulfate, and bioactive glass are several options included in this category. All of these materials are osteoconductive only. The main advantages of ceramic-based bone grafting materials are that they are plentiful, inexpensive, and do not cause additional morbidity to the patient. Ceramic-based materials work by forming a scaffold that the patient's own cells move into. Histologically, there is a greater ratio of fibrous connective tissue to bone regrowth compared to allograft when ceramic-based are used alone, making for a weaker repair.[70,71] In addition, one study reported inferior results with bioactive glass than OFD alone.[85] This was even more profound when the results were evaluated histologically, and it was found that these products support repair as opposed to true regeneration.[35]

However, other reports show these products in a more positive light, with results of calcium phosphate ceramic (CER) being comparable to allografts.[35,86–89] This was further enhanced when they combined with biologically active agents such as growth factors.[90–92] Moreover, one study has shown that combining factor-based and ceramic-based materials has similar results to allograft materials.[93] The addition of Colloss E (an equine bone protein extract) to beta-tricalcium phosphate (B-TCP) resulted in no fibrous tissue formation, which provided a much stronger repair compared to the ceramic-only group.[93] Furthermore, this same study revealed results comparable to allograft. Finally, calcium sulphate has shown positive results.[94,95]

Synthetic biomaterials have also shown promise for GTR purposes.[96] One interesting product in this class is B-TCP,[I] which has been shown to have excellent ability to regenerate bone and aid in the proliferation of dental follicle progenitor cells.[97] Furthermore, several implant studies have shown this product to be comparable to autogenous bone grafts.[98,99]

Response to treatment

Currently, our main objective in regards to periodontal surgery is the regeneration of alveolar bone. This has focused on a combination of plaque control and barrier membranes (± bone augmentation) to regenerate lost bone. While this has shown promise in the *repair* of alveolar bone, and on occasion other periodontal structures (periodontal ligament and cementum), it is not a reliable method of *regeneration* of these tissues to their predisease condition.[24] However, as mentioned above, it appears that DFDBA currently offers the best option for regrowing the attachment apparatus. Future therapies will use hormones, enzymes, and genes to repair the periodontal defects to normal architecture.[100]

The recent development of the field of tissue engineering has brought new options for the future of periodontal therapy. Tissue engineering is defined as a multidisciplinary field involving biology, medicine, and engineering that works to restore, maintain, or enhance tissue and organ function.[101] While exciting on a whole body level, this is an intense area of research that is showing some good results in the treatment of periodontitis.

Periodontal tissue regeneration depends on several basic components: blood supply, scaffolding, and the appropriate cells and signals.[45] There are numerous cells that make up the periodontal system as well as undifferentiated ones that have the potential of generating and maintaining the mineralized and unmineralized periodontal tissues.[102] Stimulatory as well as selective methods have been tested in an attempt to regrow lost periodontal tissues.[30,103]

Graft additives

There is significant research into novel additives for guided tissue regeneration. A myriad of modalities have been shown to improve performance of standard GTR materials.[104] This area of dentistry is showing great promise and is currently being called "tissue engineering."[105]

Numerous growth factors and other bioactive materials have been studied for their additive properties to regenerative materials. These growth factors are normally produced by healthy cells. However, in areas that are not designed to regenerate (i.e., the periodontium), exogenous growth factors may be beneficial.[106,107] Therefore, one of the primary strategies of regenerative periodontal tissue engineering is the addition of these factors as well as other materials to provide a superior extracellular matrix for healing.[22,108] These products are nearing release and may represent a powerful tool for periodontal regeneration in the near future.[21,109] This process of modifying an injured tissue to self-regenerate is called endogenous regenerative technology (ERT).[22]

Various products are discussed below in more detail. Note, however, that this is a quickly expanding area of dentistry and new information is consistently available. The reader is encouraged to keep up with the literature.

Bone morphogenic proteins show the greatest potential for graft additives. The huge advantage to BMPs is that they are osteoinductive and have an excellent fusion rate without the use of autogenous bone.[19,45] They appear to have a significantly positive effect in bone regeneration.[97,110,111] Furthermore, it appears that they combine very well with a new ceramic-based graft B-TCP (see above).[112] The disadvantages of BMPs are that they have to be combined with other materials in order to obtain the best results and are not currently available in the veterinary field. Other factor-based materials that are new and currently undergoing studies include growth and differentiation factor (GDF) and LIM mineralization protein (LMP).[76]

Enamel matrix derivative (EMD) is a purified acidic extract from porcine enamel matrix.[J] It contains enamel matrix proteins that play a key role in the development of tooth-supporting tissues.[22] It has been extensively studied as a regenerative product as well as a graft additive.[113,114] It is claimed that it provides periodontal regeneration by a biological approach; that is, creating a matrix on the root surfaces that promotes cementum, PDL, and alveolar bone regeneration, thus mimicking the events occurring during tooth development.[115–117] It appears to have a capacity for stimulating periodontal regeneration via positive effects on root surfaces; that is, inhibition of gingival epithelium downgrowth and also stimulation of connective tissue proliferation and attachment to the root surfaces during wound healing.[110,115,118,119] Furthermore, EMD appears to be strongly angiogenic and possesses the ability to modulate the growth of periodontal pathogens.[120,121] An acellular type of cementum regeneration and new alveolar bone formation by an accelerated osteoconductive mechanism are also achieved with application of enamel matrix proteins.[122] These positive attributes appear to be due to the fact that EMD contains multiple growth factors that may mimic the conditions during healing.[21]

In most clinical studies, the addition of EMD has improved clinical results that can be maintained over a longer period.[123–126] In fact, it is the only commercially available product that has the ability to create true regenerative responses.[127] In cases where it was added to autogenous bone, there appeared to be a mild increase in bone regeneration.[128] However, other studies found that its addition did not improve GTR success.[33,129] Additionally, at least one study revealed that EMD alone was effective at bone regeneration[130] and decreasing clinical attachment loss at a level equal to GTR.[131,132] However, most studies show that EMD alone is not as effective as GTR, especially in bone formation.[33,129,131]

Most of these studies are on the human side, and extrapolating to veterinary patients may not hold true. Regardless, the use of EMDs may be important now and will almost certainly be in the future. However, prior to widespread clinical use, there are numerous challenges associated with the use of EMDs, including short half-life, need for high concentrations, and the fact that they are unstable.[22,133] Therefore, an effective delivery medium must be developed prior to commercial release. Currently used products for delivery include PGA, PLA, PLGA,

B-TCP, as well as natural polymers such as dextran, gelatin, and collagen.[134–138]

Factors that have been studied and show promise include recombinant human growth and differentiation factor-5 (especially in combination with B-TCP);[139,140] recombinant human bone morphogenetic proteins 2, 7, and 12 ;[141–147] and fibroblast growth factors [148–151] IGF-I,[152,153] TGF-1,[154,155] and FGF-2.[156] One product that has been extensively studied is platelet-derived growth factor (PDGF), which was shown in several studies to improve bony regeneration in several species whether in graft or barrier.[123,149,157–164] This product appears to be beneficial in numerous clinical applications, including furcational defects.[165] The most effective of these products appears to be PDGF-BB, BMP 2 and 7, and IGF-1.[21]

In addition, platelet rich plasma (PRP) has shown positive effects for tissue regeneration in some studies.[166–168] The allure of this product is that it contains multiple growth factors that may mimic the natural healing process.[21,22,169] This fact may be the most important factor in its effectiveness, as no single factor can mimic the natural healing process.[109,133] In addition, it is easily obtained by simply centrifuging the patient's own blood.[21,170] It has been used in oral surgery to improve bone and soft tissue healing.[171,172] As a matter of fact, one study reported that PRP when combined with bovine porous bone mineral (BPBM) gave the same level of attachment gain whether or not a barrier was used (GTR).[173] However, both of the above studies were in combination with BPBM, and an additional study found that the addition of PRP to BPBM and GTR did not have an additive effect.[174] Thus, more research is needed prior to recommending this product on a widespread basis.

Angiogenisis (production of new blood vessels) is also an important part of periodontal tissue repair, since the periodontium is a highly vascularized tissue.[45] The blood supply is critical to periodontal regeneration, as it transports cells, nutrients, and defensins to the site, as well as provides nutrition to the newly engineered cells.[45,175] Basic fibroblast growth factor (FGF-2) has been shown to have angiogenic ability.[176] However, it appears the EMD is even more strongly angiogenic.[177]

High concentrations of these factors are typically required for periodontal regeneration.[177] It appears that one important factor in the effectiveness of all these products is related to their release rates as well as the ability to keep them in contact with the area for a long enough period to be effective.[21,123,162,178,179] This is of special concern because of their short half-lives.[45] Therefore, the development of an effective delivery vehicle is also an important factor in their use. The most promising vehicle for the sustained release of the products in the repairing defect is the scaffolding.[45] The products listed above can be incorporated into the material either during or after fabrication.[180,181] PLGA (polylactic-*co*-glycolic acid) scaffolds have been widely studied as a means of delivering growth factors and other mediators with success.[21,182,183] Additionally, purified natural biomaterials such as collagen,[184] gelatin,[185] fibrin, dextrans,[136] and alginate are attractive due to their compatibility and biodegradability.[21] Current belief holds that there is no ideal delivery medium, and a composite of several materials may produce the best effect.[21,186,187] Ideally this reservoir would be environmentally sensitive.[21,188]

An additional means to achieve the continued presence of high levels of growth factors in the defect is gene therapy.[162,189] A study with BMP-7 gene transfer showed a good ability to regenerate periodontal tissues.[190,191] Moreover, viral transfer of PDGF revealed significant improvement in periodontal wound healing models.[163]

Stem cells may provide a future means to improve periodontal regeneration.[192,193] Studies performed in rats and dogs with bone marrow stem and stromal cells have shown a positive effect in new bone formation in experimentally induced lesions.[194,195] Additionally, a canine implant model showed that both bone marrow and periodontal ligament stem cells improved HA/TCP attachment gain.[196] While more research is clearly necessary before using this methodology in a patient, this appears to be on the horizon.

Finally, it appears that we may actually be able to grow periodontal tissues in other animals and even other species that can then be transplanted to periodontal patients.[197,198] A recent study regrew human oral mucosa equivalent in rats.[199] Moreover, cloned cemetoblasts have been created, and when transplanted into PLGA carriers led to a significant level of periodontal regeneration.[200,201] Finally, BMP-7 gene transduced skin fibroblasts were shown to promote tissue engineering of periodontal structures.[190]

Several studies have looked at systemic medications as a way to improve attachment gains with GTR. To date, none have been shown to increase attachment gains, but the studies are minimal at this point. Neither systemic antibiotic nor anti-inflammatory therapy have yet been shown to improve attachment gains.[202,203]

Techniques for GTR

There are several alternatives for the technique of GTR;[7,11,19,204] this section will discuss several of them. The three main differences are

1. Infrabony pocket vs. furcational defect.
2. Whether a bone augmentation product/graft is to be used.
3. Preformed versus custom (liquid) barrier membrane.

After a suitable pocket has been diagnosed (see above) and the treatment discussed, pockets are ready to be treated. The clinician should decide prior to making the first incision what type of surgery will be performed. Below is a step-by-step description of the three most common GTR procedures: palatal aspect of the maxillary canine (Figures 18.23–18.29), distal aspect of the mandibular first molar (Figures 18.30–18.34), and class II furcational defect of a maxillary fourth premolar (Figures 18.35–18.39).

Step 1: Provide regional anaesthesia (see chapter 21).
Step 2: Create a periodontal flap appropriate for the planned surgery (Figures 18.23, 18.30, 18.35) (see chapter 16).
Step 3: Clean and treat the exposed root surface (see chapter 17) (Figures 18.24, 18.31, 18.36).
Step 4: (Optional) Place bone augmentation. The chosen product should be mixed according to package directions and placed in the defect. The defect should be completely to slightly overfilled (Figures 18.25, 18.32, 18.37).
Step 5: Place the barrier. For prefabricated membranes, the material should be cut to fit the defect and sutured in place (Figures 18.26, 18.33). Custom flowable products can be created on a glass slab, cut to size, and sutured into place (Figures 18.27, 18.38). However, most veterinary dentists prefer to make them in the defect (Figure 18.28). Note that the barrier should be overcovered by the gingiva by at least 2 mm.[223]
Step 6: Close the flap (see chapter 16 for a complete discussion on suture and suture patterns) (Figures 18.29, 18.34, 18.39).
Step 7: Expose a postoperative radiograph.

(a) (b) (c) (d)

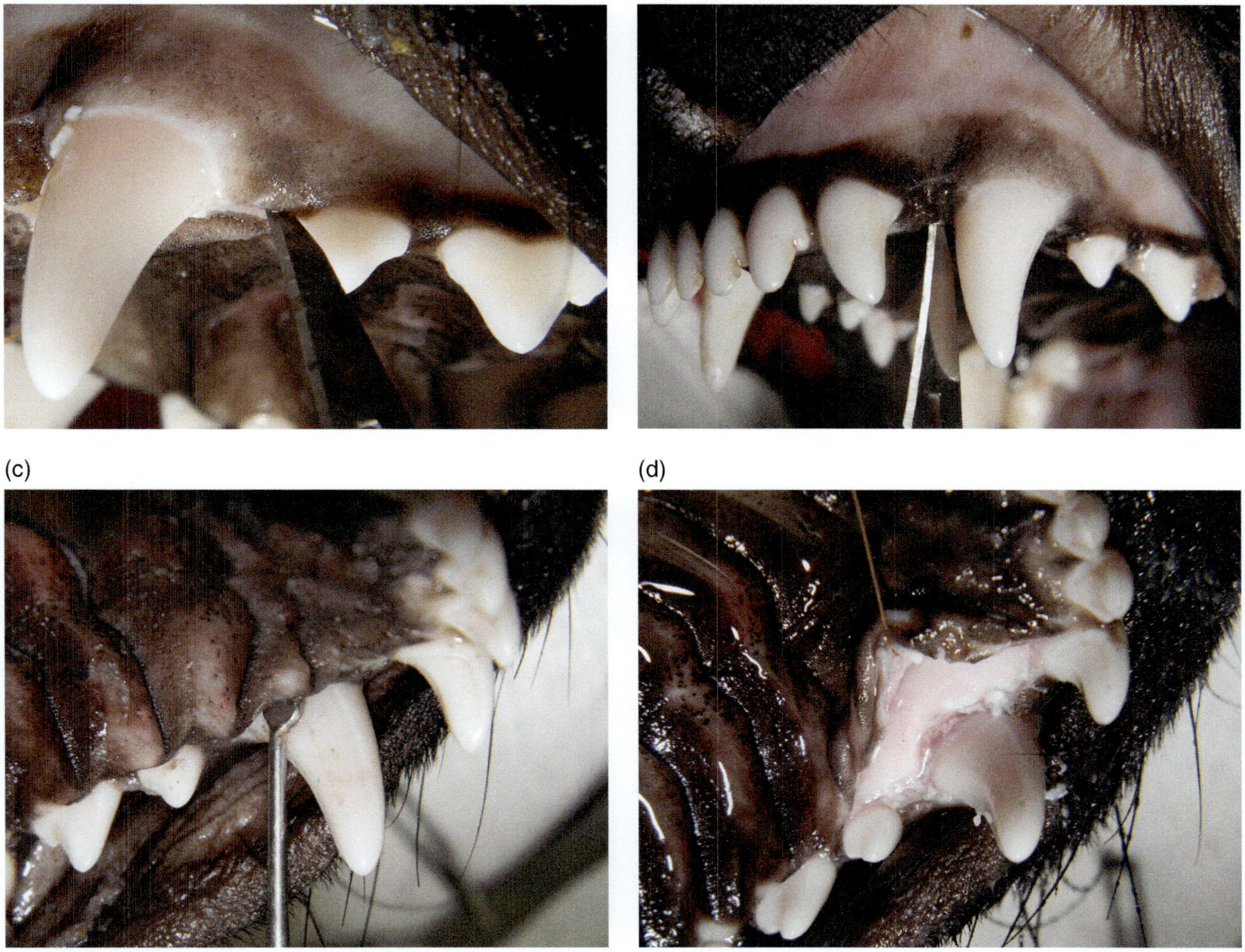

Figure 18.23 Creating a conservative (envelope) periodontal flap for pocket access (see chapter 16). Performing horizontal releasing incision (a) distal and (b) mesial to the target tooth. (c) Carefully elevating a full thickness palatine flap with a periosteal elevator. (d) Flap raised and held with a stay suture. (This is the least traumatic way to handle periodontal flaps during surgery.) Note there is adequate visualization for cleaning and grafting with a small surgical site. This minimizes surgical time and trauma as well as decreasing post-operative pain and risk of dehiscence.

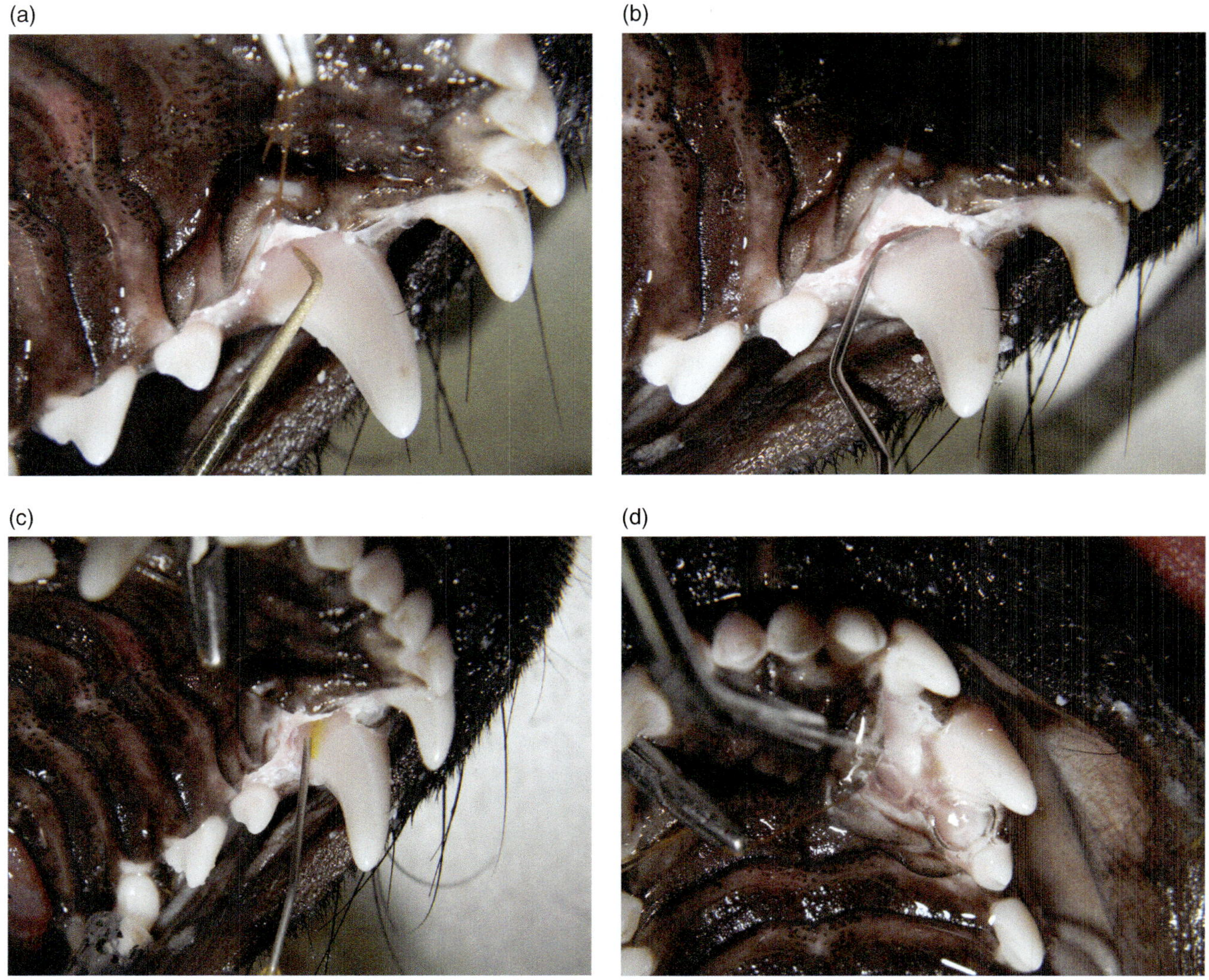

Figure 18.24 Cleaning and debriding the pocket (see chapter 17). (a) With a fine, *sub*gingival periodontal tip on an ultrasonic scaler. (b) With a curette. (c) Application of citric acid biomodification. (d) Thorough rinsing of the citric acid.

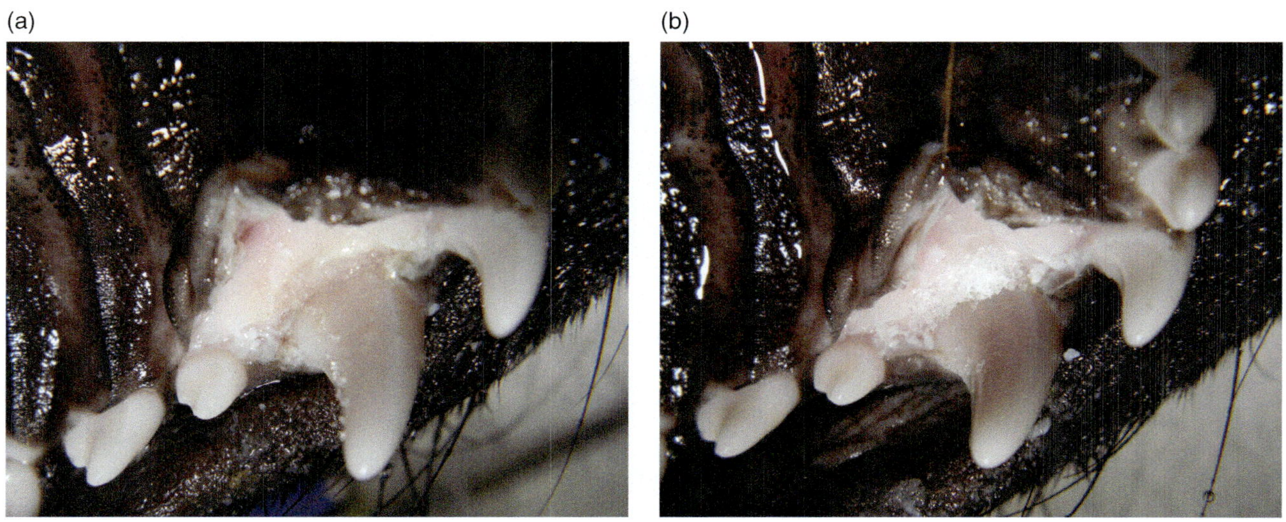

Figure 18.25 Placement of the bone augmentation. (a) Fully filled. (b) Slightly overfilled.

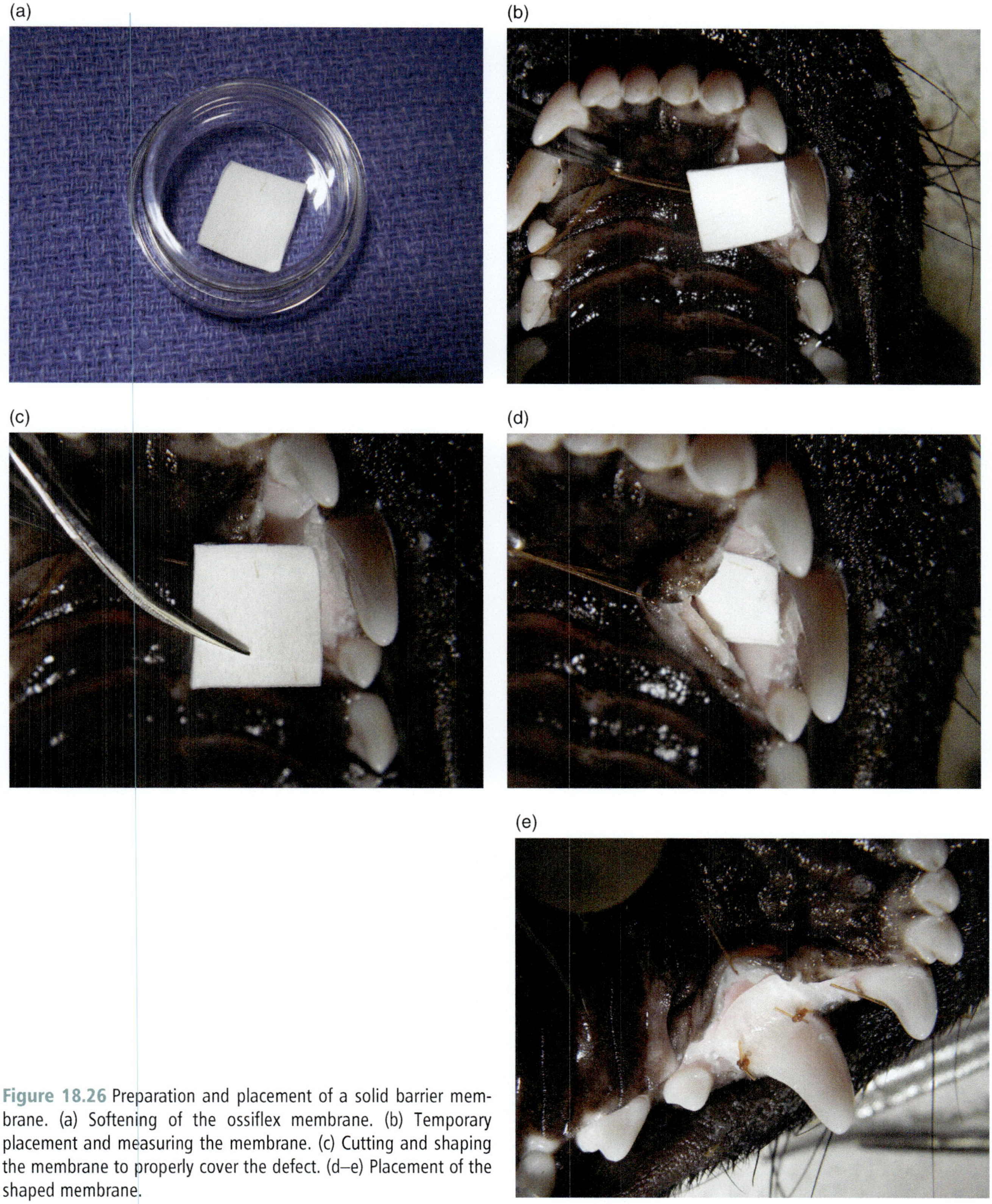

Figure 18.26 Preparation and placement of a solid barrier membrane. (a) Softening of the ossiflex membrane. (b) Temporary placement and measuring the membrane. (c) Cutting and shaping the membrane to properly cover the defect. (d–e) Placement of the shaped membrane.

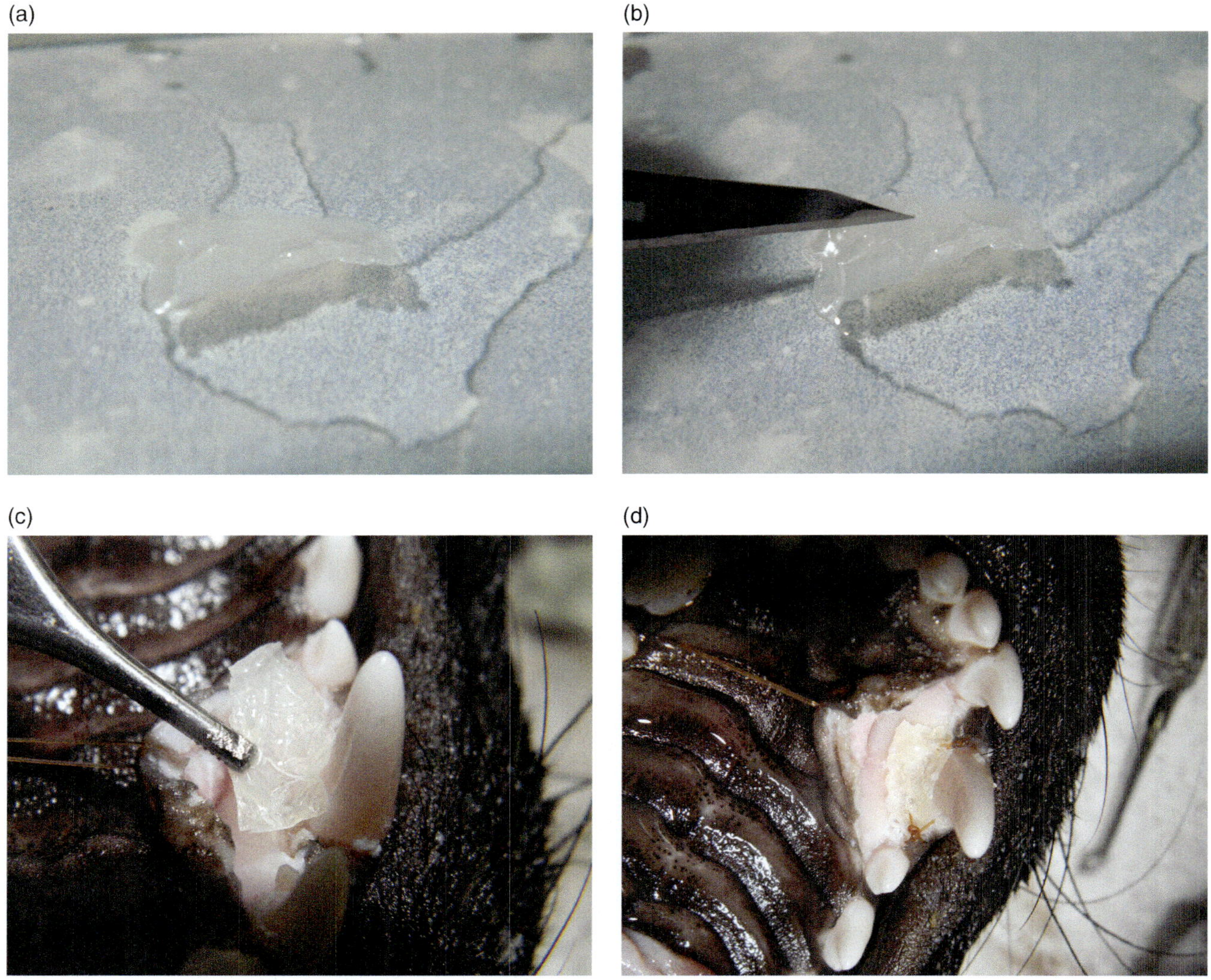

Figure 18.27 Preparation of a custom (viscous) barrier membrane prior to placement. (a) Product is placed in a thin layer on a glass slab and thoroughly wetted to harden. (b) Product is cut to the approximate size necessary for placement. It is important to *over*estimate the size needed to allow for further trimming. (c) Trial fitting, shaping, and placement. (d) Membrane sutured in place.

Determination of new attachment

As stated above, periodontal reconstruction has several possible outcomes. If regeneration fails, simple periodontal probing will elucidate it. However, more than simple probing is necessary for the determination of the type of new attachment[19] as the level of inflammation will significantly affect the probing depth.[205] These diagnostic modalities include bone probing (sounding), radiology, surgical re-entry, and histopathology.[206]

Bone probing under general anesthesia is a very effective way to determine the level of bone regrowth. In fact, it has been shown to be as accurate as surgical re-entry without the surgical trauma.[207,208] For this to be accurate, however, the pre-and postmeasurements must be done at the same point and with the probe held at the same angle.

Dental radiology is another tool to determine the alveolar bone height. However, this also requires precise placement of the tube head and film/sensor to achieve accurate comparison films.[209] Even with standardized methods,[210] radiographs are not as accurate as clinical measurements.[211,212] In fact, radiographs have been shown to consistently underestimate the level of alveolar bone.[213] This is likely due to the fact that there is a minimum level of mineralization that must be present to be radiographically evident. The most accurate way to utilize radiographs for periodontal assessment is via subtraction methods, but this is neither commonly available nor easy to perform.[214,215]

The use of radiographs is especially challenging in veterinary patients, as the bisecting angle technique is required for the vast majority of images.[216,217] Not only

(a) (b) (c)

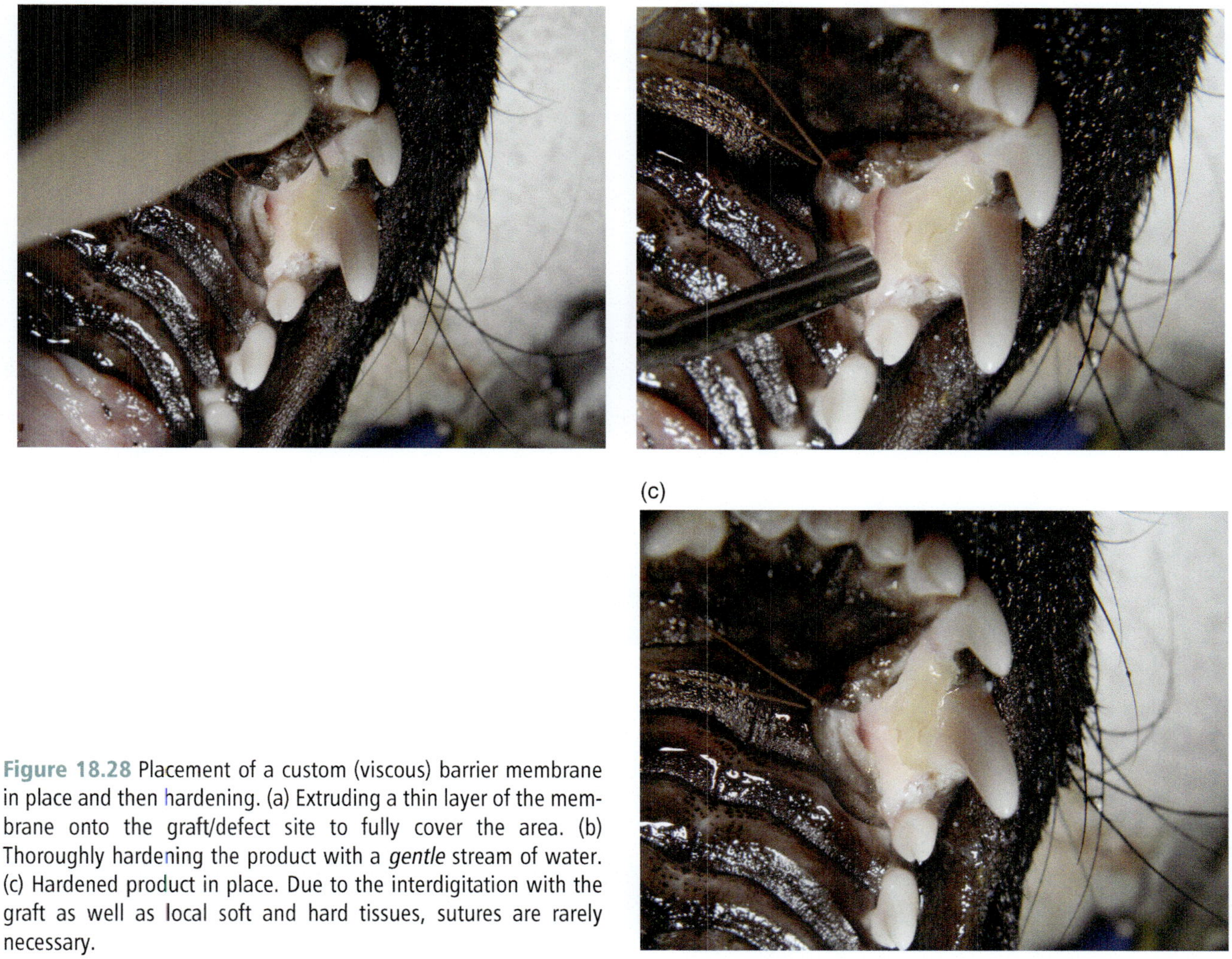

Figure 18.28 Placement of a custom (viscous) barrier membrane in place and then hardening. (a) Extruding a thin layer of the membrane onto the graft/defect site to fully cover the area. (b) Thoroughly hardening the product with a *gentle* stream of water. (c) Hardened product in place. Due to the interdigitation with the graft as well as local soft and hard tissues, sutures are rarely necessary.

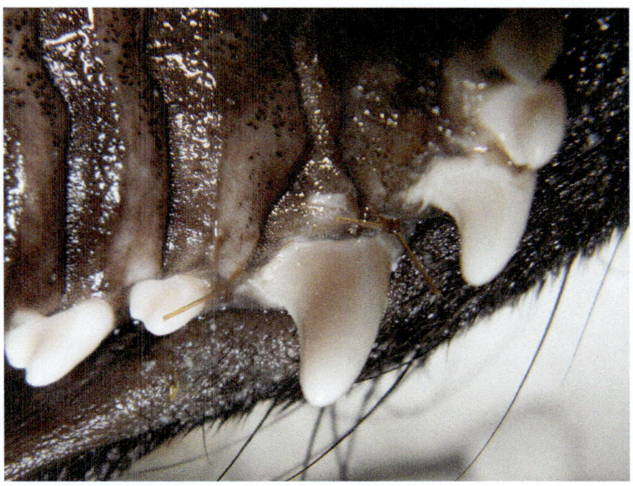

Figure 18.29 Closure of the flap. Note that this conservative flap can be closed with two simple interrupted sutures.

is exact duplication of bisecting angles more challenging (as compared to the parallel technique), the bisecting angle technique will overestimate bone loss.[218]

Histopathology is the only way to determine exactly what tissues have repopulated the area, but it is not useful for clinical success. It is, however, the gold standard for research trials.

Based on the above, the best method for evaluation of alveolar bone loss as well as response to treatment is a combination of transgingival (bone) probing (sounding) and radiography, keeping in mind the fact that radiographs will always *underestimate* the level of alveolar bone.

Periodontal splinting

Periodontal splinting[7,219,220] is designed to provide temporary stability of significantly diseased and mobile teeth during the healing period. This is because

(a) (b)

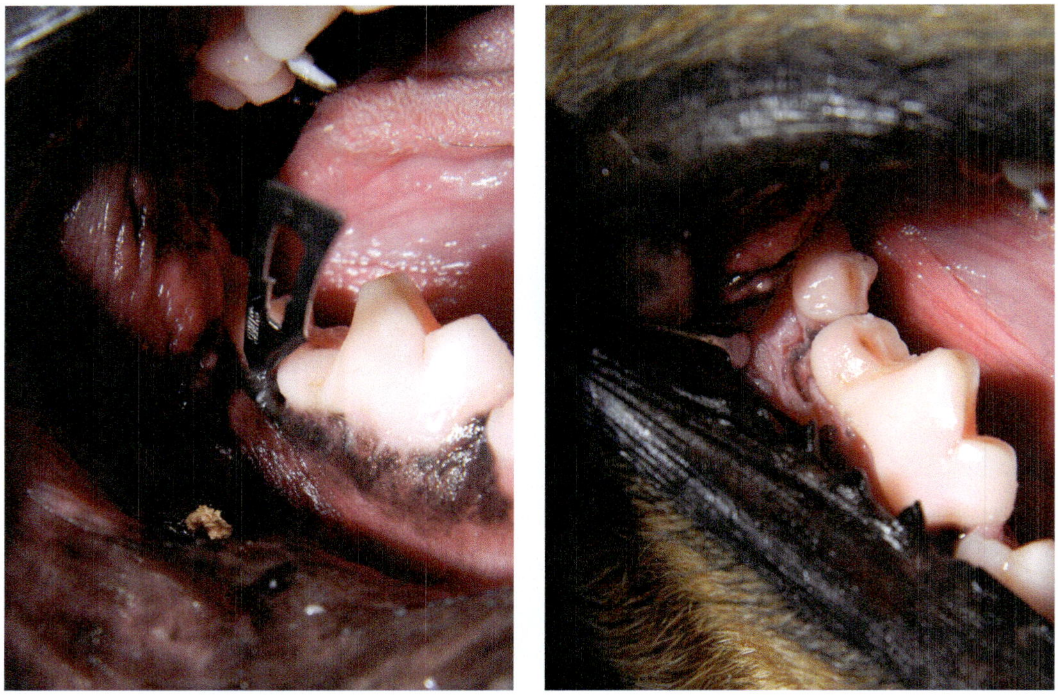

Figure 18.30 Creating an envelope flap for pocket access (see chapter 16). (a) Performing horizontal releasing incision. (b) Carefully elevating a full thickness mucogingival flap with a periosteal elevator. Note the significant granulation tissue in the pocket.

(a) (b)

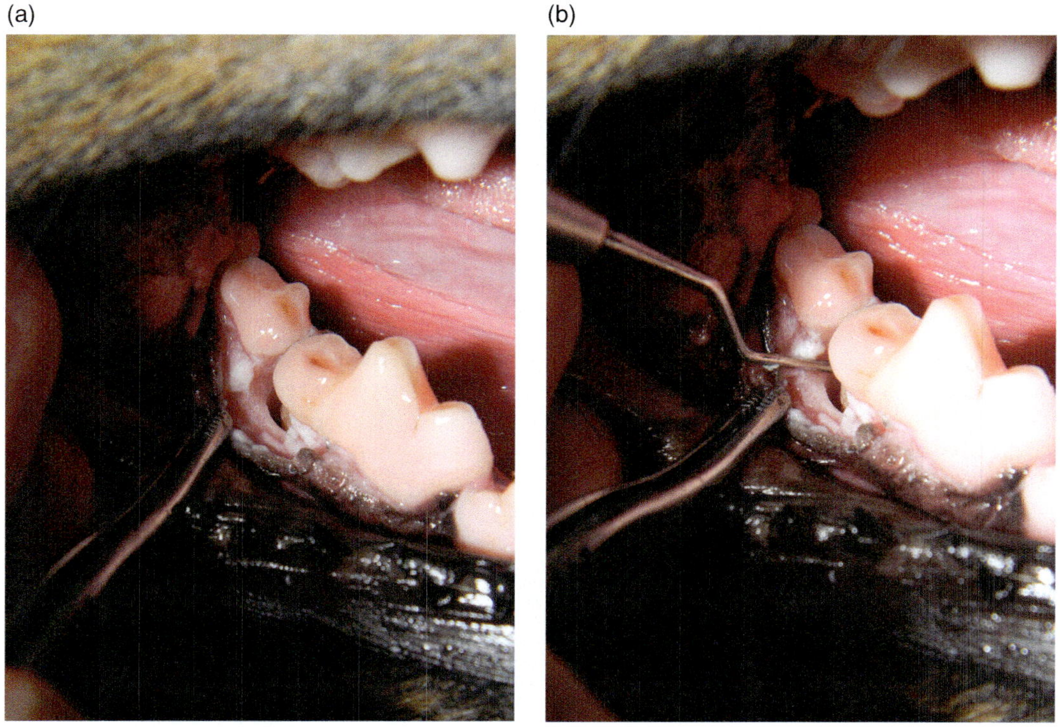

Figure 18.31 Cleaning the defect (see chapter 17). (a) Granulation tissue has been removed with a curette. This allows excellent visualization of the affected area for proper cleaning and treatment. (b) Thorough root planing of the root with a curette. (Ultrasonic scaling [not pictured] previously performed.) ***Note: Following scaling, the roots should be treated with citric acid etch (biomodification) (not pictured). See Figure 18.24.

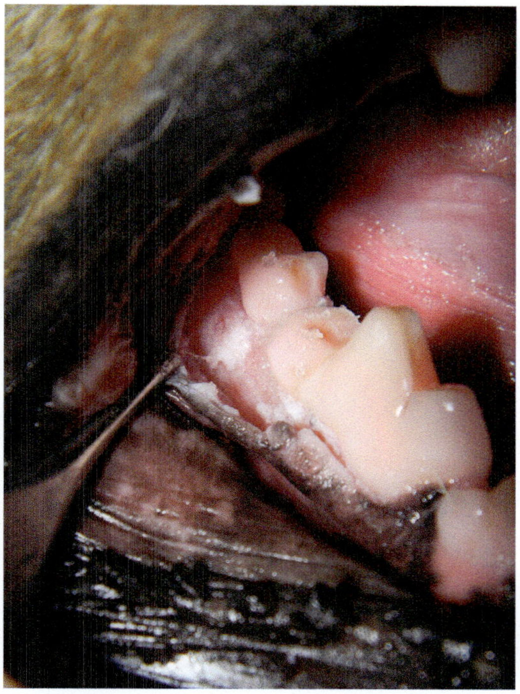

Figure 18.32 Placement of the bone augmentation.

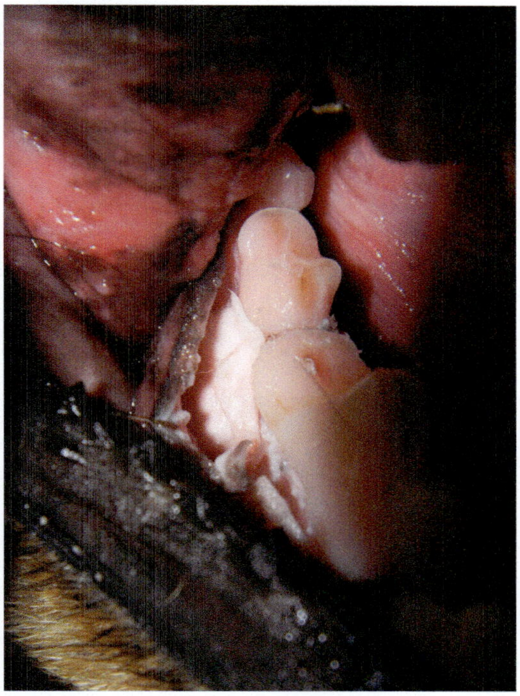

Figure 18.33 Placement of the barrier membrane. Note that sutures should be placed (not pictured).

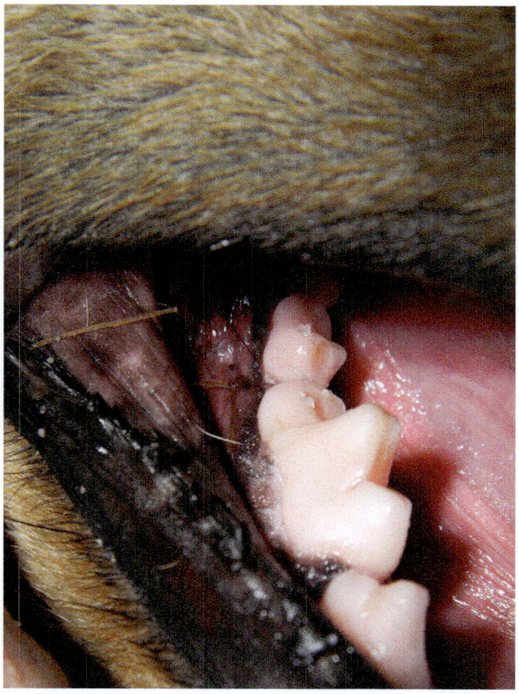

Figure 18.34 Closure. Note this envelope flap required only one suture for proper closure.

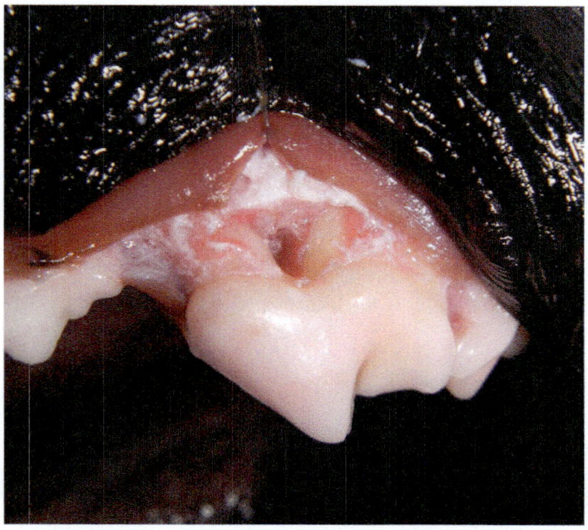

Figure 18.35 Horizontal (envelope) flap created (as in Figure 18.23 above). Flap raised and held with a stay suture. (This is the least traumatic way to handle periodontal flaps during surgery.) Note there is adequate visualization for cleaning and grafting with a small surgical site. This minimizes surgical time and trauma as well as decreasing postoperative pain and risk of dehiscence.

mobility will decrease the effectiveness of guided tissue regeneration. It does *not* directly lead to any long-term stabilization.

It is best utilized on teeth with significant angular bone loss that may respond to GTR. It may also be used to stabilize slightly mobile incisors that are not significantly infected. However, it should be noted that stabilizing the mandibular incisors across the symphysis is not recommended, especially if it is expected to be in place for a significant period of time.

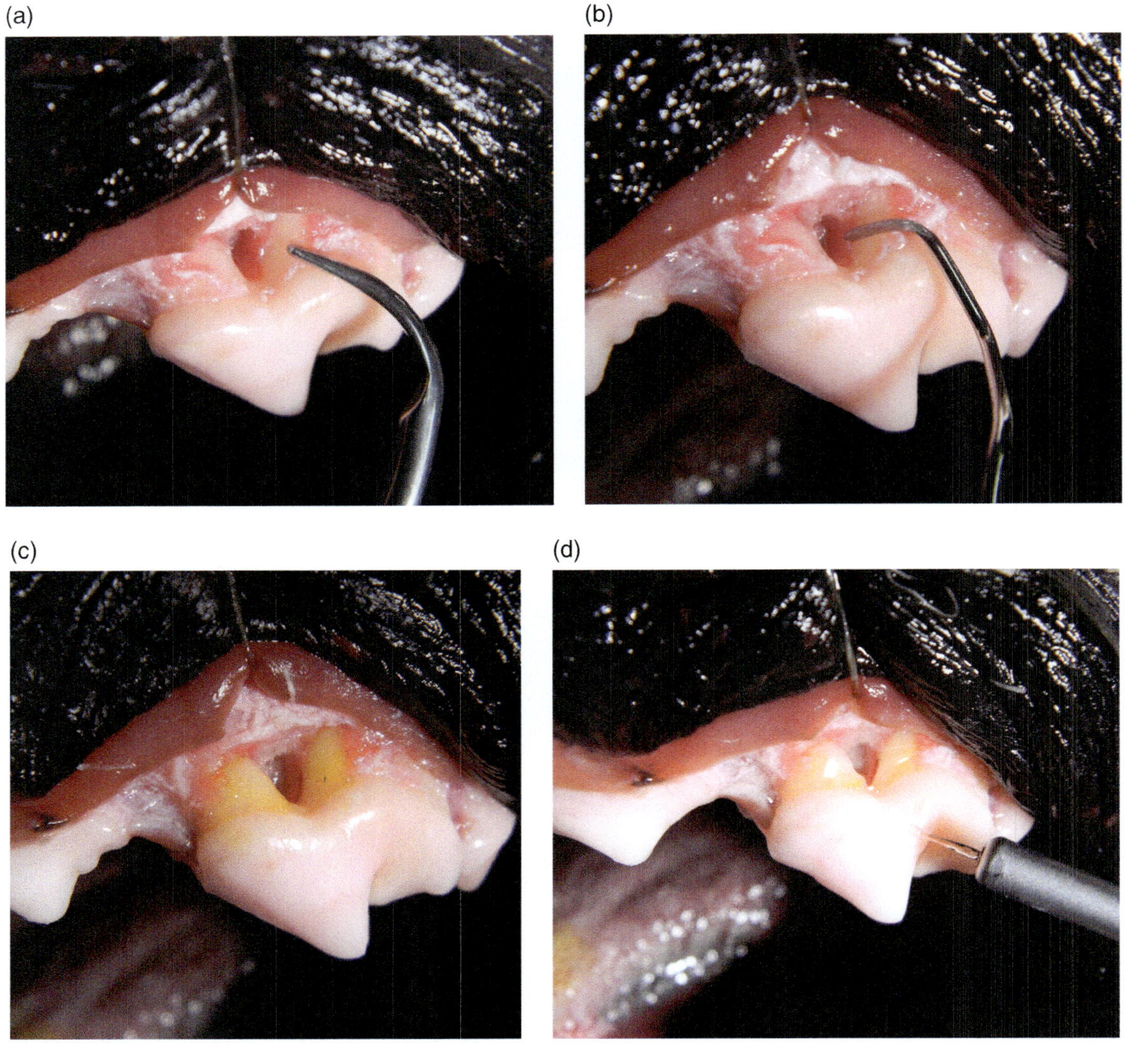

Figure 18.36 Cleaning and debriding the defect (see chapter 17). (a) With a fine, *sub*gingival periodontal tip on an ultrasonic scaler. (b) With a curette. (c) Application of citric acid biomodification. (d) Thorough rinsing of the citric acid.

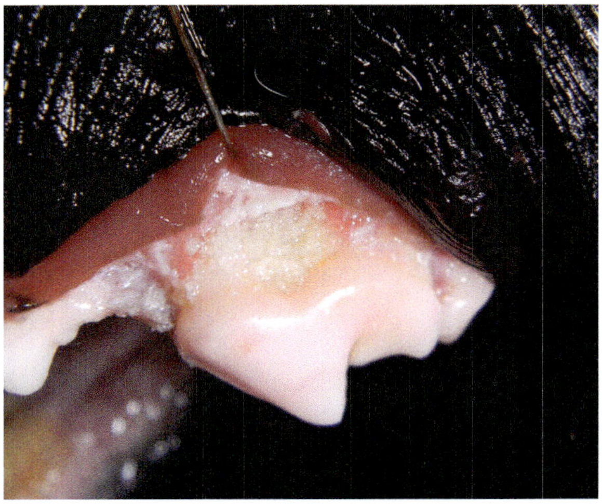

Figure 18.37 Placement of the bone augmentation.

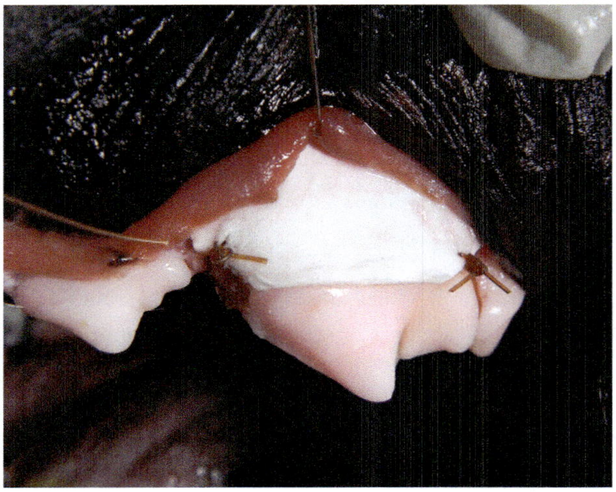

Figure 18.38 Barrier membrane in place. Note that the membrane was not softened prior to placement.

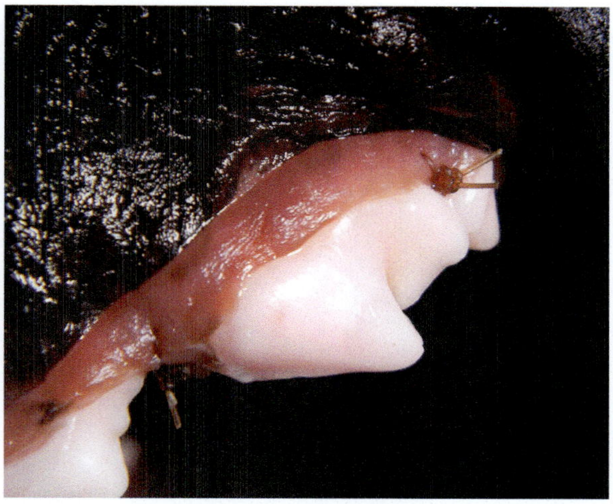

Figure 18.39 Closure. Note that this conservative envelope flap required only two sutures for proper closure.

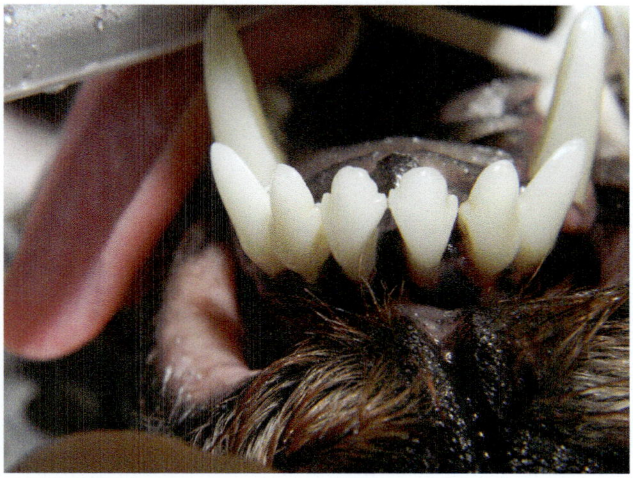

Figure 18.40 Preoperative picture from the rostral aspect showing the gingival recession. The teeth to be involved in the splint have been scaled and polished.

In some instances periodontal splinting is utilized for long-term maintenance of a tooth (particularly show dogs). This is not a recommended technique for several reasons, including:

1. It is very difficult to maintain the splint and associated teeth, as the splint interferes with homecare.
2. It keeps diseased teeth in the oral cavity, which allows for continued infection.
3. It has the potential to damage the anchor teeth.

Furthermore, periodontal splinting should not be used in cases of perio-endo involvement of non-strategic teeth, teeth with less than 20% bone remaining, and non-compliant clients.

Techniques

There are numerous options for periodontal splinting techniques, depending on temporary or permanent use. For temporary (2–4 months) splints, acrylic alone or dental composite should be used. A more aesthetic splint may result from the use of a glass fiber splint.[K] For a more permanent splint, consider adding in wire "rebar". Finally, making shallow enamel grooves will improve retention. This procedure is very similar to acrylic splints utilized for fracture repair.[221]

Acrylic or composite-only splint (Figures 18.40–18.47)

Step 1: Thoroughly clean and polish the teeth with a fluoride-free pumice (Figure 18.40).
Step 2: Etch the teeth. If the splint is to be aesthetic, only the palatal/lingual aspect is treated and it should be the entire surface. However, if aesthetics is not a concern, spot etching the entire tooth is performed (Figure 18.41).
Step 3: Rinse and dry the dentition (Figure 18.42).
Step 4: Apply the bonding agent (Figure 18.43) and then the acrylic or composite (Figure 18.44). (There are several products[L,M] available, and the choice depends on the practitioner.) Attempt to keep the acrylic off the gingiva to allow for homecare.
Step 5: After curing, the splint is shaped and smoothed with a fine diamond bur or polishing discs (Figure 18.45). If the splint encroaches on the gingiva, this is a good time to create space.
Step 6: The occlusion is checked.
Step 7: If further smoothness is desired, a layer of unfilled resin is placed on the splint (Figures 18.46 and 18.47).

Figure-8 wiring technique

This will provide significant strength but cannot be very aesthetic.

Step 1: Thoroughly clean and polish the teeth with a fluoride-free pumice.
Step 2: Use a number 1/2 or 1 bur to create a shallow defect around the teeth (Figure 18.48a).
Step 3: Place a fine wire around the teeth in a figure-8 pattern (Figure 18.48b).
Step 4: Clip and trim the end of the wire.
Steps 2–7 as above (except that the acrylic is on the facial surface as well).

(a)

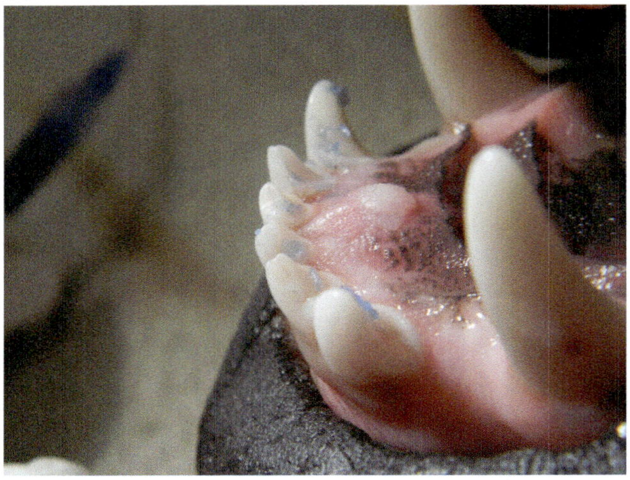

(b)

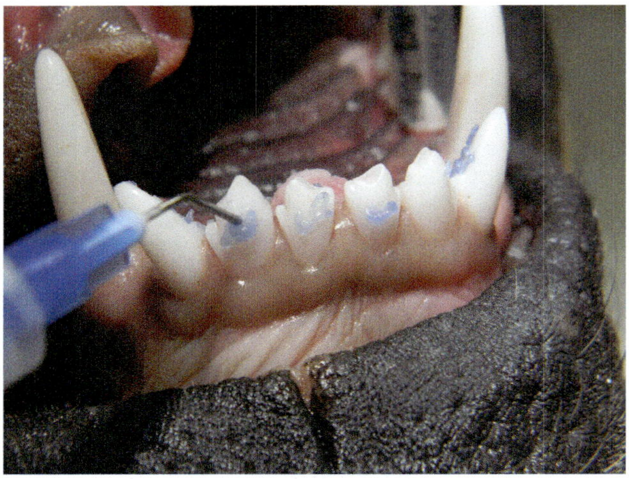

Figure 18.41 Application of the acid etch. If a cosmetic splint is planned (as in this case), only the palatal and interproximal surfaces should be etched. (a) If a circumferential splint is planned, the etch should be applied over all surfaces. (b) If unplanned surfaces are etched, placement of a bonded sealant is recommended on the involved areas.

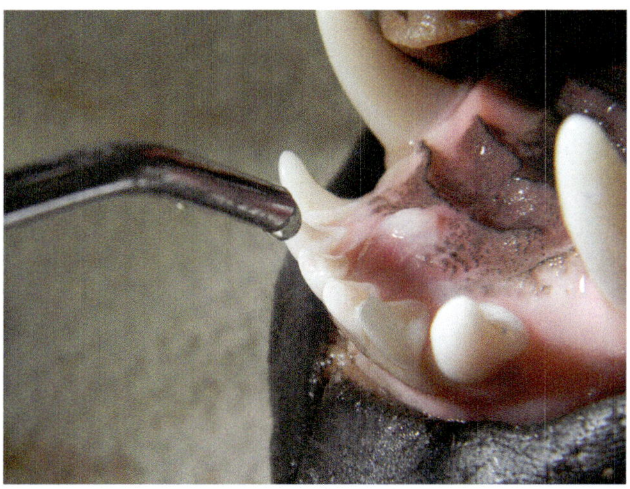

Figure 18.42 Thoroughly rinsing and drying the etch.

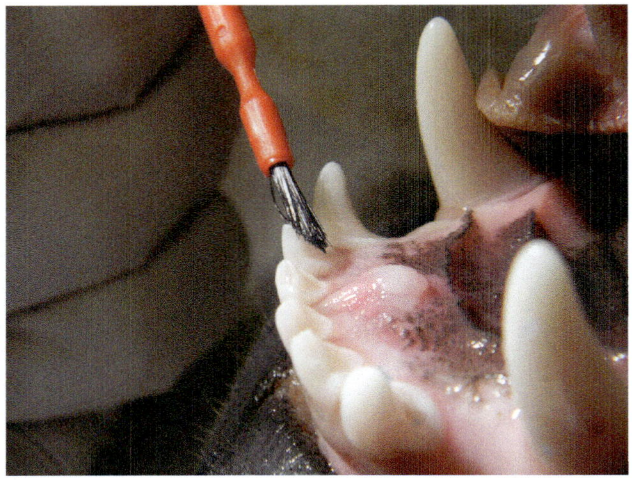

Figure 18.43 Placement of the bonding agent.

(a)

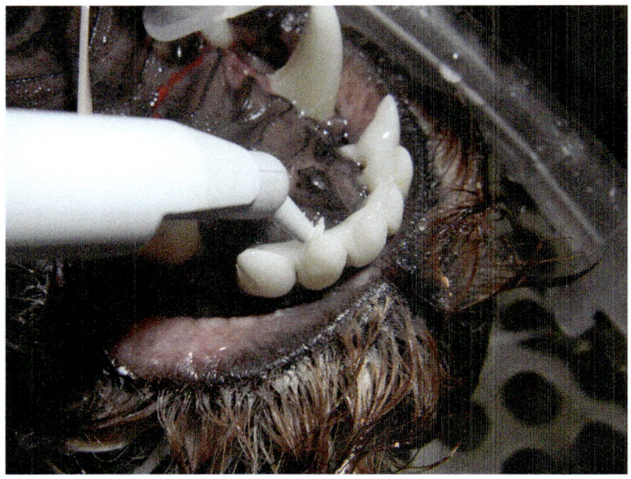

(b)

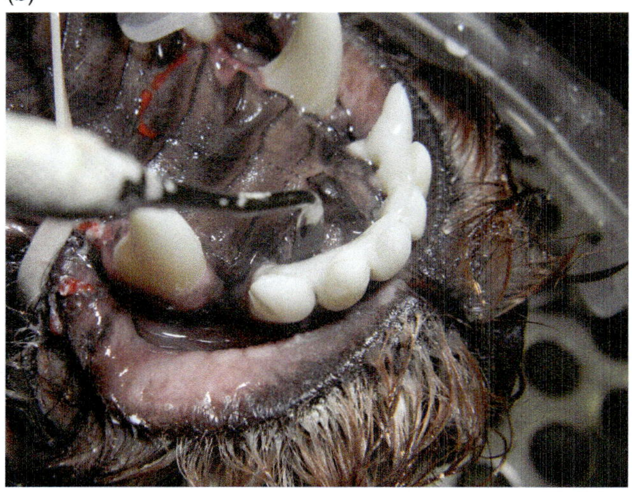

Figure 18.44 Placement and shaping of the dental composite. (a) Placement of the dental composite. (b) Shaping of the composite prior to curing with a "beaver tail." Coating the instrument with unfilled resin (bonding adhesive) will help prevent the composite sticking to the instrument during this step.

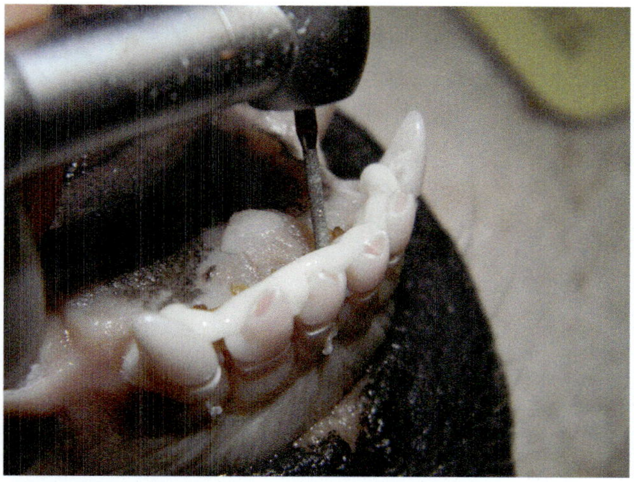

Figure 18.45 Shaping the cured composite (light curing the composite not shown) with a fine diamond bur on a water-cooled, air-driven, high-speed hand-piece.

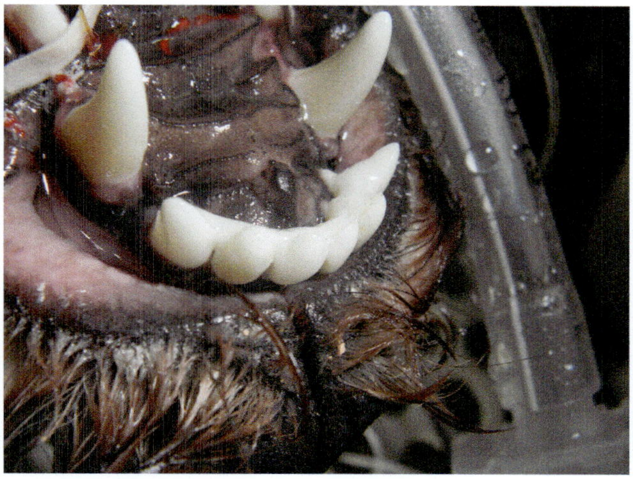

Figure 18.46 Intraoral views of the splint.

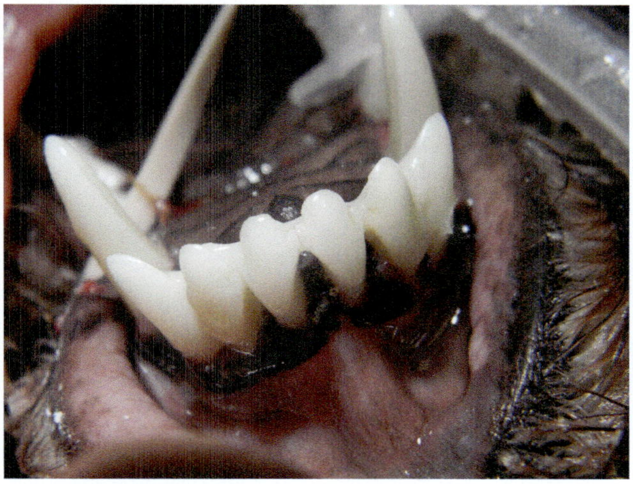

Figure 18.47 Extraoral (front) view of the splint. The splint is barely visible (compare to preoperative picture [Figure 18.40 above]).

Lingual wire technique

This is very similar to the above technique; however, only the lingual aspects are grooved (Figure 18.49a) and a wire placed in the defect (Figure 18.49b). This allows for significant strength while maintaining aesthetics.

Removal: After the healing period has occurred (approximately 6 weeks), the splint is removed. The acrylic is carefully scored and removed with extraction forceps. If necessary, a wire cutter can be used on the wires. After the acrylic (± wire) is removed, any created defects are filled with dental composite. The teeth are scaled and polished. Finally, an unfilled resin sealant is placed.

(a)

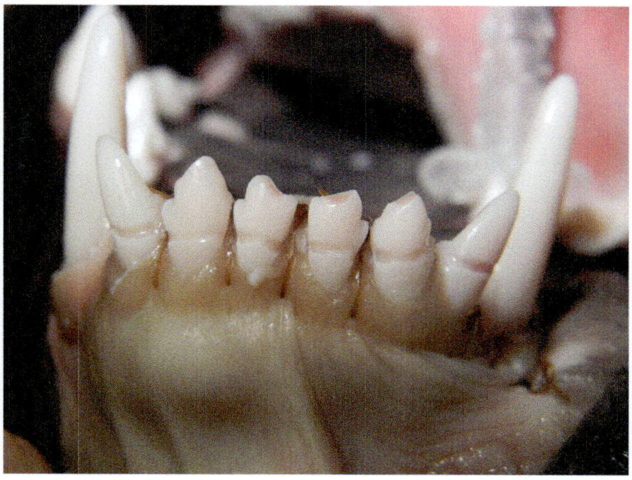

(b)

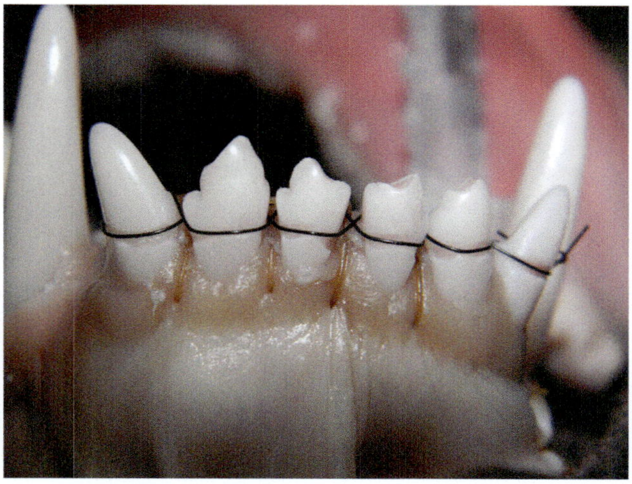

Figure 18.48 Adding a figure-8 wire to the periodontal splint. (a) Grooves have been placed circumferentially around the crowns on the teeth with a half-round bur. (b) Fine gauge wire placed figure-8 around the teeth.

(a) (b)

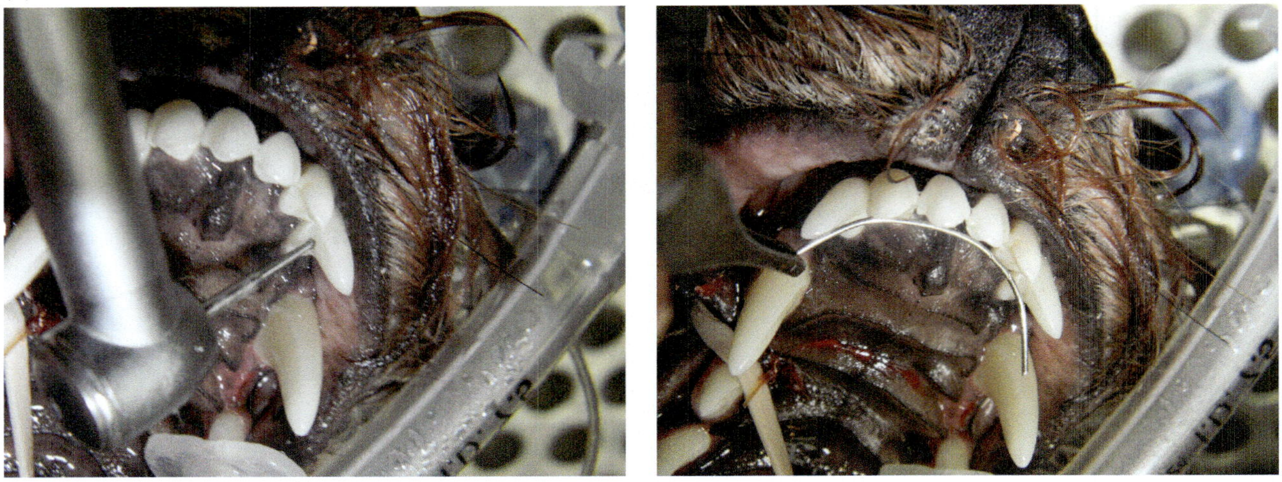

Figure 18.49 Adding a lingual/palatal bar/wire to the splint. (a) A groove is created on the lingual or palatal aspect of the teeth to be included in the splint with a number 1 round bur. (b) A wire is formed and placed in the groove.

Box 18.1 Key points

- Osseous surgery is very commonly indicated.
- In the correct presentations (i.e., 3-walled pockets), guided tissue regeneration is very effective in regaining lost attachment.
- Resective osseous surgery should be considered to reduce pocket depth in cases where regenerative techniques have a poor prognosis and sufficient bone remains.
- Second generation membranes are strongly recommended in veterinary patients.
- Bone augmentation is a rapidly changing field; the reader is encouraged to continually review the literature.
- A relatively healthy patient and motivated owner are keys to success.
- Follow-up is critical to ensure long-term maintenance.

Notes

A. GORE-TEX regenerative material, Gore-Tex.
B. OsseoQuest, Gore.
C. Bio Mend, Calcitech.
D. Bioguide, OsteoHealth.
E. Ossiflex, Veterinary Transplant Services.
F. Atrisorb, Block Drug.
G. Doxirobe, Pfizer Animal Health.
H. Osteoallograft Periomix, Veterinary Transplant Services.
I. Cerrasorb, Curasan.
J. Emdogain, Straumann AG.
K. Ribbond.
L. Maxitemp.
M. Jet Acrylic.

References

1. Sims TN, Ammons W. Resective osseous surgery. In: Carranza's Clinical Periodontology. St. Louis: Saunders, 2006, pp. 950–967.
2. Easley JR. Methods of determining alveolar osseous form. J Periodontol. 38(2):112–118, 1967.
3. Niemiec, BA. Veterinary dental radiology. In: Small Animal Dental, Oral and Maxillofacial Disease, a Color Handbook (Niemiec BA ed.). London: Manson, 2010, pp. 63–86.
4. Niemiec BA. Dental radiographic interpretation. J Vet Dent. 22(1):53–59, 2005.
5. Lyon KF, Visser CJ, Okuda A, Anthony JMG. Feline stomatitissyndrome, periodontal disease, and feline odontoclastic resorptive lesions. In: An Atlas of Veterinary Dental Radiology (DH Deforge, BH Colmery eds.). Ames: Iowa State University Press, 2000, pp. 159–170.
6. Mulligan TM, Aller MS, Williams CE. Interpretation of periodontal disease. In: Atlas of Canine and Feline Dental Radiography. Trenton, NJ: Veterinary Learning Systems, 1998, pp. 104–123.
7. Holmstrom SE, Frost PF, Eisner ER. Periodontal therapy and surgery. In: Veterinary Dental Techniques for the Small Animal Practitioner. 3rd ed. Philadelphia: Saunders, 2004, pp. 233–290.
8. Niemiec BA. Pathologies of the oral mucosa. In: Small Animal Dental, Oral and Maxillofacial Disease, a Color Handbook (Niemiec BA ed.). London: Manson, 2010, pp. 183–198.
9. Holmstrom SE, Frost P, Eisner ER. Exodontics. In: Veterinary Dental Techniques. 2nd ed. Philadelphia: Saunders, 1998, pp. 215–254.
10. Klokkevold PR, Takei HH, Carranza FA. General principles of periodontal surgery. In: Carranza's Clinical Periodontology. St. Louis: Saunders, 2006, pp. 887–901.
11. Wiggs RB, Lobprise HB. Periodontology. In: Veterinary Dentistry, Principles and Practice. Philadelphia: Lippincott-Raven, 1997, pp. 186–231.
12. Measley BL, Beybayer M, Butzin CA, et al. Use of furcal bone sounding to improve the accuracy of furcation diagnosis. J Periodontol. 65:649, 1994.

13. Carranza FA, Takei HH. Phase II periodontal therapy. In: Carranza's Clinical Periodontology. St. Louis: Saunders, 2006, pp. 881–886.
14. Kaldahl WB, Kalkwarf KL, Patil KD, Dyer JK, Bates RE Jr. Evaluation of four modalities of periodontal therapy. Mean probing depth, probing attachment level and recession changes. J Periodontol. 59(12):783–793, 1988.
15. Kaldahl WB, Kalkwarf KL, Patil KD, Molvar MP, Dyer JK. Long-term evaluation of periodontal therapy: I. Response to 4 therapeutic modalities. J Periodontol. 67(2):93–102, 1996.
16. Froum SJ, Weinberg MA, Rosenberg E, Tarnow D. A comparative study utilizing open flap debridement with and without enamel matrix derivative in the treatment of periodontal intrabony defects: A 12-month re-entry study. J Periodontol. 72(1):25–34, 2001.
17. Tibbetts L, Ochsenbein C, Loughlin D. The lingual approach to osseous surgery. J Periodontol. 20:61, 1976.
18. Ochsenbein C, Bohannan HM. The palatal approach to osseous surgery. II. Clinical application. J Periodontol. 35:54, 1964.
19. Carranza FA, Takei HH, Cochran DL. Reconstructive periodontal surgery. In: Carranza's Clinical Periodontology. St. Louis: Saunders, 2006, pp. 968–990.
20. Renvert S, Persson GR. Supportive periodontal therapy. Periodontol 2000 36:179–195, 2004.
21. Chen FM, Shelton RM, Jin Y, Chapple IL. Localized delivery of growth factors for periodontal tissue regeneration: Role, strategies, and perspectives. Med Res Rev. 29(3):472–513, 2009.
22. Chen FM, Zhang J, Zhang M, An Y, Chen F, Wu ZF. A review on endogenous regenerative technology in periodontal regenerative medicine. Biomaterials 31(31):7892–7927, 2010.
23. Needleman I, Tucker R, Giedrys-Leeper E, Worthington H. Guided tissue regeneration for periodontal intrabony defects—a Cochrane Systematic Review. Periodontol 2000 37:106–123, 2005.
24. Grzesik WJ, Narayanan AS. Cementum and periodontal wound healing and regeneration. Crit Rev Oral Biol Med. 13(6):474–484, 2002.
25. Slots J, MacDonald ES, Nowzari H, Infectious aspects of periodontal regeneration. Periodontology 2000 19:19–29, 1999.
26. Nakashima M, Reddi AH. The application of bone morphogenetic proteins to dental tissue engineering. Nat Biotechnol. 21(9):1025–1032, 2003.
27. Gottlow J, Nyman S, Lindhe J, Karring T, Wennström J. New attachment formation in the human periodontium by guided tissue regeneration. J Clin Periodontol. (6):604–616, 1986.
28. Nyman S, Gottlow J, Karring T, Lindhe J. The regenerative potential of the periodontal ligament. An experimental study in the monkey. J Clin Periodontol. 9(3):257–265, 1982.
29. Villar CC, Cochran DL. Regeneration of periodontal tissues: Guided tissue regeneration. Dent Clin North Am. 54:73–92, 2010.
30. Melcher AH. On the repair potential of periodontal tissues. J Periodontol. 47:256–260, 1976.
31. Aukhil I, Patterson E, Suggs C. Guided tissue regeneration. An experimental procedure in beagle dogs. J Periodontol. 57:7727–7734, 1986.
32. Needleman IG, Worthington HV, Giedrys-Leeper E, Tucker RJ. Guided tissue regeneration for periodontal infra-bony defects. Cochrane Database Syst Rev. 19(2), 2006.
33. Donos N, Sculean A, Glavind L, Reich E, Karring T. Wound healing of degree III furcation involvements following guided tissue regeneration and/or Emdogain. A histologic study. J Clin Periodontol. 30(12):1061–1068, 2003.
34. Murphy KG, Gunsolley JC. Guided tissue regeneration for the treatment of periodontal intrabony and furcation defects. A systematic review. Ann Periodontol. 8(1):266–302, 2003.
35. Reynolds MA, Aichelmann-Reidy ME, Branch-Mays GL, Gunsolley JC. The efficacy of bone replacement grafts in the treatment of periodontal osseous defects. A systematic review. Ann Periodontol. 8(1):227–265, 2003.
36. Sculean A, Nikolidakis D, Schwarz F. Regeneration of periodontal tissues: Combinations of barrier membranes and grafting materials—biological foundation and preclinical evidence: A systematic review. J Clin Periodontol. 35(8 Suppl):106–116, 2008.
37. Stavropoulos A, Karring T. Guided tissue regeneration combined with a deproteinized bovine bone mineral (Bio-Oss) in the treatment of intrabony periodontal defects: 6-year results from a randomized-controlled clinical trial. J Clin Periodontol. 37(2):200–210, 2010.
38. Nabers JM, Meador HL, Nabers CL, et al. Chronology, an important factor in the repair of osseous defects. Periodontics 2:304, 1964.
39. Debowes LJ. Problems with the gingiva. In: Small Animal Dental, Oral and Maxillofacial Disease, a Color Handbook (Niemiec BA ed.). London: Manson, 2010, pp. 159–181.
40. Caton J, Wagener C, Polson A, et al. Guided tissue regeneration in interproximal defects in the monkey. Int J Periodontics Restorative Dent. 12(4):266–277, 1992.
41. Claffey N, Hahn R, Egelberg J. Effect of placement of occlusive membranes on root resorption and bone regeneration during healing of circumferential periodontal defects in dogs. J Clin Periodontol. 16(6):371–379, 1989.
42. Minabe M. A critical review of the biologic rationale for guided tissue regeneration J Periodontol. 62(3):171–179, 1991.
43. Stahl SS, Froum S. Histologic healing responses in human vertical lesions following the use of osseous allografts and barrier membranes. J Clin Periodontol. 18(2):149–152, 1991.
44. Stahl SS, Froum S, Tarnow D. Human histologic responses to guided tissue regenerative techniques in intrabony lesions. Case reports on 9 sites. Clin Periodontol. 17(3):191–198, 1990.
45. Taba M Jr, Jin Q, Sugai JV, Giannobile WV. Current concepts in periodontal bioengineering. Orthod Craniofac Res. 8(4):292–302, 2005.
46. Pontoriero R, Lindhe J, Nyman S, et al. Guided tissue regeneration in degree II furcation-involved mandibular molars. A clinical study. J Clin Periodontol. 15(4):247–254, 1988.
47. Lekovic V, Kenney EB, Kovacevic K, Carranza FA Jr. Evaluation of guided tissue regeneration in Class II furcation defects. A clinical re-entry study. J Periodontol. 60(12):694–698, 1989.
48. Bottino MC, Thomas V, Janowski GM. A novel spatially designed and functionally graded electrospun membrane for periodontal regeneration Acta Biomater. 2010 Aug. 27. [Epub ahead of print.]
49. Zybutz MD, Laurell L, Rapoport DA, Persson GR. Treatment of intrabony defects with resorbable materials, non-resorbable materials and flap debridement. J Clin Periodontol. 27(3):169–178, 2000.
50. Teparat T, Solt CW, Claman LJ, Beck FM. Clinical comparison of bioabsorbable barriers with non-resorbable barriers in guided tissue regeneration in the treatment of human intrabony defects. J Periodontol. 69(6):632–641, 1998.
51. Hou LT, Yan JJ, Tsai AY, Lao CS, Lin SJ, Liu CM. Polymer-assisted regeneration therapy with Atrisorb barriers in human periodontal intrabony defects. J Clin Periodontol. 31(1):68–74, 2004.
52. Sakallioglu U, Yavuz U, Lütfioglu M, Keskiner I, Acikgöz G. Clinical outcomes of guided tissue regeneration with Atrisorb membrane in the treatment of intrabony defects: A 3-year follow-up study. Int J Periodontics Restorative Dent. 27(1):79–88, 2007.
53. Polimeni G, Koo KT, Pringle GA, Agelan A, Safadi FF, Wikesjö UM. Histopathological observations of a polylactic acid-based

device intended for guided bone/tissue regeneration. Clin Implant Dent Relat Res. 10(2):99–105, 2008.

54. Tatakis DN, Trombelli L. Adverse effects associated with a bioabsorbable guided tissue regeneration device in the treatment of human gingival recession defects. A clinicopathologic case report. J Periodontol. 70(5):542–547, 1999.
55. Froum SJ, Ortiz M, Witkin RT, Thaler R, Scopp IW, Stahl SS. Osseous autografts. III. Comparison of osseous coagulum-bone blend implants with open curetage. J Periodontol. 47(5):287–294, 1976.
56. Meadows CL, Gher ME, Quintero G, Lafferty TA. A comparison of polylactic acid granules and decalcified freeze-dried bone allograft in human periodontal osseous defects. J Periodontol. 64(2):103–109, 1993.
57. Masters LB, Mellonig JT, Brunsvold MA, Nummikoski PV. A clinical evaluation of demineralized freeze-dried bone allograft in combination with tetracycline in the treatment of periodontal osseous defects. J Periodontol. 67(8):770–781, 1996.
58. Yukna RA, Harrison BG, Caudill RF, Evans GH, Mayer ET, Miller S. Evaluation of durapatite ceramic as an alloplastic implant in periodontal osseous defects. II. Twelve month reentry results. J Periodontol. 56(9):540–547, 1985.
59. Yukna RA, Callan DP, Krauser JT, et al. Multi-center clinical evaluation of combination anorganic bovine-derived hydroxyapatite matrix (ABM)/cell binding peptide (P-15) as a bone replacement graft material in human periodontal osseous defects. 6-month results. J Periodontol. 69(6):655–663, 1998.
60. Meffert RM, Thomas JR, Hamilton KM, Brownstein CN. Hydroxylapatite as an alloplastic graft in the treatment of human periodontal osseous defects. J Periodontol. 56(2):63–73, 1985.
61. Kim CK, Choi EJ, Cho KS, Chai JK, Wikesjö UM. Periodontal repair in intrabony defects treated with a calcium carbonate implant and guided tissue regeneration. J Periodontol. 67(12):1301–1306, 1996.
62. Yukna RA. Clinical evaluation of coralline calcium carbonate as a bone replacement graft material in human periodontal osseous defects. J Periodontol. 65(2):177–185, 1994.
63. Rosenberg ES, Fox GK, Cohen C. Bioactive glass granules for regeneration of human periodontal defects. J Esthet Dent. 12(5):248–257, 2000.
64. Yukna RA. HTR polymer grafts in human periodontal osseous defects. I. 6-month clinical results. J Periodontol. 61(10):633–642, 1990.
65. Brown GD, Mealey BL, Nummikoski PV, Bifano SL, Waldrop TC. Hydroxyapatite cement implant for regeneration of periodontal osseous defects in humans. J Periodontol. 69(2):146–157, 1998.
66. Pepelassi EM, Bissada NF, Greenwell H, Farah CF. Doxycycline-tricalcium phosphate composite graft facilitates osseous healing in advanced periodontal furcation defects. J Periodontol. 62(2):106–115, 1991.
67. Kenney EB, Lekovic V, Elbaz JJ, et al. The use of a porous hydroxylapatite implant in periodontal defects. II. Treatment of class II furcation lesions in lower molars. J Periodontol. 59(2):67–72, 1988.
68. Garrett S, Gantes B, Zimmerman G, Egelberg J. Treatment of mandibular class III periodontal furcation defects. Coronally positioned flaps with and without expanded polytetrafluoroethylene membranes. J Periodontol. 65(6):592–597, 1994.
69. Calongne KB, Aichelmann-Reidy ME, Yukna RA, Mayer ET. Clinical comparison of microporous biocompatible composite of PMMA, PHEMA and calcium hydroxide grafts and expanded polytetrafluoroethylene barrier membranes in human mandibular molar Class II furcations. A case series. J Periodontol. 72(10):1451–1459, 2001.
70. Hall EE, Meffert RM, Hermann JS, Mellonig JT, Cochran DL. Comparison of bioactive glass to demineralized freeze-dried bone allograft in the treatment of intrabony defects around implants in the canine mandible. J Periodontol. 70:526–535, 1999.
71. Mellonig JT. Bone allografts in periodontal therapy. Clinical Orthopaedics Related Res. 324:116–125, 1996.
72. Bauer TW. An overview of the histology of skeletal substitute materials. Arch Pathol Lab Med. 131:217–224, 2007.
73. Greenwald AS, Boden SD, Goldberg VM, Khan Y, Laurencin CT, Rosier RN. Bone-graft substitutes: Facts, fictions, and applications. J Bone Joint Surg. 83-A(Supp 2), 2001.
74. Reynolds MA, Aichelmann-Reidy ME, Branch-Mays GL. Regeneration of periodontal tissue: Bone replacement grafts. Dent Clin North Am. 54:55–71, 2010.
75. Mellonig JT. Freeze-dried bone allografts in periodontal reconstructive surgery. Rec Periodont. 35(3):505–521, 1991.
76. Grauer JN, Beiner JM, Kwon K, Vaccaro AR. Bone graft alternatives for spinal fusion. Biodrugs 17(6), 2003.
77. Brandoff JF, Silber JS, Vaccaro AR. Contemporary alternatives to synthetic bone grafts for spine surgery. Am J Orthop. 37(8):410–414, 2008.
78. Shigeyama Y, D'Errico JA, Stone R, Somerman MJ. Commercially-prepared allograft material has biological activity in vitro. J Periodontol. 66(6):478–487, 1995.
79. Bowers GM, Chadroff B, Carnevale R, et al. Histologic evaluation of new attachment apparatus formation in humans. Part III. J Periodontol. 60(12):683–693, 1989.
80. Bowers GM, Chadroff B, Carnevale R, et al. Histologic evaluation of new attachment apparatus formation in humans. Part II. J Periodontol. 60(12):675–682, 1989.
81. Bowers G, Felton F, Middleton C, et al. Histologic comparison of regeneration in human intrabony defects when osteogenin is combined with demineralized freeze-dried bone allograft and with purified bovine collagen. J Periodontol. 62(11):690–702, 1991.
82. Sampath T, Reddi H. Homology of bone inductive-proteins from human, monkey, bovine, and rat extracellular matrix. Proc. Natl. Acad. Sci. USA 80:6591, 1983.
83. Nevins ML, Camelo M, Lynch SE, et al. Evaluation of periodontal regeneration following grafting intrabony defects with Bio-Oss collagen: A human histologic report. Int J Periodontics Restorative Dent. 23(1):9–17, 2003.
84. Camelo M, Nevins ML, Schenk RK, et al. Clinical, radiographic, and histologic evaluation of human periodontal defects treated with Bio-Oss and Bio-Gide. Int J Periodontics Restorative Dent. 18(4):321–331, 1998.
85. Ong MM, Eber RM, Korsnes MI, et al. Evaluation of a bioactive glass alloplast in treating periodontal intrabony defects. J Periodontol. 69(12):1346–1354, 1998.
86. Barnett JD, Mellonig JT, Gray JL, Towle HJ. Comparison of freeze-dried bone allograft and porous hydroxylapatite in human periodontal defects. J Periodontol. 60(5):231–237, 1989.
87. Bowen JA, Mellonig JT, Gray JL, Towle HT. Comparison of decalcified freeze-dried bone allograft and porous particulate hydroxyapatite in human periodontal osseous defects. J Periodontol. 60(12):647–654, 1989.
88. Oreamuno S, Lekovic V, Kenney EB. Comparative clinical study of porous hydroxyapatite and decalcified freeze-dried bone in human periodontal defects. J Periodontol. 61(7):399–404, 1990.
89. Richardson CR, Mellonig JT, Brunsvold MA, McDonnell HT, Cochran DL. Clinical evaluation of Bio-Oss: A bovine-derived xenograft for the treatment of periodontal osseous defects in humans. J Clin Periodontol. 26(7):421–428, 1999.

90. Välimäki VV, Aro HT. Molecular basis for action of bioactive glasses as bone graft substitute. Scand J Surg. 95(2):95–102, 2006.
91. Thomas MV, Puleo DA, Al-Sabbagh M. Bioactive glass three decades on. J Long Term Eff Med Implants. 15(6):585–597, 2005.
92. Sculean A, Windisch P, Keglevich T, Gera I. Clinical and histologic evaluation of an enamel matrix protein derivative combined with a bioactive glass for the treatment of intrabony periodontal defects in humans. Int J Periodontics Restorative Dent. 25(2):139–147, 2005.
93. Baas J, Elmengaard B, Bechtold J, Chen X, Soballe K. Ceramic bone graft substitute with equine bone protein extract is comparable to allograft in terms of implant fixation. Acta Orthopaedica. 79(6):841–850, 2008.
94. Orsini M, Orsini G, Benlloch D, Aranda JJ, Sanz M. Long-term clinical results on the use of bone-replacement grafts in the treatment of intrabony periodontal defects. Comparison of the use of autogenous bone graft plus calcium sulfate toautogenous bone graft covered with a bioabsorbable membrane. J Periodontol. 79(9):1630–1637, 2008.
95. Sukumar S, Drizhal I, Paulusová V, Bukac J. Surgical treatment of periodontal intrabony defects with calcium sulphate in combination with beta-tricalciumphosphate: Clinical observations two years post-surgery. Acta Medica (Hradec Kralove) 54(1):13–20, 2011.
96. Choi JY, Jung UW, Lee IS, Kim CS, Lee YK, Choi SH. Resolution of surgically created three-wall intrabony defects in implants using three different biomaterials: An in vivo study. Clin Oral Implants Res. 2010 Sep. 10.
97. Xu LL, Liu HC, Wang DS, E LL, Xu L, Jin ZL, Duan YZ. Effects of BMP-2 and dexamethasone on osteogenic differentiation of rat dental follicle progenitor cells seeded on three-dimensional beta-TCP. Biomed Mater. 4(6):065010, 2009.
98. Zijderveld SA, Zerbo IR, van den Bergh JP, Schulten EA, ten Bruggenkate CM. Maxillary sinus floor augmentation using a beta-tricalcium phosphate (Cerasorb) alone compared to autogenous bone grafts. Int J Oral Maxillofac Implants 20(3):432–440, 2005.
99. Szabó G, Huys L, Coulthard P, Maiorana C, Garagiola U, Barabás J, Németh Z, Hrabák K, Suba Z. A prospective multicenter randomized clinical trial of autogenous bone versus beta-tricalcium phosphate graft alone for bilateral sinus elevation: Histologic and histomorphometric evaluation. Int J Oral Maxillofac Implants 20(3):371–381, 2005.
100. Giannobile WV. Periodontal tissue engineering by growth factors. Bone 19(1 Suppl):23S–37S, 1996.
101. Sipe JD, Kelley CA, McNichol LA. Reparative medicine: Growing tissue and organs. Ann NY Acad Sci. 961, 2002.
102. Aukhil I. The potential contributions of cell and molecular biology to periodontal tissue regeneration. Curr Opin Dent. 2:91–96, 1992.
103. Urist MR. Bone: Formation by autoinduction. Science 150:893–899, 1965.
104. Elangovan S, Srinivasan S, Ayilavarapu S. Novel regenerative strategies to enhance periodontal therapy outcome. Expert Opin Biol Ther. 9(4):399–410, 2009.
105. Chen FM, Jin Y. Periodontal tissue engineering and regeneration: current approaches and expanding opportunities. Tissue Eng Part B Rev. 16(2):219–55, 2010.
106. Vasita R, Katti DS. Growth factor-delivery systems for tissue engineering: A materials perspective. Expert Rev Med Devices 3:29–47, 2006.
107. Hughes FJ, Turner W, Belibasakis G, Martuscelli G. Effects of growth factors and cytokines on osteoblast differentiation. Periodontol 2000 41:48–72, 2006.
108. Varkey M, Gittens SA, Uludag H. Growth factor delivery for bone tissue repair: An update. Expert Opin Drug Deliv. 1:19–36, 2004.
109. Kaigler D, Cirelli JA, Giannobile WV. Growth factor delivery for oral and periodontal tissue engineering. Expert Opin Drug Deliv. 3:647–662, 2006.
110. Cochran DL, Wozney JM. Biological mediators for periodontal regeneration. Periodontol 2000 19:40–58, 1999.
111. Hakki SS, Foster BL, Nagatomo KJ, et al. Bone morphogenetic protein-7 enhances cementoblast function, in vitro. J Periodontol. 2010 Aug. 3. [Epub ahead of print.]
112. Zhu M, Zeng Y, Sun T, Peng Q. [Experimental study of the effect of new bone formation on new type artificial bone composed of bioactive ceramics.] Zhongguo Xiu Fu Chong Jian Wai Ke Za Zhi. 19(3):174–177, 2005.
113. Lyngstadaas SP, Lundberg E, Ekdahl H, Andersson C, Gestrelius S. Autocrine growth factors in human periodontal ligament cells cultured on enamel matrix derivative. J Clin Periodontol. 28:181–188, 2001.
114. Esposito M, Coulthard P, Thomsen P, Worthington HV. Enamel matrix derivative for periodontal tissue regeneration in treatment of intrabony defects: A Cochrane Systematic Review. J Dent Educ. 68:834–844, 2004.
115. Sakallioglu U, Acikgöz G, Ayas B, Kirtilolu T, Sakallioglu E. Healing of periodontal defects treated with enamel matrix proteins and root surface conditioning—an experimental study in dogs. Biomaterials 25(10):1831–1840, 2004.
116. Hammarström L. Enamel matrix, cementum development and regeneration. J Clin Periodontol. 24:658–668, 1997.
117. Spahr A, Hammarström L. Response of dental follicular cells to the exposure of denuded enamel matrix in rat molars. Eur J Oral Sci. 107:360–367, 1999.
118. Sculean A, Schwarz F, Becker J, Brecx M. The application of an enamel matrix protein derivative (Emdogain) in regenerative periodontal therapy: A review. Med Princ Pract. 16:167–80, 2007.
119. Sculean A, Windisch P, Döri F, Keglevich T, Molnér B, Gera I. Emdogain in regenerative periodontal therapy. A review of the literature. Fogorv Sz. 100:220–232, 2007.
120. Yuan K, Chen CL, Lin MT. Enamel matrix derivative exhibits angiogenic effect in vitro and in a murine model. J Clin Periodontol. 30:732–738, 2003.
121. Sculean A, Auschill TM, Donos N, Brecx M, Arweiler NB. Effect of an enamel matrix protein derivative (Emdogain) on ex vivo dental plaque vitality. J Clin Periodontol. 28:1074–1078, 2001.
122. Rathe F, Junker R, Chesnutt BM, Jansen JA. The effect of enamel matrix derivative (Emdogain) on bone formation: A systematic review. Tissue Eng Part B Rev. 15:215–224, 2009.
123. Giannobile WV, Somerman MJ. Growth and amelogenin-like factors in periodontal wound healing. A systematic review. Ann Periodontol. 8(1):193–204, 2003.
124. Heden G, Wennstrom JL. Five-year follow-up of regenerative periodontal therapy with enamel matrix derivative at sites with angular bone defects. J Periodontol. 77:295–301, 2006.
125. Sculean A, Donos N, Miliauskaite A, Arweiler N, Brecx M. Treatment of intrabony defects with enamel matrix proteins or bioresorbable membranes: A four-year followup split-mouth study. J Periodontol. 72:1695–1701, 2001.
126. Saito A, Nanbu Y, Nagahata T, Yamada S. Treatment of intrabony periodontal defects with enamel matrix derivative in private practice: A long-term retrospective study. Bull Tokyo Dent Coll. 49:89–96, 2008.
127. Hirooka H. The biologic concept for the use of enamel matrix protein: True periodontal regeneration. Quintessence Int 29:621–30, 1998.

128. Cochran DL, Jones A, Heijl L, Mellonig JT, Schoolfield J, King GN. Periodontal regeneration with a combination of enamel matrix proteins and autogenous bone grafting. J Periodontol. 74(9):1269–1281, 2003.
129. Sculean A, Donos N, Brecx M, Reich E, Karring T. Treatment of intrabony defects with guided tissue regeneration andenamel-matrix-proteins. An experimental study in monkeys. J Clin Periodontol. 27(7):466–472, 2000.
130. Cochran DL, King GN, Schoolfield J, Velasquez-Plata D, Mellonig JT, Jones A. The effect of enamel matrix proteins on periodontal regeneration as determined by histological analyses. J Periodontol. 74(7):1043–1055, 2003.
131. Windisch P, Sculean A, Klein F, Tóth V, Gera I, Reich E, Eickholz P. Comparison of clinical, radiographic, and histometric measurements following treatment with guided tissue regeneration or enamel matrix proteins in human periodontal defects. J Periodontol. 73(4):409–417, 2002.
132. Sculean A, Donos N, Blaes A, Lauermann M, Reich E, Brecx M. Comparison of enamel matrix proteins and bioabsorbable membranes in the treatmentof intrabony periodontal defects. A split-mouth study. J Periodontol. 70(3):255–262, 1999.
133. Chen FM, Zhang M, Wu ZF. Toward delivery of multiple growth factors in tissue engineering. Biomaterials 31:6279–6308, 2010.
134. Takahashi D, Odajima T, Morita M, Kawanami M, Kato H. Formation and resolution of ankylosis under application of recombinant human bone morphogenetic protein-2 (rhBMP-2) to class III furcation defects in cats. J Periodontal Res. 40:299–305, 2005.
135. Cooke JW, Sarment DP, Whitesman LA, Miller SE, Jin Q, Lynch SE, et al. Effect of rhPDGF-BB delivery on mediators of periodontal wound repair. Tissue Eng. 12:1441–1450, 2006.
136. Chen FM, Wu ZF, Sun HH, Wu H, Xin SN, Wang QT, et al. Release of bioactive BMP from dextran-derived microspheres: A novel delivery concept. Int J Pharm. 307:23–32, 2006.
137. Saito A, Saito E, Handa R, Honma Y, Kawanami M. Influence of residual bone on recombinant human bone morphogenetic protein-2-induced periodontal regeneration in experimental periodontitis in dogs. J Periodontol. 80:961–968, 2009.
138. Hosokawa R, Kikuzaki K, Kimoto T, Matsuura T, Chiba D, Wadamoto M, et al. Controlled local application of basic fibroblast growth factor (FGF-2) accelerates the healing of GBR. An experimental study in beagle dogs. Clin Oral Implants Res. 11:345–353, 2000.
139. Gruber RM, Ludwig A, Merten HA, Pippig S, Kramer FJ, Schliephake H. Sinus floor augmentation with recombinant human growth and differentiation factor-5 (rhGDF-5): A pilot study in the Goettingen miniature pig comparing autogenous bone and rhGDF-5. Clin Oral Implants Res. 20(2):175–182, 2009.
140. Lee JS, Wikesjö UM, Jung UW, Choi SH, Pippig S, Siedler M, Kim CK. Periodontal wound healing/regeneration following implantation of recombinant human growth/differentiation factor-5 in a beta-tricalcium phosphate carrier into one-wall intrabony defects in dogs. J Clin Periodontol. 37(4):382–389, 2010.
141. Wikesjö UM, Sorensen RG, Kinoshita A, Jian Li X, Wozney JM. Periodontal repair in dogs: effect of recombinant human bone morphogeneticprotein-12 (rhBMP-12) on regeneration of alveolar bone and periodontal attachment. J Clin Periodontol. 31(8):662–670, 2004.
142. Chen YL, Chen PK, Jeng LB, Huang CS, Yang LC, Chung HY, Chang SC. Periodontal regeneration using ex vivo autologous stem cells engineered to express the BMP-2 gene: An alternative to alveolaplasty. Gene Ther. 15(22):1469–1477, 2008.
143. Ripamonti U, Heliotis M, Rueger DC, Sampath TK. Induction of cementogenesis by recombinant human osteogenic protein-1 (hop-1/bmp-7) in the baboon (Papio ursinus). Arch Oral Biol. 41(1):121–126, 1996.
144. Ripamonti U, Renton L. Bone morphogenetic proteins and the induction of periodontal tissue regeneration. Periodontol 2000 41:73–87, 2006.
145. Blumenthal NM, Koh-Kunst G, Alves ME, et al. Effect of surgical implantation of recombinant human bone morphogenetic protein-2 in a bioabsorbable collagen sponge or calcium phosphate putty carrier in intrabony periodontal defects in the baboon. J Periodontol. 73(12):1494–1506, 2002.
146. Sorensen RG, Wikesjö UM, Kinoshita A, Wozney JM. Periodontal repair in dogs: Evaluation of a bioresorbable calcium phosphate cement (Ceredex) as a carrier for rhBMP-2. J Clin Periodontol. 31(9):796–804, 2004.
147. Sorensen RG, Polimeni G, Kinoshita A, Wozney JM, Wikesjö UM. Effect of recombinant human bone morphogenetic protein-12 (rhBMP-12) on regeneration of periodontal attachment following tooth replantation in dogs. J Clin Periodontol. 31(8):654–661, 2004.
148. Shimabukuro Y, Terashima H, Takedachi M, Maeda K, et al. Fibroblast growth factor-2 stimulates directed migration of periodontal ligament cells via PI3K/AKT signaling and CD44/Hyaluronan interaction. J Cell Physiol. 2010 Sep 20.
149. Lee J, Stavropoulos A, Susin C, Wikesjö UM. Periodontal regeneration: Focus on growth and differentiation factors. Dent Clin North Am. 54:93–111, 2010.
150. Rossa C Jr, Marcantonio E Jr, Cirelli JA, et al. Regeneration of class III furcation defects with basic fibroblast growth factor (b-FGF) associated with GTR. A descriptive and histometric study in dogs. J Periodontol. 71(5):775–784, 2000.
151. Takayama S, Murakami S, Shimabukuro Y, Kitamura M, Okada H. Periodontal regeneration by FGF-2 (bFGF) in primate models. J Dent Res. 80(12):2075–2079, 2001.
152. Giannobile WV, Hernandez RA, Finkelman RD, Ryan S, Kiritsy CP, D'Andrea M, et al. Comparative effects of platelet-derived growth factor-BB and insulin-like growth factor-I, individually and in combination, on periodontal regeneration in Macaca fascicularis. J Periodontal Res. 31:301–312, 1996.
153. Chen FM, Zhao YM, Wu H, et al. Enhancement of periodontal tissue regeneration by locally controlled delivery of insulin-like growth factor-I from dextran-co-gelatin microspheres. J Control Release 114(2):209–222, 2006.
154. Saygin NE, Tokiyasu Y, Giannobile WV, Somerman MJ. Growth factors regulate expression of mineral associated genes in cementoblasts. J Periodontol. 71:1591–1600, 2000.
155. Mohammed S, Pack AR, Kardos TB. The effect of transforming growth factor beta one (TGF-beta 1) on wound healing, with or without barrier membranes, in a class II furcation defect in sheep. J Periodontal Res. 33(6):335–344, 1998.
156. Murakami S, Takayama S, Ikezawa K, Shimabukuro Y, Kitamura M, Nozaki T, et al. Regeneration of periodontal tissues by basic fibroblast growth factor. J Periodontal Res. 34:425–430, 1999.
157. Graham S, Leonidou A, Lester M, Heliotis M, Mantalaris A, Tsiridis E. Investigating the role of PDGF as a potential drug therapy in bone formation and fracture healing. Expert Opin Investig Drugs 18(11):1633–1654, 2009.
158. Lee YM, Park YJ, Lee SJ, Ku Y, Han SB, Klokkevold PR, Chung CP. The bone regenerative effect of platelet-derived growth factor-BB delivered with a chitosan/tricalcium phosphate sponge carrier. J Periodontol. 71(3):418–424, 2000.

159. Park YJ, Lee YM, Park SN, Sheen SY, Chung CP, Lee SJ. Platelet derived growth factor releasing chitosan sponge for periodontal bone regeneration. Biomaterials 21(2):153–159, 2000.
160. Park YJ, Ku Y, Chung CP, Lee SJ. Controlled release of platelet-derived growth factor from porous poly(L-lactide) membranes for guided tissue regeneration. J Control Release 51(2–3):201–211, 1998.
161. Nevins M, Giannobile WV, McGuire MK, Kao RT, et al. Platelet-derived growth factor stimulates bone fill and rate of attachment level gain: Results of a large multicenter randomized controlled trial. J Periodontol. 76(12):2205–2215, 2005.
162. Anusaksathien O, Webb SA, Jin QM, Giannobile WV. Platelet derived growth factor gene delivery stimulates ex vivo gingival repair. Tissue Eng. 9:745–756, 2003.
163. Jin Q, Anusaksathien O, Webb SA, Printz MA, Giannobile WV. Engineering of tooth-supporting structures by delivery of PDGF gene therapy vectors. Mol Ther. 9:519–526, 2004.
164. Anusaksathien O, Jin Q, Zhao M, Somerman MJ, Giannobile WV. Effect of sustained gene delivery of platelet-derived growth factor or its antagonist (PDGF-1308) on tissue-engineered cementum. J Periodontol. 75:429–440, 2004.
165. Nevins M, Camelo M, Nevins ML, Schenk RK, Lynch SE. Periodontal regeneration in humans using recombinant human platelet-derived growth factor-BB (rhPDGF-BB) and allogenic bone. J Periodontol. 74(9):1282–1292, 2003.
166. Camargo PM, Lekovic V, Weinlaender M, Vasilic N, Madzarevic M, Kenney EB. Platelet-rich plasma and bovine porous bone mineral combined with guided tissue regeneration in the treatment of intrabony defects in humans. J Periodontal Res. 37(4):300–306, 2002.
167. Anitua E, Sánchez M, Orive G, Andia I. The potential impact of the preparation rich in growth factors (PRGF) in different medical fields. Biomaterials 28:4551–4560, 2007.
168. Anitua E, Sánchez M, Nurden AT, Nurden P, Orive G, Andia I. New insights into and novel applications for platelet-rich fibrin therapies. Trends Biotechnol. 24:22734, 2006.
169. Anitua E, Sánchez M, Orive G, Andia I. Delivering growth factors for therapeutics. Trends Pharmacol Sci. 29:37–41, 2008.
170. Knighton DR, Ciresi K, Fiegel VD, Schumerth S, Butler E, Cerra F. Stimulation of repair in chronic, non healing, cutaneous ulcers using platelet-derived wound healing formula. Surg Gynecol Obstet. 170:56–60, 1990.
171. Mehta S, Watson JT. Platelet rich concentrate: Basic science and current clinical applications. J Orthop Trauma 22:432–438, 2008.
172. Foster TE, Puskas BL, Mandelbaum BR, Gerhardt MB, Rodeo SA. Platelet-rich plasma: From basic science to clinical applications. Am J Sports Med. 37:2259–2272, 2009.
173. Lekovic V, Camargo PM, Weinlaender M, Vasilic N, Kenney EB. Comparison of platelet-rich plasma, bovine porous bone mineral, and guided tissue regeneration versus platelet-rich plasma and bovine porous bone mineral in the treatment of intrabony defects: A reentry study. J Periodontol. 73(2):198–205, 2002.
174. Camargo PM, Lekovic V, Weinlaender M. A surgical reentry study on the influence of platelet-rich plasma in enhancing the regenerative effects of bovine porous bone mineral and guided tissue regeneration in the treatment of intrabony defects in humans. J Periodontol. 80(6):915–923, 2009.
175. McKay MS, Olson E, Hesla MA, Panyutich A, Ganz T, Perkins S et al. Immunomagnetic recovery of human neutrophil defensins from the human gingival crevice. Oral Microbiol Immunol. 14:190–193.
176. Folkman J, Klagsbrun M. Angiogenic factors. Science 235:442–447, 1987.
177. Fang J, Zhu YY, Smiley E, Bonadio J, Rouleau JP, Goldstein SA, et al. Stimulation of new bone formation by direct transfer of osteogenic plasmid genes. Proc Natl Acad Sci USA 93:5753–5758, 1996.
178. Lu L, Zhu X, Valenzuela RG, Currier BL, Yaszemski MJ. Biodegradable polymer scaffolds for cartilage tissue engineering. Clin Orthop. 391(Suppl):S251–270, 2001.
179. King GN. The importance of drug delivery to optimize the effects of bone morphogenetic proteins during periodontal regeneration. Curr Pharm Biotechnol. 2(2):131–142, 2001.
180. Whang K, Tsai DC, Nam EK, Aitken M, Sprague SM, Patel PK, et al. Ectopic bone formation via rhBMP-2 delivery from porous bioabsorbable polymer scaffolds. J Biomed Mater Res. 42:491–499, 1998.
181. Fournier N, Doillon CJ. Biological molecule-impregnated polyester: An in vivo angiogenesis study. Biomaterials 17:1659–1665, 1996.
182. Wei G, Pettway GJ, McCauley LK, Ma PX. The release profiles and bioactivity of parathyroid hormone from poly(lactic-co-glycolic acid) microspheres. Biomaterials 25:345–352, 2004.
183. Murphy WL, Peters MC, Kohn DH, Mooney DJ. Sustained release of vascular endothelial growth factor from mineralized poly(lactide-co-glycolide) scaffolds for tissue engineering. Biomaterials 21:2521–2527, 2000.
184. Wallace DG, Rosenblatt J, Collagen gel systems for sustained delivery and tissue engineering. Adv Drug Deliv Rev. 55(12):1631–1649, 2003.
185. Chen FM, Zhao YM, Sun HH, et al. Novel glycidyl methacrylated dextran (Dex-GMA)/gelatin hydrogel scaffolds containing microspheres loaded with bone morphogenetic proteins: formulation and characteristics. J Control Release 118(1):65–77, 2007.
186. Sohier J, Vlugt TJ, Cabrol N, et al. Dual release of proteins from porous polymeric scaffolds. J Control Release 111(1–2):95–106, 2006.
187. Lin CC, Metters AT. Bifunctional monolithic affinity hydrogels for dual-protein delivery. Biomacromolecules 9(3):789–795, 2008.
188. Andreadis ST, Geer DJ. Biomimetic approaches to protein and gene delivery for tissue regeneration. Trends Biotechnol. 24(7):331–337, 2006.
189. Luginbuehl V, Meinel L, Merkle HP, Gander B. Localized delivery of growth factors for bone repair. Eur J Pharm Biopharm. 58(2):197–208, 2004.
190. Jin QM, Anusaksathien O, Webb SA, Rutherford RB, Giannobile WV. Gene therapy of bone morphogenetic protein for periodontal tissue engineering. J Periodontol. 74:202–213, 2003.
191. Kofron MD, Laurencin CT. Bone tissue engineering by gene delivery. Adv Drug Deliv Rev. 58(4):555–576, 2006.
192. Shi S, Bartold PM, Miura M. The efficacy of mesenchymal stem cells to regenerate and repair dental structures. Orthod Craniofac Res. 8(3):191–199, 2005.
193. Duan X, Tu Q, Zhang J, Ye J, et al. Application of induced pluripotent stem (iPS) cells in periodontal tissue regeneration. J Cell Physiol. 2010 Jul 23. [Epub ahead of print.]
194. Kawaguchi H, Hirachi A, Hasegawa N, et al. Enhancement of periodontal tissue regeneration by transplantation of bone marrow mesenchymal stem cells. J Periodontol. 75(9):1281–1287, 2004.
195. Yang Y, Rossi FM, Putnins EE. Periodontal regeneration using engineered bone marrow mesenchymal stromal cells. Biomaterials 2010 Sep 8. [Epub ahead of print.]
196. Kim SH, Kim KH, Seo BM. Alveolar bone regeneration by transplantation of periodontal ligament stem cells and bone marrow stem cells in a canine peri-implant defect model: A pilot study. J Periodontol. 80(11):1815–1823, 2009.

197. Flores MG, Hasegawa M, Yamato M, et al. Cementum-periodontal ligament complex regeneration using the cell sheet technique. J Periodontal Res. 43(3):364–371, 2008.
198. Flores MG, Yashiro R, Washio K, et al. Periodontal ligament cell sheet promotes periodontal regeneration in athymic rats. J Clin Periodontol. 35(12):1066–1072, 2008
199. Izumi K, Feinberg SE, Iida A, Yoshizawa M. Intraoral grafting of an ex vivo produced oral mucosa equivalent: A preliminary report. Int J Oral Maxillofac Surg. 32(2):188–197, 2003.
200. Somerman MJ, Ouyang HJ, Berry JE, Saygin NE, Strayhorn CL, D'Errico JA, et al. Evolution of periodontal regeneration: From the roots' point of view. J Periodontal Res. 34:420–424, 1999.
201. Zhao M, Jin Q, Berry JE, Nociti FH Jr, Giannobile WV, Somerman MJ. Cementoblast delivery for periodontal tissue engineering. J Periodontol. 75:154–161, 2004.
202. Sculean A, Blaes A, Arweiler N, Reich E, Donos N, Brecx M. The effect of postsurgical antibiotics on the healing of intrabony defectsfollowing treatment with enamel matrix proteins. J Periodontol. 72(2):190–195, 2001.
203. Sculean A, Berakdar M, Donos N, Auschill TM, Arweiler NB. The effect of postsurgical administration of a selective cyclo-oxygenase-2 inhibitor on the healing of intrabony defects following treatment with enamelmatrix proteins. Clin Oral Investig. 7(2):108–112, 2003.
204. Beckman BW. Treatment of an infrabony pocket in an American Eskimo dog. J Vet Dent. 21(3):159–163, 2004.
205. Fowler C, Garrett S, Crigger M, et al. Histologic probe position in treated and untreated periodontal human periodontal tissues. J Clin Periodontol. 9:373, 1982.
206. Caton JC. Overview of clinical trials on periodontal regeneration. Ann Periodontol. 2:215, 1987.
207. Greensberg J, Laster L, Listgarten MA. Transgingival probing as a potential estimation of alveolar bone level. J Periodontol. 47:514, 1976.
208. Ursel MJ. Relationships between alveolar bone levels measured at surgery, estimated by transgingival probing and clinical attachment level measurements. J Clin Periodontol. 16:81, 1989.
209. Patur B, Glickman I. Clinical and roentgenographic evaluation of the post-treatment healing of infraboney pockets. J Periodontol. 33:164, 1962.
210. Tsugawa AJ, Verstraete FJ, Kass PH, Gorrel C. Diagnostic value of the use of lateral and occlusal radiographic views in comparison with periodontal probing for the assessment of periodontal attachment of the canine teeth in dogs. Am J Vet Res. 64(3):255–261, 2003.
211. Land MP, Hill RW. Radiographs in periodontics. J Clin Periodontol. 4:16, 1976.
212. Theilade J. An evaluation of the reliability of radiographs in the measurement of bone loss in periodontal disease. J Periodontol. 31:143, 1960.
213. Tonetti M, Pini Prato GP, Williams R, et al. Periodontal regeneration of human infrabony defects. III. Diagnostic strategies to detect bone gain. J Periodontol. 64:269, 1993.
214. Eikholz P, Hausmann E. Evidence for healing of class II and III furcations after GTR therapy: Digital subtraction and clinical measurements. J Periodontol. 68:636, 1997.
215. Wenzel A, Warrer K, Karring T. Digital subtraction radiography in assessing bone changes in periodontal defects following guided tissue regeneration. J Clin Periodontol. 19:208, 1992.
216. Niemiec BA, Gilbert T, Sabatino D. Equipment and basic geometry of dental radiography. J Vet Dent. 21(1):48–52, 2004.
217. DuPont G, DeBowes LJ. Atlas of Dental Radiography in Dogs and Cats. Philadelphia: Saunders, 2009, p. 232.
218. Gorrel C. Small Animal Dentistry. Philadelphia: Saunders-Elsevier, 2008, pp. 22–68.
219. DuPont G. Tooth splinting for severely mobile mandibular incisor teeth in a dog. J Vet Dent. 12(3):93–95,1995.
220. Spear FM, Cooney JP. Restorative interrelationships. In: Carranza's Clinical Periodontology. St. Louis: Saunders, 2006, pp. 1050–1071.
221. Niemiec BA. Intraoral acrylic splint application. J Vet Dent. 20(2):123–126, 2003.
222. McGinnis M, Larsen P, Miloro M, Beck FM. Comparison of resorbable and nonresorbable guided bone regeneration materials: A preliminary study. Int J Oral Maxillofac Implants 13(1):30–35, 1998.
223. Rankow HJ, Krasner PR. Endodontic applications of guided tissue regeneration in endodontic surgery. 22(1):34–43,1996.
224. Tonetti MS, Cortellini P, Suvan JE, et al. Generalizability of the added benefits of guided tissue regeneration in the treatment of deep intrabony defects. Evaluation in a multi-center randomized controlled clinical trial. J Periodontol. 69(11):1183–1192, 1998.
225. Cortellini P, Pini Prato G, Tonetti MS. Periodontal regeneration of human intrabony defects with bioresorbable membranes. A controlled clinical trial. J Periodontol. 67(3):217–223, 1996.
226. Camargo PM, Lekovic V, Weinlaender M, et al. A controlled re-entry study on the effectiveness of bovine porous bone mineral used in combination with a collagen membrane of porcine origin in the treatment of intrabony defects in humans. J Clin Periodontol. 27(12):889–896, 2000.
227. Wu SY, Chen YT, Chen CW, et al. Comparison of clinical outcomes following guided tissue regeneration treatment with a polylactic acid barrier or a collagen membrane. Int J Periodontics Restorative Dent. 30(2):173–179, 2010.
228. Owen GR, Jackson JK, Chehroudi B, Brunette DM, Burt HM. An in vitro study of plasticized poly(lactic-co-glycolic acid) films as possible guided tissue regeneration membranes: Material properties and drug release kinetics. J Biomed Mater Res A. 2010 Sep 7. [Epub ahead of print.]
229. Hanes PJ, Purvis JP. Local anti-infective therapy: Pharmacological agents. A systematic review. Ann Periodontol. 8(1):79–98, 2003.
230. Park YJ, Lee YM, Park SN, et al. Enhanced guided bone regeneration by controlled tetracycline release from poly(L-lactide) barrier membranes. J Biomed Mater Res. 51(3):391–397, 2000.
231. Chung CP, Kim DK, Park YJ, Nam KH, Lee SJ. Biological effects of drug-loaded biodegradable membranes for guided boneregeneration. J Periodontal Res. 32(1 Pt 2):172–175, 1997.
232. Scott TA, Towle HJ, Assad DA, Nicoll BK. Comparison of bioabsorbable laminar bone membrane and non-resorbable ePTFE membrane in mandibular furcations. J Periodontol. 68(7): 679–686, 1997.
233. Fugazzotto PA. The use of demineralized laminar bone sheets in guided bone regeneration procedures: report of three cases. Int J Oral Maxillofac Implants 11(2):239–244, 1996.

19

Furcation involvement and treatment

Paul Theuns

Introduction

The furcation is the anatomical area of multirooted teeth where the roots divide. Advanced periodontitis in multirooted teeth is inevitably connected to furcation involvement. The presence of furcation involvement can lead to extensive problems with regard to plaque retention, rapid progression of attachment loss, food retention, and erosive or carious lesions.[1] Furcations are some of the most difficult areas to treat due to the retention of plaque and microorganisms, and therefore regular quality homecare may not even keep the furcation free of plaque.[2,3]

Etiology

The primary cause of the development of furcation defects is bacterial plaque, as described elsewhere in this book. Both the prevalence and severity of furcation involvement increase with age.[4] Furcational bone loss can occur secondary to periodontal or pulpal disease.[5] While furcation exposure occurs late in the disease course in human periodontology owing to the significant amount of "reserve" crown, it occurs much earlier small animal patients (see Figure 5.21).[6]

Diagnosis and classification

Diagnosis is best achieved by thorough clinical examination. The extent of furcation defect is best determined by careful probing with a curved probe. Once a furcation involvement is diagnosed, radiographs can help in determining the extent of the lesion.

The most common indices used in veterinary dentistry are based upon furcation exposure as described by Hamp et al. (1975). The following is a classification of furcation exposure:[1,7,8]

F0: No furcation involvement (see Figure 5.22).

F1: Soft tissue lesion extending to the furcation level with minimal osseous destruction, 1–3 mm, or less than halfway under the crown in any direction of a multirooted tooth with attachment loss (see Figure 5.23).

F2: Soft tissue lesion combined with bone loss that permits a probe to enter the furcation from one aspect, but not to pass completely through the furcation, more than 3 mm, or greater than halfway under the crown of a multirooted tooth with attachment loss (see Figure 5.24).

F3: Lesions with extensive osseous destruction that permit through and through passage of the probe, with or without soft tissue obscuring the communication (see Figure 5.25).

Some dentists (human and veterinary) recognize a fourth stage (**F4**) where the probe passes all the way through to the other side of the furcation without soft tissue obscuring the communication (i.e. visible through and through pathway).[9]

Local anatomic factors

With regard to treatment, clinicians must consider local anatomical factors which may affect the results of therapy. Radiographs are mandatory for treatment planning.

The root trunk length (the distance between the cementoenamel junction and the entrance of the furcation) varies considerably between different individuals and different teeth. The shorter the root trunk, the more accessible the teeth are for maintenance care/procedures. Long root trunks carry a worse prognosis, as they hinder homecare efforts. In small animal patients,

Veterinary Periodontology, First Edition. Brook A. Niemiec.

essentially all teeth have short root trunks (vs. long root trunks in human teeth) (see chapter 5).

The root length also has a direct influence on the success of treatment. Longer roots are more likely to have sufficient attachment levels remaining in order to effectively treat the root.[10,11]

Another important factor in determining prognosis is the degree of divergence of the roots. There is usually a larger degree of divergence of tooth roots in small animal patients as compared to human teeth, which facilitates treatment because there is more access to reach and treat the infected furcation area.[12]

Treatment

The treatment of periodontitis with furcation involvement requires thorough cleaning and debridement of the furcation area. After the initial cleaning/scaling is performed, a thorough examination of the tooth and furcation is necessary to establish a treatment plan. A thorough evaluation includes: visual inspection, periodontal probing of the defect, sounding (see chapter 16) and dental radiographs.[13] With periodontal pockets greater than 4-mm, direct visualization is required for adequate cleaning. This visualization is best achieved via periodontal flaps (see chapter 16). In cases with no periodontal pockets, the clinician must determine if all infected areas can be reached by tooth brushing.[14] Areas that cannot be accessed need to be cleaned under general anesthesia at a suggested interval of approximately 6 months, but more frequent cleanings may be necessary.[15] If the client cannot perform sufficient, quality homecare for the teeth (see chapter 13) and/or is reluctant to comply with the required schedule of professional care, the prognosis is poor and in these cases extraction would be the treatment of choice.

Class I defects

Early (F1) lesions can be treated conservatively. Scaling and closed root planning should be effective, if followed by strict oral hygiene. After the cleaning process, homecare is critically essential (ideally on a daily basis), in order to prevent progression of the disease.

Class II and III defects

There are several options when treating teeth with advanced furcational disease including: periodontal surgery and GTR, hemisection, root resection with partial extraction, and extraction.

Periodontal flap surgery +/– guided tissue regeneration (GTR)

In most cases, the treatment of choice for these lesions (F2 and 3) involves flap surgery to provide direct vision of the furcation morphology and the depth of the involvement (Figure 19.1) (see chapter 16 for a complete discussion of periodontal flaps).

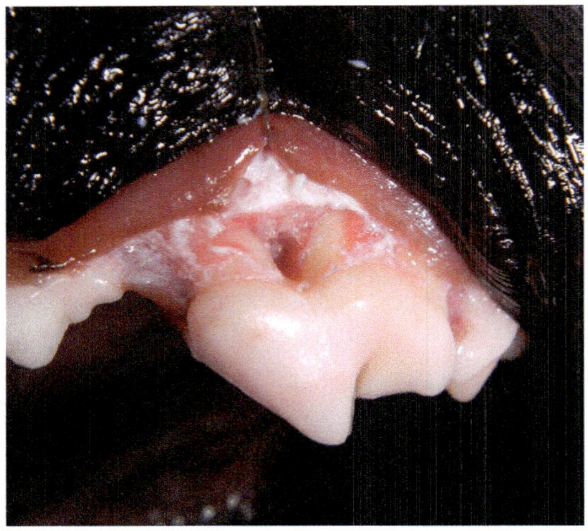

Figure 19.1 Horizontal "envelope" flap created over the right maxillary fourth premolar (108) in a dog. This gives excellent visibility of the class II furcation exposure and will allow for effective cleaning and therapy.

Proper visibility allows the surgeon to determine if the furcation should be treated with guided tissue regeneration. Conservative odontoplasty could also be considered, in order to widen the furcation entrance, making it more accessible for plaque control (see chapter 18).[16] It is important too note however, that corrective odontoplasty is a very delicate procedure removing only minimal amounts of bone.

The citric acid technique has been extensively investigated in dogs, showing encouraging results for the treatment of furcation lesions (see chapter 17).[17,18] This technique involves raising a mucoperiosteal flap and thoroughly instrumenting the root surface to remove calculus and underlying cementum (Figure 19.2). Next, citric acid (pH = 1) is applied with cotton pledgets and left on for 2–5 minutes (Figure 19.3).[19] After that time, the surface is irrigated with water (Figure 19.4). If further treatment (such as guided tissue regeneration) is deemed necessary, it is performed at this time (Figure 19.5). Guided tissue regeneration (GTR) with barriers and bone replacement grafts (see chapter 18) has been found to significantly improve attachment gain in class II and III furcations.[20–23] Attachment gains were even more significant when combined with a barrier membrane (Figure 19.6).[24,25] The final step in this technique is closure of the surgical flap (Figure 19.7).[26]

Although F2 and 3 defects are treated in a similar fashion, F3 lesions carry a worse prognosis. Regenerative methods such as GTR or hemisection may be considered for these cases. However, if the owner isn't able to perform daily oral hygiene, extraction is the treatment of choice.

(a) (b)

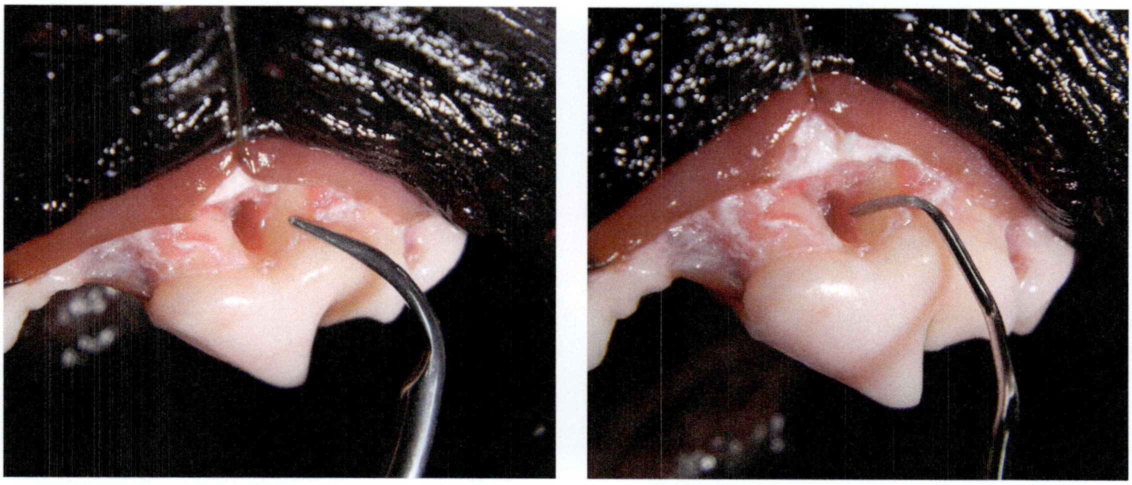

Figure 19.2 Instrumenting (scaling) the exposed root surface via ultrasonic (a) and hand (b) methods. Note the ultrasonic tip is a small, subgingival variety.

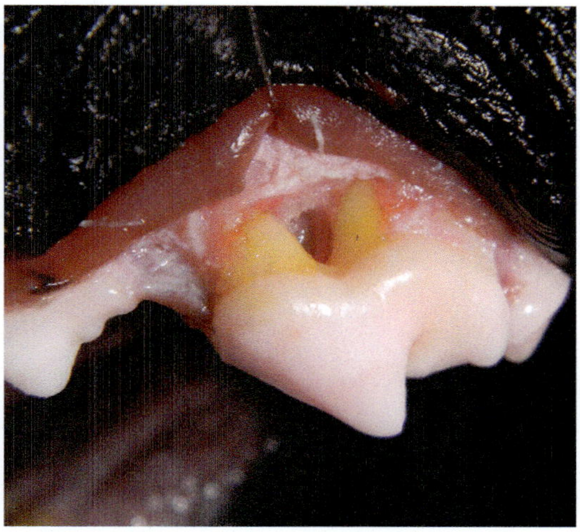

Figure 19.3 Application of the citric acid etchant to the clean and smooth root surfaces. Note that every attempt is made to avoid the soft tissues.

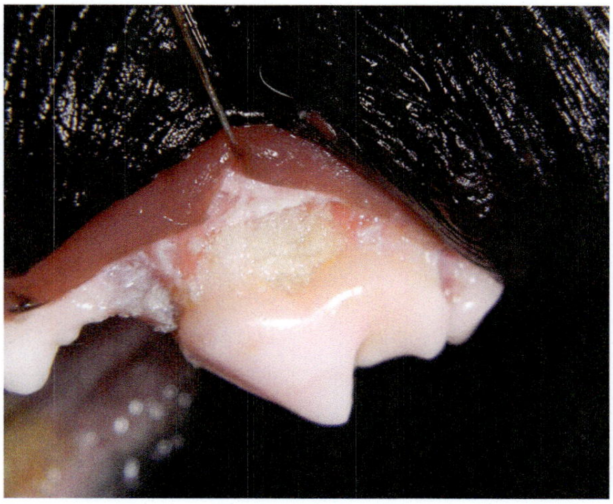

Figure 19.5 Placement of the bone augmentation product to fill the defect.

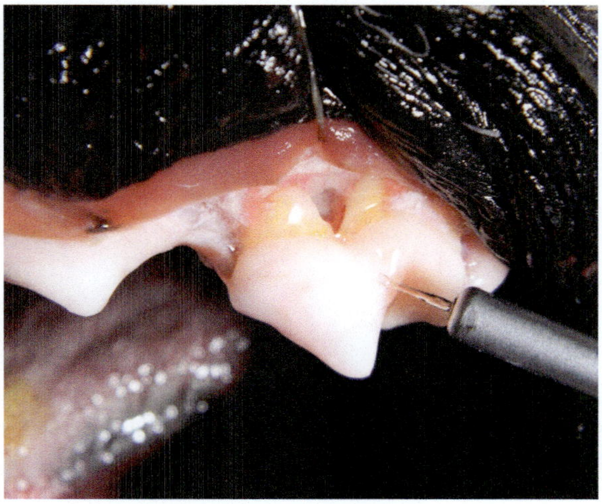

Figure 19.4 Thorough rinsing of the etch.

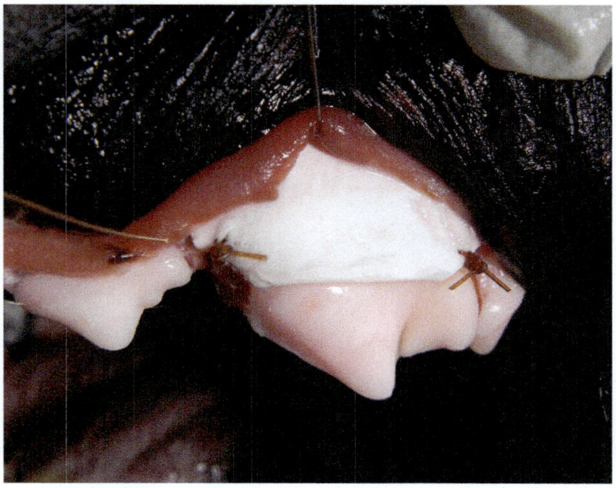

Figure 19.6 Placement of the preshaped barrier membrane.

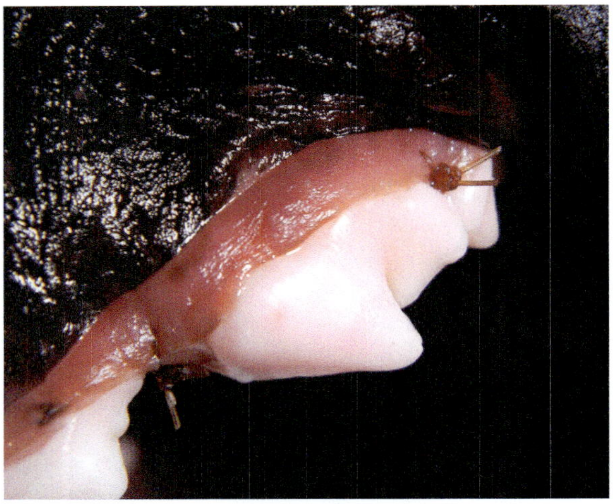

Figure 19.7 Postoperative picture demonstrating flap closure.

Hemisection

Hemisection (Figure 19.8) is the splitting of a multirooted tooth into separate portions. This procedure achieves complete removal of the furcation, allowing the area to be more effectively cleaned and managed. After the splitting procedure, the individual roots are left in place. Hemisection can be done before or after root canal treatment, but is preferably performed afterward. This procedure is rarely performed in veterinary dentistry since typically at least one of the roots has significant disease.

Tooth resection with partial extraction

When one root of a multi-rooted tooth is significantly diseased, removal of that root while maintaining the healthy/healthier root/s may be desirable[27] (Figure 19.9). The surgeon can elect to remove the whole section of the

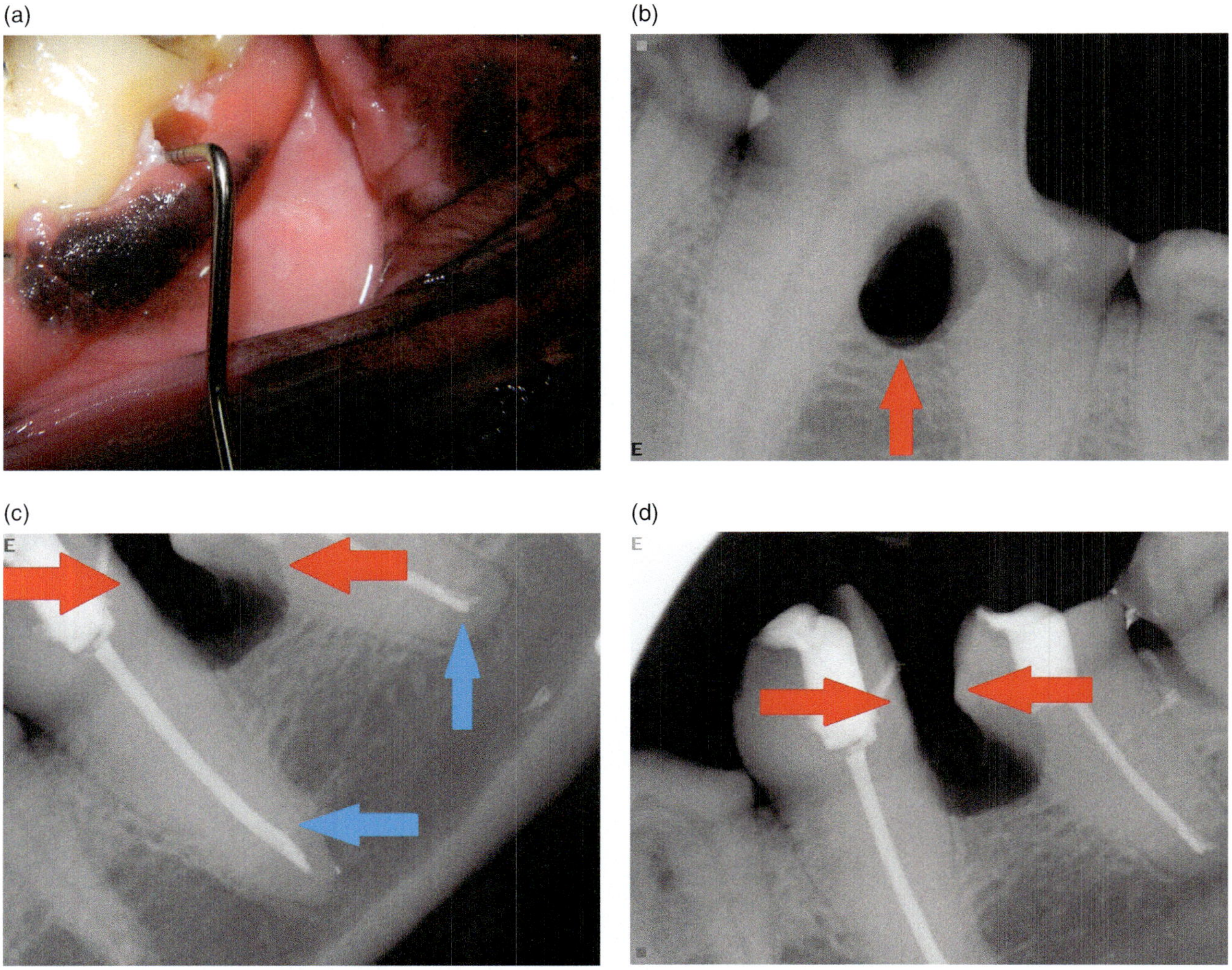

Figure 19.8 (a and b) Preoperative images of a class III furcation exposure on the left mandibular first molar (309) of a dog that had not responded to several previous regeneration attempts. (a) Intraoral dental picture demonstrating the probe through the furcation. (b) Intraoral dental radiograph confirming the complete bone loss in the furcation (red arrow). (c and d) Postoperative dental radiograph of the tooth sectioning and restoration (red arrows) and standard endodontic treatment with adequate obturation (blue arrows).

(e)

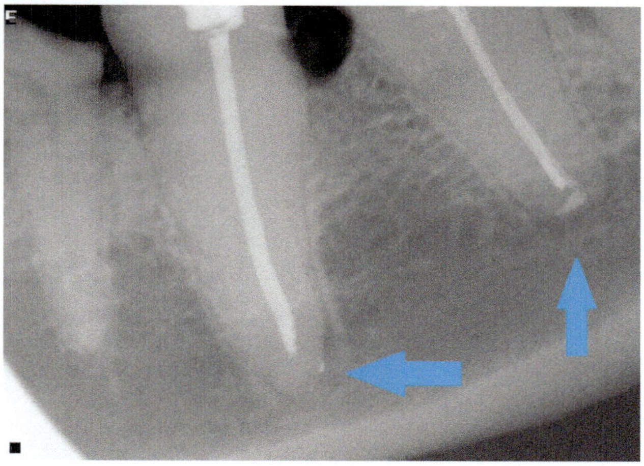

(f)

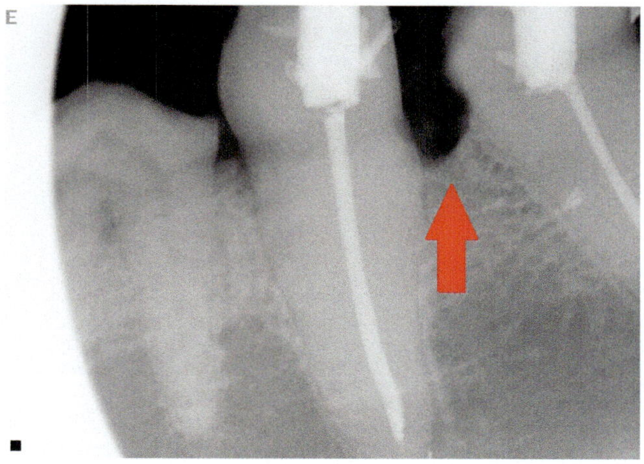

(g)

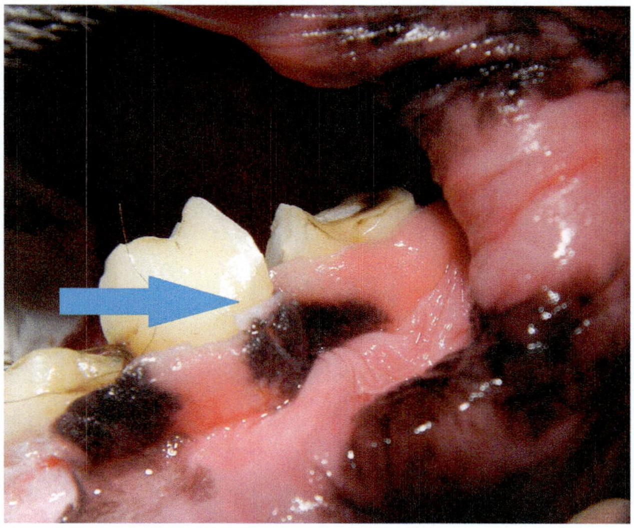

Figure 19.8 (cont'd) (e) 9-month recheck radiograph of the endodontic therapy revealing continued apical seal and lack of periapical rarefaction (blue arrows), indicating successful endodontic treatment. (f) 9-month recheck radiograph of the furcational area revealing some improvement in bone height (red arrow). This is an excellent result for this rarely done but commonly indicated procedure. (g) 9-month recheck picture of the furcational area revealing the excellent healing and lack of inflammation (blue arrow). This is an excellent result for this rarely done but commonly indicated procedure.

tooth (tooth resection) or leave the crown and remove only the root (root resection). In these cases, meticulous clinical and radiographic diagnosis is necessary to determine which root/s to extract. The goal of this procedure is to extract the diseased root, thus eliminating the furcation, while maintaining the strongest and most accessible part of the tooth.[28] The remaining root(s) must then be treated endodontically.

Regarding the maxillary fourth premolar (108, 208), it is generally advised to salvage the distal root while extracting the mesial roots. This is because the furcational area between the mesial roots is the hardest to clean. This is a generalization, and is dependent on the clinical and radiographic findings. The most common indication for root resection in veterinary dentistry is the mandibular first molar of small and toy breed dogs.[27] There is often significant disease associated with the distal root, while the mesial root is spared. There are several advantages to root resection in this presentation. First, much of the crown is maintained for mastication. Secondly, because the distal root is generally significantly diseased, its extraction is relatively atraumatic and is therefore this treatment is less invasive than complete extraction. Similarly, another advantage of root/tooth resection vs. full extraction of the mandibular first molar is the decreased risk of iatrogenic mandibular fracture. With minimal bone apical to the roots in this area, which has been further weakened by the periodontal disease, the increased force needed to extract the mesial root could result in a pathologic fracture. The option of retaining the mesial root via endodontic therapy would avoid this potential concern.

After root resection or hemisection is performed, more advanced techniques for the treatment of periodontal disease are often necessary.[29] For example, the placement of artificial bone followed by guided tissue regeneration with a membrane can be effective.

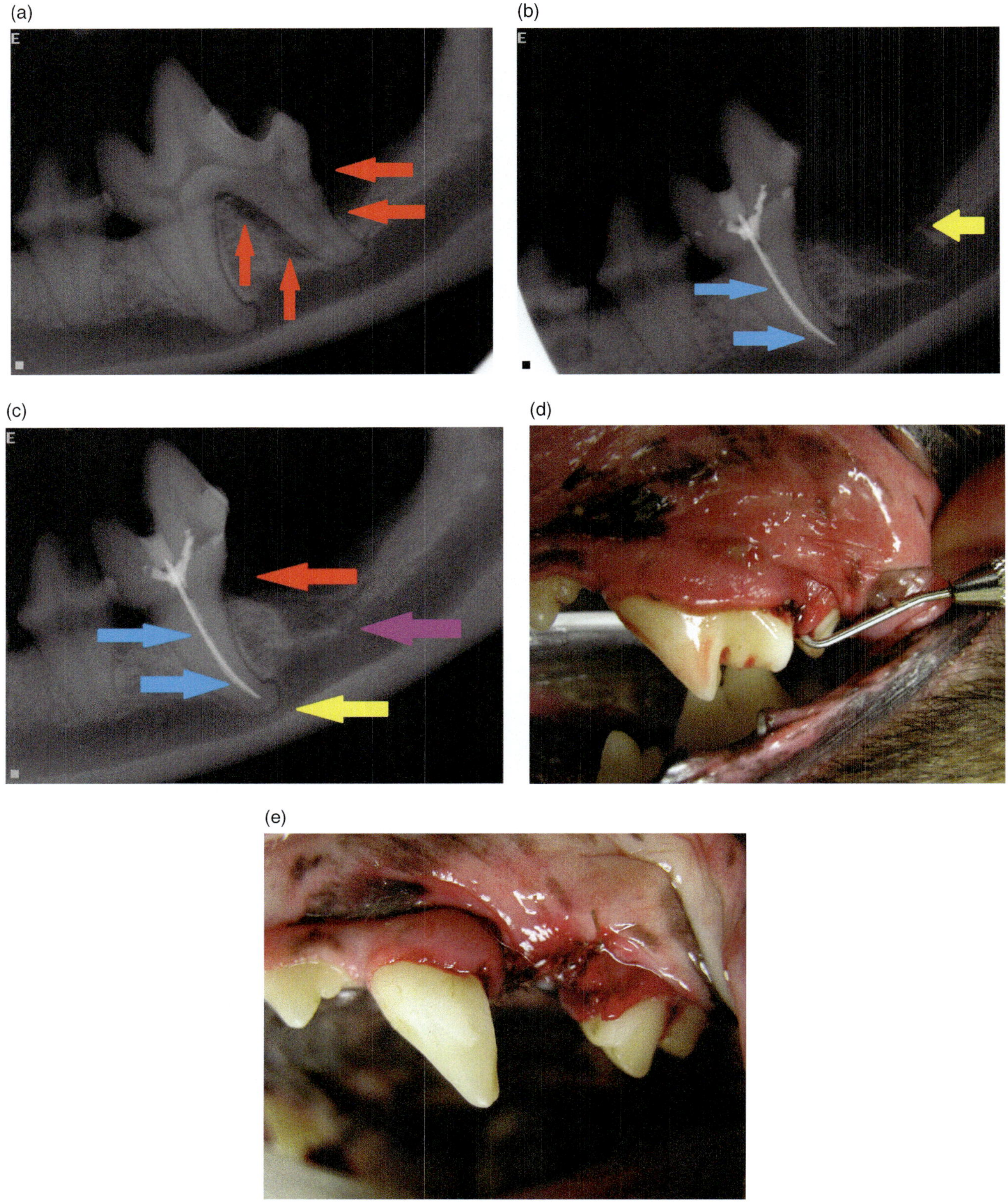

Figure 19.9 Tooth sectioning and partial extraction. (a) Preoperative intraoral dental radiograph of a left mandibular first molar (309) in a small breed dog. Notice the significant vertical alveolar bone loss on both sides of the distal root (red arrows), and early bone loss in the distal aspect of the furcation. However, note that the mesial root has normal alveolar bone height. (b) Postoperative dental radiograph of the same tooth following resection and extraction of the distal root (yellow arrow) with standard endodontic therapy performed on the mesial root (blue arrows). (c) Recheck dental radiograph of the same patient. Note the alveolus is healed (purple arrow) and there is minimal to no alveolar bone loss to the mesial root (red arrow). In addition, there is continued adequate fill of the endodontic system (blue arrows) and lack of periapical rarefaction (yellow arrow), indicating successful endodontic therapy. These findings confirm a successful therapy. (d and e) Another indication for tooth sectioning and partial extraction. (d) Preoperative image of the left maxillary fourth premolar (208) of a dog with a deep periodontal pocket on the distal aspect. (e) Postoperative picture where the distal root has been sectioned and extracted and the mesial roots treated with root canal therapy.

Prognosis

The prognosis is generally poor for maintaining a tooth with class II or III furcation exposure, but treatment can be effective.

If the problems of access for professional cleaning (SRP) and homecare can be resolved, the prognosis is no worse than that of a single rooted tooth with the same level of attachment loss.[30]

Box 19.1 Key points

- The furcation area is one of the most difficult areas to treat.
- Class II and III furcation involvement requires advanced treatment procedures.
- Post-operative oral hygiene is mandatory for successful treatment of periodontal disease with furcation involvement.
- With good oral hygiene, the prognosis for therapy of furcationally diseased teeth can be similar to single rooted teeth with the same level of attachment loss.
- Tooth resection is a viable alternative (especially in carnassial teeth) if one or more roots retain sufficient attachment.

References

1. Wiggs RB, Lobprise HB. Periodontology. In: Veterinary Dentistry, Principles and Practice. Philadelphia: Lippincott-Raven, 1997, pp. 204–205.
2. Masters DH, Hoskins SW. In: Carranza's Clinical Periodontology. St. Louis: Saunders, 2006, pp. 134–169.
3. Wolf HF, Rateitschak E, Rateitschak KH, Hassell, TM. In: Color Atlas of Dental Medicine: Periodontology. 3rd ed. Stuttgart: Thieme, 2005, pp. 172–173.
4. Kalkwarf K, Kaldahl W, Patil K, et al. Evaluation of furcation region reponse to periodontal therapy. In: Carranza's Clinical Periodontology. St. Louis: Saunders, 2006, pp. 134–169.
5. Berman LH, Hartwell GR. Diagnosis. In: Cohen's Pathways of the Pulp. 9th ed. St. Louis: Mosby Elsevier, 2006, p. 16.
6. Page RC, Schroeder HE. Spontaneous chronic periodontitis in adult dogs. A clinical and histologic survey. J Periodontol. 52: 60–73, 1981.
7. Recommendations from the AVDC Nomenclature Committee adopted by the AVDC Board.
8. Wolf HF, Rateitschak E, Rateitschak KH, Hassell, TM. In: Color Atlas of Dental Medicine: Periodontology. 3rd ed. Stuttgart: Thieme, 2005, p. 383.
9. Huffman LJ. Oral examination. In: Small Animal Dental, Oral and Maxillofacial Disease, a Color Handbook (Niemiec BA ed.). London: Manson, 2010, pp. 39–61.
10. Ammons W, Harrington GW. Furcation involvement and treatment. In: Carranza's Clinical Periodontology. St. Louis: Saunders, 2006, pp. 994.
11. Gher ME, Vernino, AR. Root morphology: Clinical significance in pathogenis and treatment of periodontal disease. J Am Dent Assoc. 101:627, 1980.
12. Carranza A, Takei H, Cochran D. Reconstructive periodontal surgery. In: Carranza's Clinical Periodontology. St. Louis: Saunders, 2006, p. 994.
13. Measley BL, Beybayer M, Butzin Ca, et al. Use of furcal bone sounding to improve the accuracy of furcation diagnosis. J Periodontol. 65:649, 1994.
14. Harvey CE, Emily PP. Periodontal disease. In: Small Animal Dentistry. St. Louis: Mosby, 1993, pp. 102–103.
15. Wiggs RB, Lobprise HB. Periodontology. In: Veterinary Dentistry, Principles and Practice. Philadelphia: Lippincott-Raven, 1997, pp. 217–231.
16. Wolf HF, Rateitschak E, Rateitschak KH, Hassell, TM. In: Color Atlas of Dental Medicine: Periodontology. 3rd ed. Stuttgart: Thieme, 2005, p. 385.
17. Crigger M, Boyle G, Nilveus R, et al. The effect of topical citric acid application on the healing of experimental furcation defects in dogs. J Periodontal Res. 13(6):538–549, 1978.
18. Nilvéus R, Bogle G, Crigger M, Egelberg J, Selvig KA. The effect of topical citric acid application on the healing of experimental furcation defects in dogs. II. Healing after repeated surgery. J Periodontal Res. 15(5):544–550, 1980.
19. Carranza FA, Takei HH, Cochran DL. Reconstructive periodontal surgery. In: Carranza's Clinical Periodontology. St. Louis: Saunders, 2006, pp. 968–990.
20. Gantes B, Martin M, Garrett S, Egelberg J. Treatment of periodontal furcation defects. (II). Bone regeneration in mandibular class II defects. J Clin Periodontol. 15(4):232–239, 1988.
21. Pepelassi EM, Bissada NF, Greenwell H, Farah CF. Doxycycline-tricalcium phosphate composite graft facilitates osseous healing in advanced periodontal furcation defects. J Periodontol. 62(2):106–115, 1991.
22. Gantès BG, Synowski BN, Garrett S, Egelberg JH. Treatment of periodontal furcation defects. Mandibular class III defects. J Periodontol. 62(6):361–365, 1991.
23. Kenney EB, Lekovic V, Elbaz JJ, et al. The use of a porous hydroxylapatite implant in periodontal defects. II. Treatment of class II furcation lesions in lower molars. J Periodontol. 59(2): 67–72, 1988.
24. Garrett S, Gantes B, Zimmerman G, Egelberg J. Treatment of mandibular class III periodontal furcation defects. Coronally positioned flaps with and without expanded polytetrafluoroethylene membranes. J Periodontol. 65(6):592–597, 1994.
25. Calongne KB, Aichelmann-Reidy ME, Yukna RA, Mayer ET. Clinical comparison of microporous biocompatible composite of PMMA, PHEMA and calcium hydroxide grafts and expanded polytetrafluoroethylene barrier membranes in human mandibular molar Class II furcations. A case series. J Periodontol. 72(10):1451–1459, 2001.
26. Carranza A, Takei H, Cochran D. Reconstructive periodontal surgery. In: Carranza's Clinical Periodontology. St. Louis: Saunders, 2006, p. 974.
27. Niemiec BA. Treatment of mandibular first molar teeth with endodontic-periodontal lesions in a dog. J Vet Dent. 18(1):21–25, 2001.
28. Ammons W, Harrington, GW. Furcation involvement and treatment. In: Carranza's Clinical Periodontology. St. Louis: Saunders, 2006, p. 996.
29. Ammons W, Harrington, GW. Furcation involvement and treatment. In: Carranza's Clinical Periodontology. St. Louis: Saunders, 2006, p. 997.
30. Ammons W, Harrington, GW. Furcation involvement and treatment. In: Carranza's Clinical Periodontology. St. Louis: Saunders, 2006, pp. 999–1004.

SECTION 5

Related topics

20

Host modulation therapies

Introduction

As stated earlier in this text, periodontal disease is initiated by plaque bacteria.[1] The bacteria and their byproducts create the inflammatory changes. These inflammatory changes may result in osteoclastic bone loss via an unknown pathway in susceptible individuals. What is known is that *the patient*, and not the bacteria directly, controls the osteoclasts that create the alveolar bone loss.

It is increasingly clear that when the host-mediated response to the biofilm is left unchecked, tissue and bone of the periodontium are destroyed. If the acute inflammatory response is resolved quickly, tissue injury is prevented. However, inadequate resolution and failure to return tissue to homeostasis results in neutrophil-mediated destruction and chronic inflammation. (See chapters 2, 4, and 5 for a complete discussion of the pathogenesis of periodontal diseases.)

There are numerous preparations that have shown promise in decreasing the amount of osteoclastic bone resorption in cases of chronic periodontitis. Many drug therapies have been shown to have good efficacy in slowing the progression of periodontal disease. However, many of them have significant side effects that make their use questionable.[2] However, an increasing number of products are nutraceuticals, with minimal to no side effects.

Box 20.1 Key clinical point

Classic periodontal therapy has concentrated on plaque control, which is still the cornerstone. However, current research is looking at methods to control the inflammation and subsequent bone loss by treating the patient. This is called "host modulation" and is currently the most popular form of "novel" periodontal therapy.

Drug therapies

Anti-inflammatories

Host-mediated immune responses to microorganisms lead to the destruction of periodontal tissues.[3,4] There is substantial evidence that the products of arachidonic acid (AA) metabolism may be pivotal in triggering and perpetuating the inflammatory changes seen in periodontitis.[5,6]

High concentrations of the AA-derived products such as leukotrieneB4 (LTB4), prostaglandinE2 (PGE2), and inflammatory cytokines (tumor necrosis factor-alpha and interleukin-1b and -6) are particularly destructive.[1,7] Manipulation of the immune response to suppress unwanted inflammatory reactions has been widely studied as a treatment for controlling such inflammatory responses in periodontal disease.[8,9] Several host response-modulating approaches have been described. However, the control of inflammation with available pharmaceutical agents is still a challenge because of the side effects associated with their chronic use.

NSAIDS

Since periodontal inflammation and subsequent bone loss is known to be an inflammatory process, anti-inflammatories are an obvious choice. Numerous NSAIDs (Cox-1 and 2) have been tested against periodontal disease and alveolar bone loss. For the most part, they are successful when administered either locally or systemically.[10] Products that showed favorable results include meloxicam,[11–13,A] celecoxib,[14] etoricoxib,[15] indomethacin,[16] ketoprofen,[17] and ibuprofen.[18] It appears that these products are most effective in the short term, however, and may not be effective for long-term therapy.[10,19]

Bisphosphonates

Another way to decrease the amount of alveolar bone loss is to directly inhibit the osteoclasts. The bisphosphonates are one class of antiresorptive medications that are designed to decrease the amount of alveolar bone loss such as that from periodontitis.

One study looked at the use of locally applied monosodium olpadronate (OPD).[20] The treated group exhibited a marked inhibition of bone loss; that is, interradicular bone volume was significantly greater than that observed in the non-treated group. The study further reported, "Osteoclasts in the OPD treated group were detached from the bone surface, were round in shape, and exhibited a loss of polarity and lack of ruffled borders." Similar findings were noted when clodronate was topically administered to rats with periodontitis.[21,22]

Furthermore, it appears that these products are effective when administered systemically.[23] A study in rats showed a statistically significant reduction in alveolar bone loss when risedronate was administered systemically.[24] An additional study, however, showed that while there is a short-term benefit with its use, long-term administration may lead to bone loss.[25]

Parathyroid hormone

Parathyroid hormone (PTH) functions as a major mediator of bone remodeling and as an essential regulator of calcium homeostasis. In addition to its well-established catabolic effects, it is now recognized that intermittent PTH administration has anabolic effects (promotion of bone formation).[26,27] Intermittent administration of PTH also has a protective factor against periodontal bone loss.[28,29] Finally, it has the ability to stimulate the proliferation of PDL fibroblasts.[30] The combination of these effects has shown positive effects in the repair of periodontally lost bone.[31]

Antimicrobials

Another group of medications with significant promise both locally and systemically are antimicrobials, in particular the tetracycline class and especially doxycycline. These are typically used below the antimicrobial dose for their anti-inflammatory properties. In addition, they appear to block cytokines, which inhibits the communication among inflammatory cells in periodontitis. The local administration of the tetracycline class of drugs is currently favored and well supported in multiple studies.[32–36] In fact, the administration of tetracyclines appears to be successful both postoperatively and long term, with numerous studies now supporting long-term administration of low-dose doxycycline.[37–43] In addition, it was found that spiramycin reaches high concentrations in saliva and also helps control periodontal infections, particularly in felines.[44] It should be noted that many of the anti-infective agents that were tested showed positive results, opening the door for other treatments.[45,46]

Statins

In addition to medications that are considered to have an obvious beneficial method of action, there are some drugs that appear to promote periodontal health as a side effect. One of these is the cholesterol-lowering drug simvastatin, which is known to have anabolic effects on bone metabolism. A recent study in rats showed that when applied topically, this drug caused a 46% reversal rate of alveolar bone loss.[47] An additional study confirmed that this product showed protective features against periodontitis-induced bone loss.[48] Likewise, atorvastatin has shown positive effects on alveolar bone height and tooth mobility.[49]

Inflammatory mediators

As stated above, the resolution of inflammation (and return to homeostasis) will prevent osteoclastic bone resorption. Control though classic anti-inflammatory pathways has been shown effective, but with significant side effects. Neutrophils are present mainly in inflamed or injured tissues and their effective elimination is a prerequisite for complete resolution of an inflammatory response.[50] Resolution of inflammation is an active, agonist-mediated, well-orchestrated return of tissue homeostasis.[51] Lipoxins, resolvins, and protectins are a new family of bioactive products of fatty acids such as arachadonic acid.[52,53] Resolvins are products of omega-3 fatty acid transformation circuits initiated by cyclooxygenase-2 to form novel small molecules.[52] These products act locally to stop leukocyte recruitment and promote resolution of inflammation.[54]

These products have a significant anti-inflammatory effect in general, as well as in relation to certain diseases.[55–61] Results indicate that neutrophils from periodontally diseased tissues respond to RvE1.[62,63] Consistent with these potent actions, topical application of RvE1 in rabbit periodontitis conferred dramatic protection against inflammation-induced tissue and bone loss associated with periodontitis.[62] An additional study showed that topical application of RvE1 had dramatic effects in the regeneration of periodontal tissues (including bone) that was destroyed by periodontal disease.[64] These products represent a powerful future option for the control of periodontal inflammation and secondary alveolar bone loss.

Neutraceuticals

Fatty acids

Fatty acids have been proposed to reduce chronic inflammation in individuals with arthritis.[65] Recent studies with dietary v-3 fatty acid use in rats resulted in reduced gingival inflammation.[66,67] The topical application of omega-3 (v-3) polyunsaturated fatty acid (PUFA) was successful in the treatment of inflammatory diseases, such as experimental periodontitis in animal models.[68,69] It was also shown that eicosapentaenoic acid (EPA) or docosahexaenoic acid (DHA) can inhibit the production of PGE2 to an extent similar to indomethacin.[70] These same products have been proven to decrease periodontal inflammation.[71]

Pilot clinical and animal studies with v-3 and v-6 PUFA supplementation also showed beneficial results on periodontal inflammation and bone loss, indicating an anti-inflammatory role for these fatty acids without any evidence of side effects.[72,73] However, the clinical studies with dietary supplements did not show significant influences on inflammation, likely due to the lack of sufficient concentration of v-3 PUFA locally. Conversely, because of the high epithelial penetration of fatty acids, topical application may be favorable for the treatment of local oral inflammatory diseases, including periodontitis.[62]

A limited number of human clinical studies with dietary fatty acids also showed improvement in some clinical parameters, especially gingival and bleeding indices. However, the results were not as profound as those in the animal studies. A recent pilot study with v-6 and v-3 fatty acids in the treatment of periodontal disease showed beneficial effects of dietary v-6 fatty acid (borage oil) on gingival inflammation and probing depth.[72]

A particular fatty acid called 1-Tetradecanol complex (1-TDC)[B] is an esterified MUFA mixture of cetylmyristoleate, cetylmyristate, cetyl palmitoleate, cetyl laureate, cetyl palmitate, and cetyl oleate. In two in vivo studies on New Zealand Rabbits,[74,75] 1-TDC stopped the progression of periodontal disease and resulted in a significant reduction in macroscopic periodontal inflammation, attachment, and bone loss (10.1% $+/-$ 1.8%). In addition, histologic assessment demonstrated that 1-TDC inhibited inflammatory cell infiltration and osteoclastic activity. Finally, it has been reported to inhibit the growth of *Actinomyces viscosus* and *Staphylococcus aureus*, as well as inhibit thromboxane A2 production.[76]

Milk basic protein

An additional neutricutical that has a positive effect on alveolar bone is milk basic protein (MBP). It has a well-known ability to improve bone formation throughout the body, and when administered at high doses can aid in the recovery of periodontally lost alveolar bone.[77,78]

Coenzyme Q10

A deficiency of this enzyme has been shown in patients with periodontal disease.[79,80] Conversely, there are reports that supplementation (systemic or topical) may have a beneficial effect on periodontal health.[81–83] While this appears promising, more controlled clinical studies are necessary before promoting this as a therapy since most reviews do not favor its use at this time.[84]

Folic acid

Studies have demonstrated that folic acid is effective in preserving gum tissue and reducing the risk of gingivitis and periodontitis.[85] Topical therapy (mouthwash) appears to be the most effective method of supplementation,[86,87] but there is evidence that systemic supplementation also has a protective effect.[88]

Nutrition

Finally, it appears that proper nutrition, including vitamin supplementation, is an important aspect of periodontal care.[89] Studies have found multivitamin supplementation to provide beneficial effects for periodontal patients,[90] and vitamin E supplementation to have positive effects on gingival healing.[91,92] In contrast, malnutrition has been shown to have a negative effect on periodontal health.[93] Therefore, proper nutrition is essential for proper periodontal health, especially in the postoperative phase.

Conclusion

Host modulation therapy is likely the future of periodontal therapy. It is also important to note that nutraceuticals, vitamins, and proper nutrition all play a

Box 20.2 Key points

- Host modulation is the act of decreasing periodontal inflammation and bone loss via regulation of the patient's immune system.
- Local and systemic administration of various medications decreases periodontal loss.
- Supplementation with various vitamins, essential fatty acids, and nutraceuticals appears to provide a safe and effective option for this method of therapy.
- Active resolution of inflammation via resolvins appears to be a future thraputic option.

role in supporting good periodontal health. These treatments, in combination with new local bone regenerating products (such as bone morphologic protein) and implantology, will dramatically change the way we treat this common problem.

Notes

A. Metacam, Boehringer Ingelheim Vetmedica, Inc.
B. EFAC, Elite Science, LLC.

References

1. Van Dyke TE, Serhan CN. Resolution of inflammation: A new paradigm for the pathogenesis of periodontal diseases. J Dent Res. 82(2):82–90, 2003.
2. Van Dyke TE. The management of inflammation in periodontal disease. J Periodontol. 79(8 Suppl):1601–1608, 2008.
3. Genco RJ. Host responses in periodontal diseases: Current concepts. J Periodontol. 63:338–355, 1992.
4. Preshaw PM, Seymour RA, Heasman PA. Current concepts in periodontal pathogenesis. Dent Update. 31(10):570–572, 574–578, 2004.
5. Kantarci A, Van Dyke TE. Lipoxin signaling in neutrophils and their role in periodontal disease. Prostaglandins Leukot Essent Fatty Acids. 73:289–299, 2005.
6. Salvi GE, Lang NP. Host response modulation in the management of periodontal diseases. J Clin Periodontol. 32(Suppl. 6):108–129, 2005.
7. Lawrence T, Willoughby DA, Gilroy DW. Anti-inflammatory lipid mediators and insights into the resolution of inflammation. Nat Rev Immunol. 2:787–795, 2002.
8. Gilroy DW, Lawrence T, Perretti M, Rossi AG. Inflammatory resolution: New opportunities for drug discovery. Nat Rev Drug Discov. 3:401–416, 2004.
9. Barros SP, Arce RM, Galloway P, Lawter R, Offenbacher S. Therapeutic effect of a topical CCR2 antagonist on induced alveolar bone loss in mice. J Periodontal Res. 2011 Jan. 18.
10. Queiroz-Junior CM, Pacheco CM, Maltos KL, Caliari MV, Duarte ID, Francischi JN. Role of systemic and local administration of selective inhibitors of cyclo-oxygenase 1 and 2 in an experimental model of periodontal disease in rats. J Periodontal Res. 44(2): 153–160, 2009.
11. Gurgel BC, Duarte PM, Nociti FH Jr, et al. Impact of an anti-inflammatory therapy and its withdrawal on the progression of experimental periodontitis in rats. J Periodontol. 75(12): 1613–1618, 2004.
12. Oliveira TM, Sakai VT, Machado MA, et al. COX-2 inhibition decreases VEGF expression and alveolar bone loss during the progression of experimental periodontitis in rats. J Periodontol. 79(6):1062–1069, 2008.
13. Buduneli N, Buduneli E, Cetin EO, Kirilmaz L, Kütükcüler N. Clinical findings and gingival crevicular fluid prostaglandin E2 and interleukin-1-beta levels following initial periodontal treatment and short-term meloxicam administration. Expert Opin Pharmacother. 11(11):1805–1812, 2010.
14. Holzhausen M, Rossa Junior C, Marcantonio Junior E, et al. Effect of selective cyclooxygenase-2 inhibition on the development of ligature-induced periodontitis in rats. J Periodontol. 73(9): 1030–1036, 2002.
15. Holzhausen M, Spolidorio DM, Muscará MN, Hebling J, Spolidorio LC. Protective effects of etoricoxib, a selective inhibitor of cyclooxygenase-2, in experimental periodontitis in rats. J Periodontal Res. 40(3):208–211, 2005.
16. Bezerra MM, de Lima V, Alencar VB, Vieira IB, Brito GA, Ribeiro RA, Rocha FA. Selective cyclooxygenase-2 inhibition prevents alveolar bone loss in experimental periodontitis in rats. J Periodontol. 71(6):1009–1014, 2000.
17. Paquette DW, Fiorellini JP, Martuscelli G, et al. Enantiospecific inhibition of ligature-induced periodontitis in beagles with topical (S)-ketoprofen. J Clin Periodontol. 24(8):521–528, 1997.
18. Offenbacher S, Williams RC, Jeffcoat MK, et al. Effects of NSAIDs on beagle crevicular cyclooxygenase metabolites and periodontal bone loss. J Periodontal Res. 27(3):207–213, 1992.
19. Nassar CA, Nassar PO, Nassar PM, Spolidorio LC. Selective cyclooxygenase-2 inhibition prevents bone resorption. Braz Oral Res. 19(1):36–40, 2005.
20. Goya JA, Paez HA, Mandalunis PM. Effect of topical administration of monosodium olpadronate on experimental periodontitis in rats. J Periodontol. 77(1):1–6, 2006.
21. Mitsuta T, Horiuchi H, Shinoda H. Effects of topical administration of clodronate on alveolar bone resorption in rats with experimental periodontitis. J Periodontol. 73(5):479–486, 2002.
22. Alencar VB, Bezerra MM, Lima V, Abreu AL, Brito GA, Rocha FA, Ribeiro RA. Disodium chlodronate prevents bone resorption in experimental periodontitis in rats. J Periodontol. 73(3): 251–256, 2002.
23. El-Shinnawi UM, El-Tantawy SI. The effect of alendronate sodium on alveolar bone loss in periodontitis (clinical trial). J Int Acad Periodontol. 5:5–10, 2003.
24. Shoji K, Horiuchi H, Shinoda H. Inhibitory effects of a bisphosphonate (risedronate) on experimental periodontitis in rats. J Periodontal Res. 30(4):277–284, 1995.
25. Cetinkaya BO, Keles GC, Ayas B, Gurgor P. Effects of risedronate on alveolar bone loss and angiogenesis: A stereologic study in rats. J Periodontol. 79(10):1950–1961, 2008.
26. Liu J, Cao Z, Li C. Intermittent PTH administration: A novel therapy method for periodontitis-associated alveolar bone loss. Med Hypotheses 72(3):294–296, 2009.
27. Miller SC, Hunziker J, Mecham M, Wronski TJ. Intermittent parathyroid hormone administration stimulates bone formation in the mandibles of aged ovariectomized rats. J Dent Res. 76: 1471–1476, 1997.
28. Barros SP, Silva MA, Somerman MJ, Nociti FH Jr. Parathyroid hormone protects against periodontitis-associated bone loss. J Dent Res. 82(10):791–795, 2003.
29. Marques MR, da Silva MA, Manzi FR, Cesar-Neto JB, Nociti FH Jr, Barros SP. Effect of intermittent PTH administration in the periodontitis-associated bone loss in ovariectomized rats. Arch Oral Biol. 50(4):421–429, 2005.
30. Lossdörfer S, Götz W, Jäger A. PTH(1e34) affects osteoprotegerin production in human PDL cells in vitro. J Dent Res. 84:634–638, 2005.
31. Lossdörfer S, Ykildiz F, Götz W, Kheralla Y, Jäger A. Anabolic effect of intermittent PTH(1–34) on the local microenvironment during the late phase of periodontal repair in a rat model of tooth root resorption. Clin Oral Investig. 14:89–98, 2010.
32. Grenier D, Roy E, Mayrand D. Modulation of Porphyromonas gingivalis proteinase activity by suboptimal doses of antimicrobial agents. J Periodontol. 74(9):1316–1319, 2003.
33. Garrett S, Johnson L, Drisko CH, Adams DF, Bandt C, Beiswanger B, Bogle G, Donly K, Hallmon WW, Hancock EB, Hanes P, Hawley CE, Kiger R, Killoy W, Mellonig JT, Polson A, Raab FJ, Ryder M, Stoller NH, Wang HL, Wolinsky LE, Evans GH, Harrold CQ, Arnold RM, Southard GL, et al. Two

multi-center studies evaluating locally delivered doxycycline hyclate, placebo control, oral hygiene, and scaling and root planing in the treatment of periodontitis. J Periodontol. 70(5): 490–503, 1999.
34. Drisko CH. The use of locally delivered doxycycline in the treatment of periodontitis. Clinical results. J Clin Periodontol. 25(11 Pt 2):947–952, 1998.
35. Machion L, Andia DC, Benatti BB, Carvalho MD, Nogueira-Filho GR, Casati MZ, Nociti FH Jr, Sallum EA. Locally delivered doxycycline as an adjunctive therapy to scaling and root planing in the treatment of smokers: A clinical study. J Periodontol. 75(3): 464–469, 2004.
36. Eickholz P, Kim TS, Bürklin T, Schacher B, Renggli HH, Schaecken MT, Holle R, Kübler A, Ratka-Krüger P. Non-surgical periodontal therapy with adjunctive topical doxycycline: A double-blind randomized controlled multicenter study. J Clin Periodontol. 29(2):108–117, 2002.
37. Emingil G, Atilla G, Sorsa T, Savolainen P, Baylas H. Effectiveness of adjunctive low-dose doxycycline therapy on clinical parameters and gingival crevicular fluid laminin-5 gamma2 chain levels in chronic periodontitis. J Periodontol. 75(10):1387–1396, 2004.
38. Gürkan A, Cinarcik S, Hüseyinov A. Adjunctive subantimicrobial dose doxycycline: Effect on clinical parameters and gingival crevicular fluid transforming growth factor-beta levels in severe, generalized chronic periodontitis. J Clin Periodontol. 32(3): 244–253, 2005.
39. Gürkan A, Emingil G, Cinarcik S, Berdeli A. Post-treatment effects of subantimicrobial dose doxycycline on clinical parameters and gingival crevicular fluid transforming growth factor-beta1 in severe, generalized chronic periodontitis. Int J Dent Hyg. 6(2):84–92, 2008.
40. Preshaw PM, Hefti AF, Jepsen S, Etienne D, Walker C, Bradshaw MH. Subantimicrobial dose doxycycline as adjunctive treatment for periodontitis. A review. J Clin Periodontol. 31(9):697–707, 2004.
41. Lee HM, Ciancio SG, Tuter G, Ryan ME, Komaroff E, Golub M. Subantimicrobial dose doxycycline efficacy as a matrix metalloproteinase inhibitor in chronic periodontitis patients is enhanced when combined with a non-steroidal anti-inflammatory drug. J Periodontol. 75:453–463, 2004.
42. Gapski R, Hasturk H, Van Dyke TE, Oringer RJ, Wang S, Braun TM, Giannobile WV. Systemic MMP inhibition for periodontal wound repair: Results of a multi-centre randomized-controlled clinical trial. J Clin Periodontol. 36(2):149–156, 2009.
43. Gapski R, Barr JL, Sarment DP, Layher MG, Socransky SS, Giannobile WV. Effect of systemic matrix metalloproteinase inhibition on periodontal wound repair: A proof of concept trial. J Periodontol. 75(3):441–452, 2004.
44. Gawor J. Antibacterial activity of the saliva after administration of Spiramycin and Metronidazole in dogs and cats. Magazyn Weterynaryjny 8(41):188–192, 1999.
45. Hanes PJ, Purvis JP. Local anti-infective therapy: Pharmacological agents. A systematic review. Ann Periodontol. 8(1):79–98, 2003.
46. Stegemann MR, Passmore CA, Sherington J. Antimicrobial activity and spectrum of cefovecin, a new extended-spectrum cephalosporin, against pathogens collected from dogs and cats in Europe and North America. Antimicrob Agents Chemother. 50(7):2286–2292, 2006.
47. Seto H, Ohba H, Tokunaga K, Hama H, Horibe M, Nagata T. Topical administration of simvastatin recovers alveolar bone loss in rats. J Periodontal Res. 43(3):261–267, 2008.
48. Vaziri H, Naserhojjati-Roodsari R, Tahsili-Fahadan N, et al. Effect of simvastatin administration on periodontitis-associated bone loss in ovariectomized rats. J Periodontol. 78(8):1561–1567, 2007.
49. Fajardo ME, Rocha ML, Sánchez-Marin FJ, Espinosa-Chávez EJ. Effect of atorvastatin on chronic periodontitis: A randomized pilot study. J Clin Periodontol. 37(11):1016–1022, 2010.
50. Ariel A, Fredman G, Sun YP, Kantarci A, Van Dyke TE, Luster AD, Serhan CN. Apoptotic neutrophils and T cells sequester chemokines during immune response resolution through modulation of CCR5 expression. Nat Immunol. 7:1209–1216, 2006.
51. Van Dyke TE. The management of inflammation in periodontal disease. J Periodontol. 79(8 Suppl):1601–168, 2008.
52. Serhan CN, Gotlinger K, Hong S, Arita M. Resolvins, docosatrienes, and neuroprotectins, novel omega-3-derived mediators, and their aspirin-triggered endogenous epimers: An overview of their protective roles in catabasis. Prostaglandins Other Lipid Mediat. 73:155–172, 2004.
53. Serhan CN. Lipoxin biosynthesis and its impact in inflammatory and vascular events. Biochim Biophys Acta. 1212(1):1–25, 1994.
54. Hasturk H, Kantarci A, Ohira T, Arita M, Ebrahimi N, Chiang N, Petasis NA, Levy BD, Serhan CN, Van Dyke TE. RvE1 protects from local inflammation and osteoclast-mediated bone destruction in periodontitis. FASEB J. 20(2):401–403, 2006.
55. Arita M, Yoshida M, Hong S, Tjonahen E, Glickman JN, Petasis NA, Blumberg RS, Serhan CN. Resolvin E1, an endogenous lipid mediator derived from omega-3 eicosapentaenoic acid, protects against 2,4,6-trinitrobenzene sulfonic acid-induced colitis. Proc Natl Acad Sci USA 102(21):7671–7676, 2005.
56. Arita M, Bianchini F, Aliberti J, Sher A, Chiang N, Hong S, Yang R, Petasis NA, Serhan CN. Stereochemical assignment, antiinflammatory properties, and receptor for the omega-3 lipid mediator resolvin E1. J Exp Med. 201(5):713–722, 2005.
57. Arita M, Ohira T, Sun YP, Elangovan S, Chiang N, Serhan CN. Resolvin E1 selectively interacts with leukotriene B4 receptor BLT1 and ChemR23 to regulate inflammation. J Immunol. 178(6):3912–3917, 2007.
58. Arita M, Clish CB, Serhan CN. The contributions of aspirin and microbial oxygenase to the biosynthesis of anti-inflammatory resolvins: Novel oxygenase products from omega-3 polyunsaturated fatty acids. Biochem Biophys Res Commun. 338(1): 149–157, 2005.
59. Serhan CN, Savill J. Resolution of inflammation: The beginning programs the end. Nat Immunol. 6:1191–1197, 2005.
60. Bannenberg GL, Chiang N, Ariel A, et al. Molecular circuits of resolution: Formation and actions of resolvins and protectins. J Immunol. 174:4345–4355, 2005.
61. Schwab JM, Chiang N, Arita M, Serhan CN. Resolvin E1 and protectin D1 activate inflammation-resolution programmes. Nature 447:869–874, 2007.
62. Hasturk H, Kantarci A, Ohira T, Arita M, Ebrahimi N, Chiang N, Petasis NA, Levy BD, Serhan CN, Van Dyke TE. RvE1 protects from local inflammation and osteoclast-mediated bone destruction in periodontitis. FASEB J. 20(2):401–403, 2006.
63. Herrera BS, Ohira T, Gao L, Omori K, Yang R, Zhu M, Muscara MN, Serhan CN, Van Dyke TE, Gyurko R. An endogenous regulator of inflammation, resolvin E1, modulates osteoclast differentiation and bone resorption. Br J Pharmacol. 155(8): 1214–1223, 2008.
64. Hasturk H, Kantarci A, Goguet-Surmenian E, et al. Resolvin E1 regulates inflammation at the cellular and tissue level and restores tissue homeostasis in vivo. J Immunol. 179(10): 7021–7029, 2007.
65. Curtis CL, Hughes CE, Flannery CR, Little CB, Harwood JL, Caterson B. n-3 fatty acids specifically modulate catabolic factors

involved in articular cartilage degradation. J Biol Chem. 275: 721–724, 2000.
66. Kesavalu L, Vasudevan B, Raghu B, et al. Omega-3 fatty acid effect on alveolar bone loss in rats. J Dent Res. 85:648–652, 2006.
67. Kesavalu L, Bakthavatchalu V, Rahman MM, et al. Omega-3 fatty acid regulates inflammatory cytokine/mediator messenger RNA expression in Porphyromonas gingivalis-induced experimental periodontal disease. Oral Microbiol Immunol. 22:232–239, 2007.
68. Vardar S, Buduneli E, Turkoglu O, et al. Therapeutic versus prophylactic plus therapeutic administration of omega-3 fatty acid on endotoxin-induced periodontitisin rats. J Periodontol. 75: 1640–1646, 2004.
69. Vardar S, Buduneli E, Baylas H, Berdeli AH, Buduneli N, Atilla G. Individual and combined effects of selective cyclooxygenase-2 inhibitor and omega-3 fatty acid on endotoxin-induced periodontitis in rats. J Periodontol. 76:99–106, 2005.
70. Nauroth JM, Liu YC, Van Elswyk M, Bell R, Hall EB, Chung G, Arterburn LM. Docosahexaenoic acid (DHA) and docosapentaenoic acid (DPAn-6) algal oils reduce inflammatory mediators in human peripheral mononuclear cells in vitro and paw edema in vivo. Lipids 45(5):375–384, 2010.
71. Naqvi AZ, Buettner C, Phillips RS, Davis RB, Mukamal KJ. n-3 fatty acids and periodontitis in US adults. J Am Diet Assoc. 110(11):1669–1675, 2010.
72. Rosenstein ED, Kushner LJ, Kramer N, Kazandjian G. Pilot study of dietary fatty acid supplementation in the treatment of adult periodontitis. Prostaglandins Leukot Essent Fatty Acids 68: 213–218, 2003.
73. Eberhard J, Heilmann F, Acil Y, Albers HK, Jepsen S. Local application of n-3 or n-6 polyunsaturated fatty acids in the treatment of human experimental gingivitis. J Clin Periodontol. 29:364–369, 2002.
74. Hasturk H, Goguet-Surmenian E, Blackwood A, Andry C, Kantarci A. 1-Tetradecanol complex: Therapeutic actions in experimental periodontitis. J Periodontol. 80(7):1103–1113, 2009.
75. Hasturk H, Jones VL, Andry C, Kantarci A. 1-Tetradecanol complex reduces progression of Porphyromonas gingivalis-induced experimental periodontitis in rabbits. J Periodontol. 78(5): 924–932, 2007.
76. http://www.imagenetix.net/articles/2006/003_06.php.
77. Seto H, Nagata T. Prevention of osteoporosis by foods and dietary supplements. Milk basic protein (MBP) induces alveolar bone formation in rat experimental periodontitis. Clin Calcium 16(10):1639–1645, 2006.
78. Seto H, Toba Y, Takada Y, Kawakami H, Ohba H, Hama H, Horibe M, Nagata T. Milk basic protein increases alveolar bone formation in rat experimental periodontitis. J Periodontal Res. 42(1):85–89, 2007.
79. Littarru GP, Nakamura R, Ho L, Folkers K, Kuzell WC. Deficiency of coenzyme Q 10 in gingival tissue from patients with periodontal disease. Proc Natl Acad Sci USA 68(10):2332–2335, 1971.
80. Nakamura R, Littarru GP, Folkers K, Wilkinson EG. Study of CoQ10-enzymes in gingiva from patients with periodontal disease and evidence for a deficiency of coenzyme Q10. Proc Natl Acad Sci USA 71(4):1456–1460, 1974.
81. Wilkinson EG, Arnold RM, Folkers K, Hansen I, Kishi H. Bioenergetics in clinical medicine. II. Adjunctive treatment with coenzyme Q in periodontal therapy. Res Commun Chem Pathol Pharmacol. 12(1):111–123, 1975.
82. Hanioka T, Tanaka M, Ojima M, Shizukuishi S, Folkers K. Effect of topical application of coenzyme Q10 on adult periodontitis. Mol Aspects Med. 15 Suppl:s241–248, 1994.
83. Wilkinson EG, Arnold RM, Folkers K. Bioenergetics in clinical medicine. VI. Adjunctive treatment of periodontal disease with coenzyme Q10. Res Commun Chem Pathol Pharmacol. 14(4):715–719, 1976.
84. Watts TL. Coenzyme Q10 and periodontal treatment: Is there any beneficial effect? Br Dent J. 178(6):209–213, 1995.
85. Stein GM, Lewis H. Oral changes in a folic acid deficient patient precipitated by anticonvulsant drug therapy. J Periodontol. 44(10):645–650, 1973.
86. Pack AR, Thomson ME. Effects of topical and systemic folic acid supplementation on gingivitis in pregnancy. J Clin Periodontol. 7(5):402–414, 1980.
87. Thomson ME, Pack AR. Effects of extended systemic and topical folate supplementation on gingivitis of pregnancy. J Clin Periodontol. 9(3):275–280, 1982.
88. Vogel RI, Fink RA, Schneider LC, Frank O, Baker H. The effect of folic acid on gingival health. J Periodontol. 47(11):667–668, 1976.
89. Indrei LL. Nutrition and periodontal disease. Rev Med Chir Soc Med Nat Iasi. 110(1):195–197, 2006.
90. Munoz CA, Kiger RD, Stephens JA, Kim J, Wilson AC. Effects of a nutritional supplement on periodontal status. Compend Contin Educ Dent. 22(5):425–428, 2001.
91. Parrish JH Jr, DeMarco TJ, Bissada NF. Vitamin E and periodontitis in the rat. Oral Surg Oral Med Oral Pathol. 44(2):210–218, 1977.
92. Kim JE, Shklar G. The effect of vitamin E on the healing of gingival wounds in rats. J Periodontol. 54(5):305–308, 1983.
93. Klokkevold PR, Mealey BL. Influence of systemic disorders and stress on the periodontium. In: Carranza's Clinical Periodontology. St. Louis: Saunders, 2006, pp. 228–310.

21

Patient management for periodontal therapy

Brett Beckman

Preoperative evaluation and assessment, intraoperative management and monitoring, and proper recovery of veterinary patients undergoing surgical procedures have been described in detail in multiple veterinary textbooks and journals. However, surgical periodontal therapy requires special demands upon patient physiology during the operative and postoperative period, necessitating focus on particular aspects of patient care. Anesthetic and analgesic management of the periodontal patient must start in the preoperative period and continue through the perioperative period to complete recovery from the anesthetic episode, including a week following the procedure.

Patient safety concerns

Anesthetic duration

Dental procedures often unexpectedly extend to considerably long anesthetic episodes due to the discovery of additional pathology. Therefore, particular attention should be paid to a proper preanesthetic diagnostic workup to ensure maximum safety prior to initiation of any periodontal procedure.[1]

Periodontal procedures require pre- and postoperative radiographs. Technicians should be adept at radiographic positioning and technique prior to anesthesia to maximize patient safety and to minimize time spent obtaining radiographs. (Hands-on training will greatly facilitate this procedure.) Definitive determination of the extent of periodontal pathology in a given patient requires periodontal probing, charting, and radiography. Therefore, therapeutic recommendations and reasonable cost estimates can only be made during anesthesia. The veterinarian must be well trained in recognition of veterinary periodontal pathology and radiographic interpretation to make efficient diagnostic and therapeutic decisions. In addition, staff in charge of generating estimates must be efficient to minimize anesthetic time. Pet guardians must be educated regarding common treatment options prior to the procedure to minimize intraoperative phone time when estimates are revised.

The two parameters that most directly affect long-term morbidity and mortality in anesthetized patients are hypothermia and hypotension.[2,3] Both of these parameters become more pronounced with extended anesthesia time.[4]

Hypothermia

Intraoperatively, hypothermia can become a clinical issue. Small patients (who are predisposed to periodontal disease) have compromisingly large surface area to body mass ratios that predispose them to accelerated heat dissipation under anesthesia.[5] Decreased perfusion accompanies lower blood pressures experienced with inhalant anesthetics contributing to hypothermia.

Furthermore, the oral cavity must remain open during the majority of oral surgical procedures, resulting in a miniature open body cavity capable of losing heat by radiation. The compressed air and water spray utilized to cool high-speed dental burs and the water used for mechanical scalers further compromises normothermia by convection loss. Cold IV fluids can also contribute to hypothermia by similar mechanisms.[6] Physiologically, hypothermia results in lower anesthetic requirements[7] predisposing to accidental anesthetic overdose. Recovery is prolonged and thermoregulation may become impaired, necessitating artificial rewarming.[7,8] Immune system compromise secondary to hypothermia may result in delayed healing or infection.[9]

Veterinary Periodontology, First Edition. Brook A. Niemiec.

Box 21.1 Key clinical point

Prevention is the key to managing hypothermia. Patient temperature maintenance should start upon admittance. Ambient temperature should be kept at a tolerable level for staff and patients. Fans should be directed away from patients and blankets and sweaters used to minimize conduction and convection losses. Warm water blankets and warm air devices[A,B] can maintain patient body temperature preoperatively. Extension of prevention in the operatory involves utilization of the above techniques combined with fluid warming.

Regional nerve blocks and continuous rate infusions allow lower inhalant levels to minimize perfusion compromise. During recovery, warm fluids and warming devices should continue to be utilized until patient temperature has stabilized and is sustainable following removal of external warming. One study suggests that warming of the extremities in dogs is more effective perioperatively than warming the torso.[10]

Patient temperature should also be closely monitored for hyperthermia both perioperatively and postoperatively, especially if opiates are included in the analgesic/anesthetic protocol. Cats are especially susceptible to opiate-induced hyperthermia particularly with hydromorphone.[11] Intervention may include a mu opiate antagonist (nalbuphine, naloxone, or butorphanol) to reverse hyperthermia should it become clinically significant.

Hypotension

Almost all anesthetic drugs have the ability to create hypotension. Furthermore, the majority of patients in need of advanced periodontal care are older to geriatric. These patients commonly have other ailments that may predispose them to this malady. Systemic or specific organ aliments may also preclude some intervention strategies for this complication (e.g., a cardiac patient may not be able to tolerate a fluid bolus).

Low blood pressure is known to cause poor perfusion, which can have numerous deleterious metabolic effects, especially if it is over a prolonged time. Therefore, blood pressure must be closely monitored during dental procedures and hypotension quickly corrected. Finally, practitioners are encouraged to have several options, including dopamine and hetastarch, available for fragile patients.

Patient manipulation

Veterinary patients with periodontal disease generally require full mouth radiography to adequately evaluate the full extent of disease. These radiographs as well as all dental procedures (including but not limited to extractions and periodontal surgery) require manipulation in numerous locations throughout the oral cavity. Consequently the patient is subject to numerous positioning changes throughout a given procedure. Care should be taken when positioning patients to avoid excessive neck manipulation that could result in endotracheal tube induction of vagal nerve stimulation and subsequent bradycardia.[3] Disengagement of the tube prior to positioning also prevents accidental tracheal tears that could result in fatal or life-threatening dyspnea and emphysema.[7,12]

Another complication of oral surgery is emphysema secondary to air from high-speed delivery systems or the air/water spray device. Emphysema generally occurs subcutaneously about the head and neck and usually resolves without treatment within 48 hours. Owners should be notified and a timely recheck scheduled to ensure resolution.

Aspiration

Periodontal therapy requires a large amount of water to be introduced into the oral cavity to cool both the mechanical scalers and high-speed hand-pieces. In addition, periodontal therapy may require removal of bone, tooth sectioning, and surgical tissue manipulation resulting in blood and debris accumulation in the oral cavity. It is therefore paramount that the endotracheal tube is secured and properly inflated prior to surgery to prevent extravasation into the patient's airway. Suction is strongly recommended to decrease this issue as well as to improve surgical visualization.

Equally important is a thorough examination of the oral cavity postoperatively to ensure no debris is present that might be aspirated upon extubation. If gauze is used to further protect the airway during surgery, it is removed and visual inspection of the epiglottis and surrounding tissue performed. If suction is not available, cotton-tipped applicators may be used to retract mucous, blood clots and debris from difficult-to-visualize areas adjacent to the epiglottis. Additional consideration for aspiration should be given to patients that undergo extractions where nasal cavity hemorrhage occurs.

Pain considerations

Periodontal disease is generally a slowly progressive chronic disease process. The human literature suggests that it is painful only in a small number of affected patients.[13] However, pain is reported consistently in areas where root exposure has occurred due to cementum destruction.[13] Some patients report dull, localized, and radiating deep jaw pain due to periodontal disease.[13] Food impaction can also cause varying degrees of discomfort.[13]

Some very important differences should be considered when assessing periodontal disease in veterinary patients. Canine small breed predilection and select individuals genetically prone to periodontal disease in the absence of consistent oral hygiene often present with profound soft tissue destruction and bone compromise. Food and debris impaction are much more likely due to severity and size of the periodontal defects in these patients. Cementum destruction resulting in root exposure creates sensitivity. Clinically, it is common to produce jaw movement upon probing even under light to moderate anesthetic depths, indicating pain associated with periodontal defects.

In humans, periodontal disease is more prevalent in compromised socioeconomic areas where oral hygiene is not routinely practiced.[14–17] From the standpoint of oral neglect, our patients resemble this human subset. A recent study revealed that 96% of the homeless people in Hong Kong had periodontal disease. The dental problems most frequently reported in this population were bleeding gums or drifting teeth (62%), dental pain (52%), and tooth trauma (38%).[16]

Another study in New Jersey showed that 55.6% of the homeless people studied had current orofacial pain and two-thirds of the participants reported having dental-related face pain during the past year.[15] Although direct assumptions of the source of pain (periodontal disease vs. caries) cannot be made, neglect likely results in a higher prevalence of pain in our animal patients as well.

Chronic pain

Veterinary patients with severe local manifestations of periodontal disease and those with unusual forms of periodontal disease have been discussed in detail in chapters 6 and 8, respectively. In many of these examples, chronic pain is a hallmark of disease. Special preparation should be strongly considered when approaching these cases surgically. Recognizing not only the pain at the site of inflammation but also the often-neglected central pain mechanisms is important when managing these patients. *Initiating acute surgical pain to chronically diseased painful tissue heightens the pain response, creating a patient that is difficult to manage postoperatively.*

The pathophysiology described above outlines the importance of pre-, peri-, and postsurgical analgesic management of patients with chronic oral pain associated with periodontal disease. This is true whether it is periodontal disease as it is classically defined or one of its local or unusual manifestations. Opiates and NSAIDs should be considered for oral pain at the site of inflammation, and centrally acting agents utilized to minimize the perpetuation of excitatory neurotransmitters in the nucleus caudalis.

Agents whose mechanisms of action alter pain modulation offer a means of attenuating the excitatory physiology responsible for this "wind-up" component of pain. Gabapentin, pregabalin, amantidine, ketamine, and lidocaine are common examples. Additional specific agents and protocols recommended by veterinary anesthesiologists for pre- and postoperative pain management can be found in current veterinary literature and anesthesia texts, and their discussion exceeds the intent of this chapter.

Box 21.2 Key clinical point

It is important to understand the pathophysiology of central pain sensitization in order to make decisions on the therapeutic approach to our chronic oral pain cases. Pain signals from the head and oral cavity are modulated within the nucleus caudalis of the brainstem, much like those from the rest of the body are modulated within the dorsal horn of the spinal cord.[18] In acute oral pain, excitatory neurotransmitters (most specifically glutamate) are released from the presynaptic neuron and enter the synapse and bind to the AMPA receptors of the postsynaptic neuron.[19] Inhibitory neurotransmitters released into the synapse from higher centers attempt to dampen this signal.[20] Sustained release of glutamate results in stimulation of NMDA receptors and subsequent Substance P release that binds to neurokinin-1 (NK-1) receptors when acute pain is not managed correctly.[21] This represents the point of transition from acute to chronic pain and the initiation of central sensitization. At this point less stimulation is needed peripherally to initiate amplification of the pain signal (allodynia), less glutamate is required to perpetuate transmission, and more descending inhibitory neurotransmitters are required to dampen pain perception.[21]

Regional nerve blocks

When correctly administered, regional nerve blocks provide not only elimination of pain perception in the innervated tissue but also positive systemic effects. Proper blockade of oral tissues prior to surgical manipulation eliminates cerebral perception, allowing anesthetic planes similar to that used with non-painful procedures. Consequently, a reduction in the percentage of inhalant anesthetic will have positive effects on intraoperative physiology, minimizing hypotension, hypoventilation, and bradycardia.[22] If perfusion is maximized, normothermia becomes easier to maintain.

This author routinely utilizes lidocaine and bupivicaine in combination for regional oral nerve blocks. Use of this combination is well documented in human medicine for a variety of applications.[23–25] The veterinary literature suggests the onset of action of bupivicaine is significantly longer than that of lidocaine. The duration of effect of lidocaine (1–2 hours)[26] does not provide adequate analgesic duration in lengthy procedures and offers very minimal if any extended effect in the postoperative period. Bupivicaine's effect is notably longer in duration (8 hours)[26] but is traditionally thought to have a longer onset of action. Studies in humans, however, suggest that the average onset may be as short as 4.4–7.7 minutes.[27–29] Bupivicaine's extended duration of effect makes it a comparatively superior choice for use alone or in combination with lidocaine. The recommended maximum total dose of local anesthetics is 2 mg/kg (whether used alone or in combination).[22]

Using a maximum patient dose of 1.0 mg/kg lidocaine 2.0% and bupivicaine 0.5%[30] results in a volume ratio of 1:4, respectively. *This maximum dose should be calculated first and not exceeded.* Recommended infusion volumes vary from 0.25–1.6 ml from small to large patients.[31]

Blood pressure, heart rate, and respiration rate should remain stable upon surgical insult if blocks have been administered properly and adequate onset time from administration has been given. Increases in these physiologic parameters indicate that the block is not effective or optimal time to onset was not allowed. The nerve block may be repeated providing that the maximum total dose is not exceeded.

No special needles or syringes are needed. Needle sizes of 27–29 gauge are too flexible to place consistently without directional deviation. Standard length 25-gauge needles are preferred.

Intravascular administration must be avoided. Aspirating prior to injection will ensure extravascular placement of the agent. Excessive systemic uptake or intravascular administration could result in CNS, cardiovascular, or vasopressive complications.[32]

This author has never experienced complications at these dosages. Clinically, prehension and mastication do not appear to be compromised postoperatively in dogs and cats receiving dental blocks even if all four quadrants are blocked.

Studies have widely demonstrated mu opiate receptor association with peripheral nerves.[21–23,33–35] Human research supports the addition of opiates to local anesthetics to extend their duration of action. Adding buprenorphine or morphine to a bupivicaine brachial plexus block in one study resulted in a duration almost twice that experienced with bupivicaine alone.[36] A similar study demonstrated analgesia from systemic buprenorphine plus a bupivicaine regional brachial plexus block to be inferior to inclusion of buprenorphine with bupivicaine locally.[37] More research is needed to explore this exciting possibility and its application in veterinary patients.

Rostral maxillary regional block (infraorbital) (Figures 21.1 and 21.2)

The rostral maxillary block affects the infraorbital nerve and the rostral maxillary alveolar nerve. The rostral maxillary alveolar nerve branches to enter the incisivomaxillary foramen within the infraorbital canal and innervates the canine and incisor teeth.[38] The infraorbital nerve courses rostrally to innervate the soft tissues of the lip and gingiva.[38]

To perform this block, manually retract the lip and the infraorbital neurovascular bundle dorsally. The

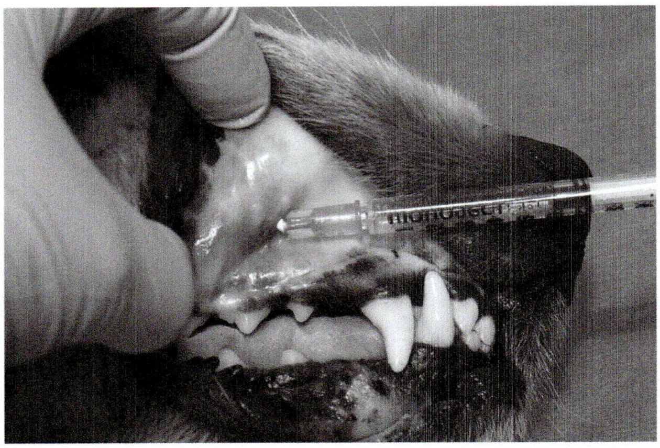

Figure 21.1 Rostral maxillary block. The infraorbital neurovascular bundle and lip are retracted dorsally and the needle is placed as shown.

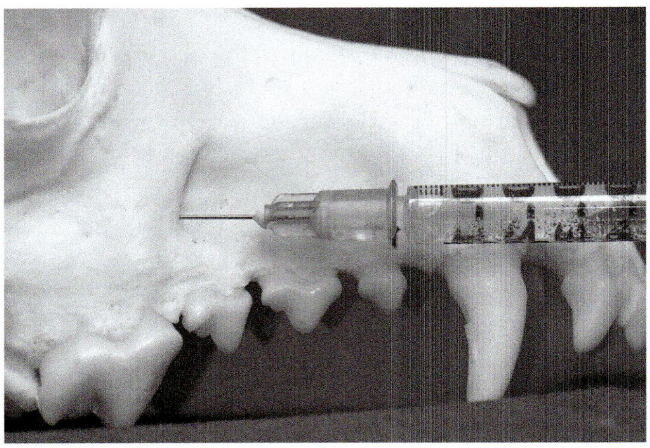

Figure 21.2 Rostral maxillary block. A cadaver skull demonstrates the location of needle placement. The needle is placed just inside the canal.

neurovascular bundle is easily palpated as a band of tissue coursing rostral and slightly dorsal from the infraorbital foramen demonstrated beneath the vestibular mucosa. Advance the needle in a caudal direction close to the maxillary bone and ventral to the retracted bundle to a point just inside the canal. The needle should pass into the canal without engaging bone. Correct placement can be confirmed if desired, by gentle lateral movement of the needle allowing it to engage the canal wall.

Caudal maxillary regional block (Figures 21.3 and 21.4)

The pterygopalatine nerve and the infraorbital nerve are branches of the maxillary nerve and supply sensory innervation to the maxilla.[38] Tissues innervated include all teeth in the quadrant, the bone surrounding the teeth, and the adjacent soft tissue to the midline. Major and minor palatine nerves leave the pterygopalatine nerve and innervate the hard and soft palatal mucosa and the palatal bone.[38] To perform this block, the mouth is opened wide and the lip commissure retracted caudally. The needle is directed in a dorsal direction, immediately behind the central portion of the maxillary second molar tooth. Advancement of the needle need not be more than 3–5 millimeters depending upon patient size. A recent study showed the caudal maxillary block may be achieved by holding direct digital pressure over the infraorbital canal for 60 seconds following the infraorbital block (see above).[39]

Rostral mandibular regional (mental) block (Figures 21.5 and 21.6)

In the rostral mandibular block, both the inferior alveolar nerve (that courses rostral within the mandibular canal) and its cutaneous branch, the middle mental nerve, are affected. The middle mental nerve exits the middle mental foramen apical to the mesial root of the second premolar in the dog, and in the diastema between the canine and third premolar in the cat, to innervate the

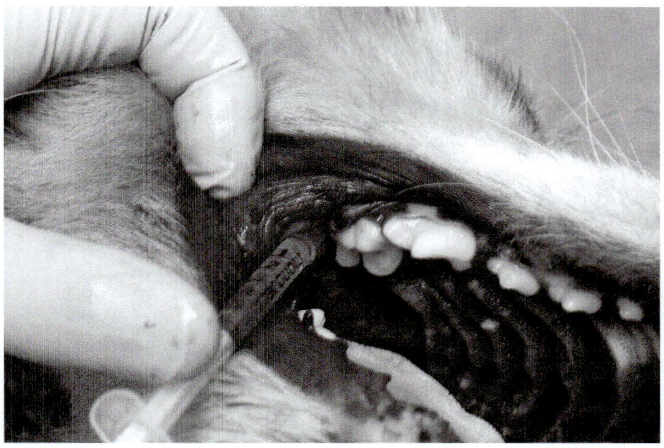

Figure 21.3 Caudal maxillary block. The needle is placed just behind the maxillary second premolar and advanced only slightly.

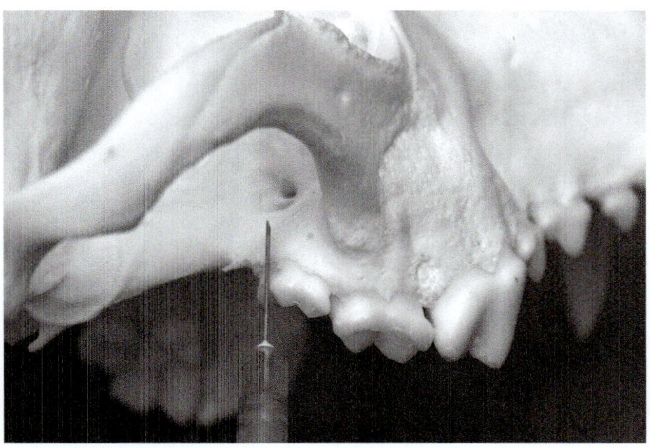

Figure 21.4 Caudal maxillary block. A cadaver skull demonstrates the location of needle placement. The needle need only advance as shown.

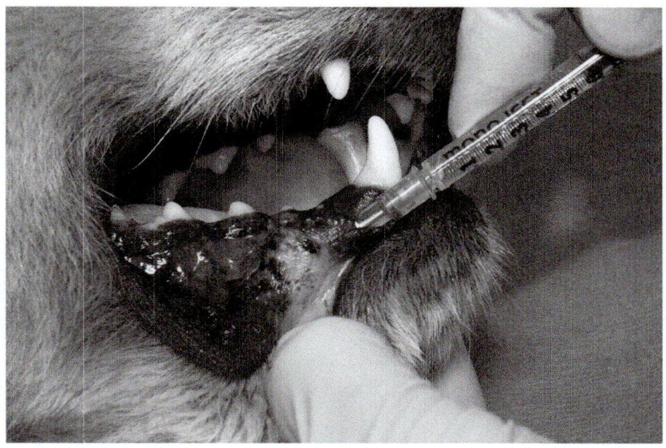

Figure 21.5 Rostral mandibular block. The mandibular labial frenulum is retracted ventrally and the needle placed as shown.

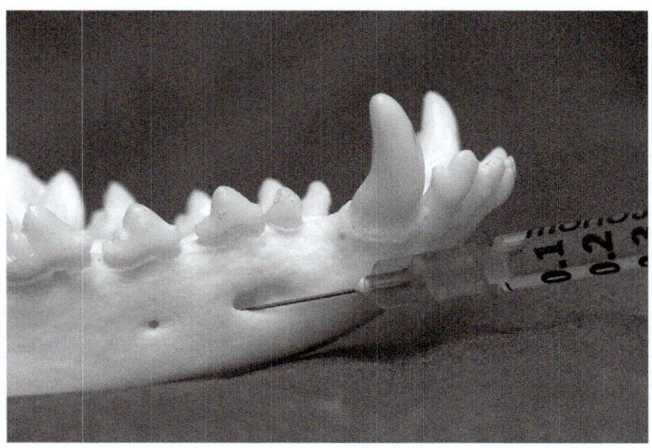

Figure 21.6 Rostral mandibular block. A cadaver skull demonstrates the location of needle placement. The needle is placed just inside the canal.

lip.[38] The canal is located one-third of the distance from the ventral to the dorsal border of the mandible. The inferior alveolar nerve continues within the canal to innervate the mandibular third premolar to the central incisor and the surrounding bone.[38] Therefore, needle placement must be within the canal to properly anesthetize all tissue.

To perform this block, the mandibular labial frenulum is retracted ventrally. The needle is inserted at the rostral aspect of the frenulum and advanced along the mandibular bone to just enter the canal. Placement can be confirmed by moving the syringe laterally to encounter the lateral aspect of the canal.

Caudal mandibular regional block (Figures 21.7 and 21.8)

The inferior alveolar nerve enters the mandibular foramen on the lingual aspect of the caudal mandibular body.[38] The caudal mandibular block is performed by infiltrating the nerve at this level prior to its entry into the canal. The administrator should visualize a line extending from the lateral canthus to the ventral mandible. The needle is then inserted at the point of intersection of this imaginary line and the lingual aspect of the ventral mandible. The needle is then advanced to a point one-third of the distance of the width of the mandible. All teeth, adjacent bone, and soft tissue are affected by this block. This block may also be performed intraorally, which is more technically demanding in some patients.

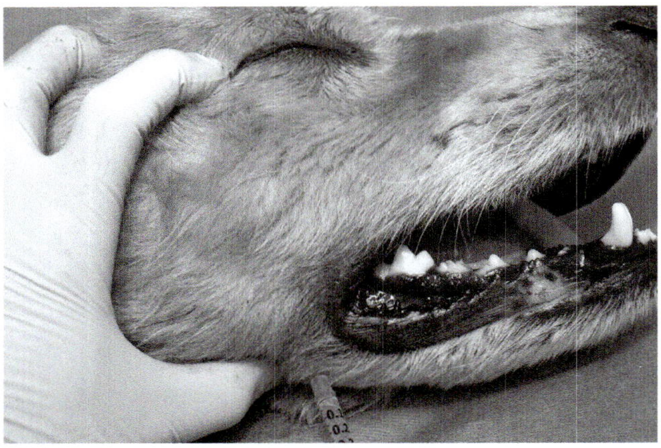

Figure 21.7 Caudal mandibular block. The lateral canthus is utilized as a landmark in determining the point of needle entry on the lingual aspect of the ventral mandibular skin.

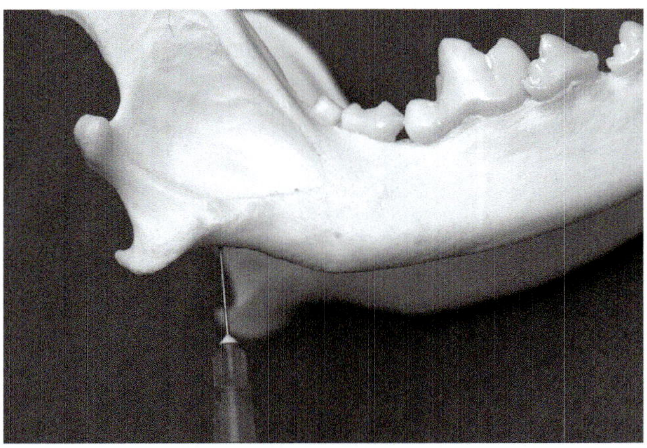

Figure 21.8 Caudal mandibular block. A cadaver skull demonstrates the location of needle placement. The agent(s) are deposited adjacent to the bone as described.

Animals that are not monitored postoperatively have been known to cause severe trauma to the tongue during the recovery period. Whether this is specifically associated with regional oral nerve blocks (particularly the caudal mandibular) or recovery from any procedure is not reflected in the literature. In any case, proper patient monitoring during recovery should preclude this problem.

Feline and brachycephalic anatomical differences

Cats and brachycephalic dogs posses similar anatomical differences that require minor variations in technique when administering nerve blocks. The rostral maxillary nerve block is performed as described; however, the entrance to the canal resides comparatively more dorsally. Careful caudal advancement should place the needle just within the canal.

The infraorbital canal in cats and brachycephalic dogs is much shorter while the foramen is relatively larger than in other dogs. Consequently, the infraorbital and pterygopalatine nerves lie just caudal to the site of administration for the rostral maxillary block. This eliminates the need for the caudal maxillary block. The orbit is closer to needle placement in these patients, so care must be taken to ensure the needle just enters the canal and is not directed too far caudally.

Postoperative care

The pain control that has been carefully provided pre- and intraoperatively is of little use if the patient is not adequately treated postop. At the end of anesthesia, the practitioner should review the pain management protocol and ensure that (1) it is appropriate for the level of surgery performed, (2) there are no gaps in the protocol (by noting the timing of administration and duration of action), and (3) the pain medications are provided for an appropriate amount of time. One week is the standard length of treatment in most periodontal cases. Finally, clients should be informed that patients will rarely show signs of pain and to administer the pain medicants as prescribed, regardless of lack of perceived pain (unless the patient is having an adverse reaction).

Pain evaluation and scoring

Pain evaluation for patients with periodontal disease both preoperatively and postoperatively should utilize oral palpation of affected tissue and behavioral observation. Patient avoidance of oral manipulation, however, may be related to pain or individual behavioral intolerance to oral manipulation unassociated with pain. Pain scales provide written documentation of pain behaviors and should be considered as a part of the pain management protocol. Additional analgesics can be given at appropriate intervals, based upon palpation and behavioral results from the pain scale evaluation, to maintain patient comfort. If questions still exist regarding pain status of a particular patient one should err on the side of assuming that pain exists. Agents for both central and peripheral pain analgesia should be utilized for patients with significant chronic periodontal pathology.

Box 21.3 Key points

- Periodontal procedures often unexpectedly turn into long anesthetics. Proper patient and client preparation and intraoperative care and monitoring will help ensure a safe anesthesia.
- Hypothermia and hypotension are serious complications and steps must be taken to prevent and/or control them.
- Periodontal patients are likely in chronic pain, which increased acutely with treatment. Pain management is mandatory for proper care.
- Regional anesthesia is a critical piece of patient management for oral care.

Notes

A. Hot Dog Patient Warming System, Augustine Biomedical & Design.
B. Gaymar TP500 T/pump, Gaymar Industries, Inc.

References

1. Huffman LJ. Oral examination. In: Small Animal Dental, Oral and Maxillofacial Disease, a Color Handbook (Niemiec BA ed.). London: Manson, 2010, pp. 39–61.
2. Torossian A. Thermal management during anaesthesia and thermoregulation standards for the prevention of inadvertent perioperative hypothermia. Best Pract Res Clin Anaesthesiol. 22(4):659–668, 2008.
3. Broadbelt DC, Pfeiffer DU, Young LE, Wood JLN. Results of the confidential enquiry into perioperative small animal fatalities regarding risk factors for anesthetic-related death in dogs. JAVMA 233(7):1096–1103, 2008.
4. Hall LW, Clarke KW, Trim CM. Veterinary Anesthesia. 10th ed. London: Saunders, 2001.
5. Muir WW, Hubbell JAI, Skarda RT, Bednarski RM. Handbook of Veterinary Pain Management. 3rd ed. St. Louis:Mosby, 2002, pp. 177–179.
6. Marietta M, Facchini L, et al. Pathophysiology of bleeding in surgery. Transplant Proc. 38(3):812–814, 2006.
7. Paddleford RR. Manual of Small Animal Anesthesia. 2nd ed. Philadephia: Saunders, 1999, p. 144.
8. Pottie RG, Dart CM, et al. Effect of hypothermia on recovery from general anaesthesia in the dog. Aust Vet J. 85(4):158–162, 2007.
9. Kurosawa S, Kato M. Anesthetics, immune cells, and immune responses. J Anesth 22(3):263–277, 2008.
10. Cabell LW, Perkowski SZ, et al. The effects of active peripheral skin warming on perioperative hypothermia in dogs. Vet Surg 26(2):79–85, 1997.
11. Niedfeldt RL, Robertson SA. Postanesthetic hyperthermia in cats: A retrospective comparison between hydromorphone and buprenorphine. Vet Anaesth Analg. 33(6):341–342, 2006.
12. Mitchell SL, McCarth R, Rudloff E, Pemell RT. Tracheal rupture associated with intubation in cats: 20 cases (1996–1998). JAVMA 216(10):1592–1595, 2000.
13. Nagy RJ, Novak MJ. Chronic periodontitis. In: Carranza's Clinical Periodontology. St. Louis: Saunders, 2006.
14. Luo Y, McGrath C. Oral health status of homeless people in Hong Kong. Spec Care Dentist 26(4):150–1504, 2006.
15. Conte M, Broder HL, Jenkins G, Reed R, Janal MN. Oral health, related behaviors and oral health impacts among homeless adults. J Public Health Dent. 66(4):276–278, 2006.
16. Luo Y, McGrath C. Oral health and its impact on the life quality of homeless people in Hong Kong. Community Dent Health 25(3):137–142, 2008.
17. Cunha-Cruz J, Hujoel PP, Kressin NR. Oral health-related quality of life of periodontal patients. J Periodontal Res. 42(2):169–176, 2007.
18. Hargreaves KM, Hutter JW. Endodontic pharmacology. In: Pathways of the Pulp (Cohen S, Burns RC eds.). 8th ed. St Louis: Mosby, 2002.
19. Tony L Yaksh. Central pharmacology of nociceptive transmission. In: Wall and Melzack's Textbook of Pain (McMahon S, Koltzenburg M eds.). 5th ed. China: Elsevier, 2006.
20. Fields HL, Basbaum AI, Heinricher MM. Central nervous system mechanisms of pain modulation. In: Wall and Melzack's Textbook of Pain (McMahon S, Koltzenburg M eds.). 5th ed. China: Elsevier, 2006, pp. 130–135.
21. Brookoff D. Chronic pain: A new disease? Hospital Pract. 35(7):45, 2000.
22. Holmstrom SE, Frost P, Eisner ER. Dental prophylaxis. In: Veterinary Dental Techniques. 2nd ed. Philadelphia: Saunders, 1998, pp. 492–493.
23. Lee-Elliott CE, Dundas D, Patel U. Randomized trial of lidocaine vs lidocaine/bupivacaine periprostatic injection on longitudinal pain scores after prostate biopsy. J Urol. 171(1):247–250, 2004.
24. Kaukinen S, Kaukinen L, Eerola R. Epidural anaesthesia with mixtures of bupiviacaine-lidocaine and etidocaine-lidocaine. Ann Chir Gynaeco. l69(6):281–286, 1980.
25. Price DD, Long S, Wilsey B, Fafii A. Analysis of peak magnitude and duration of analgesia produced by local anesthetics injected into sympathetic ganglia of complex regional pain syndrome patients. Clin J Pain. 14(3):216–226, 1998.
26. Khursheed R. Local Anesthetics. In: Handbook of Veterinary Pain Management (Gaynor JS, Muir W III eds.). St. Louis: Mosby, 2002, p. 232.
27. Gross R, McCartney M, Reader A, Beck M. A prospective, randomized, double-blind comparison of bupivacaine and lidocaine for maxillary infiltrations. J Endod. 33(9):1021–1024, 2997.
28. Lai F, Sutton B, Nicholson G. Comparison of L-bupivacaine 0.75% and lidocaine 2% with bupivacaine 0.75% and lidocaine 2% for peribulbar anaesthesia. Br J Anaesth. 90(4):512–514, 2003.

29. Valvano M, Leffler S. Comparison of bupivacaine and lidocaine/bupivacaine for local anesthesia/digital nerve block. Ann Emerg Med. 27(4):490–492, 1996.
30. Stein R, Thompson D. Veterinary Anesthesia Support Group. www.VASG.org.
31. Beckman BW. Pathophysiology and management of surgical and chronic oral pain in dogs and cats. J Vet Dent. 23(1):50–60, 2006.
32. Khursheed R. Local anesthetics. In: Handbook of Veterinary Pain Management (Gaynor JS, Muir W III eds.). St. Louis: Mosby, 2002, p. 232.
33. Ko MC, Butleman ER, Woods JH. The role of peripheral mu opioid receptors in the modulation of capsaicin-induced thermal nociception in rhesus monkeys. J Pharmacol Exp Ther. 286(1):150–156, 1998.
34. Obara I, Przewlocki R, Przewlocka B. Local peripheral effects of mu-opioid receptor agonists in neuropathic pain in rats. Neurosci Lett. 360(1–2):85–89, 2004.
35. Houghton AK, Valdez JG, Westlund KN. Peripheral morphine administration blocks the development of hyperalgesia and allodynia after bone damage in the rat anesthesiology. Anesthesiology 89(1):190–201, 1998.
36. Bazin JE, Massoni C, Bruelle P, Fenies V, Groslier D, Schoeffler P. The addition of opioids to local anaesthetics in brachial plexus block: The comparative effects of morphine, buprenorphine and sufentanil. Anaesthesia 52(9):858–862, 1997.
37. Candido KD, Winnie AP, Ghaleb AH, Fattouh MW, Franco CD. Buprenorphine added to the local anesthetic for axillary brachial plexus block prolongs postoperative analgesia. Reg Anesth Pain Med. 27(2):162–167, 2002.
38. Evans HE, Christensen GC. Miller's Anatomy of the Dog. 2nd ed. Philadelphia: Saunders, 1979, pp. 914–920.
39. Klima, L. Intraoral nerve blocks: Expectations and delivery. Proceedings Veterinary Dental Forum, 2007, pp. 381–383.

SECTION 6

Periodontal instrumentation

22

Periodontal hand instruments

There are various types of hand instruments available for periodontal therapy. These include instruments designed for collecting diagnostic information as well as performing scaling and surgery. This chapter will provide information on the majority of instruments currently available along with brief descriptions of proper usage. More detailed attention is provided on hand instruments designed for scaling.

Instruments for diagnosis

Periodontal probes (Figure 22.1)

Periodontal probes are primarily used to measure sulcal or pocket depth, as well as to determine their anatomic configuration.[1] In addition, they can be used to measure oral masses as well as gingival enlargement and recession. These probes are tapered rod-like instruments with blunt rounded tips that are measured and marked in millimeters.[1–3] There are numerous designs of periodontal probes currently available. The majority of probes require manual measurements, but there are options for instruments that measure pocket depth mechanically.[4]

Standard periodontal probes fall into two major categories: notched and anodized (or color-coded).[2,5] In addition, they can be obtained in a variety of cross-sectional shapes such as round, oval, or flat.[3] The notched types are made with mechanically produced indentations at selected intervals. These may or may not have coloration within the indented markings. While perfectly suitable for diagnosis, they are usually slightly thicker than color-coded probes. Regardless of the type selected, it is strongly recommended to choose a probe with markings at every millimeter for more accurate measurements. A longer style of probe is also recommended, as dogs commonly have pockets in excess of 10 mm. This author's probe of choice is the UNC-15 probe, which is 15 mm long and has markings every mm (Figure 22.1a). The marquis probe with markings every 3 mm and measures up to 18 mm is another good option, but any probe can be effective (Figure 22.1b).

Specialized probes are also available. One style employs a latch that will collapse if too much pressure is applied. This helps avoid false positives that may occur if the probe is forced through the gingival attachment, as inflamed periodontal tissues are friable and can easily be penetrated by the thin metal probes. Another specialized selection is a curved #2 Nabers probe that is used for furcation detection[1] (Figure 22.1c).

Recently, a veterinary-specific probe[A] has become available that is color-coded for canine and feline patients. This probe allows for inexperienced operators to consistently diagnose periodontal pockets in cats and dogs (Figure 22.1d).

Many periodontal probes (including the veterinary probe above) are combined with an explorer that is placed on the opposite end of the instrument. This creates an "expro," which is the most efficient instrument for periodontal/oral evaluation (Figure 22.1e).

Dental explorers (Figure 22.2)

These are sharp, relatively fine instruments that are used to evaluate for tooth surface irregularities such as residual calculus, caries, resorptive lesions, fractures, and inconspicuous pulp exposure.[1–3] These instruments are generally used supragingivally but with care can be used subgingivally (e.g., evaluating for tooth resorption).

Veterinary Periodontology, First Edition. Brook A. Niemiec.

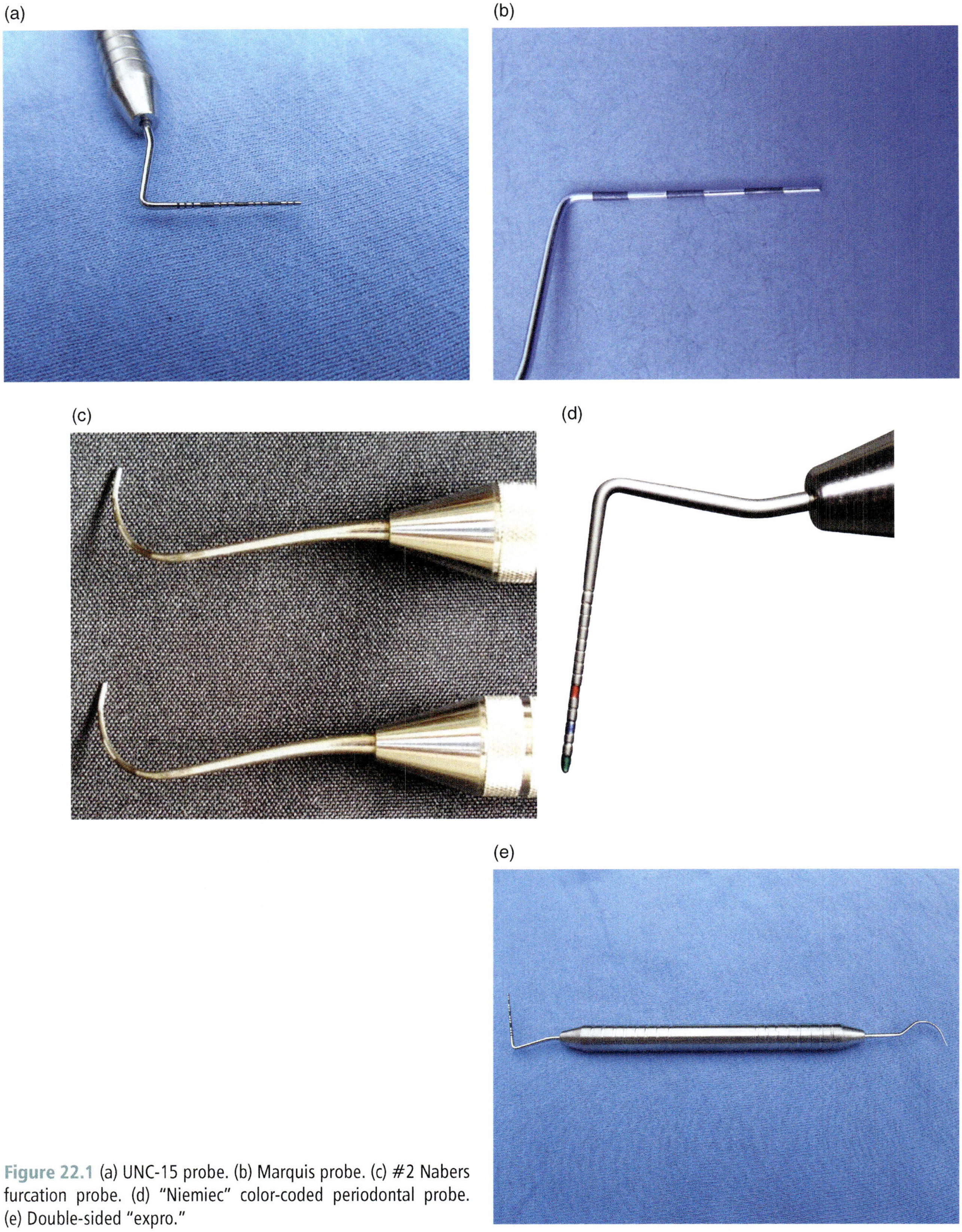

Figure 22.1 (a) UNC-15 probe. (b) Marquis probe. (c) #2 Nabers furcation probe. (d) "Niemiec" color-coded periodontal probe. (e) Double-sided "expro."

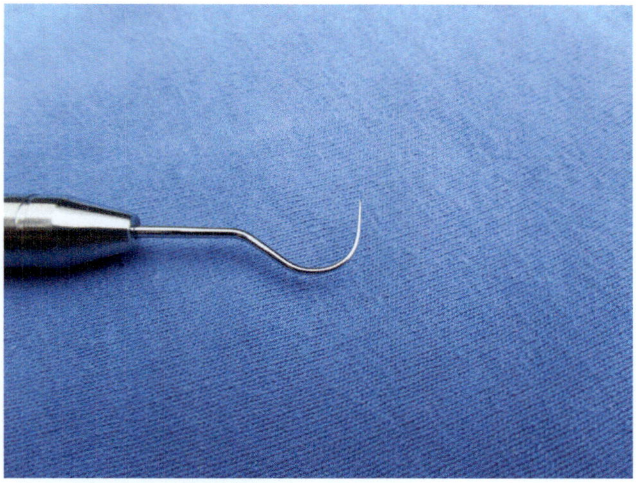

Figure 22.2 Classic sickle explorer.

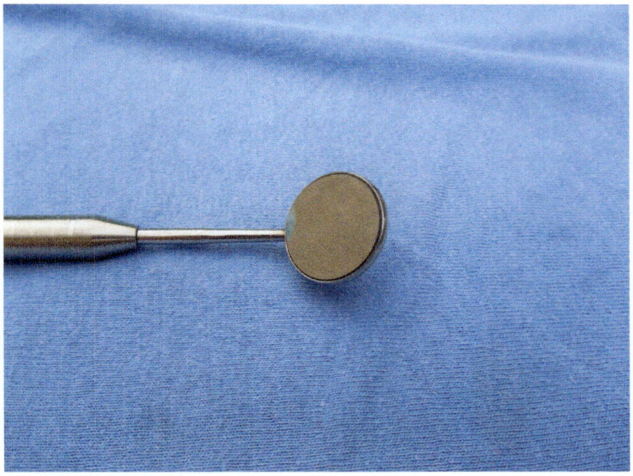

Figure 22.3 Front surface mirror.

The classic explorer is sickle-shaped (#23),[2] but many fine styles are available for increased tactile sensitivity. This author recommends that practitioners have a "pigtail" (#3CH) explorer to evaluate feline dentition.

Dental mirrors (Figure 22.3)

Mirrors are helpful to evaluate the distal areas of the teeth/mouth. They can also be a useful aid in illumination, transillumination, and retraction.[2,6] There are numerous types of dental mirrors, each with various positive attributes and scenarios for different indications. The front surface mirror provides the best image and is thus likely the best choice for use in veterinary dentistry.[2]

Box 22.1 Instruments for scaling

Note that periodontal hand instruments are only effective when sharp. This means they need to be sharpened on a regular basis (at least weekly if used regularly). If a curette or scaler has not been sharpened in over a few months, it will likely need to be professionally sharpened or replaced. For sharpening instructions please see appendix 3.

Scalers (Figure 22.4)

Scalers have three sharp edges (both sides and the bottom), a sharp tip, and are flat across the top (Figures 22.4a and b).[2,3,5] There are numerous sizes and shapes of scalers available, with the same basic architecture. Large-sized scalers include the Ball and Indiana University types, as well as the classic sickle (Figure 22.4c).[1] In contrast, Jacquette scalers are medium-sized and straight (Figure 22.4d). There are also smaller posterior scalers,[1] but these are not commonly used in veterinary medicine. This author recommends a combination of a large- and medium-sized scaler, which can be obtained in one instrument (U15/30) (Figure 22.4e).

Most scalers are "universal," meaning they can be used anywhere in the mouth. These instruments have their cutting edge perpendicular to the handle[3] (Figure 22.4f) and therefore are most effective when the handle is parallel to the tooth. Area-specific scalers are another option; they add an additional angle to the terminal end or shank of the instrument (see curettes below). Scalers with straight shanks are designed to be used rostrally in the mouth, while those with an additional (contra) angle are used more distally.[1]

While these instruments are very effective at calculus removal, they are designed for *supra*gingival scaling only.[3,5] If introduced under the gingival margin they may result in tearing/cutting the gingival tissues, because all contact surfaces (the sides, bottom, and tip) of scalers are sharp.[1]

Hoe scalers (Figure 22.5)

These instruments are actually rarely used in veterinary dentistry, but the standard hoe scalers are the McCall's series. Hoe scalers are very thin instruments that are designed to be used in a pull manner. The blade is bent at a 99- to 100-degree angle, with the cutting edge beveled at 45 degrees.[2] It is also slightly bowed to allow a two-point contact with the tooth surface, resulting in superior control.[1] The blade is very thin to allow for excellent access to the roots in narrow pockets.

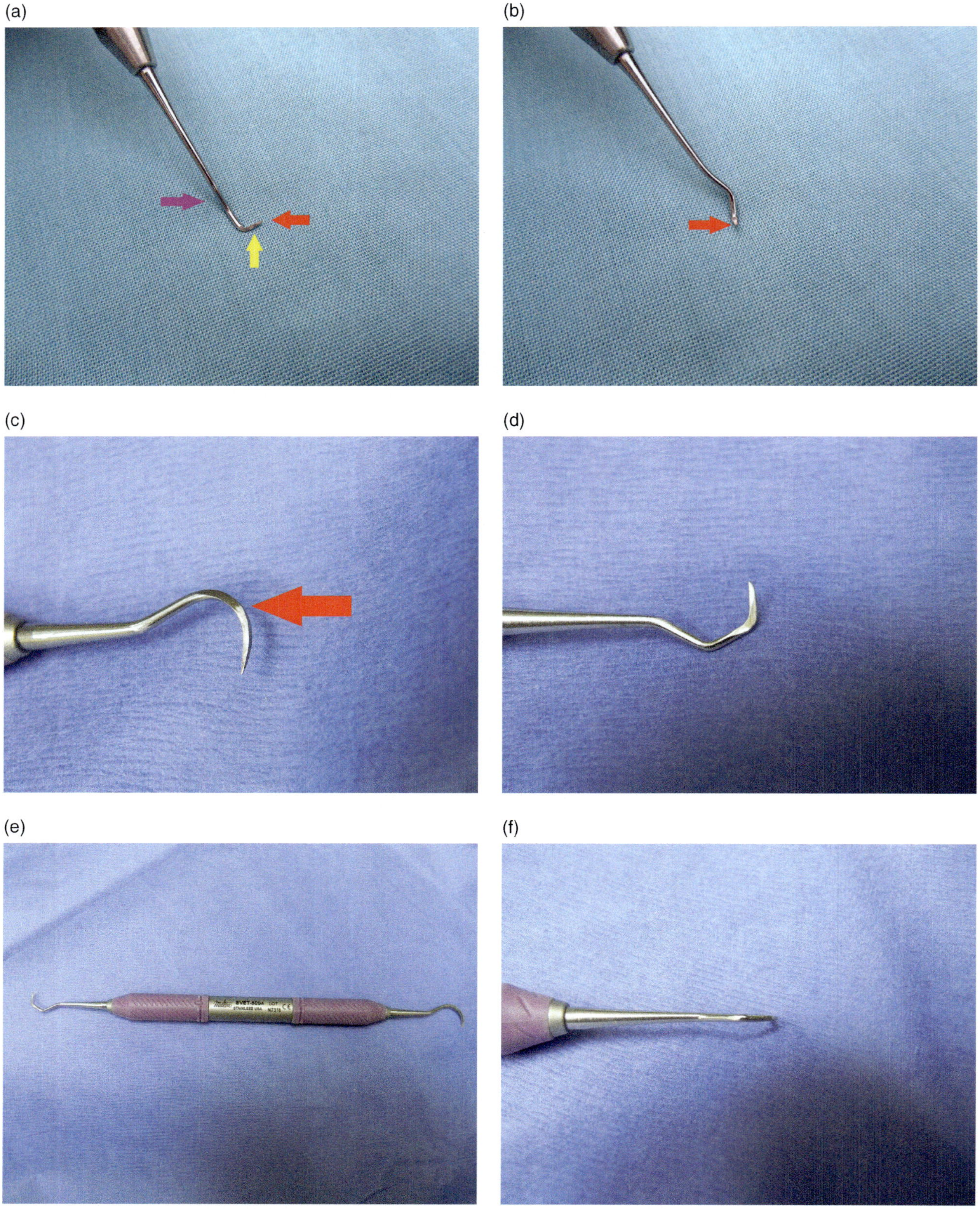

Figure 22.4 Scalers. (a) Side view. (b) Top view. Notice the sharp edges (yellow arrows) and tip (red arrow). In addition, there is a mild accessory bend (purple arrow). (c) Sickle scaler (for large calculus accumulations). Note sharp back (red arrow). (d) Jacquette scaler (for smaller spaces). (e) Double-ended Jacquette/sickle scaler. (f) Back view: showing lack of secondary angle of a "universal" scaler.

(a)

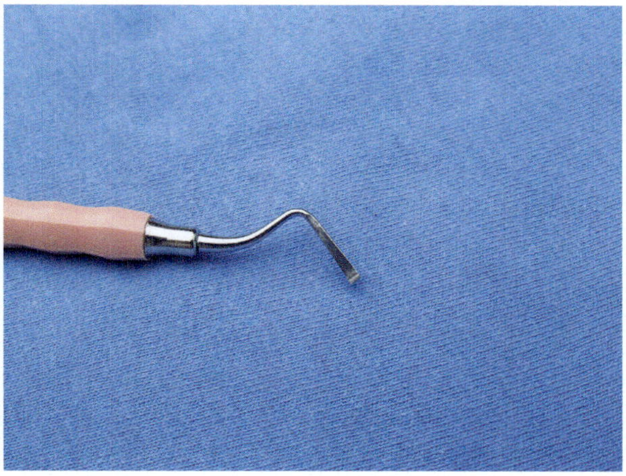

(b)

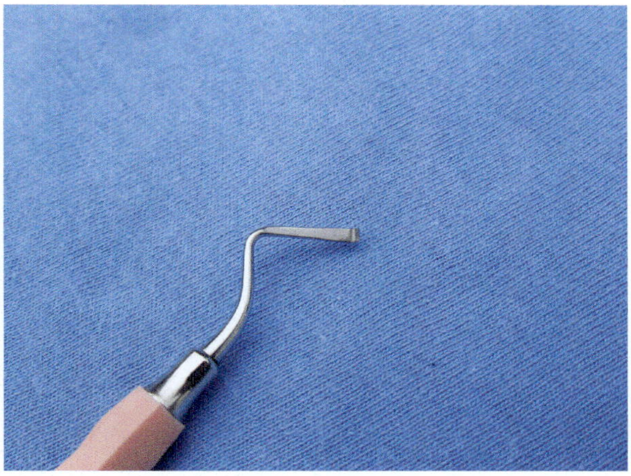

(c)

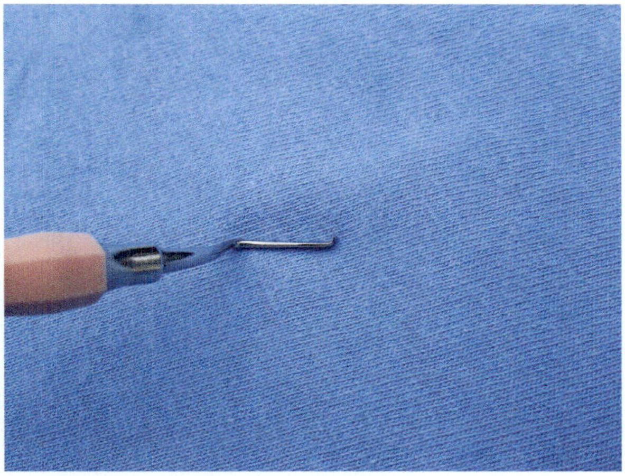

Figure 22.5 Hoe scaler. (a) Front. (b) Face. (c) Side.

Curettes

Curettes are the instruments of choice for subgingival calculus removal, root planing, and subgingival curettage.[1] A curette has two cutting edges and a blunted toe and bottom (Figure 22.6).[2,7] These instruments are semicircular in cross section with a convex base.[1] When properly utilized they will not cut through the delicate periodontal attachment or lacerate the gingiva,[2] and they can be safely utilized within periodontal pockets. There are two major types of curettes, universal and area-specific.[1]

(a)

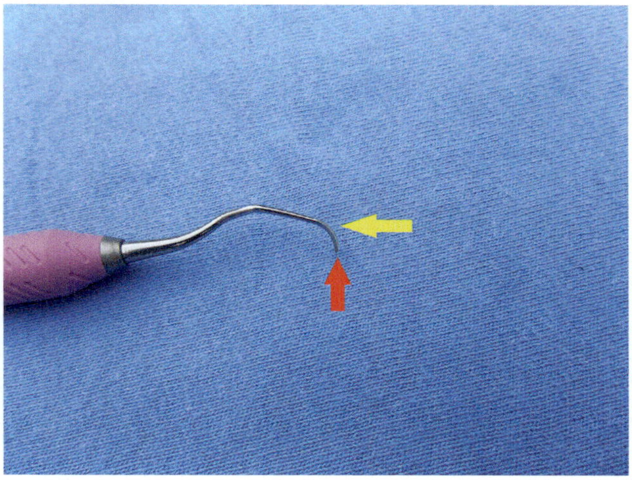

(b)

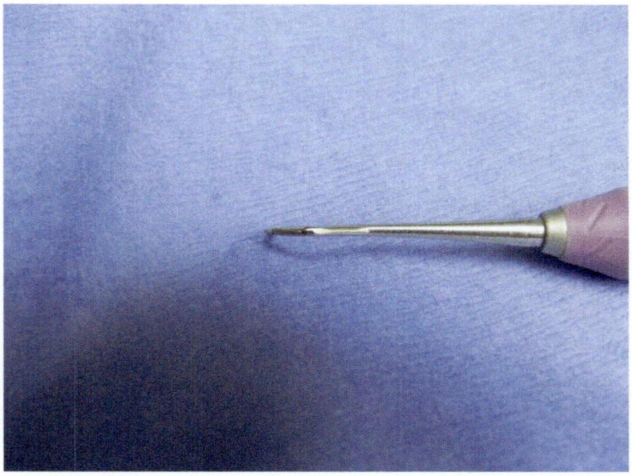

Figure 22.6 Gracey curette. (a) Side view showing curved face (yellow arrow) and blunted toe (red arrow). (b) Back view showing blunted surface.

Universal curettes (Figure 22.7)

Universal curettes typically have a blade at a 90-degree angle to the terminal shank.[1,3] This design allows them to be used throughout the mouth, providing that the instrument is adapted to the tooth correctly.[7] Various manufacturers offer options of angulation and blade size.[1] Colombia and Barnhart are the most common types of universal curettes. These instruments generally have what is known as "handle parallelism."[2] Handle parallelism means that when the handle of the instrument is parallel to the tooth, the blade is in proper position for calculus removal.

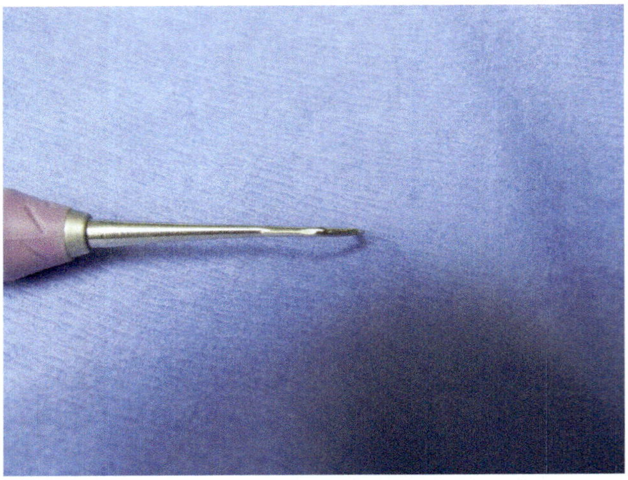

Figure 22.7 Universal curette (from behind). No accessory bend.

Area-specific curettes (Figure 22.8)

Gracey curettes are the classic area-specific curette. They are designed with different angles to provide superior adaptation to specific areas of the dentition.[1] The primary angle or bend allows the instrument to gain access to different areas of the mouth. (Figure 22.8a) Additionally, these instruments are created with an offset blade that is at a 60- to 70-degree angle to the terminal shank.[3] (Figure 22.8b) The blade itself is also curved.[1] These instruments have only one cutting edge,[2] but these blade modifications allow the instrument to be adapted to precise positions on the tooth for proper cleaning. Thus, these instruments have what is called "shank parallelism."[2] Shank parallelism means that the blade is in proper position for calculus removal when the terminal shank (as opposed to the handle) is parallel to the tooth.[1] A major advantage of this design is that the

(a)

(b)

(c)

(d)

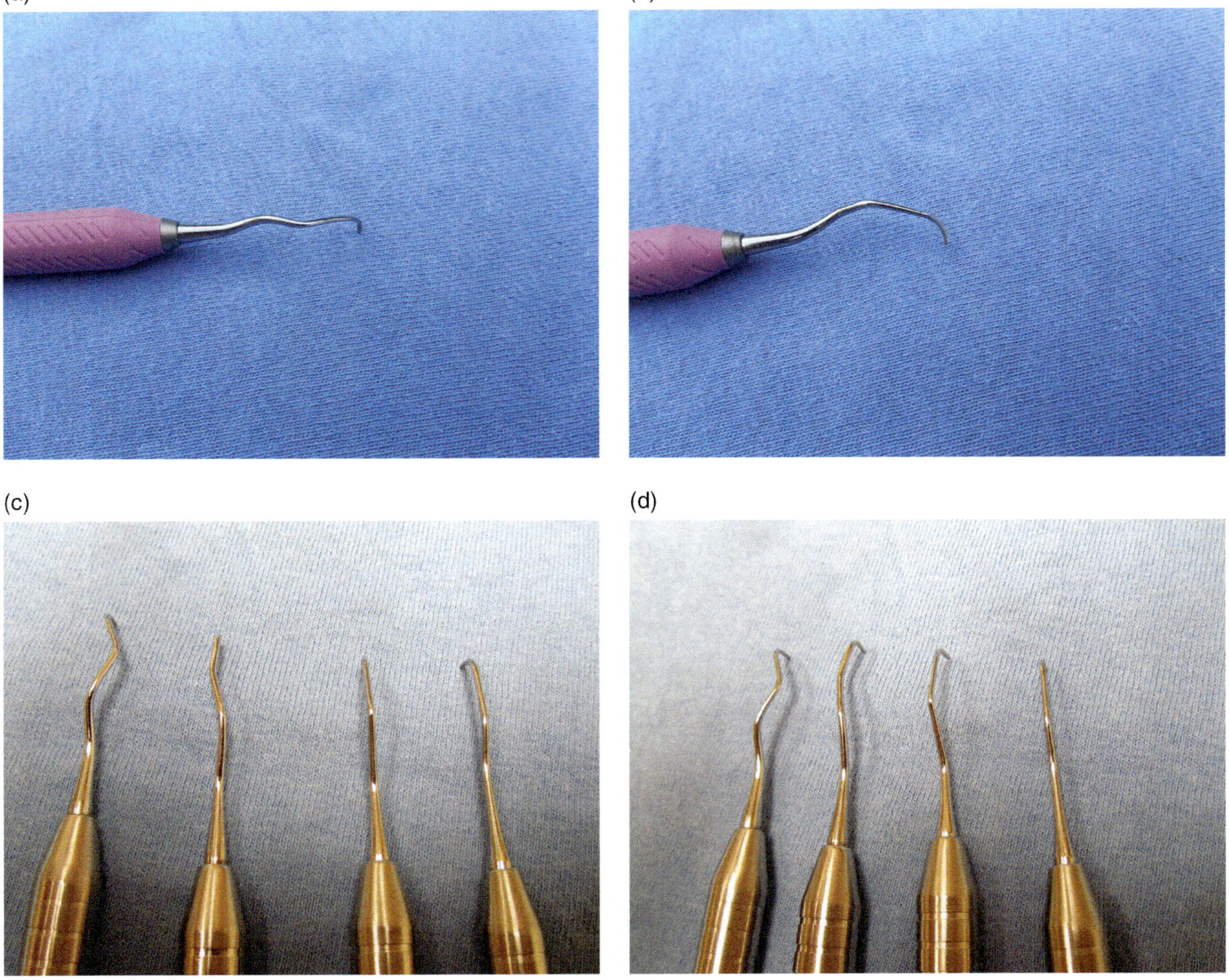

Figure 22.8 Gracey curette. (a) 45-degree view: reveals accessory bend. (b) Side view showing curved face and blunted toe. (c and d) Various curettes demonstrating the difference in angulation. From right: 1/2, 7/8, 12/13, 15/16. The bigger the bend, the higher the number, and the further distal it is designed to be used.

operator's hand can stay outside of the mouth, allowing for easier manipulation.

The proper curette should be selected based on its angulation. Curettes are labeled by numbers that correlate to the angle of the blade in relation to the shaft of the instrument (Figure 22.8 c and d). The lower the number (i.e., 1/2) the smaller the angle of the blade, and the more rostral in the mouth the instrument is used.[1] Conversely, larger numbers (e.g., 13/14) have a larger angle and are designed to be utilized more distally in the mouth.[7] Keep in mind that these numbers were designed in association with human dentition, and therefore may not correlate well with the same area of the mouth in veterinary patients. Regardless of the position in the mouth, the operator should choose the curette that best adapts to the tooth. This author recommends a minimum armatarium of a 1/2, 7/8, and 13/14 curette, as this selection will cover the vast majority of presentations in veterinary patients. These have been packaged along with diagnostic equipment for the convenience of veterinary professionals[B,C] (Figure 22.9).

There are two types of Gracey curettes, "rigid" and "finishing."[1] The rigid curettes have a larger, stronger, and less flexible shaft than the finishing type. This means that they are better suited for removing heavy calculus deposits but lack the tactile sensitivity of the finishing type.[2] Due to the level of calculus encountered in veterinary patients, rigid shafts are recommended for use in general practice. A dental practice (or a general practice with a strong dental interest) should also consider adding some finishing curettes to their armatarium.

In addition to the standard Gracey curettes (as described above), there are two other varieties of modified Gracey curettes in common usage.

Extended shank curettes

These curettes are designed with a terminal shank 5 mm longer than the standard Gracey, which allows usage in deeper periodontal pockets (deeper than 5 mm).[1] It is for this reason that one brand name of extended shank curettes is called the *After-Five*.[7] In addition, these curettes have a thicker, tapering shaft and a thinner blade for superior cleaning in deep pockets. Since 5 mm + pockets are very common in veterinary medicine, it is strongly recommended that all practices have a supply of these instruments.

Mini-bladed curettes (Figure 22.10)

These are basically "after-five" curettes that have a blade that is half the length of standard Gracey curettes.[1] This shorter blade allows insertion into deep/narrow pockets, furcations, developmental grooves, and areas of unusual root morphology.[7] These "*mini-five*" curettes along with

(a)

(b)

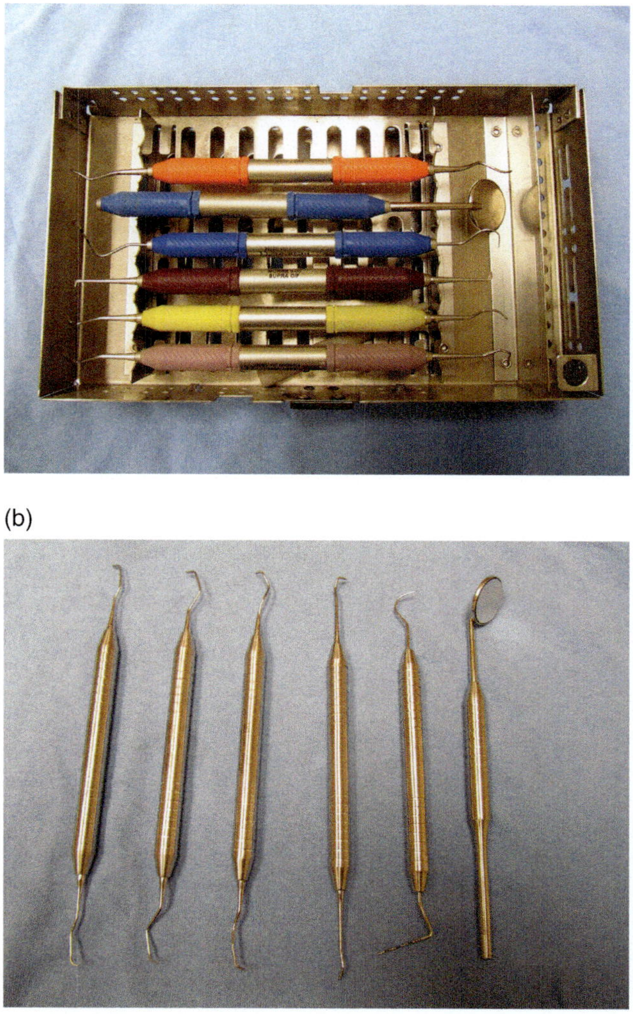

Figure 22.9 Basic periodontal kits. (a) Weldin periodontal kit (Miltex). (b) Diplomate kit (Dentalaire products).

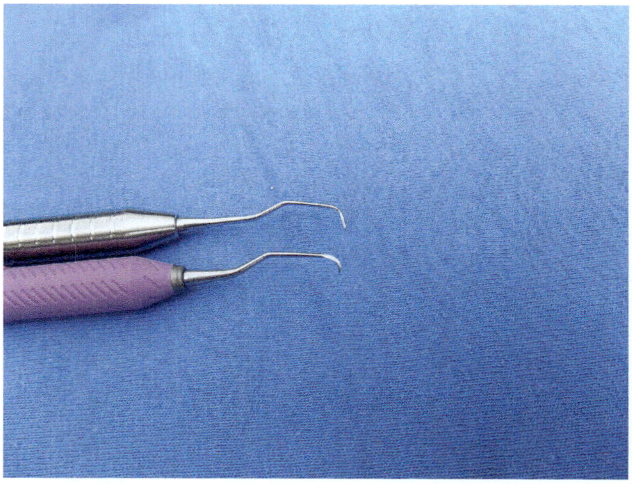

Figure 22.10 Comparison between standard (top) and petite (bottom) curettes. Note how much smaller the petite version is; this is for deep pockets and tight spaces.

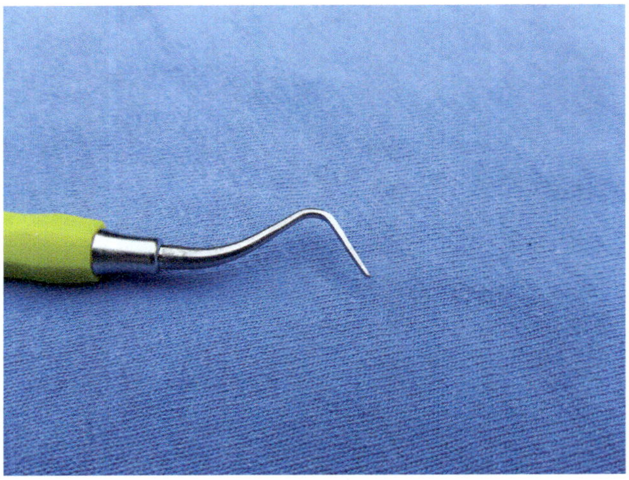

Figure 22.11 Periodontal chisel.

other short-bladed instruments allow for instrumentation of these previously unreachable areas. Consequently, mini-bladed instruments provide superior cleaning ability in hard to reach areas.

Chisels (Figure 22.11)

Chisels are designed for very tight proximal spaces,[1] such as between the maxillary fourth premolar and first molar, or between the mandibular first and second molars. Standard curettes and scalers may not effectively access these tight areas. Chisels are double-ended, with one straight end and one curved end. They have slightly curved blades with a straight cutting edge beveled at 45 degrees. Chisels are used in a push motion while the side of the blade is held firmly against the tooth root. Ideally, they should be used in a horizontal direction to avoid potential gingival laceration if the instrument is inadvertently pushed into the sulcus.[2]

Files (Figure 22.12)

Files have a series of small blades on a wider base. They are designed to break large deposits of tough calculus.[2] They are very effective at removing calculus, but their design makes them prone to damaging the tooth surface. They are rarely used today because ultrasonic scalers are safer and more efficient and are therefore a superior choice for these presentations.

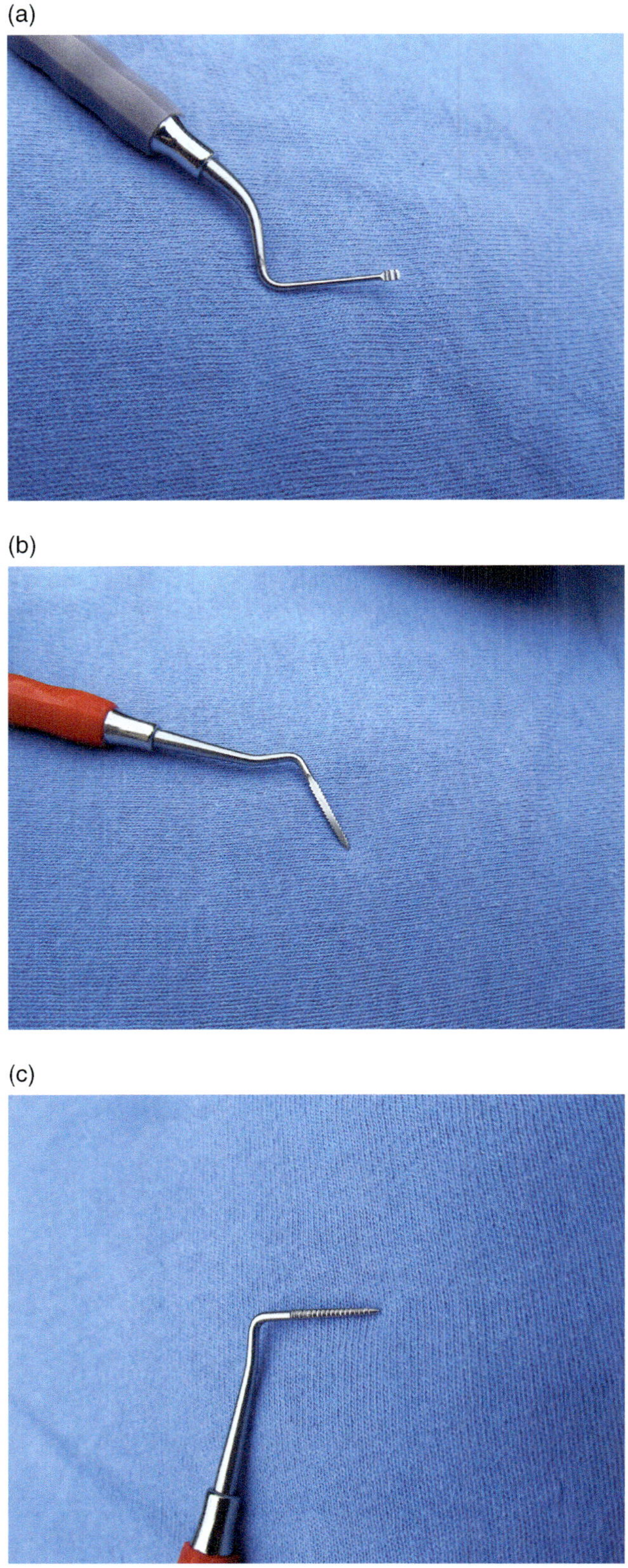

Figure 22.12 Files. (a) Orban file. (b and c) Sugarman file.

Quetin furcation curettes

These curettes[1] are hoe-type instruments that are extremely fine and have a very shallow half-moon shape. They are primarily designed for use in furcational defects but are also very effective in cleaning developmental grooves. The very small/fine design makes this types of curette the best hand instrument for these presentations.[1] However, even the smallest/finest mini-curette often results in damage to the furcation. Consequently, the practitioner should always use extra caution in furcational areas.

(a)

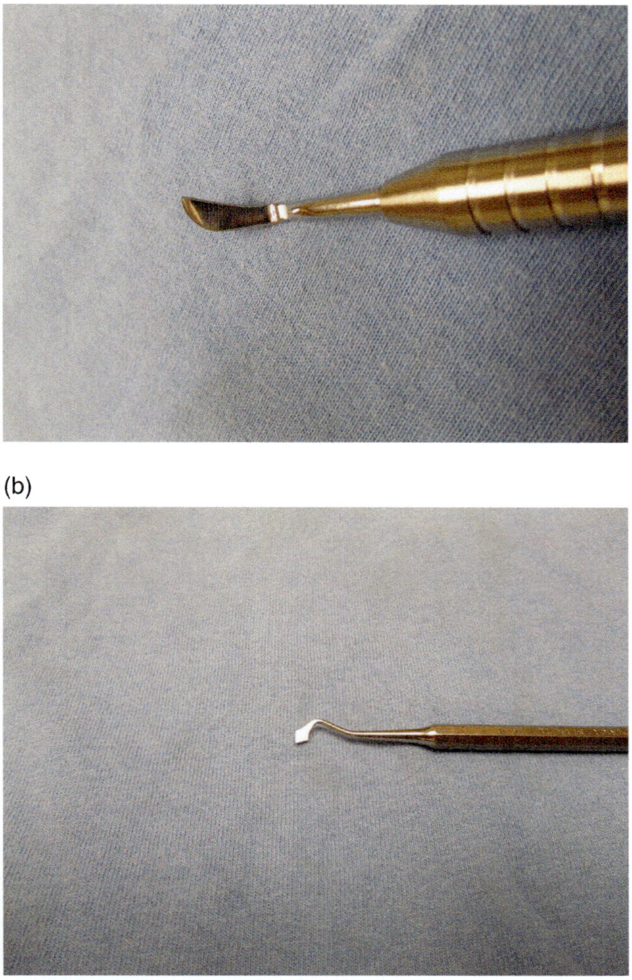

(b)

Figure 22.13 Knives. (a) Kirkland. (b) Orban.

Diamond-coated files

These files[1] are very fine instruments that are designed for the final cleaning/finishing of root surfaces. They do not have cutting edges but instead are coated with very fine grit diamonds. When new, these instruments are very sharp and must be used very carefully and with a light touch. Standard curettes are used first to remove the vast majority of the calculus. Following the removal of the gross calculus, the diamond-coated files are used like sandpaper to remove the minute deposits of residual calculus.[1] This creates a perfectly clean and smooth tooth. Care must be taken with these files, as overinstrumentation is easily done and will damage the root surface.

Knives (Figure 22.13)

There are two main types of knives[8] commonly used in periodontal surgery.

The Kirkland knife is generally used for gingivectomy in human dentistry. The entire outer edge of the kidney-shaped knife is the cutting edge. While excellent for fine surgeries with mild gingival enlargement, they are somewhat less effective when dealing with the large deposits of fibrous hyperplasia seen commonly in veterinary dentistry.

The other type in common use is the interdental knife (Orban, Goldman-Fox, and Merrifield). These instruments are spear-shaped and have cutting edges on both sides. They come in various sizes.

Box 22.2 Key points

- Scalers are used for supragingival areas and curettes for subgingival areas.
- *Gracey* curettes are the best choice for instrumenting periodontal pockets because they adapt well to the teeth and generally keep the operator's hand out of the patient's mouth.
- Periodontal instruments must be kept sharp for proper performance.

Notes

A. Niemiec Periodonal Probe, Dentalaire Products.
B. Diplomate periodontal kit, Dentalaire Products.
C. Weldin Periodontal Kit, Miltex.

References

1. Pattison AM, Pattison GL. Scaling and root planning. In: Carranza's Clinical Periodontology. St. Louis: Saunders, 2006, pp. 749–797.
2. Wiggs RB, Lobprise HB. Dental equipment. In: Veterinary Dentistry, Principles and Practice. Philadelphia: Lippincott-Raven, 1997, pp. 1–28.
3. Bellows J. Equipping the dental practice. In: Small Animal Dental Equipment, Materials, and Techniques, a Primer. Ames, IA: Blackwell, 2004, pp. 13–55.
4. Debowes LJ. Problems with the gingiva. In: Small Animal Dental, Oral and Maxillofacial Disease, a Color Handbook (Niemiec BA ed.). London: Manson, 2010, pp. 159–181.
5. Niemiec BA: Periodontal therapy. Top Companion Anim Med. 23(2):81–90, 2008.
6. Huffman LJ. Oral examination. In: Small Animal Dental, Oral and Maxillofacial Disease, a Color Handbook (Niemiec BA ed.). London: Manson, 2010, pp. 39–61.
7. Holmstrom SE, Frost P, Eisner ER. Dental equipment and care. In: Veterinary Dental Techniques for the Small Animal Practitioner. 3rd ed. Philadelphia: Saunders, 2004, pp. 31–106.
8. Klokkevold PR, Takei HH, Carranza FA. General principles of periodontal surgery. In: Carranza's Clinical Periodontology. St. Louis: Saunders, 2006, pp. 887–901.

23
Mechanical scalers

Historically, all scaling was performed by hand, and this is still the case in many human dental offices. However, veterinary patients (especially large breed dogs) have a much greater tooth surface area compared to human patients. Furthermore, there is typically a significantly higher larger accumulation of dental calculus in most of our patients in comparison to the average human being. Finally, general anesthesia is required for adequate scaling of veterinary patient's teeth. The combination of these factors makes the use of mechanical scalers necessary in veterinary hospitals, as their use can greatly decrease anesthetic time and increase safety and efficiency for dental scaling in animal patients.[1–6]

Mechanical scalers come in both sonic and ultrasonic types.[4,6,7] These instruments were originally designed with big and bulky tips for removal of large deposits of supragingival calculus.[6,8] Recently, however, there has been significant interest in using mechanical scalers subgingivally, resulting in the development of thinner, more delicate tips, which are typically found on ultrasonic equipment.[8,9] Mechanical scaling with these specialized tips has been shown to be at least as effective as hand scaling for plaque and calculus removal, as well as providing a positive clinical response to therapy.[1,10–20]

Ultrasonic scalers

The most common type of mechanical scaler used in veterinary dentistry today is the ultrasonic scaler. These instruments are electrically powered and the oscillations are run by the alternating electrical current.

Ultrasonic scalers are very efficient and provide an additional benefit of creating a bactericidal effect in the coolant spray (cavitation).[7,8,21,22] Cavitation results from vacuum bubbles created by the motion of the ultrasonic scaler that quickly burst and release energy.[6,23] The cavitational effect has been one of the arguments for the use of ultrasonic scalers over sonic scalers. However, this long-held theory is currently being challenged by recent studies that demonstrate that it is the heat produced, not the vibrational energy that creates the antibacterial effects.[24] In fact, the acoustic microstreaming produced by all mechanical scalers has been shown to break up the bacterial biofilm.[25] Furthermore, the water spray delivered by all mechanical scalers serves to flush plaque, calculus, and other debris from the sulcus/pocket,[8,26] which decreases bacterial numbers and improves subgingival periodontal health.[27] Consequently, sonic scalers may be as antibacterial as ultrasonic scalers and therefore can be used as subgingival instruments, as long as the appropriate appropriate ultrasonic subgingival attachments are used.

There are two main types of ultrasonic scalers, magnetostrictive and piezoelectric.[7,26] These instruments are electrically powered; the oscillations are a result of the alternating electrical current. Both types of ultrasonic scalers are effective at calculus removal because they produce vibration at a frequency of approximately 20,000–45,000 Hz.[7,8,26] Some ultrasonic scalers have a limited effective working surface involving the last few mm from the tip, while others have an effective working surface for up to 12 mm.[4] Regardless, the area of maximum vibration (and therefore efficiency) for all mechanical scalers is 1–2 mm from the tip.[28–30] The very tip of the instruments should not be used, as the tips are not effective for calculus removal and can potentially damage the tooth.[8]

Veterinary Periodontology, First Edition. Brook A. Niemiec.

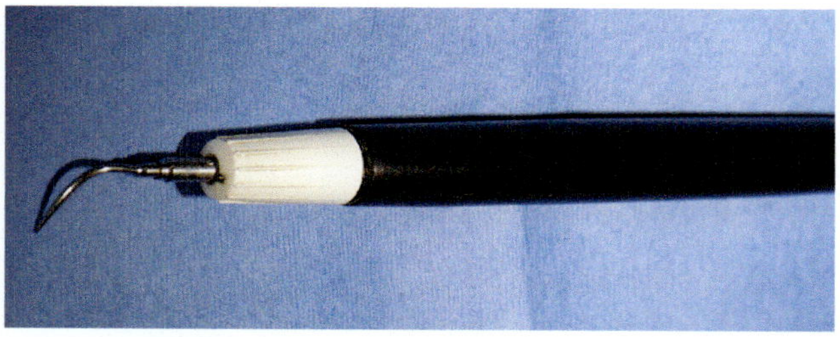

Figure 23.1 Magnetostrictive scaler, external view.

(a)

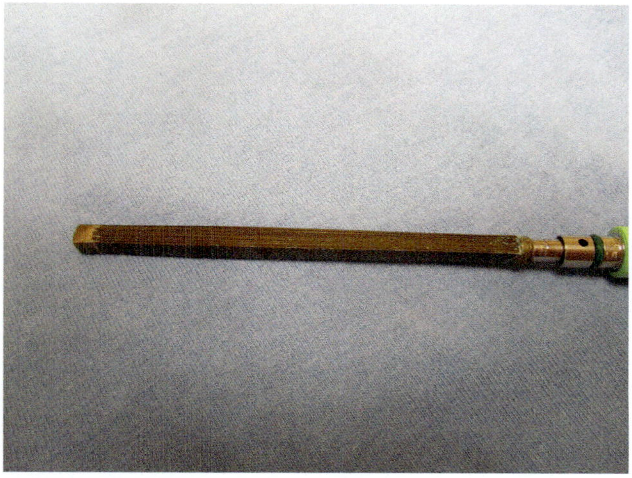

(b)

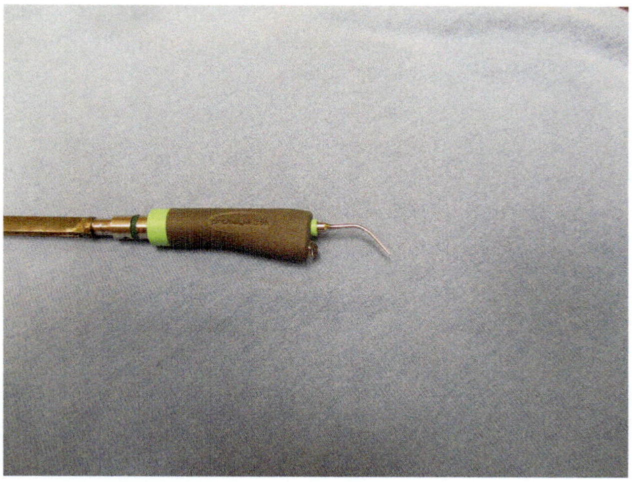

Figure 23.2 Magnetostrictive scaler, ferromagnetic stack type, internal view. (a) Close-up view of the strips of laminated nickel. (b) Close-up view of the connection between the strips and the tip.

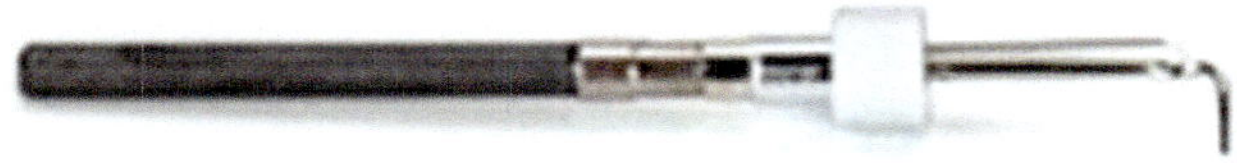

Figure 23.3 Magnetostrictive scaler, ferrite rod type, internal view.

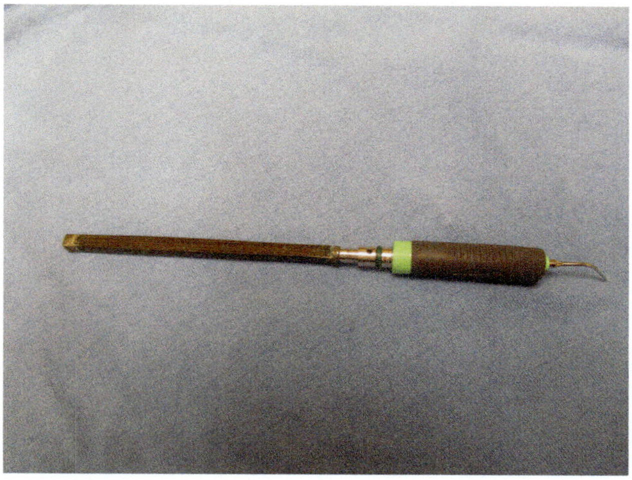

Figure 23.4 Magnetostrictive scaler, ferromagnetic stack type, internal view; revealing the permanent connection between the stack and the tip. The entire apparatus must be changed when it wears out.

Magnetostrictive units (Figure 23.1) generate their activity from either ferromagnetic stacks or a ferrite rod in the handle.[4,7,26] Ferromagnetic stacks are strips of laminated nickel (Figure 23.2) that lengthen and shorten approximately 0.001 inches when stimulated by alternating current (AC) electricity.[7] The ferrite rod type has a titanium tip attached to the cleaning end (Figure 23.3). Generally, for either of these units, the entire rod/tip unit must be replaced when worn out or damaged[7] (Figure 23.4). Although the replacements for these magnetostrictive units are more expensive than are the tips for piezoelectric scalers (see below), they do not need to be replaced as often.

Magnetostrictive scalers have an elliptical or figure-8 pattern of vibration, so all sides of the working end are effective, especially the ferrite rod style.[4,7,8] Moreover, it has been shown that the ferrite rod has a more elliptical motion than the ferromagnetic stacks, which results in less "dead strikes" (oscillations that are not effective at cleaning) and thus may be more efficient.[4,7] Finally, the ferrite rods are effective over the full 12 mm of their working tip as opposed to the metal stack, which is effective at the last 4 mm, and piezoelectric, which is effective only over the terminal 3 mm.[4] One potential drawback of the magnetostrictive scalers is that these instruments generate significant heat and therefore require the water spray for cooling and creation of the cavitation effect.[7] Examples of magnetostrictive scalers include Scalex 830,[A] Cavitron,[B] Odontoson,[C] and Vetroson.[D]

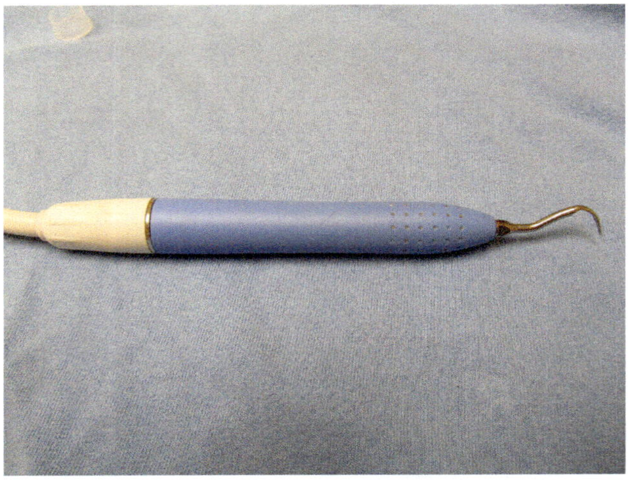

Figure 23.5 Piezoelectric scaler, eternal view. Note the short and thick handle.

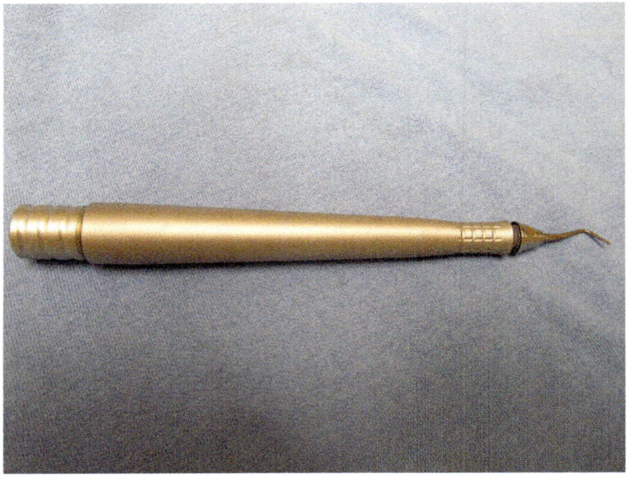

Figure 23.6 Sonic scaler, external view.

Piezoelectric systems operate as a result of the expansion and contraction of quartz crystals in the handle.[4,7] Consequently, their handles are thicker but shorter than those of the magnetostrictive systems (Figure 23.5). As they "wear out," only the tip needs to be replaced, but this occurs more frequently than with magnetostrictive units.[26]

In contrast to magnetostrictive scalers, piezoelectrics were reported to have a curvilinear pattern of vibration[7] and thus only the sides (not the front or back) of the instrument were reportedly effective at plaque removal.[6] However, a recent study has shown that piezoelectrics also demonstrate an elliptical motion, suggesting that they therefore can be used on all surfaces.[31] Until this information is further substantiated, it is recommended to continue utilizing the sides of piezoelectric scalers. Other than this potential limitation, these units are equally effective at plaque removal, do not generate as much heat, and are less damaging to the enamel. Consequently, piezoelectric scalers may be safer than magnetostrictive systems.[28,32] Examples of piezoelectric scalers include the Megasonic 2000,[E] Petpiezo,[F] and the Piezon Master 400.[G]

Sonic scalers (Figure 23.6)

In contrast to ultrasonic scalers, sonic scalers are powered by compressed air.[4,7] The air running through a hole at the end of the shaft turns a rotor causing it to spin, resulting in an oval-elliptical tip oscillation.[6,26] These instruments vibrate at a slow speed of only 2,000–6,500 Hz,[6,8] although speeds of up to 9,000 Hz have been reported.[4] Most reports indicate that this slower speed results in longer scaling time compared to ultrasonics.[33] However, some studies show equal scaling time[34] and at least one report indicated that sonic scalers are actually faster.[35] An additional advantage is that they do not generate heat like most ultrasonic systems do, thereby reducing the chance of pulp damage.[26]

Due to their lower speed and power, they have long been thought to not offer cavitation, although this is also being challenged (as above). However, they do offer the same advantage of lavage, which may be the critical part of all the mechanical scalers' ability to decrease bacterial loads in the pocket/sulcus.[8,27] Several studies have shown sonic scalers to be as effective as ultrasonics in bacterial reduction and clinical success.[18,36] Another disadvantage of sonic scalers is that they have a higher amplitude (10 times or more as compared to ultrasonics), which may be more damaging to the root surface.[4,37] Finally, these instruments require a significant amount of air pressure to be effective, which may be an issue with smaller compressor systems.[5] Sonic scalers are available from Star Dental,[H] KaVo,[I] and Miltex.[J]

Tips (Figure 23.7)

There are numerous choices of tips available for periodontal therapy. They can be divided into two main categories, supragingival and subgingival.

Supragingival tips

Supragingival tips tend to be thicker and wider than subgingival and are designed to be utilized on a higher power setting.[4,6,8] This allows for more efficient scaling on the comparatively more robust enamel. Another difference is that the water coolant typically exits the tip relatively high on the instrument. Supragingival tips must *not* be utilized under the gingival margin, as they will damage the cementum and potentially overheat the tooth (especially when using the magnetostrictive systems).[4,6–8]

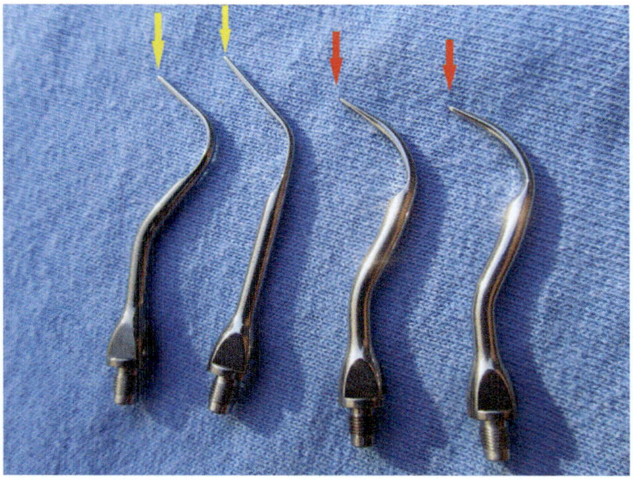

Figure 23.7 A selection of ultrasonic tips for a piezoelectric ultrasonic scaler. On the right are two shorter/thicker scalers for *supra*gingival scaling (red arrows). On the left are longer, thinner instruments for careful *sub*gingival scaling (yellow arrows).

Subgingival tips

There has been a tremendous surge in the development and usage of subgingival ultrasonic tips.[6] This is driven by the fact that these instruments (when properly designed and employed) were found to be as effective (or more so) as hand scaling. Subgingival tips are generally significantly thinner than supragingival tips.[4,6,7] This is an important aspect that allows them to work in the tight periodontal or furcational spaces.[6,7] In addition, these tips are designed to be utilized on lower power settings so as to not damage the delicate cementum on the root surface.[6,8] Finally, and probably most importantly, the water port for coolant is very near the tip of the instrument.[7] This is critical because the coolant must be able to get to the area where the instrument is working. The water spray provides not only cooling effects but also flushes the pocket/sulcus and delivers the lavage, which decreases bacterial numbers.[27]

Tip replacement (Figure 23.8)

All mechanical scaling instruments must be carefully inspected on a regular basis to ensure that they have not been damaged or become worn, as small changes will greatly affect the efficiency of the instrument. In fact, it has been shown that a loss of the last 1 mm of the tip causes a 25% loss of efficiency, and with a 2 mm loss it increases to 50% loss. Worn or damaged tips will thus markedly slow the cleaning procedure.[4] Most mechanical scalers come with a chart to measure the wear of the instrument, which is a great visual aid for evaluations over time.

(a)

(b)

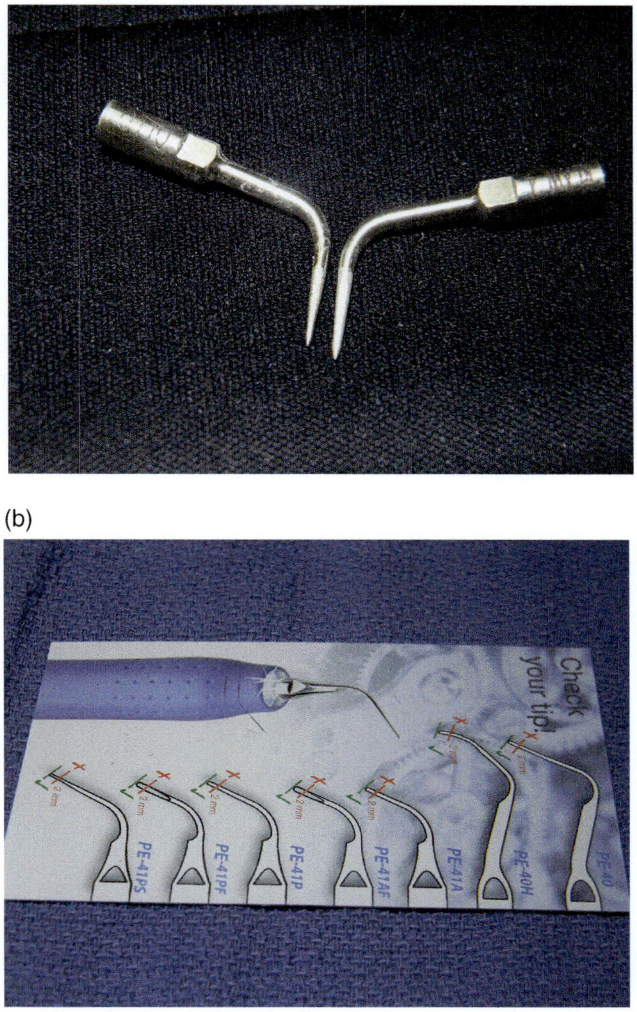

Figure 23.8 Measuring tip wear. (a) Image showing a new (right) and used (left) ultrasonic tip. Note that the used tip has lost approximately 2 mm of its tip/point. This decreases its efficiency by approximately 50%. (b) Commercial tip wear guide.

Rotary scalers

These are soft-sided, non-cutting, soft steel burs that run on a high-speed hand-piece.[7] At a standard high-speed rotation (300,000 rpm) with six sides to the bur, these scalers run at approximately the same frequency as ultrasonic scalers (30 kHz).[7] Rotary scalers can be very effective for calculus removal but are by far the *most damaging* instrument for this purpose.[7,28,38] Therefore, these instruments are *not* recommended for routine scaling.[4]

Conclusions

There have been significant advances in mechanical periodontal instrumentation in the last decade. This has resulted in the development of exceedingly thin and delicate subgingival tips. These new tips are equal, or superior to, hand scaling for supra- and subgingival debridement. The lavage created by the water spray further decreases bacterial load. Finally, mechanical scalers are somewhat less technique-sensitive and significantly more efficient than hand scaling.

For all these reasons, mechanical scaling is becoming a mainstay of periodontal therapy and should be utilized in all veterinary facilities. That being said, studies that have shown these instruments to be invaluable adjuncts to periodontal therapy have utilized only *new and highly specialized tips*. Veterinary practices with older/outdated units will *not* enjoy these benefits and may in fact cause greater damage to the root surface. Practitioners are strongly recommended to invest in a late-model ultrasonic scaler with a fine subgingival tip for performing mechanical subgingival debridement.

Box 23.1 Key points

- Ultrasonic and sonic scaling is very effective and efficient.
- Supragingival tips are large and bulky, whereas subgingival tips are thinner and finer.
- Subgingival tips are ***required*** for subgingival use.
- Sonic scalers are likely as effective as ultrasonic varieties.
- Rotosonic scaling is ***not*** recommended!
- The use of mechanical scalers can greatly decrease anesthetic time and increase safety and efficiency for dental scaling in animal patients.
- The acoustic microstreaming produced by all mechanical scalers (including sonic) has been shown to break up the bacterial biofilm.
- The area of maximum vibration (and therefore efficiency) for all mechanical scalers is 1–2 mm from the tip.
- The loss of the last 1 mm of the tip causes a 25% loss of efficiency, and with a 2 mm loss it increases to 50% loss.
- Supragingival ultrasonic tips must ***not*** be used under the gingival margin.
- The properties that define subgingival tips are
  - Thinner to allow for work in the subgingival space.
  - Lower power setting.
  - Most importantly, the water coolant reaches the very tip.

Notes

A. Scalex 830, Dentalaire Products.
B. Cavatron, Densply.
C. Odontoson, Hørsholm.
D. Summit Hill.
E. Megasonic 2000, Dentalaire Products.
F. Petpiezo, Inovadent.
G. Piezon Master 400, Electro Medical Systems.
H. BlisSonic Ergonomic Scaler.
I. KaVo SONICflex scaler, KaVo.
J. Mx Esonic Scaler, Miltex.

References

1. Copulos TA, Low SB, Walker CB, et al. Comparative analysis between a modified ultrasonic tip and hand instruments on clinical parameters of periodontal disease. J Periodontol. 64:694, 1993.
2. Dragoo MR. A clinical evaluation of hand and ultrasonic instruments on subgingival debridement. Part 1. With unmodified and modified ultrasonic inserts. Int J Periodont Restor Dent. 12:311, 1992.
3. Kocher T, Rühling A, Momsen H, Plagmann HC. Effectiveness of subgingival instrumentation with power-driven instruments in the hands of experienced and inexperienced operators. A study on manikins. J Clin Periodontol. 24(7):498–504, 1997.
4. Bellows J. Equipping the dental practice. In: Small Animal Dental Equipment, Materials, and Techniques, a Primer. Ames, IA: Blackwell, 2004, pp. 13–55.
5. Tunkel J, Heinecke A, Flemmig TF. A systematic review of efficacy of machine-driven and manual subgingival debridement in the treatment of chronic periodontitis. J Clin Periodontol. 29 Suppl 3:72–78, 2002.
6. Jahn CA. Sonic and ultrasonic instrumentation. In: Carranza's Clinical Periodontology. St. Louis: Saunders, 2006, pp. 828–835.
7. Wiggs RB, Lobprise HB. Dental equipment. In: Veterinary Dentistry, Principles and Practice. Philadelphia: Lippincott-Raven, 1997, pp. 1–28.
8. Pattison AM, Pattison GL. Scaling and root planning. In: Carranza's Clinical Periodontology. St. Louis: Saunders, 2006, pp. 749–797.
9. Holbrook T, Low S. Power driven scaling and polishing instruments. In: Clarke's Clinical Dentistry. Philadelphia: Lippincott, 1991.
10. Breininger DR, O'Leary TJ, Blumenshine RV. Comparative effectiveness of ultrasonic and hand scaling for the removal of subgingival calculus. J Periodontol. 58:9, 1987.
11. Santos FA, Pochapski MT, Leal PC, Gimenes-Sakima PP, Marcantonio E Jr. Comparative study on the effect of ultrasonic instruments on the root surface in vivo. Clin Oral Investig. 12(2):143–150, 2008.
12. Stende GW, Schaffer EM. A comparison of ultrasonic and hand scaling. J Periodontol. 32:312, 1961.
13. Torfason T, Kiger R, Selvig KA, et al. Clinical improvement of gingival conditions following ultrasonic verses hand instrumentation of periodontal pockets. J Clin Periodontol. 6:165, 1979.
14. Oosterwall PJ, Matee MI, Mikx FHM, et al. The effect of subgingival debridement with hand and ultrasonic instruments on subgingival microflora. J Clin Periodontol. 14:528, 1987.
15. Drisko CH. Root instrumentation. Power-driven versus manual scalers, which one? Dent Clin North Am. 42(2):229–244, 1998.
16. Dragoo MR. A clinical evaluation of hand and ultrasonic instruments on subgingival debridement. 1. With unmodified and modified ultrasonic inserts. Int J Periodont Restor Dent. 12(4): 310–323, 1992.
17. Gagnot G, Mora F, Poblete MG, et al. Comparative study of manual and ultrasonic instrumentation of cementum surfaces: Influence of lateral pressure. Int J Periodont Restor Dent. 24:137, 2004.
18. Derdilopoulou FV, Nonhoff J, Neumann K, Kielbassa AM. Microbiological findings after periodontal therapy using curettes, Er:YAG laser, sonic, and ultrasonic scalers. J Clin Periodontol. 34(7):588–598, 2007.
19. Obeid PR, D'Hoore W, Bercy P. Comparative clinical responses related to the use of various periodontal instrumentation. J Clin Periodontol. 31(3):193–199, 2004.
20. Thornton S, Garnick J. Comparison of ultrasonic to hand instruments in the removal of subgingival plaque. J Periodontol. 53(1):35–37, 1982.

21. Felver B, King DC, Lea SC, Price GJ, Damien Walmsley A. Cavitation occurrence around ultrasonic dental scalers. Ultrason Sonochem. 16(5):692–697, 2009.
22. Walsley AD, Laird WR, Williams AR. Dental plaque removal by cavitational activity during ultrasonic scaling. J Clin Periodontol. 15:539, 1988.
23. Bellows J. Periodontal equipment, materials, and techniques. In: Small Animal Dental Equipment, Materials, and Techniques, a Primer. Ames, IA: Blackwell, 2004, pp. 115–173.
24. Schenk GY, Flemmig T, Lob S, Ruckdeschel G, Hickel R. Lack of antimicrobial effect on periodontopathic bacteria by ultrasonic and sonic scalers in vitro. J Clin Periodontol. 27:116–119, 2000.
25. Khambay BS, Walmsley AD. Acoustic microstreaming: Detection and measurement around ultrasonic scalers. J Periodontol. 70(6):626–631, 1999.
26. Holmstrom SE, Frost P, Eisner ER. Dental equipment and care. In: Veterinary Dental Techniques for the Small Animal Practitioner. 3rd ed. Philadelphia: Saunders, 2004, pp. 31–106.
27. Baehni PY, Thilo B, Chapuis B, Pernet D. Effects of ultrasonic and sonic scalers on dental plaque microflora in vitro and in vivo. J Clin Periodontol. 19:455, 1992.
28. Holmstrom SE, Frost P, Eisner ER. Dental prophylaxis. In: Veterinary Dental Techniques. 2nd ed. Philadelphia: Saunders, 1998, pp. 133–166.
29. Niemiec BA. Periodontal therapy. Top Companion Anim Med. 23(2):81–90, 2008.
30. Debowes LJ. Problems with the gingiva. In: Small Animal Dental, Oral and Maxillofacial Disease, a Color Handbook (Niemiec BA ed.). London: Manson, 2010, pp. 159–181.
31. Lea SC, Felver B, Landini G, Walmsley AD. Three-dimensional analyses of ultrasonic scaler oscillations. J Clin Periodontol. 36(1):44–50, 2009.
32. Bellows J. Equipping the dental practice. In: Small Animal Dental Equipment, Materials, and Techniques, a Primer. Ames, IA: Blackwell, 2004, pp. 45–80.
33. Loose B, Kiger R. An evaluation of basic periodontal therapy using sonic and ultrasonic scalers. J Clin Periodontol Res. 14:29–33, 1987.
34. Lie T, Leknes KN. Evaluation of the effect on root surfaces of air turbine scalers and ultrasonic instrumentation. J Periodontol. 56(9):522–531, 1985.
35. Clinical Research Associates. Sonic and Ultrasonic Scalers. Provo, UT. 6:1, 1982.
36. Hermann JS, Rieder C, Rateitschak KH, Hefti AF. Sonic and ultrasonic scalers in a clinical comparison. A study in non-instructed patients with gingivitis or slight adult periodontitis. Schweiz Monatsschr Zahnmed. 105(2):165–170, 1995.
37. Jacobson L, Blomlöf J, Lindskog S. Root surface texture after different scaling modalities. Scand J Dent Res. 102(3):156–160, 1994.
38. Brine EJ, Marretta SM, Pijanowski GJ. Comparison of the effects of four different power scalers on enamel tooth surface in the dog. J Vet Dent. 17(1):17–21, 2000.

24

Other power equipment used in periodontology

There are a few mechanical instruments other than ultrasonic scalers that practitioners performing periodontal therapy should be familiar with. The most important of these is the prophy polishing cup on a low-speed (sometimes referred to as slow-speed) hand-piece. In addition, practitioners should have a basic familiarity with the different varieties of dental burs and the high-speed hand-pieces that run them. Air abrasion dentistry will also be discussed in this chapter.

Hand-pieces

The vast majority of dental equipment other than ultrasonic scalers is powered by compressed air (typically 30–40 psi).[1,2] This is a very efficient and relatively clean source of power. Ideally, these are the newer "oil-less" compressors. If further cleanliness is desired, these hand-pieces can be powered with nitrogen.[3] An additional advantage to nitrogen is the fact that less hand-piece maintenance is required due to the increased cleanliness of the gas.[1,3] Those practices that perform significant amounts of advanced oral surgery may consider switching to nitrogen power. Finally, the use of a water filter or distilled water is strongly recommended for both infection control and for hand-piece maintenance.[2,3]

Most dental machines have three attachments in addition to the ultrasonic scaler. These include a high-speed hand-piece, low-speed hand-piece, and three-way air-water syringe. High-speed drills (Figure 24.1) operate at a very high rate of speed (generally 300–400,000 but up to 800,000 rpm[1]) but are generally low torque.[2,3] This means that they will stall if excessive pressure is placed on the instrument. These high-speed instruments are very efficient in tooth and bone removal but do not have good tactile sensitivity. High-speed hand-pieces have an aperture for water coolant directed on the bur's working surface that helps prevent the hard tissues from overheating.[1,3] The speed at which the high-speed hand-piece operates is typically governed by the amount of pressure placed by the operator on the foot pedal.

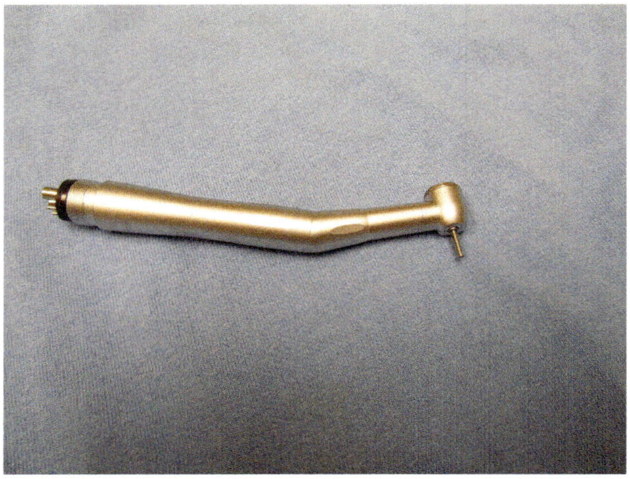

Figure 24.1 High-speed air-driven hand-piece.

A low-speed hand-piece (Figure 24.2) is preferred when precision is required. Low-speed hand-pieces have a ring dial that controls their speed (Figure 24.3). Low-speed hand-pieces are generally run in the 5,000–20,000 rpm range;[2,3] however, they can be run at speeds up to 100,000 rpm.[1] In addition, the head attachments such as "contra angles" and "reduction angles" have the ability to further regulate the speed of rotation up or down through a fixed reduction with internal gears.[2]

Veterinary Periodontology, First Edition. Brook A. Niemiec.

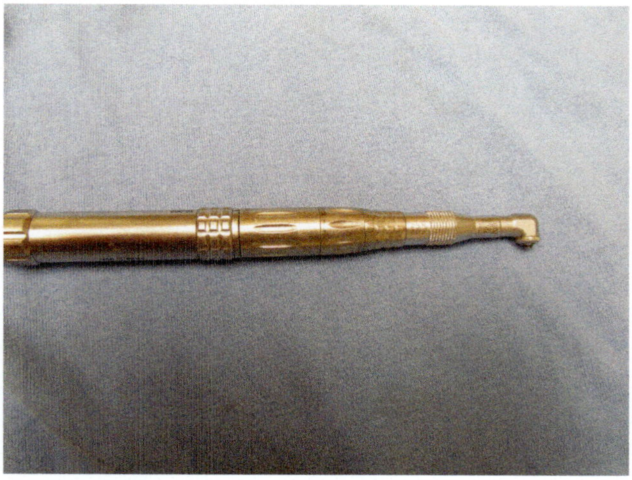

Figure 24.2 Slow-speed air-driven hand-piece.

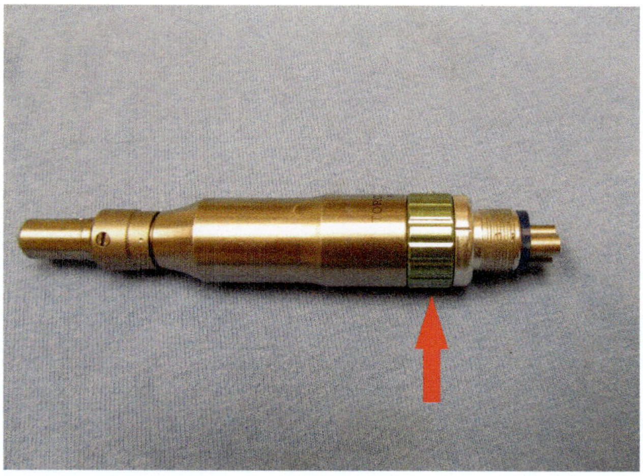

Figure 24.3 Close-up view of a slow-speed air-driven hand-piece demonstrating the speed control dial (red arrow).

While these instruments can be used to remove tooth tissue (particularly carious dentin), they do not provide coolant and therefore care must be taken when using them, especially for prolonged periods.[2] In veterinary periodontology, low-speed hand-pieces are typically only used for polishing (see below).

Dental burs

There are several types of dental burs.[1–3] They include high-speed, low-speed, and laboratory types. The main differences in the bur itself are the diameter of the shank as well as attachment to the hand-piece. Laboratory and slow-speed burs tend to have a larger diameter than high-speed burs. Additionally, low-speed burs tend to have a latch type of attachment as opposed to the friction grip of high-speed (see below). Since low-speed and laboratory burs are not typically indicated for periodontal work, they will not be discussed herein.

(a)

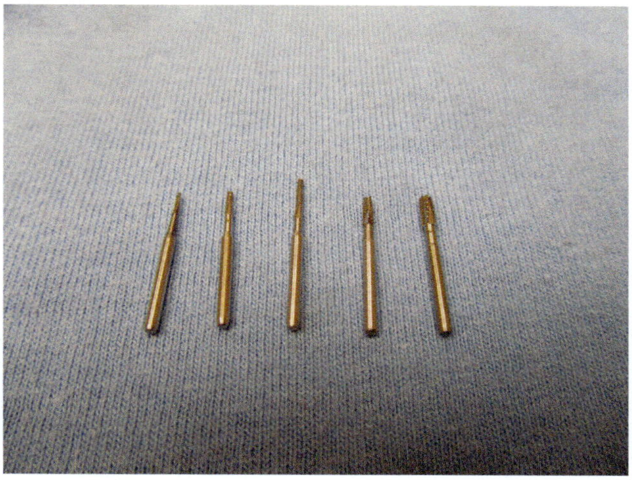

(b)

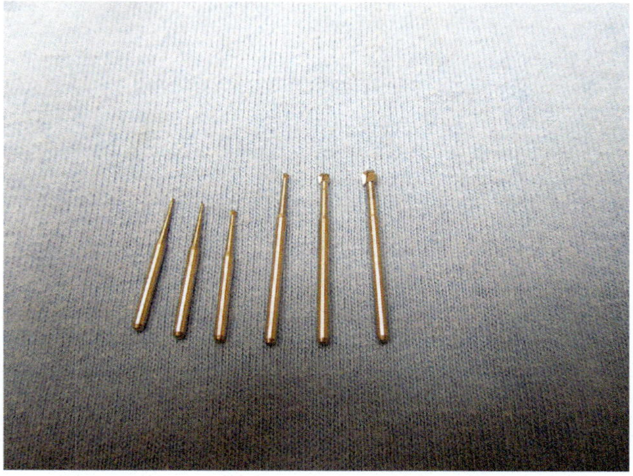

Figure 24.4 Cutting burs. (a) Cross-cut taper fissure burs; from left: 699, 701, 701L, 702, 703. (b) Round burs; from left: 1/4, 1/2, 1, 2L, 4L, 8L.

Cutting burs (Figure 24.4)

These are rotary dental instruments with cutting blades typically used on high-speed hand-pieces. In veterinary periodontics they are used for cutting teeth (for extractions or tooth resection) and removing bone (alveoplasty). The vast majority of dental burs in common use are carbide steel, which maintains its cutting ability better than other metals.[1] In regards to the method of attachment to the hand-piece, dental burs are available in several different types, with friction grip (FG) being the most common. Dental burs come in numerous shapes and sizes for various purposes. This author recommends that all practitioners have at a minimum a supply of taper fissure (699–703), round (1/4–2), and pear-shaped (330) burs. In addition, short shank (S or SS) and surgical length (SL or SU) burs can be helpful in managing certain presentation. Note that SS or SL burs may not have the

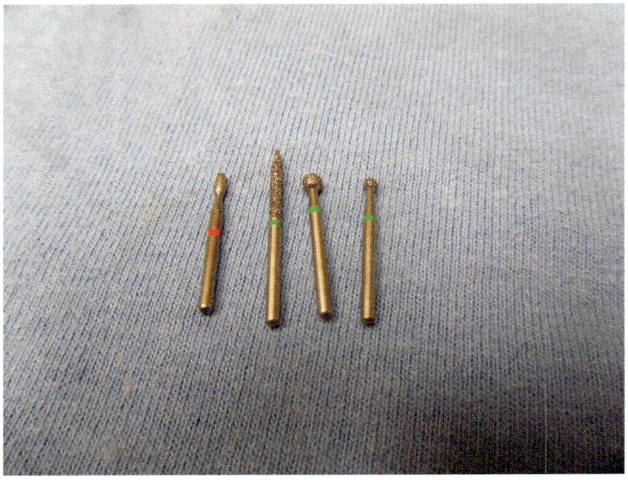

Figure 24.5 Diamond-coated burs (or abrasive points). On the left is a "football"-shaped fine diamond bur as demonstrated by the red line. The other three burs are various shaped/sized coarse diamonds as labelled by the green line.

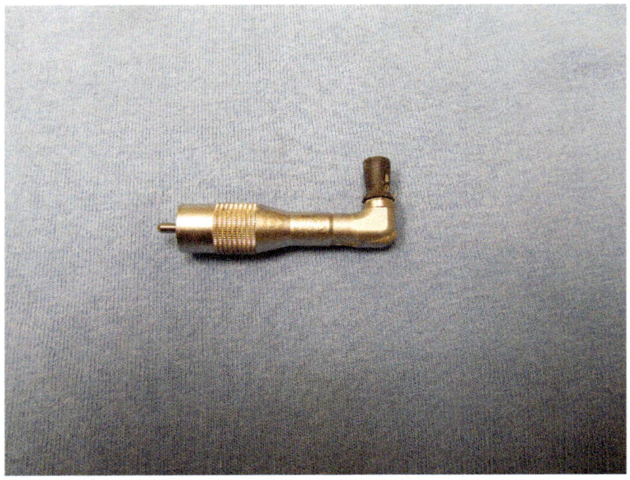

Figure 24.6 A 90-degree "prophy" angle that is attached to a slow-speed hand-piece.

coolant appropriately targeted to the working end of the bur. Therefore, consider using conventional-length burs with traditional high-speed hand-pieces to avoid this problem.

Abrasive points (Figure 24.5)

In contrast to cutting burs, diamond burs are considered to be abrasive points. They are generally used for gingivectomy or bone smoothing. These are created from various shaped and sized blanks onto which diamonds have been electroplated. Like sandpaper, these electroplated industrial diamonds vary in their coarseness, depending on the size of diamond particles. Coarse grit diamond burs are best utilized for gingivectomy procedures or coarse removal of bone or tooth structure. Finer grits are used for final tooth preparation and finishing restorations. One important point with diamond burs is that they have increased continuous surface contact and therefore generate more heat, thus increasing the chance of thermal damage to vital pulps.[4]

Instruments for polishing

Prophy angles (Figure 24.6)

Prophy angles[1–3,5] provide the attachment to the low-speed hand-piece for the prophy cup. There are numerous designs available; however, the 90-degree prophy angle is the most common choice.

When using standard prophy angles, the rubber prophy cup attaches at the tip as a separate disposable piece. However, the newer disposable prophy angles with attached cups[A,B] are gaining popularity, as they decrease the spread of infection. Standard prophy angles operate by continuously rotating the prophy cup, but other prophy angles are available that are designed to oscillate rather than continually rotate.[C,D] These are equally effective for polishing as continually rotating ones but are slightly more expensive. However, they do not require lubrication, generate less heat, and avoid hair catching.

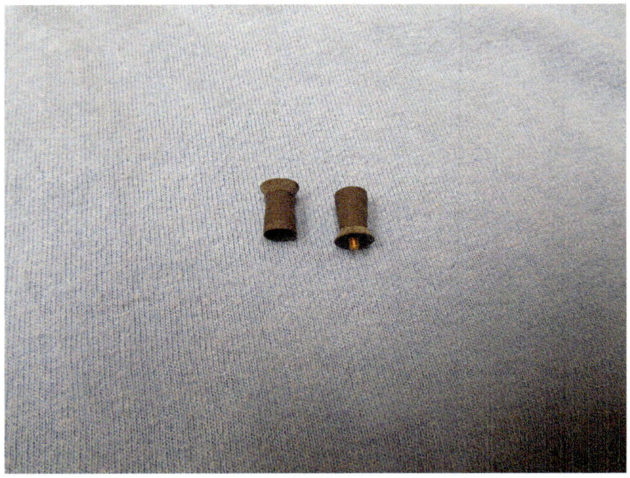

Figure 24.7 Gray "soft" screw-on style prophy cups.

The polishing hand-piece should be run at a slow speed, no greater than 3,000 rpm. Faster rotation will not improve the speed or quality of the procedure but may result in overheating the tooth. Remember that in contrast to the high-speed hand-piece, the slow-speeds do not provide water coolant.

Prophy cups (Figure 24.7)

Tooth polishing is typically performed with a rubber prophy cup.[1–3] These can be attached to a disposable prophy angle (as above) or separate and attached by snap or screw to a metal multiuse angle. There are numerous types and brands of prophy cups available. The soft (gray) cups that are designed to be used with prophy paste are generally recommended.[6] With the softer rubber texture, it takes less pressure to flare the edges of these cups when subgingival polishing is performed. Additional products include the standard "white" prophy cups, which are suitable but require more downward pressure to flare under the gingiva. Finally, pasteless prophy cups have been developed[E] and provide another option.

Regardless of which style of cup is used (except pasteless), plenty of polish paste should always be employed.[6] This is important because it is the polish that smoothes the tooth, while the prophy cup only serves to move the paste. The use of polish provides additional advantages, as it not only helps to smooth the tooth but also lubricates the cup to decrease the amount of frictional heat buildup.

Finally, cups should be changed between each patient. This avoids the use of a damaged cup (which lowers its efficacy) and also decreases the transmission of infectious organisms.

Air abrasion units

Air abrasion units[3,7,8,F] can be used for polishing or minor cleaning of the teeth (mostly stain removal). These units employ compressed air to spray a mixture of water and abrasive powder onto the teeth. The most common abrasive is fine sodium bicarbonate powder. This provides a "sandblasting" effect that may allow access into developmental grooves as well as interproximal areas. An additional advantage is that these units do not generate heat.

Note that care must be taken when utilizing these instruments, as improper usage can result in several deleterious effects. First, significant damage can occur if the spray is inadvertently directed toward the oral soft tissues. In addition, barotraumas have been reported with these instruments when directed into a salivary duct. Subcutaneous emphysema has been reported subsequent to their use. The use of these units may be contraindicated in some patients, as they can cause an increase in the serum sodium level. This may be of particular concern in patients with renal or cardiac disease.

Box 24.1 Key points

- High-speed hand-pieces have water coolant but low-speed generally do not; therefore you need to be careful when using low-speed burs to not overheat the structure being worked on.
- High-speed burs are very low torque, which means that if excessive pressure is placed on the structure stalling will occur and bur fracture may result.
- Long and short burs (as opposed to traditional length) may not have the coolant directed toward the correct place, so be careful using them.
- Plenty of polish paste should always be employed as the polish smoothes the tooth, while the prophy cup only serves to move the paste.

Notes

A. Upgrade Disposable Prophy Angle, Sultan Healthcare.
B. Disposable Standard Prophy Angles, Keystone Vet.
C. CROSSTEX TWIST PROPHY ANGLE, New Line Medical, Inc.
D. Disposable Oscillating Prophy Angles, Keystone Vet.
E. Butler Paste-Free Prophy pasteless disposable prophylaxis angle, Sunstar Americas, Inc.
F. Plaque Sweep, Dentsply.

References

1. Wiggs RB, Lobprise HB. Dental equipment. In: Veterinary Dentistry, Principles and Practice. Philadelphia: Lippincott-Raven, 1997, pp. 1–28.
2. Holmstrom SE, Frost P, Eisner ER. Dental equipment and care. In: Veterinary Dental Techniques for the Small Animal Practitioner. 3rd ed. Philadelphia: Saunders, 2004, pp. 31–106.
3. Bellows J. Equipping the dental practice. In: Small Animal Dental Equipment, Materials, and Techniques, a Primer. Ames, IA: Blackwell, 2004, pp. 13–55.
4. Reder BS, Eames WB. The cutting rates and durability of diamond stones. J Dent Res. 55(B):186, 1976.
5. Bellows J. Periodontal equipment, materials, and techniques. In: Small Animal Dental Equipment, Materials, and Techniques, a Primer. Ames, IA: Blackwell, 2004, pp. 115–173.
6. Niemiec BA. Periodontal therapy. Top Companion Anim Med. 23(2):81–90, 2008.
7. Wiggs RB, Lobprise HB. Periodontology. In: Veterinary Dentistry, Principles and Practice. Philadelphia: Lippincott-Raven, 1997, pp. 186–231.
8. Debowes LJ. Problems with the gingiva. In: Small Animal Dental, Oral and Maxillofacial Disease, a Color Handbook (Niemiec BA ed.). London: Manson, 2010, pp. 159–181.

Appendix 1
AVDC-Approved abbreviations

		Definition
AB		abrasion
APG		apexogenesis
APX		apexification
AT		attrition
B		biopsy
	B/E	biopsy excisional
	B/I	biopsy incisional
BG		bone graft (includes placement of bone substitute or bone stimulant material)
C		canine
CA		caries
CBU		core build up
CFL		cleft lip
	CFL/R	cleft lip repair
CFP		cleft palate
	CFP/R	cleft palate repair
CMO		cranio-mandibular osteopathy
CR		crown
	CR/M	crown metal
	CR/P	crown preparation
	CR/PFM	crown porcelain fused to metal
CRA		crown amputation
CRL		crown lengthening
CRR		crown reduction

Veterinary Periodontology, First Edition. Brook A. Niemiec.

		Definition
CS		culture/susceptibility
DT		deciduous (primary) tooth
DTC		dentigerous cyst
E		enamel
	E/D	enamel defect
	E/H	enamel hypocalcification or hypoplasia
F		flap
	F/AR	apically repositioned periodontal flap
	F/CR	coronally repositioned periodontal flap
	F/L	lateral sliding periodontal flap
FB		foreign body
FGG		free gingival graft
FRE		frenoplasty (frenotomy, frenectomy)
FX		fracture (tooth or jaw)
		For tooth fracture abbreviations, see under T/FX.
	FX/R	repair of jaw fracture
	FX/R/P	pin repair of jaw fracture
	FX/R/PL	plate repair of jaw fracture
	FX/R/S	screw repair of jaw fracture
	FX/R/WIR	wire repair of jaw fracture
	FX/R/WIR/C	cerclage wire repair of jaw fracture
	FX/R/WIR/ID	interdental wire repair of jaw fracture
	FX/R/WIR/OS	osseous wire repair of jaw fracture
G		granuloma
	G/B	buccal granuloma (cheek-chewing lesion)
	G/E/L	eosinophilic granuloma—lip
	G/E/P	eosinophilic granuloma—palate
	G/E/T	eosinophilic granuloma—tongue
	G/L	sublingual granuloma (tongue-chewing lesion)
GH		gingival hyperplasia/hypertrophy
GR		gingival recession
GTR		guided tissue regeneration
GV		gingivoplasty (gingivectomy)
I1,2,3		incisor teeth
IM		impression and model
IMP		implant
IO		interceptive (extraction) orthodontics
	IO/D	deciduous (primary) tooth interceptive orthodontics

(*continued*)

		Definition
	IO/P	permanent (secondary) tooth interceptive orthodontics
IP		inclined plane
	IP/AC	acrylic inclined plane
	IP/C	composite inclined plane
	IP/M	metal (i.e., lab-produced) inclined plane
LAC		laceration
	LAC/B	laceration buccal (cheek)
	LAC/L	laceration lip
	LAC/T	laceration tongue
M1,2,3		molar teeth
MAL		Malocclusion—see definitions in Nomenclature document
	MAL/1	class 1 malocclusion (neutroclusion—normal jaw relationship, specific teeth are incorrectly positioned)
	MAL/2	class 2 malocclusion (mandibular distoclusion—mandible shorter than maxilla)
	MAL/3	class 3 malocclusion (mandibular mesioclusion—maxilla shorter than mandible)
	MAL/1–3/BV	buccoversion
	MAL/1–3/CXB	caudal crossbite
	MAL/1–3/DV	distoversion
	MAL/1–3/LABV	labioversion
	MAL/1–3/LV	linguoversion
	MAL/1–3/MV	mesioversion
	MAL/1–3/OB	open bite
	MAL/1–3/RXB	rostral crossbite
	MAL/1–3/XB	Crossbite—see CXB or RXB
		(use of the term "*wry bite*" is not recommended, and WRY is not an AVDC-approved abbreviation)
MN		mandible or mandibular
	MN/FX	mandibular fracture
MX		maxilla or maxillary
	MX/FX	maxillary fracture
OA		orthodontic appliance
	OA/BKT	bracket orthodontic appliance
	OA/BU	button orthodontic appliance
	OA/EC	elastic (power chain) orthodontic appliance
	OA/WIR	wire orthodontic appliance
OAA		adjust orthodontic appliance
OAI		install orthodontic appliance
OAR		remove orthodontic appliance

		Definition
OC		orthodontic/genetic consultation
OM		oral mass
	OM/AD	adenocarcinoma
	OM/EPA	acanthomatous ameloblastoma (epulis)
	OM/EPF	fibromatous epulis
	OM/EPO	osseifying epulis
	OM/FS	fibrosarcoma
	OM/LS	lymphosarcoma
	OM/MM	malignant melanoma
	OM/OS	osteosarcoma
	OM/PAP	papillomatosis
	OM/SCC	squamous cell carcinoma
ONF		oronasal fistula
	ONF/R	oronasal fistula repair
OR		orthodontic recheck
OST		osteomyelitis
PC		pulp capping
	PC/D	direct pulp capping
	PC/I	indirect pulp capping
PDI		periodontal disease index
	PD0	normal periodontium
	PD1	gingivitis only
	PD2	$<25\%$ attachment loss
	PD3	25–50% attachment loss
	PD4	$>50\%$ attachment loss
PE		pulp exposure
PM1,2,3,4		premolar teeth
PRO		periodontal prophylaxis (examination, scaling, polishing, irrigation)
R		restoration of tooth
	R/A	restoration with amalgam
	R/C	restoration with composite
	R/CP	restoration with compomer
	R/I	restoration with glass ionomer
RAD		radiograph
RC		root canal therapy
	RC/S	surgical root canal therapy
RD		retained deciduous (primary) tooth
		RL is no longer used for resorptive lesion. See TR for tooth resorption.
RPC		root planning—closed

(*continued*)

		Definition
RPO		root planning—open
RR		internal root resorption
RRT		retained root tip
RRX		root resection (crown left intact)
RTR		retained tooth root
S		surgery
	S/M	mandibulectomy
	S/P	palate surgery
	S/X	maxillectomy
SC		subgingival curettage
SN		supernumerary
SPL		splint
	SPL/AC	acrylic splint
	SPL/C	composite splint
	SPL/WIR	Wire-reinforced splint
ST		stomatitis
	ST/CU	Stomatitis—contact ulcers
	ST/FFS	Stomatitis—feline faucitis-stomatitis
SYM		symphysis
	SYM/S	symphyseal separation
	SYM/WIR	wire repair of symphyseal separation
T		tooth
	T/A	avulsed tooth
	T/FX	fractured tooth (see next seven listings for fracture types)
	T/FX/EF	enamel fracture
	T/FX/EI	enamel infraction
	T/FX/CCF	complicated crown fracture
	T/FX/RF	root fracture
	T/FX/UCF	uncomplicated crown fracture
	T/FX/CCRF	complicated crown-root fracture
	T/FX/UCRF	uncomplicated crown-root fracture
		For further information on the tooth fracture definitions, see the Tooth Fracture section on the Nomenclature web page.
	T/I	impacted tooth
	T/LUX	luxated tooth
	T/NE	near pulp exposure
	T/NV	non-vital tooth
	T/PE	pulp exposure
	T/V	vital tooth

		Definition
TMJ		temporomandibular joint
	TMJ/C	temporomandibular joint condylectomy
	TMJ/D	TMJ dysplasia
	TMJ/FX	TMJ fracture
	TMJ/LUX	TMJ luxation
	TMJ/R	reduction of TMJ luxation
TP		treatment plan
TR		tooth resorption
	TR1	TR stage 1: mild dental hard tissue loss (cementum or cementum and enamel)
	TR2	TR stage 2: moderate dental hard tissue loss (cementum or cementum and enamel with loss of dentin that does not extend to the pulp cavity)
	TR3	TR stage 3: deep dental hard tissue loss (cementum or cementum and enamel with loss of dentin that extends to the pulp cavity); most of the tooth retains its integrity
	TR4	TR stage 4: extensive dental hard tissue loss (cementum or cementum and enamel with loss of dentin that extends to the pulp cavity); most of the tooth has lost its integrity (TR4a) crown and root are equally affected (TR4b) crown is more severely affected than the root (TR4c) root is more severely affected than the crown
	TR5	TR stage 5: remnants of dental hard tissue are visible only as irregular radiopacities, and gingival covering is complete
TRX		tooth partial resection (e.g., hemisection)
VP		vital pulp therapy
X		simple closed extraction of a tooth
XS		extraction with tooth sectioning, non-surgical
XSS		surgical (open) extraction of a tooth

This list is current as of April 11, 2012. The list is revised periodically by AVDC. For the current list, browse to http://www.avdc.org/abbreviations.pdf. Changes are made periodically in these AVDC-approved abbreviations. These abbreviations were adopted by AVDC to facilitate entry of information in AVDC case logs; inclusion of AVDC-approved abbreviations on this list does not imply that the abbreviations will be recognized by or made use of by journals and textbook publishers.

Appendix 2

Dental charts

Southern California Veterinary Dental Specialties
Brook Niemiec, DVM, Dip. AVDC, Fellow AVD

Name: ______________________________ Date: ____________

Anesthetic Protocol:

Pre-Medication
Atropine________
Buprenorphine____

Induction
Valium _________
Propoflo________
O Sevoflurane/O_2

Maintenance
O Oxygen
O Isoflurane
O Sevoflurane

Occlusion
O Scissors
O Brachygnathic
O Even
O Anterior Crossbite
O Posterior Crossbite
O Prognathic
O Wry
O Endentulous

Skull Type
O Brachycephalic
O Mesocephalic
O Dolichocephalic

Mandibular Symphysis
O Intact
O Luxated

Temporomandibular Palpation
O Normal
O Pain
O Crepitus
O Clicking
O Inhibited
O Luxated

Prophylaxis:

Crown Scaling
O Hand
O Ultra-sonic

Subgingival
O Exploration
O Subgingival Curettage
O Root Planing

Polishing
O Chlorhexidine + Pumice
O Fluoride Tx
O Oravet

Exodontia
O Crown Amputation
O Routine Extraction
O Sectioning
O Buccal Cortical Bone Removal
O Alveoloplasty
O Suture
O Chromic Gut___
O Monocryl___
O PDS ___

Diagnostic
O Biopsy
O Culture

	109	108	107	106	104	103	102	101	201	202	203	204	206	207	208	209
Mobility/Furcation																
Perio Pocket																
Attachment Loss																

Right **Left**

Buccal →

Palatal →

Lingual →

Buccal →

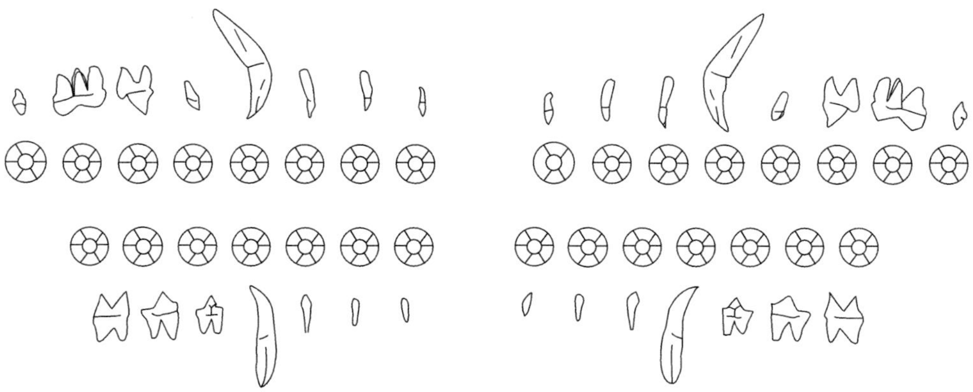

	409	408	407	404	403	402	401	301	302	303	304	307	308	309
M/F														
P														
AL														

ED-Enamel Defect
F-Furcation Exposure
CCF-Complicated crown Fracture
GR-Gingival Recession
GV-Gingivectomy

GH-Gingival Hyperplasia
M-Mobility
O-Missing Tooth
OM-Oral Mass
P-Periodontal Pocket
R-Rotated Tooth

PD-Persistent Deciduous
RC-Root Canal Therapy
R/C-Restoration/Composite
R/GI-Restoration/Glass Ionomer
RPC-Root Planing Closed
RPO-Root Planing Open
RR-Retained Root

SI-Intrinsic Staining
TR-Tooth Resorption
UCF-Uncomplicated Crown Fracture
VPT-Vital Pulp Therapy
W-Worn
X-Extracted

Southern California Veterinary Dental Specialties
Brook Niemiec, DVM, Dip. AVDC, Fellow AVD

Name:______________________________ **Date:**__________

Skull Type
O Brachycephalic
O Mesocephalic
O Dolichocephalic

Mandibular Symphysis
O Intact
O Luxated

Occlusion
O Scissors
O Brachygnathic
O Even
O Anterior Crossbite
O Posterior Crossbite
O Prognathic
O Wry
O Endentulous

Temporomandibular Palpation
O Normal
O Pain
O Crepitus
O Clicking
O Inhibited
O Luxated

Prophylaxis:

Crown Scaling
O Hand
O Ultra-sonic

Subgingival
O Exploration
O Subgingival Curettage
O Root Planing
O Doxirobe

Polishing
O Chlorhexidine + Pumice
O Fluoride Tx

Exodontia
O Crown Amputation
O Routine Extraction
O Sectioning
O Buccal Cortical Bone Removal
O Alveoloplasty
O Suture
  O Chromic Gut___
  O Monocryl___

Periodontal Surgery
O Gingivectomy
O Open Curettage
O Periodontal Flap
  O Reverse Bevel
  O Apically repositioning
  O Coronal repositioning
  O Lateral Sliding
O Guided Tissue Regeneration

Restoration
O Fillings
  O Bonded Sealant

Diagnostic
O Biopsy
O Culture

	110	109	108	107	106	105	104	103	102	101	201	202	203	204	205	206	207	208	209	210
Mobility/Furcation																				
Perio Pocket																				
Attachment Loss																				

Right

Buccal →

Palatal →

Lingual →

Buccal →

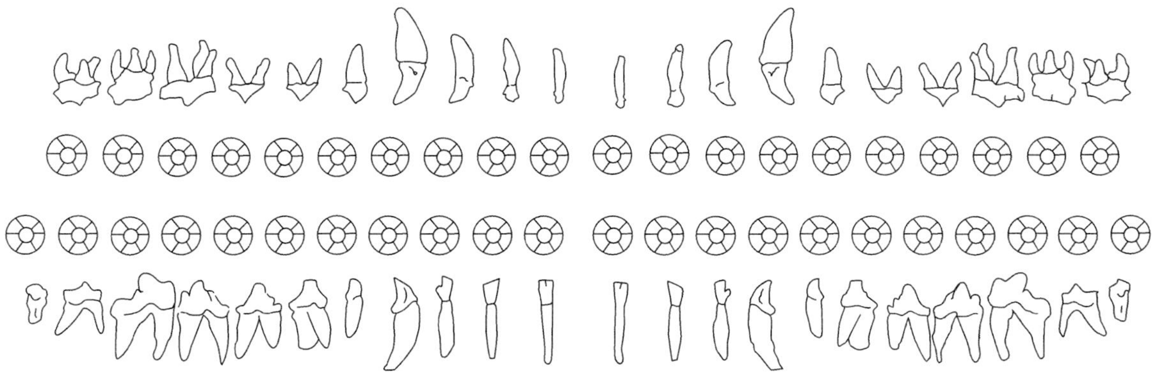

	411	410	409	408	407	406	405	404	403	402	401	301	302	303	304	305	306	307	308	309	310	311
M/F																						
P																						
AL																						

CA-Caries
CR-Crown Restoration
CWD-Crowding
Dox-Doxirobe
EH-Enamel Hypoplasia
F-Furcation Exposure
CCF-Complicated Crown Fx

GH-Gingival Hyperplasia
GR-Gingival Recession
GV-Gingivectomy
LUX-Luxated tooth
M-Mobility
O-Missing Tooth
PD-Persistent Deciduous

PE-Pulp Exposure
R-Rotated Tooth
R/C-Restoration/Composite
R/BS-Rest/Bonded Sealant
RC-Root Canal Therapy
RPC-Root Plane Closed

RPO-Root Planed Open
RR-Retained Root
TR-Tooth Resorption
UCF-Uncomplicated Crown Fracture
W-Worn
VPT-Vital Pulp Therapy
X-Extracted

Appendix 3

Sharpening

REFERENCE

Dental Hand Instrument Sharpening Instructions

How to sharpen instruments?

The sharpening stone moves while the instrument is held stationary.

1. Place 1 drop of Miltex® Honing Oil on the Arkansas or India sharpening stone. No lubrication is required on ceramic stones. (Apply oil only if it was not previously applied to stone or if more lubrication is needed).
2. Hold the instrument in one hand while applying the stone to the lateral surface of the point of the instrument, forming a 110° angle with the face of the blade of the instrument.
3. Position the sharpening stone to contact the heel of the instrument blade and work toward the tip, keeping the stone in contact with the blade throughout the sharpening procedure
4. Move the sharpening stone up and down along the instrument with short strokes, placing more pressure on the down stroke. (Continue to keep the instrument still).
5. Finish sharpening the instrument with a down stroke, which prevents a rough edge from forming on the instrument.

a) Metal particles and lubricant will accumulate on the blade and can be wiped off with sterile gauze. (This accumulation is also an indication that the proper angulation was maintained during the sharpening process).

6. For sickle scalers, continue sharpening to the point of the scaler. For curettes, continue around the toe to maintain its curved shape.
7. Test for sharpness with a plastic Miltex® test stick. If the blade of the instrument is sharp, it will grab into the stick. If the blade is dull, it will slide over the stick without grabbing. If the blade of the instrument is still dull after sharpening, re-evaluate the angle of the stone and repeat the sharpening procedure (steps 2-6).
8. Repeat the procedure to sharpen the other side of sickle scalers and universal curettes.

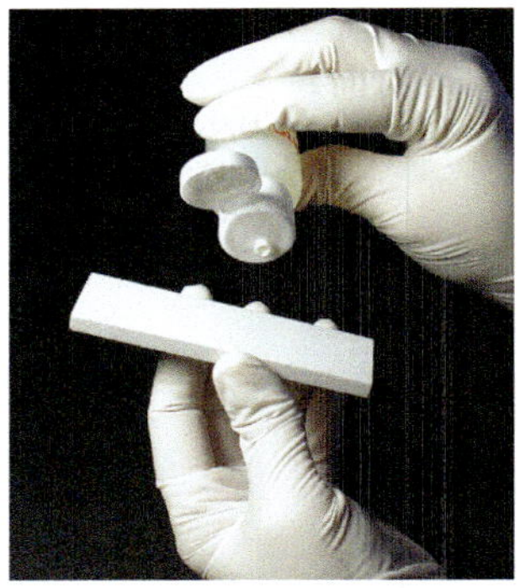

STEP 1

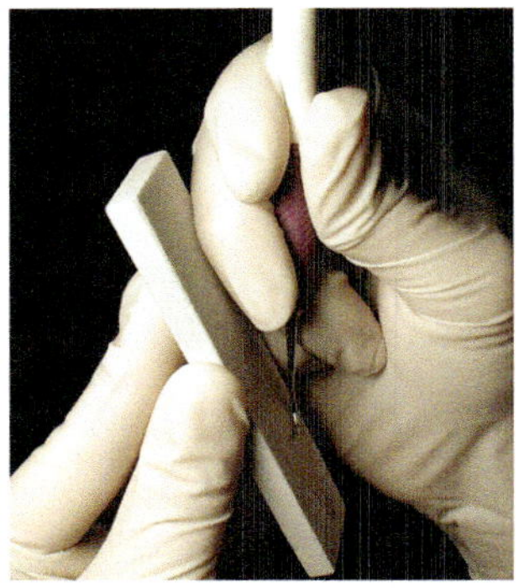

STEPS 2 & 4

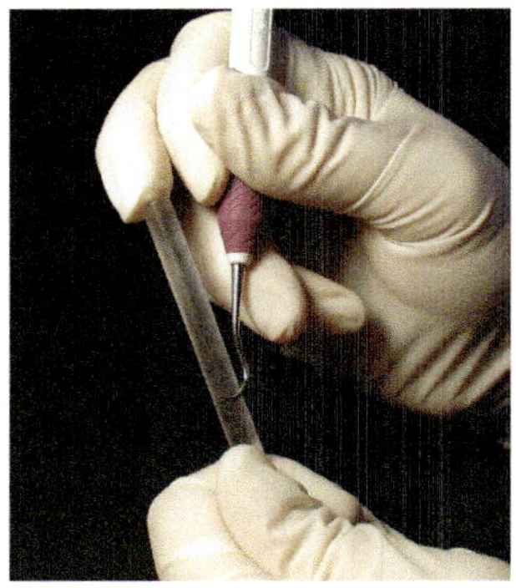

STEP 7

REFERENCE

Dental Hand Instrument Sharpening Instructions

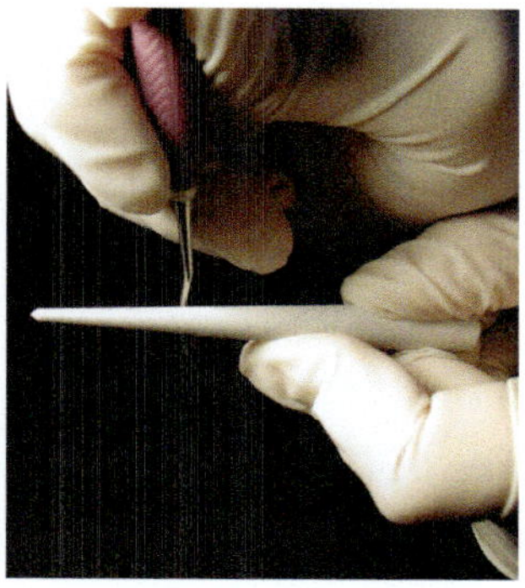

ROUNDING THE TOE
CURVED SICKLE

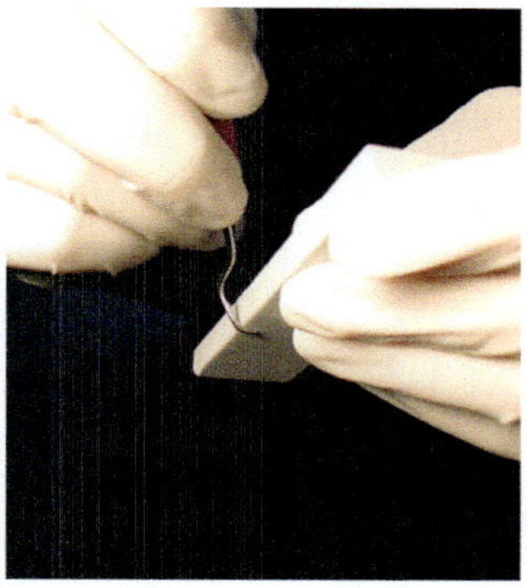

ROUNDING THE TOE
STRAIGHT SICKLE

Rounding the toe of curettes

1. Place 1 drop of Miltex® Honing Oil on the Arkansas or India sharpening stone. No lubrication is required on ceramic stones. (Apply oil only if it was not previously applied to stone or if more lubrication is needed).
2. Place the sharpening stone at a 45° angle to the face of the instrument.
3. Using downward strokes, rotate the sharpening stone around the toe of the instrument.

Sharpening the face of dental instruments

Sharpening the face of periodontal instruments is only recommended for removing a roughened edge. Extraneous grinding of the face can weaken the instrument blade.

For curettes and curved sickles, use a conical or cylindrical sharpening stone (Arkansas Conical, part number: STN-ARK-CON or India No. 309 part number: STN-IND-CON-309)

1. Place 1 drop of Miltex® Honing Oil on the Arkansas or India sharpening stone. No lubrication is required on ceramic stones.

   (Apply oil only if it was not previously applied to stone or if more lubrication is needed).
2. Place the stone at the junction between the face of the instrument and the shank of the instrument.
3. Roll the sharpening stone across the face of the instrument, moving toward the toe of the instrument.
4. Use as few strokes as possible and light, even pressure.

For straight sickle instruments, use a flat sharpening stone (Arkansas No. 4 flat, part number: STN-ARK-FLT-4 or India No.1, part number STN-IND-FLT-1).

1. Place 1 drop of Miltex® Honing Oil on the Arkansas or India sharpening stone. No lubrication is required on ceramic stones.

   (Apply oil only if it was not previously applied to stone or if more lubrication is needed).
2. Place the stone on the entire facial surface of the instrument.
3. Move the stone across the facial surface of the instrument in a back and forth motion.
4. Use as few strokes as possible and light, even pressure.

Appendix 4
Resources

Resources—dental radiology techniques and interpretation

www.vetdentalrad.com

The premier full-service veterinary dental radiology company. Offers telemedicine consulting services including STAT readings (within 20 minutes), enabling patient treatment within the same anesthetic episode. Educational DVDs are also available as a valuable training resource on dental radiographic exposure and interpretation. In addition, equipment prepurchase consults are available to help practitioners choose the right dental equipment for their needs and practice.

Resources—client education

www.vetdentalrad.com

Increasing dental compliance DVD

This is a live recording of a powerful marketing lecture presented by the author. This presentation offers tips and techniques to get your clients to comply with your dental recommendations and is appropriate for the entire staff to view. Involving the entire staff in this learning experience will help take your practice's dental services to the next level.

"The importance of dental radiographs" client educational poster

"A picture is worth 1,000 words." This high-quality laminated poster demonstrates the importance of dental radiology in common diseases. Pathologies include periodontal disease, fractured teeth, tooth resorptive lesions, and oral neoplasia. Displaying this poster for clients to view and read will greatly increase utilization of your dental radiology equipment and services.

Resources—hands-on dental training

San diego veterinary dental training center

Classes taught by the author are held in a state-of-the-art 700 sq. ft. training facility specifically designed for veterinary dentistry. We offer regularly scheduled hands-on dental training weekend seminars covering periodontal therapy and surgery, in addition to extractions, dental radiology, and restorations. Class sizes are small, providing excellent student:teacher ratios and learning opportunities.

For more information, please contact us:
(858) 279-2108
dsabatino@SCDVS.com
www.vetdentaltraining.com

American veterinary dental forum

This is a large annual meeting held in the fall season and organized by the AVDC, AVD, and AVDS. The meeting changes locations around the county and is regularly attended by most veterinary dentists. All facets of veterinary dentistry are taught in this 3-day meeting.

www.AVDF.org

Training centers from other diplomates

Colorado Pet Dental Training Center
Dr. Tony Woodward
www.vetdentalclasses.com

Punta Gorda Veterinary Dental Training
Dr. Brett Beckman
www.veterinarydentistry.net

Animal Dental Training Center
Dr. Iral Luskin
www.animaldentalcenter.com/html/adtc-frameset.html

Veterinary Periodontology, First Edition. Brook A. Niemiec.

Fox Valley Veterinary Dentistry
Dr. Cindy Charlier
http://www.fvvds.com/dentalce.html

Further reading on veterinary dentistry

From the author

- Small Animal Dental, Oral and Maxillofacial Disease, a Color Handbook. London: Manson, 2010.
- Veterinary Dentistry Applications in Emergency Medicine and Compromised and Critical Patients. San Diego: Practical Veterinary Publishing, 2012.
- Veterinary Endodontics. San Diego: Practical Veterinary Publishing, 2011.
- Veterinary Orthodontics. San Diego: Practical Veterinary Publishing, 2012.
- Veterinary Restorative and Operative Dentistry. San Diego: Practical Veterinary Publishing, 2012.

From other sources

- Atlas of Dental Radiography in Dogs and Cats. Philadelphia: Saunders, 2008. Dupont G, Debowes LJ.
- Blackwell's Five-Minute Veterinary Consult Clinical Companion Small Animal Dentistry. Ames, IA: Wiley-Blackwell, 2007. Lobprise HB.
- Carranza's Clinical Periodontology. St. Louis: Saunders, 2006. Newman MG, Takei HH, Klokkevald PR, Carranza FA.
- Feline Dentistry: Oral Assessment, Treatment, and Preventative Care. Ames, IA: Wiley-Blackwell, 2010. Bellows J.
- Veterinary Dental Techniques for the Small Animal Practitioner. 3rd ed. Philadelphia: Saunders, 2004. Holmstrom SE, Frost PF, Eisner ER.
- Veterinary Dentistry, Principles and Practice. Philadelphia: Lippincott-Raven, 1997. Wiggs RB, Lobprise HB.

Appendix 5

Plaque and calculus indices

Plaque index (PI) (Silness and Loe)

PI 0: No observable plaque
PI 1: A thin film of plaque is detected at the gingival margin by running a probe or explorer across the tooth surfaces
PI 2: A moderate amount of plaque is detected along the gingival margin. Plaque is visible clinically.
PI 3: Heavy plaque accumulation is detected at the gingival margin and in the interdental spaces.

Calculus index (CI)

CI 0: No observable calculus
CI 1: Scattered calculus covering less than 1/3 of the buccal surface of the tooth.
CI 2: Calculus covering between one- and two-thirds of the buccal tooth surface with minimal subgingival calculus.
CI 3: Calculus covering greater than two-thirds of the buccal tooth surface and extending subgingivally.

Veterinary Periodontology, First Edition. Brook A. Niemiec.

Index

Veterinary Periodontology, First Edition. Brook A. Niemiec.